CARDIOLOGY AND CO-EXISTING DISEASE

CARDIOLOGY AND CO-EXISTING DISEASE

Edited by

Elliot Rapaport, M.D.

Professor
Department of Medicine
William Watt Kerr Professor
of Clinical Medicine
Associate Dean for
San Francisco General Hospital
University of California,
San Francisco
School of Medicine
San Francisco, California

Churchill Livingstone
New York, Edinburgh, London, Madrid, Melbourne, Milan, Tokyo

Library of Congress Cataloging-in-Publication Data
Cardiology and co-existing disease / edited by Elliot Rapaport.
   p. cm.
  Includes bibliographical references and index.
  ISBN 0-443-08887-X
  1. Cardiological manifestations of general diseases. 2. Heart—
Diseases—Complications. I. Rapaport, Elliot, date.
  [DNLM: 1. Heart—physiology. 2. Heart Diseases—complications.
WG 202 C26985 1994]
RC682.C395 1994
616.1′2—dc20
DNLM/DLC
for Library of Congress   94-15544
                                      CIP

© Churchill Livingstone Inc. 1994

Distributed in the United Kingdom by Churchill Livingstone, Robert Stevenson House, 1–3 Baxter's Place, Leith Walk, Edinburgh EH1 3AF, and by associated companies, branches, and representatives throughout the world.

The Publishers have made every effort to trace the copyright holders for borrowed material. If they have inadvertently overlooked any, they will be pleased to make the necessary arrangements at the first opportunity.

Assistant Editor: *Shireen Dunwoody*
Copy Editor: *Paul Bernstein*
Production Supervisor: *Laura Mosberg Cohen*
Cover Design: *Paul Moran*

Printed in the United States of America

First published in 1994   7 6 5 4 3 2 1

Contributors

Thomas P. Bersot, M.D., Ph.D.
Associate Professor, Department of Medicine, University of California, San Francisco, School of Medicine; Chief, Lipid Clinic, San Francisco General Hospital; Scientist, Gladstone Institute of Cardiovascular Disease, San Francisco, California

Simon Chakko, M.D.
Associate Professor, Department of Medicine, University of Miami School of Medicine; Director, Non-Invasive Cardiac Laboratory, Miami Veterans Affairs Medical Center, Miami, Florida

H. Cecil Coghlan, M.D.
Professor and Deputy Director, Division of Cardiology and Director, Uihlein Autonomic Research Laboratory, Department of Medicine, University of Alabama School of Medicine, University of Alabama at Birmingham, Birmingham, Alabama

Denton A. Cooley, M.D.
Clinical Professor, Department of Surgery, University of Texas Medical School at Houston; Surgeon-in-Chief, Texas Heart Institute, Houston, Texas

Alan D. Guerci, M.D.
Associate Professor, Department of Medicine, Columbia University College of Physicians and Surgeons, New York, New York

Robert J. Hall, M.D.
Clinical Professor, Department of Medicine, University of Texas Medical School at Houston; Clinical Professor, Department of Medicine, Baylor College of Medicine; Acting Chief, Department of Adult Cardiology, St. Luke's Episcopal Hospital; Director, Cardiology Education, St. Luke's Episcopal Hospital and Texas Heart Institute, Houston, Texas

Laurence A. Harker, M.D.
Blomeyer Professor and Director, Division of Hematology and Oncology, Department of Medicine, Emory University School of Medicine, Atlanta, Georgia

Judith Hsia, M.D.
Associate Professor, Division of Cardiology, Department of Medicine, George Washington University School of Medicine and Health Sciences, Washington, D.C.

Willa A. Hsueh, M.D.
Professor and Chief, Division of Endocrinology, Diabetes, and Hypertension, Department of Medicine, University of Southern California School of Medicine, Los Angeles, California

Barry J. Materson, M.D., M.B.A.
Professor, Department of Medicine, University of Miami School of Medicine; Associate Chief of Staff for Education, Miami Veterans Affairs Medical Center, Miami, Florida

Hugh A. McAllister, Jr., M.D.
Clinical Professor, Department of Pathology, University of Texas Medical School at Houston; Clinical Professor, Department of Pathology, Baylor College of Medicine; Chief, Department of Pathology, St. Luke's Episcopal Hospital and Texas Heart Insitute, Houston, Texas

Joseph K. Perloff, M.D.
Streisand/American Heart Association Professor, Division of Cardiology, Department of Medicine and Department of Pediatrics, University of California, Los Angeles, UCLA School of Medicine, Los Angeles, California

Richard A. Preston, M.D.
Associate Clinical Professor, Department of Medicine, University of Miami School of Medicine; Chief, Renal Clinic, Miami Veterans Affairs Medical Center, Miami, Florida

Elliot Rapaport, M.D.
Professor, Department of Medicine, William Watt Kerr Professor of Clinical Medicine, and Associate Dean for San Francisco General Hospital, University of California, San Francisco, School of Medicine, San Francisco, California

Mohammed F. Saad, M.D.
Associate Professor, Division of Endocrinology, Diabetes, and Hypertension, Department of Medicine, University of Southern California School of Medicine, Los Angeles, California

Steven M. Scharf, M.D., Ph.D.
Associate Professor, Department of Medicine, Albert Einstein College of Medicine of Yeshiva University, Bronx, New York; Section Head, Pulmonary Research, Division of Pulmonary and Critical Care Medicine, Long Island Jewish Hospital, New Hyde Park, New York

Julio F. Tubau, M.D.
Associate Professor, Division of Cardiology, Department of Medicine, University of Southern California School of Medicine, Los Angeles, California

Preface

Cardiovascular disease remains the major cause of mortality in the United States despite the significant decline (more than 50 percent) that has occurred over the past three decades. In addition to the diseases of the heart and circulatory system, there are a number of other organ system diseases in which the heart and vascular system may be prominently involved and contribute significantly to morbidity and even death of the patient. The primary care physician and the internist/cardiologist, as well as the cardiologist, must continually be alert to signs and symptoms that point to primary cardiovascular disease but, in reality, are a manifestation of a systemic process or disease arising elsewhere.

Cardiology and Co-Existing Disease is devoted to examining and emphasizing the more important secondary causes of cardiovascular morbidity. These range from endocrine disorders, including diabetes, to neuromuscular disease, hematologic disorders, diseases of the liver, autonomic nervous system dysfunction, end-stage renal disease, pulmonary heart disease, AIDS, and finally neoplastic disease. Although it was necessary to be selective in choosing what could be incorporated within this volume, I believe we have identified the major diseases of other organs in which cardiovascular involvement may be a prominent feature and that may be the direct cause of significant morbidity and mortality.

I want to express my deep appreciation to those who have contributed to *Cardiology and Co-Existing Disease* for sharing their expertise. The time and effort that they have expended has created a volume that I believe will materially assist readers not only in understanding better how disease in other organs may alter myocardial and circulatory function, but also in presenting practical ways in which they may recognize and manage these abnormalities within their own practices.

I wish to acknowledge the invaluable editorial assistance of Sally Eccleston and Judy Serrell, here in San Francisco, and to thank the editorial staff of Churchill Livingstone for their encouragement, which led to this undertaking. In particular, I wish to thank Jennifer Mitchell, Shireen Dunwoody, and Paul Bernstein for their patience and help during the period that was required to put this volume together. I am most grateful as well to my wife for her support and patience during times when preparation of this book took precedence over other priorities in our lives.

Elliot Rapaport, M.D.

Contents

Pregnancy and the Heart

Alan D. Guerci

CARDIOVASCULAR PHYSIOLOGY DURING PREGNANCY

Pregnancy, labor, and the immediate postpartum period are accompanied by profound circulatory changes. These changes place the normal heart under severe stress and may prove intolerable to a woman with a diseased heart or aorta.

Progesterone, produced in large quantities by the corpus luteum during the first trimester of pregnancy and by the placenta later, is a moderately potent vasodilator. The hypotensive action of progesterone stimulates compensatory fluid retention. Intravascular volume expansion is further augmented by high circulating levels of estrogen, which stimulate renin secretion, aldosterone production, and, ultimately, sodium retention. The overall result is, on average, a 50 percent increase in intravascular volume.[1]

Red blood cell mass also increases during pregnancy, but by a lesser amount. Hemoglobin and hematocrit may fall to levels as low as 11 g and 33 percent, respectively.

Heart rate increases by 10 to 20 bpm. Cardiac output begins to rise in the middle of the first trimester and reaches a plateau at 30 to 50 percent above pre-gravid levels early in the third trimester.[1,2] Despite the increases in intravascular volume and cardiac output, blood pressure typically declines slightly during the first trimester, remains low throughout the second trimester, and then gradually returns toward pregravid levels in the weeks before term. Diastolic blood pressure usually falls by more than systolic blood pressure, with the net result of a widened pulse pressure.

Exercise capacity is reduced by 20 percent or more during pregnancy, probably as a result of impedance of venous return by the gravid uterus. In the later stages of pregnancy, the uterus may also interfere with venous return in the supine position by compressing the inferior vena cava. Dizziness and even syncope may result. Venous return is best maintained by lying in the left lateral recumbent position.

During labor and delivery, cardiac output increases by an additional 50 percent.[3] Moderate sinus tachycardia and systolic hypertension are the norm. Although the cardiovascular stress of labor may be reduced partially by coaching the patient and by adequate analgesia, it cannot be eliminated.

The uterus contracts and shears off the placenta immediately after delivery. This action returns 500 ml or more of blood to the central circulation. Whereas this redistribution of blood is easily accommodated by the normal heart, it poses a threat to the diseased heart. Heart rate and cardiac output return to normal levels within a day or two of delivery.

All obstetricians understand that they are responsible for the welfare of two patients: the pregnant woman and the fetus. Any cardiologist involved in the care of a pregnant woman must share this realization. Normal umbilical vein PO_2 is only about 40 mmHg, and oxygen delivery to the umbilical vein (which carries oxygenated blood from the placenta to the fetus) is limited by blood flow to the uterus. Any maternal condition associated with cyanosis imperils the fetus. Furthermore, uterine blood flow declines during maximal exercise.[4] Maximal exercise may therefore place the fetus at unnecessary and unpredictable risk and probably should be avoided.[5,6]

Uterine blood flow is abolished by uterine contractions; hence the current practice of fetal monitoring. Fetal heart rate typically declines during uterine contractions but should rebound promptly at the end of each contraction.

To the extent that modern analgesics induce vasodilatation, fetal welfare may be jeopardized. This is particularly true of epidural anesthesia, which may lead to profound material hypotension and fetal distress. This complication of anesthetic technique is ordinarily prevented by vigorous volume expansion immediately prior to anesthesia induction. It is not uncommon for the obstetrician or anesthesiologist to infuse a liter or more of normal saline over several minutes, prior to the administration of anesthesia. Managing the fluid requirements of a woman with impaired ability to dispose of venous return, or one with a right-to-left shunt likely to be made worse by peripheral vasodilatation, presents obvious challenges.

Symptoms and Signs of Normal Pregnancy

Fatigue, exertional breathlessness, and palpitations are common symptoms during pregnancy. Mild to moderate lower extremity edema usually develops late in pregnancy.

By the second trimester, arterial pulses are hyperdynamic, and the point of maximal impulse is prominent but not sustained. The point of maximal impulse may be displaced slightly leftward. S_1 is loud and may be physiologically split. S_2 may be widely split. A systolic flow murmur, loudest along the left sternal border, is almost always present. A third heart sound is common.[7]

Two continuous murmurs may develop during pregnancy. A venous hum may be audible above or just below either clavicle.[8] The mammary souffle, a systolic or continuous sound audible over the breast, is more common in lactating women but may be heard in the late stages of pregnancy. In most instances, it can be obliterated by applying pressure to the stethoscope.[9]

Laboratory Findings

A number of electrocardiographic changes are common during pregnancy. The frontal plane QRS axis typically shifts leftward, and nonspecific ST-T changes may develop. Sinus tachycardia and premature atrial beats occur frequently, and premature ventricular beats may be present.

If possible, chest x-rays should be avoided. When chest radiography is necessary, the abdomen and pelvis should be shielded. As a result of elevation of the diaphragm, the left ventricle may be prominent. Indeed, echocardiography performed with the patient in the left lateral position may demonstrate increased end-diastolic dimensions in both ventricles due to increased intravascular volume.

CARDIOVASCULAR DISEASES AND PREGNANCY

General Approach

In general, women with congenital or acquired heart disease and New York Heart Association class I or II symptoms can survive pregnancy and deliver a healthy baby. However, it behooves the physician to obtain a detailed and specific history of physical activity, for many persons with chronic heart disease are not completely aware of how sedentary they have become.

Maternal cyanosis imposes a substantial burden on the fetus. Rates of fetal loss approaching 50 percent have been reported among women with cyanotic congenital heart disease, and premature birth and low birth weight are also common.[10,11]

Rheumatic Heart Disease

Mitral Stenosis

Two of the basic circulatory changes in pregnancy, increased cardiac output and increased heart rate, present a direct threat to the patient with mitral stenosis. Increased flow across a stenotic mitral valve raises left atrial and pulmonary pressures. This problem is exacerbated by the increased heart rate, which occurs principally at the expense of the time spent in diastole. Time available for flow across the valve is therefore reduced, fur-

ther increasing left atrial and pulmonary pressures.[12]

Pulmonary congestion may occur gradually or suddenly. In the latter case, atrial fibrillation with rapid ventricular response is the usual cause. The onset of atrial fibrillation during pregnancy represents an extreme case of the normal physiology of pregnancy, because stretch of atrial tissue and elevated catecholamine levels increase phase 4 depolarization and predispose toward premature atrial beats. However, the result in a woman with mitral stenosis may be catastrophic, with immediate and severe pulmonary edema.

The therapeutic approach to atrial fibrillation in pregnancy is similar to that for the nonpregnant patient. Oxygen is given to raise arterial PO_2, and digitalis preparations and β-blockers are given to control the ventricular rate. Verapamil is sometimes given to control ventricular rate, but experience with verapamil is not sufficient to establish its long-term safety in pregnancy. Quinidine sulfate or procainamide may then be given to restore sinus rhythm. If these measures fail to restore sinus rhythm, DC cardioversion may be employed. The fetal heart rate should be monitored during cardioversion, for there is a theoretical risk of inducing an arrhythmia in the fetus. Recurrent atrial fibrillation may be prevented by sharply restricting physical activity and by the chronic administration of β-blockers. Mild diuretics may also be employed, but it is important to avoid severe volume depletion.

Vaginal delivery is usually tolerated by women with mild to moderate mitral stenosis.[13,14] Invasive hemodynamic monitoring with a pulmonary artery catheter is advised during labor and delivery and for another 24 hours after delivery in patients with moderate to severe mitral stenosis (calculated valve area less than 1.5

cm^2), or in patients with lesser degrees of mitral stenosis who develop symptoms of lung congestion during pregnancy. Epidural anesthesia is recommended, as its vasodilating effects usually have a favorable impact on left atrial pressure.

Percutaneous balloon mitral valvuloplasty may be performed in pregnant women with mitral stenosis and uncontrollable lung congestion. The major risk of the procedure is radiation exposure to the fetus. Careful shielding of the mother's abdomen and pelvis is essential.

Mitral valve replacement during pregnancy is associated with fetal death rates in excess of 10 percent.[15,16] If surgery becomes unavoidable, closed commissurotomy is preferred over either open commissurotomy or valve replacement, both of which require extracorporeal circulation. Even with high flow rates, extracorporeal circulation is associated with low levels of uterine perfusion.

Mitral Regurgitation

Mitral regurgitation is generally well tolerated during pregnancy, presumably because the systemic vasodilatation of pregnancy reduces the regurgitant volume.[12] Digitalis preparations and diuretics are first-line treatments for lung congestion. Unfortunately, adverse effects on the fetus have been reported in connection with the use of several vasodilators. Hydralazine may be given to control blood pressure (and afterload) during labor.

Other Rheumatic Conditions

Rheumatic lesions of the aortic or tricuspid valves are usually overshadowed by coexistent mitral disease. Aortic valve disease may predominate, however. Severe aortic stenosis has been associated with fetal and maternal mortality rates each around 20 percent.[17] If bed rest, digitalis preparations, and diuretics do not control symptoms, valve replacement must be considered. Aortic regurgitation is usually tolerated, for the same reason that mitral regurgitation is usually tolerated: peripheral vascular resistance is reduced during pregnancy.

Acyanotic Congenital Heart Disease

Survival to childbearing age is common in patients with bicuspid aortic valve, atrial septal defect, patent ductus arteriosus, pulmonic stenosis, ventricular septal defect, and coarctation of the aorta.[18]

Congenital Aortic Stenosis

The principles of care of patients with congenital aortic stenosis are outlined in the section on rheumatic heart disease. Patients with severe aortic stenosis should be advised against pregnancy. If such patients do become pregnant, abortion or valve replacement should be recommended in an effort to save the life of the mother.

Atrial Septal Defect

Pulmonary hypertension poses the major risk to pregnant women with atrial septal defect. Since pulmonary hypertension usually does not develop until middle age, atrial septal defect is not ordinarily a threat to the mother or fetus. In the absence of pulmonary hypertension, even moderate left-to-right shunts are usually well tolerated, again because peripheral resistance declines during pregnancy.

Patent Ductus Arteriosus

In the absence of pulmonary hypertension, maternal mortality is rare in patent ductus. Patients with heart failure should be treated with bed rest, digitalis, and diuretics. Catheter or surgical closure should be attempted only in patients who fail to respond to these measures. The left-to-right shunt of patent ductus arteriosus with moderate to severe pulmonary hypertension may reverse during the induction of anesthesia or immediately after delivery. This problem can be treated with fluids and pressors.

Pulmonic Stenosis
Women with valvular pulmonic stenosis usually tolerate pregnancy. If heart failure persists despite the usual conservative measures (bed rest, digitalis, and diuretics), balloon or surgical valvotomy should be considered.

Ventricular Septal Defect
Isolated ventricular septal defect is usually tolerated during pregnancy. As in the case of patent ductus arteriosus, the left-to-right shunt of ventricular septal defect may reverse if the patient becomes hypotensive.

Coarctation of the Aorta
The risks of coarctation to the mother include severe hypertension, congestive heart failure, aortic rupture, and aortic dissection.[19] In addition to the obvious danger of aortic catastrophes to the fetus, the treatment of hypertension and heart failure may imperil the fetus because both may reduce an already low distal aortic pressure. Bed rest is therefore an important part of the management of coarctation. Successful surgical correction has been reported in cases of uncontrollable heart failure or hypertension.

Cyanotic Congenital Heart Disease

Women with uncorrected cyanotic heart disease should not become pregnant, for the risks of maternal and especially fetal mortality are high. The incidence of cardiac and extracardiac malformations is also high in these fetuses. If already begun, pregnancy should be interrupted.

If a woman with complex cyanotic heart disease refuses to terminate her pregnancy, she must be followed closely for the development of heart failure and arrhythmias. Physical activity should be sharply curtailed. Supplemental oxygen, invasive hemodynamic monitoring, and antibiotic prophylaxis are all recommended during labor and delivery. The use of regional anesthetics, which reduce peripheral resistance and exacerbate right-to-left shunting, should be avoided. If the cyanotic heart disease has been corrected and the patient is functional class I or II, pregnancy is usually tolerated.

Eisenmenger Syndrome
Eisenmenger syndrome is produced by obliterative pulmonary arterial changes in patients with long-standing and severe left-to-right shunts. Severe pulmonary hypertension, shunt reversal, and cyanosis are characteristic features.

The risk of maternal mortality in pregnant women with Eisenmenger syndrome is as high as 50 percent.[20] Premature delivery, intrauterine growth retardation, and neonatal death are common. For these reasons, women with Eisenmenger syndrome are best counseled against becoming pregnant or, in the event of pregnancy, for early abortion. Should a woman with Eisenmenger syndrome refuse abortion, bed rest is advisable and close medical follow-up mandatory. In order to prevent pulmonary or paradoxical embolism, anticoagulation with intermittent subcutaneous heparin is usually recommended during the final trimester of pregnancy. Electrocardiographic, invasive hemodynamic, and arterial blood gas monitoring are essential during labor and delivery.[21] The use of anesthetic agents and techniques with minimal negative inotropic and arterial dilating effect is important in order to prevent sudden cardiovascular collapse or worsening of right-to-left shunting.

Ischemic Heart Disease

Ischemic heart disease is rare among women of childbearing age. Diabetes, familial hypercholesterolemia, and the combination of cigarette smoking and oral contraceptive use are important risk factors.

If a pregnant woman develops chest, neck, arm, or back discomfort typical of myocardial ischemia, low-level exercise testing, with or without echocardiography, should be performed. Maximal stress testing should be avoided, as fetal distress has been observed during maximal exercise.[4-6] On the other hand, submaximal exercise testing appears to be safe.[6] Radionuclide exercise testing is contraindicated because of radiation exposure to the fetus. Cardiac catheterization should be undertaken only if the information it will provide is vital to therapeutic decisions. The safety of prolonged therapy with nitrates or calcium antagonists in pregnancy is unknown. Therefore, β-blockers are the drugs of choice for the management of angina pectoris during pregnancy.

Acute myocardial infarction occurring during the third trimester or during labor is associated with high mortality rates.[22] Invasive hemodynamic monitoring is indicated, as are generous amounts of analgesia and supplemental oxygen. Elective cesarean section may be appropriate.

Cardiomyopathy

Peripartum Cardiomyopathy
Although peripartum cardiomyopathy may develop at any time during the third trimester or in the 6 months following de-

livery, most patients become symptomatic in the first month or two postpartum.[23,24] The clinical presentation is that of a dilated cardiomyopathy. Myocarditis is present in most cases, but the cause is unknown.[25] Approximately one-half of women with peripartum cardiomyopathy will recover over the next 6 months. In the remainder, chronic congestive heart failure or death ensue.[26]

Acute heart failure should be treated in conventional fashion with digitalis and diuretics. If vasodilators are needed during pregnancy, converting enzyme inhibitors and nitroprusside should be avoided because of fetal toxicity. Hydralazine may be used safely. Aortic balloon counterpulsation may be used to support a patient with critical left ventricular dysfunction. Myocarditis developing after delivery may resolve spontaneously, and the role of immunosuppressive therapy in these patients has not been defined. Patients who recover from peripartum myocarditis may experience relapse in subsequent pregnancies.[27] These patients should therefore be advised not to become pregnant again.

Hypertrophic Cardiomyopathy
The published literature reveals a generally favorable outcome in women with hypertrophic cardiomyopathy who become pregnant.[28] Shortness of breath is common but usually responds to β-blockers. If high-grade ventricular arrhythmias are present and persist despite β-blockage, they may be treated with quinidine or procainamide without endangering the fetus. Amiodarone should be used only as a drug of last resort, as its safety is unknown.

Vaginal delivery is safe in hypertrophic cardiomyopathy. In fact, the route of delivery is less important than careful management of fluids and anesthetic agents. Profound reductions of preload and afterload must be avoided.

Diseases of the Aorta

Marfan Syndrome
Favorable outcome is possible in patients with Marfan syndrome, provided that the aorta is not dilated.[29] Patients should understand, however, that aortic dissection may occur even when aortic dimensions are normal.[30] Furthermore, there is a 50 percent chance that the condition will be inherited. The risk of aortic dissection and death is high when the aorta is dilated.

Aortic Dissection
Even in the absence of Marfan syndrome or coarctation of the aorta, there seems to be a slight risk of dissection of the aorta during the third trimester or during labor. The diagnosis can be made safely and accurately with transesophageal echocardiography or with magnetic resonance imaging. β-Blockers and hydralazine should be used to reduce blood pressure. If at all possible, the child should be delivered by cesarean section before attempted repair of a dissection involving the ascending aorta (type A dissection).

Miscellaneous Problems

Prosthetic Valves
Patients with prosthetic valves and good exercise capacity can tolerate pregnancy.[31] The major problem in management involves anticoagulation. Coumadin is teratogenic and should not be given when the patient is trying to become pregnant or at any time during the first trimester.[32] Instead, intermittent subcutaneous heparin should be given in doses sufficient to raise the activated partial thromboplastin time. A dose of 10,000 units, two or three times daily, is usually sufficient.[33,34] Intravenous heparin should be substituted for subcutaneous heparin at the onset of labor. Therapy may be reinstituted 24 hours after delivery.

Arrhythmias
Isolated premature atrial and ventricular beats are common in pregnant women and do not require evaluation unless something else in the history or physical examination suggests structural heart disease. Exacerbation of pre-existing supraventricular tachycardia is common in pregnancy. β-Blockers, procainamide, and low doses of quinidine may be used safely.

Newly occurring supraventricular or ventricular tachycardia requires formal evaluation. Exogenous causes (alcohol, caffeine), thyroid disease, structural heart disease, and even coronary disease must be considered.

Antibiotic Prophylaxis
The American Heart Association recommends routine antibiotic prophylaxis for patients with prosthetic valves. The customary dose is ampicillin, 2 g IM or IV, and gentamicin, 1.5 mg/kg, 30 to 60 minutes before cesarean section or at 8-hour intervals during labor and delivery. An additional dose may be given 8 hours after delivery. Vancomycin, 1 g, may be substituted for ampicillin in allergic individuals.

Many authorities recommend that this same regimen be given during delivery to any woman with a structural disorder (e.g., mitral stenosis) or jet lesion (e.g., small ventricular septal defect or hypertrophic cardiomyopathy with mitral regurgitation).[35] However, the incidence of bacteremia during uncomplicated vaginal delivery is less than 4 percent, and some have questioned this recommendation.[36]

REFERENCES

1. Ueland K: Maternal cardiovascular dynamics: VII. Intrapartum blood volume changes. Am J Obstet Gynecol 126:671, 1976
2. Robson SC, Hunter S, Boys RJ et al: Serial study of factors influencing changes in cardiac output during human pregnancy. Am J Physiol 256:H1060, 1989
3. Robson SC, Dunlop W, Boys RJ et al: Cardiac output during labour. Br Med J 295:1169, 1987
4. Artal R: Cardiopulmonary responses to exercise in pregnancy. p. 25. In Elkayam U, Gleicher N (eds): Cardiac Problems in Pregnancy: Diagnosis and Management of Maternal and Fetal Disease. 2nd Ed. Alan R Liss, Inc, New York, 1990
5. Artal R, Romem Y, Paul RH et al: Fetal bradycardia induced by maternal exercise. Lancet 2:258, 1984
6. Carpenter MW, Sady SP, Hoegsberg B et al: Fetal heart rate response to maternal exertion. JAMA 259:3006, 1988
7. Cutforth R, MacDonald CB: Heart sounds and murmurs in pregnancy. Am Heart J 71:741, 1966
8. Perloff JK: Normal or innocent murmurs. p. 8. In Perloff JK (ed): The Clinical Recognition of Congenital Heart Disease. 3rd Ed. WB Saunders, Philadelphia, 1987
9. Tabaznik B, Randall TW, Hersch C: The mammary souffle of pregnancy and lactation. Circulation 22:1069, 1960
10. Whittemore R, Hobbins JC, Engle MA: Pregnancy and its outcome in women with and without surgical treatment of congenital heart disease. Am J Cardiol 50:641, 1982
11. Whittemore R: Congenital heart disease: its impact on pregnancy. Hosp Pract 18:65, 1983
12. Ueland K: Rheumatic heart disease and pregnancy. In Elkayam U, Gleicher N (eds): Cardiac Problems in Pregnancy. 2nd Ed. Alan R Liss, Inc, New York, 1990
13. Jacobi P, Adler Z, Zimmer EZ et al: Effect of uterine contractions on left atrial pressure in pregnant women with mitral stenosis. Br J Med 298:27, 1989
14. Clark SL, Phelan JP, Greenspoon J et al: Labor and delivery in the presence of mitral stenosis: central hemodynamic observations. Am J Obstet Gynecol 152:984, 1985
15. Bernal JM, Miralles PJ: Cardiac surgery with cardiopulmonary bypass during pregnancy. Obstet Gynecol Surv 41:1, 1986
16. Becker RM: Intracardiac surgery in pregnant women. Ann Thorac Surg 36:453, 1983
17. Arias F, Pineda J: Aortic stenosis and pregnancy. J Reprod Med 4:229, 1978
18. Elkayam U, Cobb T, Gleicher N: Congenital heart disease and pregnancy. p. 73. In Elkayam U, Gleicher N (eds): Cardiac Problems in Pregnancy. 2nd Ed. Alan R Liss, Inc, New York, 1990
19. Barash PG, Hobbins JC, Hook R et al: Management of coarctation of the aorta during pregnancy. J Thorac Cariovasc Surg 69:781, 1975
20. Gleicher N, Midwall J, Hochberger D et al: Eisenmenger's syndrome and pregnancy. Obstet Gynecol Surv 34:721, 1979
21. Midwall J, Jaffin H, Herman MV et al: Shunt flow and pulmonary hemodynamics during labor and delivery in the Eisenmenger's syndrome. Am J Cardiol 42:299, 1978
22. Goldman ME, Meller J: Coronary artery disease in pregnancy. p. 153. In Elkayam U, Gleicher N (eds): Cardiac Problems in Pregnancy. 2nd Ed. Alan R Liss, Inc, New York, 1990
23. O'Connell JB, Rosa Costanzo-Nordin M, Subramanian R et al: Peripartum cariomyopathy: clinical, hemodynamic, histologic and prognostic characteristics. J Am Coll Cardiol 8:52, 1986
24. Lee W, Cotton DB: Peripartum cardiomyopathy: current concepts and clinical management. Clin Obstet Gynecol 32:54, 1989
25. Midei MC, DeMent SH, Feldman AM et al: Peripartum myocarditis and cardiomyopathy. Circulation 81:922, 1990
26. Carvalho A, Brandao A, Martinez EE et al: Prognosis in peripartum cariomyopathy. Am J Cardiol 64:540, 1989
27. St. John Sutton M, Cole P, Saltzman D et

al: Risks of cardiac dysfunction in peripartum cardiomyopathy (PPCM) with subsequent pregnancy. Circulation 80:II-320, 1989

28. Shah DM, Sunderji SG: Hypertrophic cardiomyopathy and pregnancy: report of the maternal mortality and review of the literature. Obstet Gynecol Surv 40:444, 1985

29. Pyeritz RE: Maternal and fetal complications of pregnancy in the Marfan syndrome. Am J Med 71:784, 1981

30. Rosenblum NG, Grossman AR, Mennuti MT et al: Failure of serial echocardiographic studies to predict aortic dissection in pregnant patient with Marfan's syndrome. Am J Obstet Gynecol 146:470, 1983

31. Matorras R, Reque JA, Usandizaga JA et al: Prosthetic heart valve and pregnancy. A study of 59 cases. Gynecol Obstet Invest 19:21, 1985

32. Sareli P, England MJ, Berk HR et al: Maternal and fetal sequelae of anticoagulation during pregnancy in patients with mechanical heart valve prosthesis. Am J Cardiol 63:1462, 1989

33. Wang RYC, Lee PK, Chow JSF et al: Efficacy of low dose subcutaneously administered heparin in the treatment of pregnant women with artificial heart valves. Med J Aust 2:126, 1983

34. Elkayam U, Gleicher N: Anticoagulation in pregnant women with artificial heart valves. N Engl J Med 316:1663, 1987

35. Cesario TC: Antibiotic therapy in pregnancy. p. 437. In Elkayam U, Gleicher N (eds): Cardiac Problems in Pregnancy. 2nd Ed. Alan R Liss, Inc, New York, 1990

36. Sugrue D, Blake S, Troy P et al: Antibiotic prophylaxis against infective endocarditis after normal delivery. Is it necessary? Br Heart J 44:499, 1980

2

Pulmonary Heart Disease

Steven M. Scharf

The heart and the respiratory system are intimately connected. Disorders of one system produce disordered function of the other. In the 1800s Laennec[1] described patients with pulmonary emphysema and associated right heart enlargement. In 1930, Paul White was credited with recognizing that enlargement of the right ventricle (RV) can result from lung disease; he also coined the term *cor pulmonale*. Since that time, but especially with the advent of technological advances in cardiovascular physiology and diagnosis, a great deal has been learned about the manner in which disordered respiratory function affects the heart, especially the RV. Uniform pathologic-clinical criteria for defining cor pulmonale do not exist; hence, precise estimates of prevalence are hard to come by. However, heart failure on the basis of cor pulmonale probably constitutes 15 to 20 percent of all cases of heart failure[2] and 7 to 10 percent of all heart disease.[3]

DEFINITIONS

Cor pulmonale, or pulmonary heart disease (PHD), is heart disease caused by dysfunction of the lungs leading to dysfunction of the pulmonary vascular system. McGinn and White[4] used the term "acute cor pulmonale" to describe right heart strain resulting from acute pulmonary hypertension, as from massive pulmonary embolism. This form contrasts to chronic cor pulmonale, which is defined by the World Health Organization as "an alteration in structure and function of the RV resulting from disease affecting the structures and function of the lung except when this alteration results from left disease of the heart or congenital heart disease."[5] The presence of PHD is associated with decreased survival in patients with lung disease. Only one-third of patients with lung disease and PHD will be alive 4 years after disease onset as opposed to 64 percent of those without PHD. There has been no appreciable change in these figures over the last 25 years.[6,7]

In this chapter we review some of the factors that characterize PHD, both acute and chronic. First, since PHD is essentially disease of the RV, we briefly describe normal RV functional anatomy and physiology. We then discuss characteristics of the normal and abnormal pulmonary circulation relevant to alteration of RV function. With this background, we return to the pathophysiologic and clinical features of acute and chronic PHD.

NORMAL RIGHT VENTRICLE

The RV develops embryologically from two separate components of the primitive cardiac tube. The *bulbus cordis* is incorporated into the *conus* (outflow tract), and the *sinus venosus* is incorporated into the *sinus* (inflow tract).[8] The RV preserves the functional distinction of its dual embryologic origin.[9–11] Normal RV contraction is almost peristaltic in nature, with a wave of contraction beginning in the sinus and ending in the conus portion of the RV. Thus, the RV is ideally suited to be a low-pressure, high-volume pump. While dysfunction of the left ventricle (LV) is clearly recognized as a threat to life, under normal resting conditions the RV appears to have little importance in regulation of cardiac output. However, when pulmonary arterial pressure is elevated, or cardiac output increases, the RV is necessary for normal homeostasis.

The normal RV is a thin (less than 0.5 cm thick) crescent-shaped structure with a large surface area. When the RV dilates, it changes its shape to become more ellipsoid. Thus, accurate determination of RV volume from measurement of a limited number of dimensions using a simple geometric model is more difficult than for corresponding measurements of the LV. The interaction between the RV and the low pulmonary vascular impedance produces pulmonary arterial pressures of less than one-fourth those of the LV. Hence, the work capacity of the RV is considerably less than that for the LV. Data like those shown in Figure 2-1 are often used to illustrate the idea that the RV is a "volume pump," while the LV is a "pressure pump."[12] However, the determinants of ventricular function (preload, afterload, and contractility) are the same for LV and RV, and there is no fundamental difference between the ventricles.[13] This is illustrated in Figure 2-2, showing that for the same relative in-

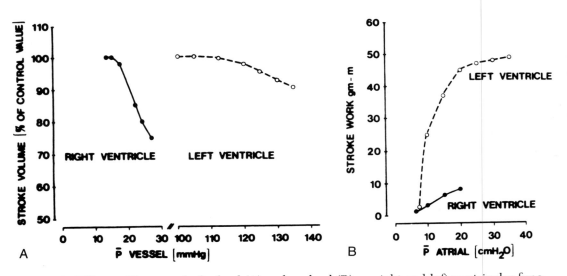

Fig. 2-1. Effects of increased afterload (**A**) and preload (**B**) on right and left ventricular function. The data in the left panel were obtained by constriction of the main pulmonary artery or aorta in dogs. Note for any given increase in afterload (left) stroke volume falls more rapidly in the right than in the left ventricle. (From McFadden and Braunwald,[12] with permission.)

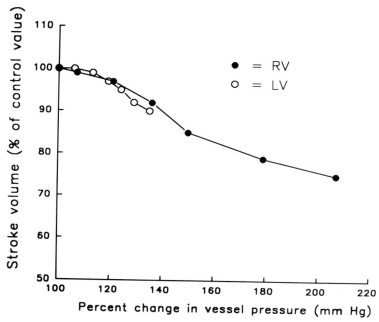

Fig. 2-2. Data from Figure 2-1A redrawn as a function of the percent change in afterload rather than as absolute change. Note that for the same percent increase in afterload, the RV responds with the same percent decrease in stroke volume, and right ventricular afterload increases to a greater degree than left ventricular afterload. RV, right ventricle; LV, left ventricle.

crease in afterload, the RV has the same load tolerance as the LV.

PULMONARY AND RIGHT HEART PRESSURE

Normally, pulmonary and RV pressures are measured relative to atmospheric pressure and are "zero" referenced to a level 5 cm below the angle of Louis in the supine patient (the approximate level of the right atrium). Normal pulmonary hemodynamic values are shown in Table 2-1 and pulmonary and RV pressure contours in Figure 2-3. All right-sided pressures are subject to transmitted changes in intrathoracic pressure. Normally, these are small. However, in the presence of airway obstruction, a common cause of

PHD, these may be considerable.[14] Thus, the true pressure across the wall of the cardiac or vascular structure will be quite different from that recorded by referring the pressure to atmospheric. In these cases, intravascular pressure may be referred to intrathoracic pressure, often measured with an esophageal balloon to obtain measurements of *transmural pressure*. Finally, local changes in juxtacardiac pressure, as could occur with pulmonary hyperinflation, especially of the lower lobes, will be reflected in recorded intravascular pressures.[15] In such cases, constraint within the cardiac fossa could impede cardiac filling and elevate intracardiac pressures. The measurement of increased "filling pressure" without taking these factors into account could lead to erroneous conclusions regarding the state of ventricular filling.

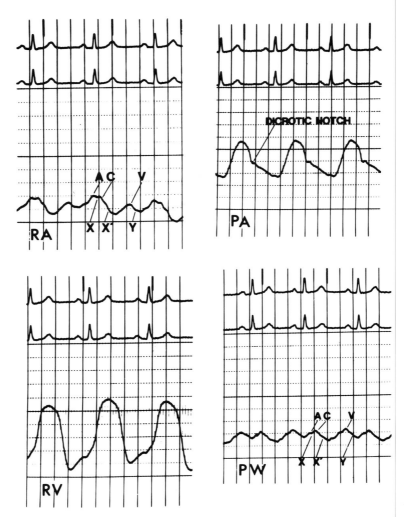

Fig. 2-3. Normal right-sided pressure traces. Full scale = 40 torr. See text for discussion. (Courtesy of Gary Friedman, M.D., Division of Cardiology, Long Island Jewish Medical Center, New Hyde Park, NY.)

Pulmonary venous pressure is normally equal to left atrial pressure. Both left and right atrial pressures exhibit the pressure waves denoted as *a*, *c*, and *v*, waves (Fig. 2-3). The *a* wave corresponds to atrial contraction, and the *v* wave corresponds to atrial filling during ventricular systole. The origin of the *c* wave is still unclear but is probably related to bulging of the atrioventricular valves into the atria at the onset of ventricular systole. The pressure descent following the *a* wave is called the *x* descent, that following the *v* wave the *y* descent, and that following the *c* wave the *x'* descent. The RV pressure wave is characterized by gradual diastolic upsloping with rapid upstroke at the onset of systole. RV end-

Table 2-1. Normal Pulmonary Hemodynamics

Variable	Value
Cardiac index	2.4–4.4 L/min/m²
Cardiac output	4–7 L/min
Pulmonary artery pressure	
Systolic	20–30 mmHg
Diastolic	5–10 mmHg
Mean	12–15 mmHg
Wedge	6–12 mmHg
Pulmonary blood volume	290 ± 50 ml/m²
Pulmonary vascular resistance	
Absolute	150–250 dyne-sec/cm⁵
Index	50–220 dyne-sec/cm⁵/m²
Right atrial pressure (mean)	−2–+5 mmHg
RV pressure	
Systolic	20–30 mmHg
Diastolic	0–5 mmHg
RV stroke work index	7–12 g-m/beat/m²

diastolic pressure is equal to mean right atrial pressure, and normally there is no systolic flow across the tricuspid valve. During diastole there is normally no flow across the pulmonary vascular bed, hence pulmonary arterial diastolic pressure is equal to left atrial pressure. Similarly, since the pulmonary arteries are normally end arteries, a catheter wedged into a small pulmonary artery, or a balloon-tipped catheter with its balloon inflated in a medium-sized vessel such that no flow occurs, will measure pulmonary venous and therefore left atrial pressure, provided that pulmonary venous pressure is greater than the critical closing pressure of the pulmonary vascular bed (see discussion below). Such pressure recordings are often called the "capillary wedge" pressure, although it has very little to do with actual capillary pressure, and should more properly be called the "pulmonary wedge" pressure. Pulmonary capillary pressure actually provides the hydrostatic pressure for pulmonary microfiltration and hence regulates the formation of pulmonary edema. The reader is referred elsewhere for a de-

tailed review of pulmonary edema formation.[16]

NORMAL PULMONARY VASCULATURE

The pulmonary circulation must accommodate large increases in gas transport to meet changing demands. At rest, 250 to 300 ml of O_2/min are transported across the lungs. With maximum exercise, this figure increases to 3,000 to 4,000 ml. The lungs receive the entire cardiac output, which ranges from 4 to 5 L/min at rest to as much as 25 L/min with vigorous exercise.

Several differences between the pulmonary and systemic circulations should be noted.[17] In the systemic circulation the major flow resistance is in the precapillary vessels, whereas in the pulmonary circulation it is in the alveolar capillaries. Second, systemic microvascular pressures are generally fairly uniform within an organ. In the lungs, these are quite variable, depending on the anatomic location within the lung (i.e., dependent vs. nondependent regions; body position; the site of the vessel within the pulmonary parenchyma—intra- versus extra-alveolar; and the state of lung inflation). Third, the systemic circulation within the lung, the bronchial and pleural vessels, drains into the same venous bed as the pulmonary vessels. This is done via a network of anastomoses that constitute potential shunts from one bed to the other at all levels: arterial, capillary, and venous.

Morphometric analysis of the pulmonary vasculature reveals that there are more arteries than airways.[18–20] After a few generations, pulmonary arteries lose their muscular media, and the most peripheral branches consist only of endothelium and internal elastic membrane. This flimsy structure is fairly susceptible to direct mechanical interactions with surrounding lung parenchyma, either compression or tethering open. Extension of muscular coats from arterial generations that normally have them (100 to 500 μm in diameter), to smaller vessels that normally do not is one of the prime histologic manifestations of vascular remodeling in disease states associated with pulmonary hypertension and ultimately chronic PHD. The muscular coat of pulmonary arterioles is relatively smaller than that in systemic arterioles, 3 to 4 percent compared with 40 to 50 percent. The pulmonary circulation has no valves, and pulmonary veins are relatively thinner walls than systemic veins of the same size.[20] These factors interact to allow the pulmonary circulation an enormous capacity to accommodate increased flow and oxygen and carbon dioxide transport. Further, the enormous capacity of the pulmonary vasculature allows large increases in cardiac output with little change in pulmonary arterial pressures, which in turn constitute part of the afterload placed on the RV.

EFFECTS OF LUNG INFLATION ON PULMONARY VASCULATURE

It is useful to distinguish three types of intraparenchymal pulmonary microvessels: *intra-alveolar*, *extra-alveolar*, and *alveolar corner* vessels. Intra-alveolar vessels are contained within and fill the walls between adjacent alveoli. They are subject to changes in intra-alveolar pressure, being compressed when alveolar pressure rises relative to pleural surface pressure (lung inflation) and vice versa. They are also subject to effects of alveolar surface tension[21] and presumably change their morphology in conditions such as respiratory distress syndrome when surface forces change. Extra-alveolar vessels are small vessels not exposed to alveolar pressure, surrounded by a connective tissue sheath. They are subject to interstitial pressure that *decreases* with lung inflation and *increases* with decreased lung volume. Hence, *lung inflation* acts in an opposite manner on intra- and extra-alveolar vessels.

The interaction between these two types of vessels explains the biphasic behavior of pulmonary vascular capacitance and resistance with lung inflation.[22–24] As lung volume increases from residual volume (the lowest achievable volume) to functional residual capacity (FRC, end-expiration), pulmonary vascular resistance (PVR) normally decreases and vascular capacitance increases, reflecting the influence of extra-alveolar vessels. With increases in lung volume from FRC to total lung capacity, PVR increases and capacitance decreases, reflecting the influence of intra-alveolar vessels (Fig. 2-4). Finally, alveolar corner vessels are found at the junction of three alveoli and are contained within folds, or pleats, of endothelium beneath sharp curvatures of

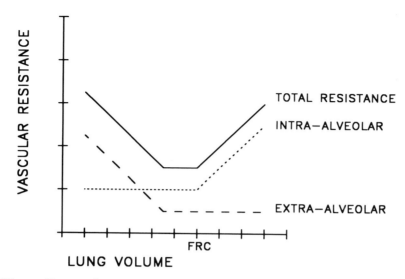

Fig. 2-4. Effects of lung inflation on the resistance of different types of pulmonary vessels and the end result on overall PVR. In this model, total PVR is the algebraic sum of the resistance of intra- and extra-alveolar vessels in series. Lung inflation decreases the resistance of the extra-alveolar and increases the resistance of the intra-alveolar vessels. Note that the minimum value of overall PVR occurs at functional residual capacity (i.e., lung volume at end-expiration).

the alveolar surface film.[17] These vascular pleats protect corner vessels from changes in alveolar pressure, and may thus buffer the effects of increased lung volume, allowing arterial to venous flow even at high alveolar pressures.

With increased PVR, pulmonary arterial pressure increases with high levels of positive end-expiratory pressure (PEEP), especially if cardiac output is maintained.[25,26] These effects are exaggerated in the presence of concomitant pulmonary edema[27] and with lung hyperinflation such as asthma and emphysema.[28,29]

PULMONARY VASCULAR RESISTANCE—NEWER CONCEPTS

The pulmonary vascular bed is often modeled as a simple rigid tube that obeys Poiseuille's law for flow resistance. In such a system flow (Q) is laminar and is determined by the gradient between mean pulmonary arterial pressure (P_{PA}) and pulmonary venous or left atrial pressure (P_{LA}) and a simple laminar flow resistance (PVR):

$$Q = \frac{(P_{PA} - P_{LA})}{PVR}$$

By rearranging:

$$PVR = \frac{(P_{PA} - P_{LA})}{Q} \times 79.9$$

When pressures are measured in torr and flow in L/min, multiplying by 79.9 converts to absolute resistance units, dyne-sec/cm⁵.

The concept of PVR being a simple laminar flow resistance is a useful clinical approximation, but has certain limitations and can lead to misleading conclusions. For one thing, it assumes that P_{LA} is the back pressure to pulmonary flow. According to the classic model of West and

Dollery,[30] this is true only when P_{LA} is greater than alveolar pressure (Zone 3 lung). When alveolar pressure is greater than P_{LA}, alveolar pressure is the true back pressure to pulmonary blood flow (Zone 2). Further, when alveolar pressure is greater than P_{PA}, there is no flow through the lung (Zone 1). Thus, at first approximation, the lung acts as a series of Starling resistors, whose surrounding pressure or critical closing pressure is equal to alveolar pressure, with inflow and outflow pressures equal to P_{PA} and P_{LA}, respectively.

Even this approach, more accurate though it is, is only an approximation.

First, it has been known for years that pulmonary blood flow can increase enormously with little change in pulmonary arterial pressures in normal lungs.[31] Thus, calculated PVR decreases with increased blood flow. The usual explanation for this is that there is dilatation of pulmonary vessels and/or recruitment of previously closed vessels. While this is undoubtedly true, the result also in part stems from the assumption that PVR is calculated using P_{LA} as the outflow pressure. If one plots the actual pressure-flow relationship of the pulmonary vascular bed, a curve such as that seen in Figure 2-5 occurs.[32] The curve extrapolates to

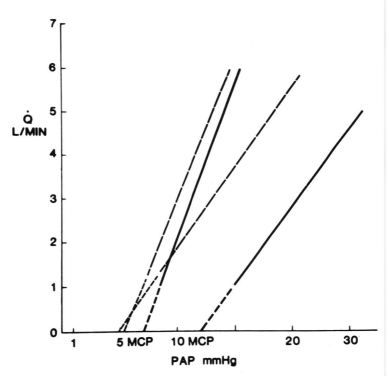

Fig. 2-5. Mean pressure-flow curves before and after oleic acid-induced pulmonary edema. Dashed lines represent controls at time zero and at 5 hours. Solid lines represent before and after 5 hours of pulmonary edema formation. In the time control experiments there was a decrease in the slope (conductance) of the pressure-flow curves, but no change in the critical closing pressure (zero intercept). With pulmonary edema, a similar decrease occurred in the conductance (solid lines). However, there was also an increase in the criticial closing pressure (zero flow intercept). (From Prewitt and Ducas,[32] with permission.)

zero flow at a positive pressure, the critical closing pressure of the pulmonary vascular bed, often considerably higher than alveolar pressure. This suggests that there are other sources of critical closure in the pulmonary bed such as smooth muscle tone or pulmonary edema. Furthermore, vasodilators (e.g., hydralazine) may affect either PVR (the actual slope of the pressure-flow curve) and/or the critical closing pressure.[32]

The presence of a critical closing pressure substantially higher than P_{LA} can yield inaccurate conclusions based on the usual method of calculation of changes in vessel diameter with a given maneuver.[32,33] Critical closing pressure in the pulmonary vascular bed also has possible clinical implications for understanding the effects of vasodilators commonly given for PHD. For example, when pulmonary hypertension is produced by increased critical closing pressure, then fluctuations in P_{LA} have little influence on pulmonary arterial flow. However, a drug that acts to decrease critical closing pressure would make pulmonary arterial flow and pressure *more* sensitive to fluctuation in P_{LA}, and hence in left heart function. Many maneuvers have been shown to affect the critical closing pressure of the pulmonary vascular bed including edema formation (Fig. 2-5), pulmonary embolization, and endotoxin.[34]

Finally, since pulmonary flow is pulsatile, calculations of PVR based on laminar flow assumptions may not reflect the load placed on the RV very well. It has been suggested that calculation of *input impedance* yields a better approximation of RV afterload.[35,36] This approach, which takes into account the capacitative as well as the resistive properties of the pulmonary bed, helps to explain changes in RV function not readily interpreted by the simplified Poiseuille's law approach for rigid tubes. For example, for the same

increase in mean P_{PA}, occlusion of the mainstem pulmonary artery constitutes a greater increase in RV afterload than occlusion of small pulmonary vessels by microembolization.[37] This is probably because with proximal pulmonary occlusion there is a greater decrease in the capacitative component of pulmonary vascular impedance than with distal occlusion.

PULMONARY VASOMOTION

Since treatment of PHD is often undertaken with drugs that affect pulmonary vasomotor tone, a brief review of this vast topic is in order. The normal pulmonary vascular bed has little resting vasomotor tone. However, there are many endogenous and exogenous substances that act on the pulmonary bed (Table 2-2). Some

Table 2-2. Pulmonary Vasoactive Substances

Vasoconstrictors
α-Adrenergic agonists—norepinephrine, phenylephrine
Angiotensin II
Thromboxane A_2
Serotonin
Histamine (from relaxed pulmonary bed)
Prostaglandins F_{2a}, E_2, and D_2
Leukotrienes C_4 and D_4
Interleukin-2
Tumor necrosis factor
Endothelin
Vasodilators
Histamine (preconstricted bed)
β-Agonists—isoproterenol
Bradykinin
Prostaglandins E_2 and E_1 (neonates)
Platelet activating factor (preconstricted bed)
Endothelium-derived relaxing factor
Acetylcholine
Adenosine

of these act globally to affect the entire pulmonary bed (e.g., norepinephrine) and some act regionally when certain local conditions apply (e.g., hypoxic pulmonary vasoconstriction). The state of initial vasomotor tone may influence the action of an agent. An example is histamine, which acts as a constrictor on dilated vessels and a dilator on constricted vessels.[38,39] An important substance whose impact is only now being fully appreciated is endothelial-derived relaxing factor (EDRF), now known to be nitric oxide (NO).[40] This endothelial-derived substance is the final common pathway by which a number of substances, such as acetylcholine, act to dilate the pulmonary vascular bed.[41] NO in turn probably acts by stimulating guanylate cyclase, leading to increased intracellular levels of cyclic guanosine $3'5'$ monophosphate, which is the agent acting directly on smooth muscle cells.[42]

There are many cell types present in the lung that are capable of producing vasoactive *mediators*. These include mast cells, neutrophils, macrophages, and vascular endothelium. Many mediator substances are hypothesized to be released during pulmonary injury (e.g., respiratory distress syndrome, infection, and pulmonary embolism); they cause pulmonary vasoconstriction and in turn raise RV afterload.[43,44] Arachidonic acid metabolism via the cyclooxygenase pathway leads to the production of the prostenoids, some of which have vasoconstrictor and some of which have vasodilator properties. This pathway is blocked by the nonsteroidal anti-inflammatory agents. Arachidonic acid metabolism by the lipooxygenase pathway leads to the production of the leukotrienes, which are also vasoactive. Thus, the possibility arises of considerable cross-talk between endothelial-derived vasoactive substances such as prostenoids and neutrophil-derived vasoactive substances such as leukotrienes in the regulation of pulmonary vasomotion and vascular permeability.[43] Presently, as will be seen below, the treatment of pulmonary hypertension and PHD with pulmonary vasodilators is far from ideal. An understanding of these complex properties will undoubtedly lead to improvement in the pharmacologic therapy of severe pulmonary hypertension. One example of this is the use of prostacyclin, a cyclooxygenase pathway product, in the treatment of primary pulmonary hypertension.[45]

The autonomic innervation of the pulmonary bed is less well understood than the systemic circulation. There are considerable interspecies differences, and the understanding of human pulmonary autonomic physiology is not far advanced. Both α- and β-adrenergic responses with appropriate blocking by the usual blocking substances can be demonstrated. Vagal stimulation is complex since the vagus nerve contains parasympathetic as well as sympathetic fibers. In addition, there are a number of poorly understood brain-pulmonary vascular connections that may play a role in regulating pulmonary microvascular pressures and may be partially responsible for changes in pulmonary fluid balance with cranial disease.[46]

EFFECTS OF ALTERED GAS EXCHANGE ON PULMONARY CIRCULATION

Pulmonary vascular reaction to altered gas exchange is a local event that acts to preserve optimum ventilation-perfusion relationships. For example, when a local area of the lung has decreased ventilation and becomes hypoxic and acidotic, local pulmonary vasoconstriction acts to shunt blood away from the affected area and prevents the formation of a local area of low ventilation-perfusion ratio.

Hypoxic pulmonary vasoconstriction is probably the most important mechanism producing pulmonary hypertension and subsequent PHD. The most common cause of hypoxia is hypoventilation, hence hypercarbic and acidotic pulmonary vasoconstriction probably play a role in these states as well. Vasoconstriction on exposure to hypoxia is not an intrinsic property of pulmonary vessels. When stripped of adventitia, pulmonary arteries dilate in response to hypoxia, like systemic vessels. Thus, hypoxic vasoconstriction results from the interaction of pulmonary vessels with secondary mediators produced in conjunction with surrounding tissue. A number of substances have been proposed as the mediators of pulmonary hypoxic vasoconstriction. Much interest has been focused on endothelial-derived substances.[47–49] The "substance" responsible may in fact be species dependent. In some species, inhibition of the cyclooxygenase pathway of arachidonic acid metabolism inhibits hypoxic vasoconstriction, whereas in others inhibition of the lipooxygenase pathway has the same effect.[48] The endothelial-derived vasoconstrictor endothelin may also play a role in some species.[47]

PULMONARY VASCULAR REMODELING

Increased pulmonary arterial pressure or flow, as well as chronic hypoxemia due to pathologic conditions, is often associated in the initial stages with active pulmonary vasoconstriction. At this stage, therapy with vasodilating substances, oxygen being prominent among these, is often associated with decreased PVR and clinical improvement. With chronicity, how-

ever, structural changes occur in the pulmonary bed that are often considered to be irreversible. The progressive nature of these histologic changes was recognized and classified by Heath and Edwards in 1958 in a study of congenital heart disease.[50] They proposed a classification of these progressive vascular alterations ranging from mild and potentially reversible (stages I and II) to severe and irreversible (stages IV and V) (Table 2-3). The major feature of remodeled vessels is an extension of smooth muscle into vessels that are normally thin and nonmuscular and an increase in the smooth muscle layers of normally muscularized arteries. Other changes include damage to intimal endothelium resulting in intimal hyperplasia and fibrosis. With a more prolonged course, proliferation of fibrous tissue in periadventitial regions is seen. Eventually, thrombus formation and fibrosis obliterate the vessels.

It has been hypothesized that vascular remodeling is triggered by endothelial cell injury, either chemical, inflammatory, or mechanical. Mediators released from damaged endothelial cells may initiate smooth muscle proliferation. Alternatively, intact endothelial cells may produce proliferation-inhibiting substances,

Table 2-3. Heath and Edwards Classification of Progressive Pulmonary Vascular Changes in Pulmonary Hypertension

Grade	Histologic Feature
I	Medial hypertrophy
II	Cellular intimal proliferation
III	Luminal occlusion due to intimal hyperplasia ("onionskinning")
IV	Plexiform lesions with dilation and bypass channels around occluded vessels
V	Angiomatoid formation
VI	Fibrinoid necrosis

(Adapted from Heath and Edwards,[50] with permission.)

possibly heparin-like,[51] which are not produced from damaged endothelial cells. Although remodeling has been traditionally considered to be irreversible, recent studies in rats exposed to hypoxia have shown that removal of the inciting stimulus can lead to the onset of proteolysis and reversal of structural changes.[52] In the future, therapy for pulmonary hypertension and PHD may take advantage of these factors.

PULMONARY HYPERTENSION

The most common cause of pulmonary hypertension is left heart dysfunction. However, strictly speaking, this does not constitute PHD and will not be considered here, except to note that many of the features of PHD are shared by RV failure on the basis of LV dysfunction. Pulmonary hypertension on the basis of lung disease is sometimes called *active* pulmonary hypertension, implying that pulmonary hypertension develops in response to changes in pulmonary vessels. In these disorders, pulmonary diastolic arterial pressure exceeds LV end-diastolic pressure (= P_{LA}) and the resulting pressure gradient reflects increased PVR.[53] Table 2-4 lists some of the major causes of PHD in this category.

The natural history of pulmonary hypertension depends on its cause and its response to treatment. Such factors as associated systemic illness, the reversibility of inciting stimuli (e.g., hypoxia), and the presence of PHD all influence the ultimate prognosis of a given patient. In any patient with heart failure in whom LV failure is not clearly demonstrable, it behooves the clinician to consider the major categories of pulmonary hypertension in an organized fashion, as there are

a number of easily treatable and potentially reversible processes that can lead to pulmonary hypertension. A good example is obstructive sleep apnea, which is often easily treated with the application of nasal continuous airway pressure (CPAP). The level of pulmonary hypertension can be helpful in favoring certain causes of PHD.

Table 2-5 lists some representative hemodynamics in various conditions. The greatest levels of pulmonary arterial pressure are usually seen in chronic primary diseases of the pulmonary vasculature, as exemplified by primary pulmonary hypertension. With systemic levels of systolic pulmonary arterial pressure, it is unusual for the cause to be, for example, chronic bronchitis. In addition, note the role of exercise in bringing out pulmonary hypertension. As noted above, the pulmonary vascular bed normally has an enormous reserve for handling increased blood flow with exercise. Patients with early or borderline increases in PVR may exhibit normal or near-normal pulmonary hemodynamics at rest. However, increasing blood flow results in substantial elevations in pulmonary arterial pressures since the reserve of the pulmonary bed for passive dilatation in response to increased blood flow is limited.

Pulmonary Airway and Parenchymal Diseases

Hypoxia and direct obliteration of the pulmonary vascular bed, as part of the disease process, cause pulmonary hypertension. Hypoxia may be caused by hypoventilation, ventilation-perfusion imbalance, or occasionally anatomic right-left shunting. The most common cause of chronic PHD, chronic obstructive pulmonary disease (COPD), is in this category, followed by diseases leading to pulmonary fibrosis.[54–57]

Table 2-4. Diseases Associated With Pulmonary Hypertension and/or Pulmonary Heart Disease

Diseases affecting airways and lung parenchyma
    Chronic obstructive pulmonary disease
    Chronic bronchial asthma
    Cystic fibrosis
    Congenital developmental defects
    Infiltrative or granulomatous defects
        Idiopathic pulmonary fibrosis
        Sarcoidosis
        Tuberculosis
        Pneumoconioses
        Scleroderma
        Mixed connective tissue disease
        Systemic lupus erythematosus
        Rheumatoid arthritis
        Dermatomyositis
        Eosinophilic granuloma
        Radiation
        Diffuse malignant infiltration
    Upper airways obstruction
    Pulmonary resection (provided the remaining lung is abnormal)
    High altitude pulmonary edema
Diseases affecting the thoracic cage
    Kyphoscoliosis
    Thoracoplasty
    Neuromuscular disease causing muscle weakness
        Amyotrophic lateral sclerosis
        Muscular dystrophy
        Quadriplegia

Diseases affecting pulmonary vasculature
    Primary pulmonary hypertension
    Pulmonary veno-occlusive disease
    Polyarteritis (pulmonary arteritis)
    Rheumatoid arthritis
    Scleroderma
    Systemic lupus erythematosus
    Acute pulmonary thromboembolism
        Air embolism
        Amniotic fluid embolism
        Fat embolism
    Chronic pulmonary thromboembolic disease
    Cirrhosis of the liver (associated with primary pulmonary hypertension-like syndrome)
    Filariasis
    Schistosomiasis
    Sickle cell disease
    Tumor emboli
    Congenital peripheral pulmonary artery stenosis
    Toxin-induced pulmonary hypertension
        Aminorex fumarate
        Intravenous drug abuse
    Mediastinal tumor—external pressure and direct invasion
    Acquired immune deficiency syndrome (AIDS)

Causes of hypoventilation
    Sleep apnea syndrome
    Idiopathic alveolar hypoventilation syndrome (Ondine's curse)
    Obesity—hypoventilation syndrome

Table 2-5. Typical Pulmonary Hemodynamics

Disease	P_{RA}	mPAP	P_w	CI	PVR
Mitral stenosis[218]					
Rest	—	33.5 ± 12.5	20.3 ± 6.3	2.9 ± 0.8	—
Exercise	—	56.7 ± 23.3	33.0 ± 8.9	4.0 ± 1.2	—
Interstitial lung disease[192]					
Rest	—	26.8 ± 9.0	4.7 ± 2.7	3.6 ± 0.8	7.1 ± 4.5[a]
Exercise	—	40.5 ± 13.8	—	5.5 ± 1.4	8.3 ± 4.5[a]
Chronic obstructive pulmonary disease[219]					
Rest	5.0 ± 0.7	27.5 ± 2.3	8.6 ± 0.6	3.4 ± 0.2	433 ± 41.4[b]
Primary pulmonary hypertension[98]					
Rest	10.4 ± 6.3	60.7 ± 19.7	8.7 ± 3.9	2.4 ± 11.2	23.9 ± 11.2[a]

Abbreviations: P_{RA}, right atrial pressure (mmHg); mPAP, mean pulmonary artery pressure; P_w, pulmonary wedge pressure (mmHg); CI, cardiac index (L/M/m²); PVR, pulmonary vascular resistance.
[a] mmHg/L/min (multiply by 79.9 to convert to absolute units).
[b] Absolute resistance units (dyne-sec/cm⁵).

In COPD, the strongest predictor of pulmonary hypertension is hypoxemia due to altered ventilation-perfusion distribution. In patients with chronic bronchitis, alveolar ventilation is reduced in large sections of the lung, with subsequent development of alveolar and arterial hypoxemia. Pulmonary hypoxic vasoconstriction is enhanced by concomitant acidosis,[58,59] which may be the result of hypercapnia. Similar mechanisms are at work in other diseases of the airways such as asthma, cystic fibrosis, and bronchiectasis. Patients with the emphysematous form of COPD who are not hypoxic generally do not develop pulmonary hypertension unless the disease is advanced, although pulmonary hypertension is usually demonstrable on exercise.[60] In "pure" emphysema, pulmonary hypertension may develop as a result of obliteration of pulmonary vessels by the disease process, although this remains controversial, and most patients with COPD who develop pulmonary hypertension and subsequent PHD have a component of airway disease and hypoxemia.[61] There is a loose relationship between the degree of airflow obstruction as measured by forced expired volume in 1 second (FEV_1) and pulmonary arterial pressure; pulmonary hypertension is unusual in patients with COPD whose FEV_1 is greater than 1.0 L or greater than 50 percent of predicted.[62] A far stronger correlation is found between resting room air arterial oxygen content and pulmonary arterial pressure. As arterial O_2 saturation falls below 90 percent ($PaO_2 <$ 50 to 55 mmHg), there is an inverse correlation between arterial saturation and pulmonary artery pressure and PVR.[63]

Chronic Interstitial Lung Disease

Chronic lung diseases, such as idiopathic pulmonary fibrosis and the pneumoconioses probably leads to pulmonary artery hypertension through direct compression and obliteration of pulmonary blood vessels by the pathologic process as well as by hypoxemia. When vital capacity (VC) is reduced to between 50 and 80 percent of predicted, pulmonary hypertension is generally demonstrable only during exercise, although baseline calculated PVR is increased.[63,64] With further reductions in VC, pulmonary hypertension may appear at rest. Since carbon monoxide diffusion capacity (DLCO) reflects pulmonary capillary volume, this measure also decreases with obliteration of pulmonary vasculature. Indeed, DLCO is a better predictor of pulmonary hypertension in diseases in which the vasculature is preferentially affected. One example is sarcoidosis, in which DLCO, but not VC, correlates with the degree of pulmonary hypertension.[63] In the early stages of interstitial lung disease, hypoxemia is generally demonstrable only during exercise and is not likely to be a cause of pulmonary hypertension. However, with disease progression, rest hypoxemia may ensue and may contribute to the development of pulmonary hypertension and PHD.

Collagen Vascular Disorders

Pulmonary hypertension is often observed in collagen vascular disorders, which can affect the interstitium of the lung (interstitial pneumonitis and fibrosis) and/or pulmonary vessels directly (vasculitis). Up to 40 percent of patients with lupus erythematosus have evidence of pulmonary hypertension,[65] and the incidence in scleroderma is even higher.[66] Patients with collagen disorders developing pulmonary hypertension are often young women with a history of Raynaud's phenomenon.[67] DLCO is a sensitive predictor of pulmonary hypertension in patients with collagen diseases, even in the absence of marked reductions in VC and normal chest roentgenograms.[68]

Sleep Disordered Breathing

Usually found in middle-aged men, in whom the prevalence is 1 to 4 percent,[69] sleep disordered breathing can affect all age groups, weight categories, and both sexes. The most common disorder is obstructive sleep apnea syndrome (OSA), in which recurrent episodes of upper airway obstruction occur at night, leading to large decreases in intrathoracic pressure and often severe intermittent hypoxemia. Chronic awake pulmonary hypertension can be found in up to 12 to 20 percent of OSA patients.[70,71] In most of these patients, daytime hypoxemia can be demonstrated as well.[72] In many of the patients with normal daytime pulmonary arterial pressures, pulmonary hypertension is demonstrable during exercise.[70] Primary alveolar hypoventilation while awake may accompany sleep disordered breathing in a subset of these patients with pickwickian syndrome.[73] Such patients appear to be the most prone to the development of clinically evident heart failure.

Pulmonary Thromboembolic Disease

Acute or chronic pulmonary hypertension and PHD can follow pulmonary thromboembolic disease. It is generally accepted that in normals, one-half to two-thirds of the pulmonary vascular bed must be obliterated before pulmonary hypertension develops.[74] Chronic recurrent pulmonary embolism, sickle cell disease, schistosomiasis, fat, tumor, and amniotic fluid embolism are examples of other disorders in which foreign particles can lodge in and obstruct the pulmonary vasculature. In patients with prior cardiopulmonary disease, as little as 30 percent obliteration of the pulmonary vasculature can result in substantial increases in PVR, suggesting altered pressure-flow characteristics in this setting.[75,76]

Chronic PHD is not a common sequela of acute pulmonary embolism since angiographic evidence of clot retraction and fibrinolysis is apparent by 10 to 14 days after an event, and resolution is usually almost complete, as shown by radionuclide scanning, at 21 to 30 days.[77] However, decreased DLCO may persist for 6 to 12 months afterwards,[78] demonstrating continued microvascular occlusion.

Fewer than 2 percent of patients who are properly treated continue to have showers of emboli or fail to lyse the emboli and pass into a chronic phase of sustained pulmonary hypertension with the possibility of developing PHD.[79] Some controversy exists as to whether clot persistence in the pulmonary bed represents continued showers of emboli, retrograde propagation of in situ thrombi,[80] or diffuse thrombosis.[81] Chronic clots become fibrotic and adherent to the arterial wall, thus causing obstruction. Such lesions may be removable,[82] resulting in substantial hemodynamic improvement. These patients usually do not present with acute episodes suggestive of acute pulmonary embolism, but exhibit the insidious onset of symptoms suggestive of chronic PHD.

Primary Pulmonary Hypertension

No underlying etiologic factor can be found for primary pulmonary hypertension. The greatest prevalence is in women in the third and fourth decades, with a female to male ratio of 1.7:1.[83] However, cases in patients more than 60 years of age have been reported, and the disorder cannot be ruled out in any age group. The syndrome carries a poor prognosis, with a median survival of 3 years from time of diagnosis in patients presenting with New York Heart Association (NYHA) functional class III. Patients presenting with NYHA functional class IV status have a median survival of only 6

months.[83] Evidence of PHD such as increased right atrial pressure, decreased cardiac index, decreased DLCO, and Raynaud's phenomenon are other poor prognostic indicators.

Many etiologic factors have been posited and have been reviewed elsewhere.[84] There is evidence suggesting that microthromboembolic disease is important. Thrombosis probably occurs *in situ*, since no identifiable source of recurrent emboli is demonstrable in most cases[84]; thrombosis is probably the result of endothelial damage.[85] The role of thromboembolism in primary pulmonary hypertension is still debated. Evidence of improved prognosis with anticoagulation[86,87] suggests that microthromboembolism, no matter what the etiology, plays a role in the dismal outcome of this disease. However, the role of anticoagulation in this disorder still remains controversial.

We now consider the pathophysiology, clinical presentation, diagnosis and treatment of acute and chronic PHD.

DIAGNOSTIC TOOLS

The clinical history and physical examination are critical in the evaluation of PHD, but, with some exceptions, they may be nonspecific. A number of noninvasive techniques are extremely useful for evaluating PHD and may make invasive evaluation via cardiac catheterization unnecessary in many cases. In this review we will concentrate on some of these noninvasive techniques.

Pulmonary Function Testing

Pulmonary function testing is very useful in the evaluation of patients with pulmonary hypertension, not because pulmonary function tests can, per se, lead to the diagnosis of PHD, but rather because they can aid in categorizing the type and severity of pulmonary impairment. Initial evaluation should consist of spirometry, lung volume measurements, DLCO, and arterial blood gas tensions at rest and possibly during exercise. Ventilatory impairment can indicate loss of lung volume (restrictive ventilatory defect), decrease in maximum flow rates (obstructive ventilatory impairment), or both. The single most useful measurement is the FEV_1, which is a general assessment of ventilatory function and is directly correlated with the maximum voluntary ventilation. Oximetry during exercise testing may reveal exercise-induced hypoxemia unsuspected in patients with normal resting blood gas tensions. In certain cases, exercise testing to evaluate aerobic capacity (maximum oxygen consumption and carbon dioxide production) may be useful for quantitating symptomatology, but this cannot be a general recommendation.

Electrocardiogram

The electrocardiographic (ECG) abnormalities in PHD depend on its etiology. Patients with COPD, especially those with emphysema, have ECG abnormalities that reflect structural changes in the thorax.[88-90] These are superimposed on the changes due to PHD.[91] Table 2-6 lists some combinations of these criteria that suggest PHD. In general ECG criteria are fairly specific, but not terribly sensitive for the detection of PHD. In an autopsy series[92] ECG criteria were shown to have a sensitivity of 75 percent for cases with isolated RV hypertrophy and 53 percent with biventricular hypertrophy. The absence of all criteria correctly excluded 96 percent of cases with no RV hypertrophy. In a recent study, esophageal electrocardiography demonstrated

Table 2-6. ECG Evidence of Pulmonary Heart Disease

Without COPD
  Right axis deviation—mean QRS axis to the right of $+110°$
  R/S amplitude ratio in $V_1 > 1$
  R/S amplitude ratio in $V_6 < 1$
  Clockwise rotation of the electrical axis
  P-pulmonale pattern (increased P wave amplitude II, III, and AVF)
  S_1Q_3 or $S_1S_2S_3$ pattern
  Normal voltage QRS
  Incomplete (or rarely complete) right bundle branch block

With concomitant COPD
  Isoelectric P waves in lead I or right axis deviation of the P-wave vector ($> +60°$
  P-pulmonale pattern
  Tendency for right axis deviation in QRS
  R/S amplitude ratio in $V_1 > 1$
  R/S amplitude ratio in $V_6 < 1$
  Low-voltage QRS (in emphysema)
  S_1Q_3 or $S_1S_2S_3$ pattern
  Incomplete (or rarely complete) right bundle branch block
  Marked clockwise rotation of the electrical axis
  Occasional large Q wave or QS in the inferior or midprecordial leads, suggesting healed myocardial infarction

even higher sensitivity and 100 percent specificity.[93]

One problem with the ECG diagnosis of RV hypertrophy is that the electrical activity of the LV is usually much greater than that of the RV. Thus, small changes in the size of the RV may not greatly affect the ECG. An increase in anterior-directed forces may occur with RV hypertrophy, but this may be a sign of posterior LV infarction as well. Mitral stenosis and PHD may meet the QRS criteria for apical, lateral, and posterior infarction.[94] Severe RV hypertrophy may result in Q waves in the precordial leads, falsely suggesting anterior myocardial infarction.

Many rhythm disturbances have been noted in PHD, especially in the chronic state. These range from premature atrial contractions to supraventricular tachycardias of all types, including paroxysmal atrial tachycardia, multifocal atrial tachycardia, atrial fibrillation, atrial flutter, and junctional tachycardias. These arrhythmias are frequently found in patients undergoing acute exacerbations of preexisting lung disease such as COPD, and are frequently related either to the disease process, acute RV overload, electrolyte abnormalities, hypoxemia or acidosis, or to therapy with β-agonists, methylxanthines, and diuretics. The reported incidence of supraventricular arrhythmias ranges from 20 to 71 percent.[95] The incidence of ventricular arrhythmias is probably lower (7 to 24 percent).[95,96] In patients with primary pulmonary hypertension (a "pure" cause of PHD), ventricular tachyarrhythmias and atrioventricular junctional block are unusual.[97]

Chest X-Rays

Routine chest x-rays can be useful for detecting and estimating the extent of certain types of parenchymal lung disease, as well as for finding signs of LV dysfunction. They may also be useful for detecting signs of advanced pulmonary hypertension. On a posteroanterior film, a right descending pulmonary artery greater than 16 mm in diameter or a left descending pulmonary artery greater than 18 mm in diameter on the lateral view is indicative of pulmonary hypertension.[95] RV enlargement seen on the posteroanterior view results in displacement and increased transverse diameter of the heart shadow to the right. In the lateral view RV enlargement leads to filling of the retrosternal air space (Fig. 2-6). Changes in mediastinal and chest wall configuration may render the correlation of x-ray signs with RV weight unreliable. However, in patients with primary pulmonary hypertension or chronic pulmonary

thromboembolic disease, the National Institutes of Health (NIH) registry[98] of 187 patients demonstrated that enlarged main pulmonary arteries were present in 90 percent, enlarged hilar pulmonary arteries in 80 percent, and peripheral pulmonary vascular pruning in 51 percent of the patients. Normal heart size was present in only 6 percent of these patients.

Echocardiography

Echocardiography is an extremely powerful tool in evaluating the function of the RV and detecting and quantitating pulmonary hypertension and consequent PHD. M-mode echocardiography is of limited value in evaluating RV function, since the right-sided cardiac structures are situated posteriorly to the echo-dense sternum. Pulmonary hyperinflation and excessive chest motion in patients with COPD also impose limitations on the use of M-mode echocardiography.[99]

Two-dimensional echocardiography provides multiple cross-sectional views of the heart and improves visualization of the right heart. While RV free wall thickness and mass are less easy to assess, good evaluation is available of the thickness, configuration, and motion of the interventricular septum.[100,101] While RV volume is not easily calculated from measurements of a few axes, multiple cross-sectional views can be used to obtain relatively accurate estimates of RV volume using the Simpson's rule approximation technique. Bommer et al.[102] confirmed the correlation of right atrial and RV size from echocardiography with RV volume as measured in eight autopsy cases and in 50 patients undergoing cardiac catheterization.

There have been a number of echocardiographic techniques proposed for estimating RV systolic pressure. Danchin et

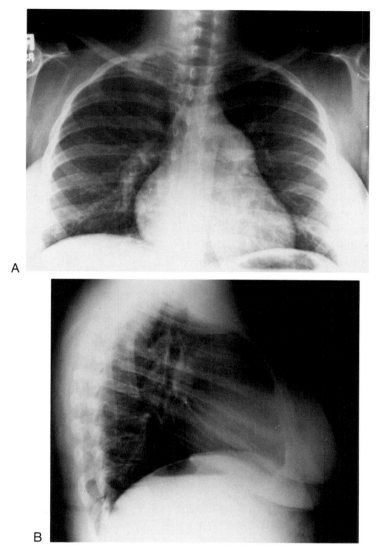

Fig. 2-6. Chest x-ray of a 32-year-old woman with primary pulmonary hypertension and pulmonary systolic pressure of 65 torr. **(A)** Posteroanterior (PA) projection. **(B)** Lateral projection. Note enlargement of the mainstem and right pulmonary arteries on PA view. There is enlargement of the RV on PA projection and loss of the retrosternal airspace on lateral projection.

al.[103] obtained a loose but significant (r = 0.63) correlation between RV diameters and mean pulmonary artery pressure (mPAP). Zenker et al.[104] obtained a closer correlation (r = 0.95) between mPAP and an RV index = (TA × RV + AW/BSA),

where TA = tricuspid annulus, RV = RV short axis dimensions, AW = RV anterior wall thickness, and BSA = body surface area.

The technique of Doppler echocardiography has proved to be a convenient tool for estimating RV systolic pressure. Pressure gradients across a valve can be calculated from the modified Bernoulli equation:

$$PG = 4 \ (V^2)$$

where PG = pressure gradient and V = maximum velocity across the valve. Using the maximum velocity of systolic regurgitant jets across the tricuspid valve, the peak systolic pressure gradient between RV and right atrium may be estimated.[105,106] If right atrial pressure is measured by another technique (e.g., by physical examination), then the calculated RV systolic pressure gradient is added to the estimated right atrial pressure, and RV systolic pressure may be reliably estimated (Fig. 2-7). A number of investigators have used variations of this technique to demonstrate good correlation between echo Doppler-based estimations of RV systolic pressure and actual measured pressures.[107–109] Another approach using echo Doppler techniques is to measure the mean time interval from onset to peak velocity of pulmonary artery flow, which correlates well with the logarithm of pulmonary artery pressure.[110]

Chronic overload of the RV leads to RV dilatation, an effect especially prominent during inspiration because of increased venous return. These changes can result in configurational changes in impaired LV diastolic filling, due to the effects of interventricular interdependence.[111] These effects are mediated through the pericardium and the interventricular septum. Configurational changes in the septum have echocardiographic manifestations. Normally the septum is concave toward the LV, resulting in a relatively circular LV shape in the axial plane during diastole. During systole there is symmetrical inward motion of the ventricular walls resulting in constriction of the LV

while maintaining its circular shape. Thus, the septum functions as part of the LV during systole.

With RV volume overload, the septum may become flattened or even reverse its curvature so as to become concave toward the RV.[112] In extreme cases, the septum may bulge into the LV in diastole. During systole, the septum may demonstrate so-called paradoxical motion,[113,114] defined as motion away from the LV posterolateral wall and toward the RV free wall (that is, the septum may function as part of the RV).

Radioisotope Lung Scanning

Radioisotope scanning is useful in the initial evaluation of patients with unexplained pulmonary hypertension. Patients with segmental perfusion defects, especially when accompanied by normal regional ventilation scans, should be considered for further evaluation for chronic thromboembolic disease. In these patients consideration should be given to selective pulmonary angiography for definitive diagnosis before initiating chronic therapy with anticoagulation or before performing vena cava interruption procedures.

Radionuclide Techniques for Evaluation of RV Function

Equilibrium-gated blood pool imaging allows continuous monitoring of the RV by labeling erythrocytes with technetium-99m. Ejection fraction is calculated by comparing counts at end-systole with those at end-diastole[99] collected at approximately 10 minutes. RV dimensions are difficult to measure with this technique because of the obscuring of the RV

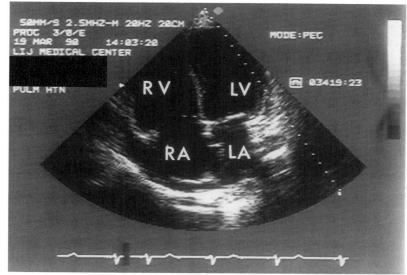

A

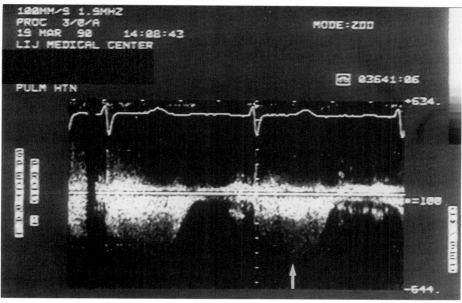

B

Fig. 2-7. Systolic two-dimensional echocardiogram from a patient with pulmonary hypertension on the basis of COPD. **(A)** Four-chamber view. Note dilatation of the right atrium (RA) and ventricle (RV) with flattening and even some bowing into the left ventricle (LV) of the interventricular septum. Note also an interatrial aneurysm probably apparent because of increased right atrial/left atrial pressure gradient. **(B)** M-mode Doppler velocity profile across the tricuspid valve. The peak regurgitant flow (downward direction, *arrow*) was estimated as 4 m/sec. This gives an estimated RV systolic pressure of 64 torr greater than the right atrial pressure. Right atrial pressure was clinically estimated as 5 mmHg, giving an estimated RV systolic pressure of 69 mmHg. (Courtesy of Scott Roth, M.D., Division of Cardiology, Long Island Jewish Medical Center, New Hyde Park, NY.)

borders by background radiation in other cardiac chambers and the lungs.[115] The first-pass technique also involves radiolabeling with technetium-99m, but is based on principles of indicator dilution therapy. Counting is done sequentially over each ventricle.[99,101] The advantage of this technique is that large numbers of counts are gathered over only a few heart beats. The greater contrast between cardiac and background counts allows better definition of cardiac borders and hence estimation of dimensions. While decrease ejection fraction and RV dilation may be detected by the first-pass technique,[116] the prediction of pulmonary arterial pressure and the detection of mild pulmonary arterial hypertension is not good.[117] Exercise studies may enhance the detection of decreased RV ejection fraction by radionuclide techniques.[116]

Thallium-201 is another radionuclide used for imaging the RV. Thallium is taken up by myocardial tissue and thus contrasts to technetium, which images the blood pool. While visualization of the RV at rest is not common in normals, the thickened RV myocardium present in patients with chronic PHD makes RV visualization common in these patients.[118] The thallium imaging technique is most sensitive for detecting RV hypertrophy when mean pulmonary arterial pressure is greater than 30 torr.[119]

Magnetic Resonance Imaging

Magnetic resonance imaging (MRI) is an exciting development in the noninvasive evaluation of PHD. This technique allows evaluation of RV free wall mass.[120,121] Mean RV free wall mass has been shown to be greater in patients with chronic PHD than in normals by this technique, and interobserver agreement has been reported to be good. Further

evaluation of this technique will define its role in the early diagnosis of chronic PHD.

Lung Biopsy

The role of open lung biopsy in the evaluation of pulmonary hypertension is still being debated. Open lung biopsy may diagnose unsuspected causes of pulmonary hypertension such as vasculitis, primary pulmonary hypertension, or interstitial fibrosis. However, high-resolution computed tomography (CT) scanning may yield evidence of interstitial lung disease not apparent on chest x-ray. Further, with a typical clinical presentation, it is rare to demonstrate histologic findings other than those of primary pulmonary hypertension. Finally, qualitative analysis of histology fails to predict the response to therapy.[84] Thus, considering the morbidity of this procedure, it is probably advisable only for those cases in which the possibility of secondary pulmonary hypertension still exists after noninvasive evaluation.

ACUTE PULMONARY HEART DISEASE

While massive pulmonary embolism is the best known cause of acute PHD, the same syndrome can be seen in any patient in whom PVR acutely and severely increases. Other causes include ventilation at high lung volume in patients with acute respiratory distress syndrome,[27] which increases PVR as a result of compression of overdistended alveoli; and the probable resultant effects of vasoconstrictor substances and edema fluid on critical closing pressures and on the diameters of pulmonary resistance vessels.

Pathophysiology

Numerous animal studies have demonstrated that a previously normal RV can tolerate an acute rise in systolic pressure produced by pulmonary vascular occlusion up to approximately 55 to 60 torr (mean, 40) without engendering circulatory collapse.[11] These levels are associated with decreased cardiac output and blood pressure and mild increases in right atrial pressure and RV dimensions (reviewed in Scharf et al.[11]). If there are concomitant decreases in systemic arterial pressure to less than approximately 60 torr, circulatory collapse ensues even though the degree of pulmonary artery constriction is unchanged. Conversely, if systemic arterial pressure is increased, either pharmacologically with vasoconstrictors or mechanically by occlusion of the descending aorta, the degree to which RV systolic pressure can be increased without producing overt circulatory collapse is greater (i.e., the afterload tolerance of the RV increases).[11,122–124]

The interaction between systemic and circulatory responses to RV occlusion has direct relevance for the mechanism by which circulatory collapse ensues and the therapy of acute RV failure. Indeed, RV failure probably results from an imbalance between myocardial oxygen demand and supply.[125] As RV work increases, and RV dilatation occurs, RV oxygen demand increases. However, as systemic arterial pressure falls with decreased cardiac output, the pressure for coronary, including RV coronary, perfusion decreases. This, plus the fact that increased RV wall pressures may limit coronary perfusion even further, leads to a limitation on the degree to which RV myocardial blood flow can increase to compensate for increased RV oxygen demand.

Some have postulated actual RV ischemia at the point of failure,[124–126] while others believe this is not a necessary precondition for failure.[11] A recent experimental study by Calvin and Ascah[126] explored the relationship of RV ischemia to changes in RV configuration during acute increases in RV systolic pressure. They found that RV dilatation with reversal of the transeptal RV-LV pressure gradient and leftward septal shift were associated with the onset of RV ischemia as measured by adenosine triphosphate/creatine phosphate depletion. This occurred when RV systolic pressure had tripled and cardiac output decreased by 30 percent. As cardiac output decreases further, systemic arterial pressure decreases, which further exacerbates RV dysfunction and decreases cardiac output. Thus a vicious cycle ensues leading to circulatory collapse and death.

These ideas have a direct bearing on the mode of cardiovascular support chosen for acute pulmonary hypertension and shock. At a point close to the maximum load tolerable, massive fluid infusion, beyond the point of adequate RV filling, could, by increasing RV dilation, increase RV oxygen demand and worsen the situation. The administration of positive inotropic agents could have the same effect. In experimental massive pulmonary embolization, vasoconstrictors, which raise systemic arterial pressure, were shown to be superior to either inotropic stimulation or fluid infusion[127,128] for improving survival and circulatory support. Few data exist in humans; however, it is probably prudent to consider vasoconstrictors in the circulatory support of shock associated with massive pulmonary embolism once adequate RV filling pressures are ensured.

Clinical Features

As is usual in clinical medicine, the most important diagnostic cues are to be found in the history. Since massive pulmonary embolization is by far the most common cause of acute PHD, elements in the history that suggest the possibility of embolism should be sought. These include prolonged periods of immobilization, disorders associated with a hypercoagulable state, obesity, and the presence of foreign bodies (e.g., chronically placed catheters) in the venous system. The clinical manifestations of acute PHD may be nonspecific and include dyspnea, orthopnea, and cough. Shock, tachycardia, and sweating may be nonspecific signs of stress. Physical exam may reveal distended neck veins with prominent *a* and *v* waves, pulsus paradoxus, and peripheral cyanosis. Inspection of the precordium may demonstrate RV lift along the left sternal border or subxiphoid region. Auscultation may reveal a gallop (S$_3$ or S$_4$) and a loud pulmonic second sound. A holosystolic murmur, accentuated during inspiration along the left sternal border, suggests tricuspid regurgitation. Auscultation of the lung fields may be normal or may reveal bilateral crackles.

Diagnostic studies with lung scanning or pulmonary angiography are usually initiated promptly once the diagnosis is suspected and the circulatory system is stabilized. Occasionally a large saddle embolus is visualized on echocardiography or MRI.

Treatment

Principles of circulatory support have been discussed above. Definitive treatment of severe acute PHD depends on the etiology. Since the most common cause is massive pulmonary embolism, modern therapy usually employs thrombolytic agents in patients with no contraindication for their use. A number of regimes have been employed, including streptokinase 250,000 units followed by infusion of 100,000 units/hr for 12 to 24 hours; urokinase 4,400 units/kg/hr for 12 to 24 hours; and recombinant tissue plasminogen activator (TPA), 80 to 100 mg over 2 hours.[77,129,130] Contraindications to thrombolytic therapy include recent surgery, bleeding diathesis, severe hypertension, and severe anemia.

While the diagnostic work-up of pulmonary embolism is beyond the scope of this chapter, there is controversy as to whether one ought to demand the definitive diagnosis of pulmonary embolism in a patient with acute right heart strain and shock. If the clinical background is relatively stable, and no other contraindications exist, many clinicians administer thrombolytic agents immediately, since the situation is life-threatening. Surgical embolectomy has been used in selected cases of acute massive pulmonary embolization. Patients often stabilize with cardiocirculatory support and anticoagulation, obviating the need for thrombolysis or embolectomy.

CHRONIC PULMONARY HEART DISEASE

Right Ventricle

As noted above, chronic PHD is defined on the basis of changes in RV structure. Uniform hypertrophy of the RV (wall thickness > 5.0 mm) is the result of chronic pulmonary hypertension. Therefore, RV weight is increased. Upper limits for normal RV weights in men have varied from 60 to 80 g, although 65 g in men and 50 g in women are probably reasonable criteria.[95] The cross-sectional area through the ventricular wall increases, as does myocardial fiber thickness.[131-133] Baseline RV myocardial blood flow increases proportionally to muscle mass.[133] RV end-diastolic pressure increases only in the later stages of pulmonary hypertension and RV hypertrophy.

Because of increased muscle mass and RV chamber size, RV myocardial oxygen demand increases. This probably renders the RV more susceptible to demand/supply imbalance along the lines discussed for acute PHD. In chronic PHD, RV systolic pressures may be quite high, even approaching systemic levels. Thus, RV systolic pressures of greater than approximately 55 to 60 torr suggest a chronic problem in which RV hypertrophy has been an adaptive change.

Cardiac output at rest is usually normal or even elevated in many patients with chronic PHD.[134] Patients with poor prognosis demonstrate progressively decreasing cardiac output over time. Thus, maintenance of peripheral blood flow is an important adaptive response to chronic tissue hypoxemia. Polycythemia augments peripheral oxygen delivery, especially in those patients with decreased cardiac output. However, polycythemia may be a maladaptive response since increasing blood viscosity also increases PVR, and may further decrease cardiac output.[125]

Pathophysiology

A number of studies have investigated the changes in hemodynamic parameters with time in patients with COPD.[135–140] Weitzenblum et al.[135] studied pulmonary hemodynamics in two groups of patients, a less severe group (mPAP < 20 mmHg) and a more severe group (mPAP > 20 mmHg). Both groups demonstrated roughly the same small increase in mPAP over 5 years (0.65 and 0.39 torr/year respectively). Pulmonary wedge pressures, RV end-diastolic pressure, and cardiac output were unchanged. No patients received oxygen or pulmonary vasodilators. In 27 patients with progressive hypoxemia, mPAP deteriorated more rapidly (5 mmHg/year). Thus, progression of mPAP was associated with progressive hypoxe-

mia in this study. Boushy and North[136] reported essentially similar findings in a larger study of 136 patients. The inverse correlation between arterial PO_2 and mPAP suggests that hypoxic vasoconstriction and/or vascular remodeling are primarily responsible for deteriorating pulmonary hemodynamics and the development of chronic PHD.[115]

Mahler et al.[137] studied patients with COPD during exercise and demonstrated increased PVR, RV afterload, and increased RV end-diastolic and end-systolic dimensions. These findings suggest that RV function deteriorates during exercise, which may contribute to exercise limitation in these patients. In contrast, in a study on patients with pulmonary hypertension at rest, Stein et al.[141] failed to show a correlation between changes in RV contractile function and clinical features of heart failure such as peripheral edema, ascites, and elevated right atrial pressure. This suggests that factors in addition to altered contractile function contribute to the clinical syndrome of heart failure.

The study of Schrijen et al.[138] showed progressive decreases in systemic arterial pressure in patients with pulmonary hypertension (mPAP > 20 mmHg). These authors postulated that decreased LV afterload could buffer against increases in mPAP with time. These studies were performed primarily in patients with the bronchitic form of COPD. Although one study in patients with the emphysematous form of COPD showed lower cardiac outputs in severe than in mild disease,[139] other studies have failed to demonstrate a correlation between cardiac output and severity of disease.[135,138,140]

Left Ventricle

With acute RV dilatation, ventricular interdependence acts to inhibit LV filling through the mechanisms of ventricular interdependence[111,142] and is mediated through a leftward shift in the interventricular septum and the pericardium. Indeed, decreased compliance of the LV has been demonstrated in patients with chronic PHD.[143] There has been a great deal of debate in the literature as to whether chronic RV overloading leads to structural and functional changes in the LV as well. In experimental animals, chronic banding of the pulmonary artery can lead to LV as well as RV hypertrophy,[132] supporting the "whole heart" concept of chronic PHD. Rao et al.[144] first reported depressed LV function in some patients with COPD in the absence of identifiable causes of LV failure. Others have reported decreased LV function as measured by systolic time intervals[145] and LV ejection fraction.[146,147]

On the other hand, a number of authors have failed to find evidence of LV dysfunction in patients with COPD and PHD, when no identifiable cause of LV failure is found.[148–151] Recently, Kohama et al.[152] demonstrated myocardial fibrosis and cellular hypertrophy in the LV in patients with COPD who died of heart failure, in whom there was no identifiable cause of LV dysfunction. These authors suggested that such changes might be related to hypoxemia, hypercarbia/acidosis, and possibly increased catecholamine levels associated with these blood gas alterations.

Patients with air flow obstruction may generate large negative swings in intrathoracic pressure, especially during inspiration. Such swings increase venous return, which further dilates the RV and leads to greater decreases in LV compliance, as demonstrated in experimental animals[14] and humans.[153] This probably explains the inspiratory decrease in preload usually seen during inspiration.[14] Patients with COPD also often demonstrate pulmonary hyperinflation. By direct mechanical heart-lung interactions,

increased lung volume, especially of the lower lobes, can act to hinder LV filling further.[14,15] Hypoxemia itself impairs LV relaxation and can decrease effective compliance.[154] Finally, decreased intrathoracic pressure, when sustained, can lead to impairment of LV ejection (i.e., increased LV afterload), since if intrathoracic pressure decreases more than LV systolic pressure, the *transmural* pressure across the LV wall actually increases. The role of increased LV afterload during the breath to breath decreases in intrathoracic pressure associated with air flow obstruction has been suggested as a mechanism contributing to LV dysfunction as well, although considerable controversy exists as to the importance of this mechanism.[14]

Clinical Presentation

Patients with chronic PHD exhibit signs and symptoms of the underlying disease. Dyspnea is a frequent symptom. While dyspnea often occurs concurrently with hypoxemia, in many patients, especially those with infiltrative or fibrotic lung disease or vascular obstruction, dyspnea is not associated with hypoxemia, is not completely relieved with oxygen therapy, and may be on a reflex basis.[155]

Patients with chronic PHD frequently present with syncope, especially related to exercise. Increased venous return with exercise can lead to increased RV pressure and volume, hence increasing RV oxygen demand. However, if cardiac output does not increase in proportion to increased oxygen demand, a myocardial supply/demand imbalance can result, leading to RV failure and circulatory collapse by the mechanisms discussed above. Further, during exercise peripheral arterial vasodilatation occurs, which might be unmatched by increased cardiac output. This can lead to decreased systemic blood pressure and result in syncope. In some patients syncope may be associated with coughing fits, probably because of decreased venous return, although Valsalva-type reflexes cannot be excluded.

A type of chest pain called "pulmonary artery pain" has been described in patients with chronic PHD.[156,157] It is described as anginal in character, but longer lasting and not responsive to nitrates. It has been attributed to stretching of the pulmonary artery or to actual RV ischemia. However, Zimmerman and Parker[158] have questioned the existence of such a symptom separate from typical coronary artery disease.

Hemoptysis may be associated with pulmonary hypertension due to leakage of blood from vascular to alveolar space in dilated pulmonary capillaries that rupture. However, hemoptysis should not be attributed to pulmonary hypertension until other diagnoses, such as tumor, bronchiectasis, or pulmonary infarction are excluded.

Right upper quadrant fullness, early satiety, and nausea and vomiting may be exhibited. These symptoms have been attributed to liver distension, with distension of the capsule in cases of RV failure. The liver may be tender. Neurologic symptoms such as headache and mental obtundation are often seen in patients with PHD, changes attributable to decreased cardiac output and altered arterial blood gas tensions. Occasionally, hoarseness is seen, which can be attributed to enlargement of the left main pulmonary artery where it passes contiguous to the aorta.

Tachypnea (respiratory rate >24) at rest is often found in patients with chronic pulmonary vasculopathy, chronic pulmonary fibrosis, or infiltrative disease, but usually not in patients with chronic bronchitis.[159] As in acute PHD, there may be a loud pulmonary component of the

second heart sound and a right ventricular heave and gallop. A holosystolic murmur along the left sternal border that is exacerbated on inspiration (called Carvallo's sign) may be present with tricuspid regurgitation. Elevated neck veins with prominent *a* and *v* waves are associated with congestive heart failure.

Peripheral edema is part of the congestive heart failure syndrome; it may extend into the abdominal wall and sacrum. In most cases edema results from chronic elevation of venous pressure with transudation of fluid into the extravascular space. However, increased venous pressure is not demonstrable in all patients with peripheral edema.[160] This finding has led to the hypothesis that chronic hypoxemia[161] and/or hypercapnia[162] can alter renal handling of sodium and water, leading to fluid retention.

THERAPY

Oxygen Therapy

Short-Term Effects

Degaute et al.[163] studied the short-term hemodynamic effects of administration of oxygen in patients with acute exacerbations of COPD. Arterial blood gas tensions and total peripheral oxygen delivery were recorded on room air and while patients breathed 28 percent oxygen. Fifteen severely hypoxic patients (PaO_2 = 40 torr) demonstrated increased arterial oxygen content, but no change in cardiac output. Twenty moderately hypoxemic patients (PaO_2 = 49 torr) also demonstrated increased arterial oxygen content but a decrease in cardiac output, possibly due to withdrawal of hypoxic induced sympathoadrenal stimulation. In the latter group of patients, oxygen delivery did not change with oxygen administration. Mean PAP remained increased in spite of oxygen administration, suggesting that hypoxic vasoconstriction was not the sole cause of pulmonary hypertension.

McNee et al.[164] studied the effects of oxygen administration on RV hemodynamics in patients with stable and decompensated PHD on the basis of COPD. Mean PAP for nonedematous and edematous patients was similar (30 and 33 torr, respectively). Even though mPAP was similar, RV ejection fraction was lower in decompensated than in compensated patients (0.23 versus 0.47, respectively). Cardiac output was normal in both groups. Oxygen therapy did not significantly change RV or LV ejection fraction or RV end-systolic pressure-volume relationships. Thus, oxygen administration does little to improve RV function acutely, and increases oxygen delivery by virtue of increased arterial oxygen content. The beneficial effects probably derive from effects of oxygen on the periphery.

Long-Term Effects
Studies demonstrating beneficial effects of long-term oxygen administration in pulmonary hypertension and PHD have generally been carried out in those patients with COPD. There are two large controlled trials demonstrating improved survival rate with oxygen administration in patients with COPD. In fact, oxygen has been the only therapeutic agent to date to improve patient survival definitively, although lung transplantation (see below) appears to be of great potential benefit for patients with end-stage lung disease, as experience with this mode of therapy accumulates.

The British domiciliary oxygen trial[165] consisted of 87 patients with severe COPD randomized to oxygen therapy (treated group = 42 patients) or not (untreated = 45 patients). The 2 groups were clinically matched and had similarly severe pulmonary function. The mortality for treated men was lower than that for untreated men (11.9 percent/year versus 29.4 percent/year). The differences for women was even more impressive (5.7 percent/year for treated versus 36.5 percent/year for untreated patients). The different mortality for men and women was not explained, since pulmonary function was matched between the sexes. Long-term oxygen therapy also prevented the progressive decreases in room air PaO_2 seen in untreated patients. Cooper and Howard[166] analyzed the sequential changes in pulmonary function and room air gas exchange in patients over 5 years of long-term oxygen therapy. These patients demonstrated rapid decline in FEV_1 and in room air PaO_2. The severity of pulmonary function at the time of initiation of therapy was a predictor of length of survival, and patients with FEV_1 of less than 0.6 L had little apparent survival benefit from oxygen administration. This finding underscores the need to combine oxygen therapy with bronchodilators, antibiotics, and steroid therapy as indicated for treatment of the primary disease process. These authors pointed out that prevention of severe hypoxemia may be the mechanism by which oxygen improves survival, and that alleviation of pulmonary hypertension has not been demonstrated to be of therapeutic benefit per se.[134,167,168]

The American nocturnal oxygen therapy trial (NOTT)[169–171] randomized hypoxemic COPD patients to 12 hours of nocturnal oxygen or to continuous oxygen therapy (mean 17.7 hr/day) for at least 12 months. The overall mortality in the nocturnal alone group was twice that of the continuous group.[170] PVR increased by 6.5 percent in the nocturnal therapy group, while the continuous therapy group demonstrated an 11 percent *decrease*. Exercise tolerance failed to improve in either group.

MacNee[172] recently reviewed the factors predicting survival in patients receiving long-term oxygen therapy. Elevated mPAP more than 28 torr, arterial PO_2 less than 46.5 torr, and FEV_1 less than 0.45 L were successful predictors of decreased survival in patients receiving long-term oxygen therapy. Timms et al.[171] showed that an initial PVR of less than 400 dyne-sec/cm^5 was a predictor of survival. Ashutosh et al.[173] demonstrated that patients whose mPAP fell by 5 mmHg more after 24 hours of therapy with 28 percent oxygen had improved survival on long-term therapy. These data suggest that poor prognosis is related to increased severity of disease at the onset of therapy, and they raise the question as to whether patients with very severe disease benefit at all from long-term oxygen therapy.

There are inconsistent findings on the effect of oxygen therapy on RV function. Olvey et al.[174] reported improvement in the RV ejection fraction response to exercise with oxygen, while others[171,119] failed to demonstrate significant changes in other indices of RV function. Finally, the beneficial survival effects of oxygen therapy in other forms of hypoxic pulmonary disease have not been demonstrated, although oxygen should clearly be used to treat any form of hypoxic lung disease. Table 2-7 shows recommended guidelines for the chronic administration of oxygen as agreed by two consensus

TABLE 2-7. Guidelines for Administration of Long-Term Oxygen Therapy

---

$PaO_2 \leq 55$ mmHg on room air at rest in nonrecumbent position

$PaO_2 > 55$ mmHg with evidence of secondary pulmonary hypertension, polycythemia, RV hypertrophy, impaired mental or cognitive function

$PaO_2 \leq 55$ mmHg during exercise with demonstrable improvement in exercise performance with oxygen therapy

$PaO_2 \leq 55$ mmHg during sleep especially associated with fragmentation of sleep, cardiac arrhythmias or ischemia, or pulmonary hypertension

---

committees.[169,175] The latter[175] also reaffirmed that oxygen given during ambulation increases endurance and reduces dyspnea. Oximetry is an acceptable method for demonstrating hypoxemia during exercise and sleep, as well as for follow-up and for monitoring the results of long-term therapy. Finally, optimal therapy with antibiotics, steroids, and bronchodilators may improve lung function and obviate the need for chronic oxygen administration.

Pulmonary Vasodilator Therapy

Theoretically, pharmacologic dilatation of the pulmonary vascular bed could reverse many of the pathophysiologic sequelae of pulmonary hypertension and could lead to improved hemodynamics and RV function. A meaningful response to vasodilators should include a rise in cardiac output associated with reductions of calculated PVR and mPAP and improvement in exercise tolerance. The assessment of pulmonary vasodilators is often performed acutely to determine responsiveness of the pulmonary circulation and to predict results of chronic therapy.

A number of different specific criteria have been proposed, and there is no universal agreement as to what constitutes a meaningful response to pulmonary vasodilators. For example, Rich and Brundage[176] defined a positive response to high-dose calcium channel blockers as a 50 percent decrease in PVR, accompanied by a 33 percent fall in mPAP. Weir et al.[177] defined a positive response as a 10 percent decrease in cardiac output accompanied by a 5 torr decrease in mPAP, a 20 percent reduction in PVR, and a decrease in the ratio of PVR to systemic vascular resistance. A decrease in PVR accompanied by increased cardiac output and no change in mPAP is not universally accepted as a positive therapeutic response. This is because with persistently elevated mPAP shear stresses imposed on the pulmonary vasculature could conceivably continue to produce histologic damage. In addition, if mPAP fails to decrease with vasodilator therapy, one could argue that RV afterload may not have decreased.

Vasodilator therapy is not without significant risk. All pulmonary vasodilators are systemic vasodilators as well and can lead to substantial reductions in blood pressure, if cardiac output does increase sufficiently to offset decreased systemic vascular resistance. Vasodilators may blunt pulmonary hypoxic vasoconstriction, leading to worsening of ventilation-perfusion distributions within the lung and thus exacerbating hypoxemia.

Finally, there is a question of the ability of the acute response to predict the response to long-term therapy. Improved long-term survival has been predicted by the acute response to vasodilators. However, this may be a function of the stage at which the disease is diagnosed rather than any therapeutic efficacy on the part of the drug.[178]

In 1989, Dantzker et al.[179] published results in six patients with primary pulmonary hypertension in whom acute hemodynamic improvement was demonstrated with either nifedipine or hydralazine. Their long-term therapy was interrupted to determine if hemodynamic changes could be correlated with the administration of drugs. No patients showed a rise in mPAP or PVR following withdrawal of vasodilator drugs, and none showed a decrease when drugs were restarted. Either vasodilator drugs caused long-term remission of the disease, or long-term hemodynamic changes were spontaneously variable in spite of drug administration. The authors stressed the need for long-term *controlled* trials of vasodilator therapy before

this mode could be definitively recommended. All of the patients evaluated by Dantzker et al. reported feeling improved, in spite of observed hemodynamic changes, and the placebo effect needs to be considered. At the present time, therapy with pulmonary vasodilators should be considered to be in the trial stage; careful hemodynamic and clinical evaluation as well as follow-up are needed, preferably from a center that is gathering data.[180]

Vasodilator Therapy in COPD

In general, vasodilator therapy has failed to demonstrate sustained therapeutic benefits in patients with COPD (beyond those of long-term oxygen administration) and cannot be recommended for routine use.[115] Theophylline is a commonly administered bronchodilator. However, the methylxanthines have also been shown to improve RV performance in patients with COPD[180,181] and is a pulmonary vasodilator.[181] These effects persist when slow-release preparations are used,[182] which may explain part of the therapeutic benefit of these preparations. β_2-Specific agonists also act as pulmonary vasodilators,[182–184] although sustained efficacy has not been demonstrated.[183] Other vasodilators evaluated in COPD include calcium channel blockers,[185–190] hydralazine,[191–193] nitrates,[194] nitroprusside,[184] α_1-blockers,[195,196] and angiotensin-converting enzyme inhibitors.[197,198]

Vasodilators in Primary Pulmonary Hypertension

Predicting the response to pulmonary vasodilators on the basis of histologic classification or baseline hemodynamics is not possible.[84] A number of vasodilators have been evaluated for this disease. These include calcium channel blockers, hydralazine, acetylcholine, isoproterenol, and recently prostenoids such as prostacyclin and prostaglandin E₁.[176–179,199–204]

Prostacyclin has been shown to be a useful pulmonary vasodilator drug with a short half-life that can predict the acute response to other vasodilator drugs such as hydralazine and nifedipine.[205] Prostacyclin also inhibits platelet aggregation that may be induced by endothelial injury. Recently, continuous IV prostacyclin infusion by portable pump was shown to result in sustained (8-week) hemodynamic improvement compared with conventional treatment with oral vasodilators, anticoagulation, oxygen, cardiac glycosides, and diuretics.[45] The use of prostacyclin is obviously inhibited by the necessity of long-term IV administration; however, long-term trials using implanted pumps and chronic access lines are being evaluated.

Rich and Brundage[176] have evaluated long-term, high-dose calcium channel blocker therapy titrated using right heart catheterization. Nifedipine or diltiazem is administered in an initial test dose of 20 or 60 mg, respectively. Oral doses are repeated hourly until a favorable hemodynamic response is achieved or there are adverse effects (primarily systemic hypotension). The cumulative dose is then administered every 6 to 8 hours chronically. In four of five patients receiving this regime, a sustained reduction in mPAP and PVR with regression of RV hypertrophy was noted after 1 year.

CARDIAC GLYCOSIDES

The utility of cardiac glycosides in PHD has been demonstrated only when there is concomitant LV dysfunction, and there are few data to support therapeutic benefit from cardiac glycosides in PHD.[206–208] This plus the fact that acute hypoxia may increase toxicity[208] makes it difficult to recommend cardiac glycosides for routine treatment of PHD.

Phlebotomy and Diuretics

Reduction in intravascular volume could lead to improved functional status. Extravascular lung water may increase during exacerbations of PHD with edema[209,210] and regress with remission. Reduction of extravascular lung water using diuretics may, therefore, be of significant benefit to gas exchange. Too great a reduction in vascular volume could reduce mean circulatory pressure and lead to unwanted reductions in cardiac output. In addition, care must be taken to avoid hypokalemia and alkalosis, which may blunt respiratory drive.

Blood viscosity sharply increases as hematocrit increases above 55. This may increase PVR. Polycythemia may be a sign of chronic hypoxemia and should theoretically be preventable with adequate oxygen administration. However, with persistently elevated hematocrit (> 55) phlebotomy should be considered. Chetty et al.[211] demonstrated that therapeutic phlebotomy improved exercise tolerance in polycythemic patients with COPD. This was associated with improved cardiac output and stroke volume.

LUNG TRANSPLANTATION

Although lung transplantation was originally introduced for treatment of end-stage restrictive lung disease, the indications and eligible age range for this procedure are continuing to expand. Patients with end-stage obstructive and vascular lung disease are now considered eligible for transplantation.

Although *en bloc* heart-lung transplantation was the original procedure proposed for patients with end-stage pulmonary hypertension,[212] the scarcity of donor organs necessitated the growing popularity of single lung transplantation. Bolman et al.[213] described their experience with single lung and heart-lung transplantation. Both groups showed marked decreases in mPAP from near systemic levels to normal. Similarly, Pasque et al.[214] noted similar results in their patients with single lung transplantation. Recent studies have shown impressive 2-year survival rates (70 to 75 percent).[213–215] These improved survival rates are no doubt partly due to improved immunosuppressive regimens.[216]

Finally, patients with PHD who undergo lung transplantation may demonstrate improvement in RV function with resolution of their pulmonary hypertension.[64,217] For example, Pasque et al.[214] noted marked increase in RV ejection fraction, from 22 to 51 percent in their patients following single lung transplant. Studies have not yet been done to address the issue of whether hypertrophic changes in the RV are reversible with single or double lung transplantation, although clinically and functionally RV function can be markedly improved.

With advances in organ preservation and post-transplant immunosuppression, it is to be expected that the prognosis in cases of end-stage pulmonary vasculopathy with single lung transplant will offer new hope to patients otherwise doomed to early death. Eligibility criteria are changing for lung transplantation and may vary from center to center. Therefore, physicians considering patients for lung transplantation should contact a transplant center when this consideration becomes serious, to facilitate cooperation among the referring physician, the transplant center, and the patient. Finally, this mode of therapy, promising as it is, will no doubt always be limited by organ donor availability.

REFERENCES

1. Laennec, RTH: A Treatise on the Disease of the Chest and on Mediate auscultation. p. 91. T and G Underwood, London, 1827
2. Fishman AP: Pulmonary Diseases and Disorders. McGraw-Hill, New York, 1980
3. Feldman NT, Ingram RH, Jr: Chronic cor pulmonale. p. 1485. In Hurst JW, Logue RB, Schlant RC et al (eds): The Heart, Arteries and Veins. 4th Ed. McGraw-Hill, New York, 1978
4. McGinn S, White PD: Acute cor pulmonale resulting from pulmonary embolism. JAMA 104:1473, 1935
5. World Health Organization: Definition of chronic cor pulmonale: a report of the expert committee. Circulation 27:594, 1963
6. Renzetti AD, McClement JH, Litt BD: The Veterans Administration co-operative study of pulmonary function. III: Mortality in relation to respiratory function in chronic obstructive lung disease. Am J Med 41:115, 1966
7. France AJ, Prescott RJ, Biernacki W et al: Does right ventricular function predict survival in patients with chronic obstructive pulmonary disease? Thorax 43:621, 1988
8. March HW, Ross JK, Lower RR: Observations on the behavior of the right ventricular outflow tract, with reference to its development origins. Am J Med 32:835, 1962
9. Armour JA, Pace JB, Randell WC: Interrelationships of architecture and function of the right ventricle. Am J Physiol 218:174, 1970
10. Pace JB, Keefe WF, Armour JA, Randall WC: Influence of sympathetic nerve stimulation on right ventricular outflow

tract pressure in anesthetized dogs. Circ Res 24:397, 1969

11. Scharf SM, Warner KG, Josa M et al: Load tolerance of the right ventricle: effect of increased aortic pressure. J Crit Care 1:163, 1986

12. McFadden ER, Braunwald E: Cor pulmonale. p. 1581. In Braunwald E (ed): Heart Disease—A Textbook of Cardiovascular Medicine. WB Saunders, Philadelphia, 1992

13. Maughan WL, Oikawa RY: Right ventricular function. p. 179. In Scharf SM, Cassidy SS (eds): Heart-Lung Interactions in Health and Disease. Marcel Dekker, New York, 1989

14. Scharf SM: Cardiovascular effects of airways obstruction. Lung 169:1, 1991

15. Marini JJ, O'Quin R, Culver BH, Butler J: Estimation of transmural cardiac pressures during ventilation with PEEP. J Appl Physiol 53:384, 1982

16. Oppenheimer L, Goldberg HS: Pulmonary circulation and edema formation. p. 93. In Scharf SM, Cassidy SS (eds): Heart-Lung Interactions in Health and Disease. Marcel Dekker, New York, 1989

17. Gil J: The normal pulmonary microcirculation. p. 3. In Fishman AP (ed): The Pulmonary Circulation: Normal and Abnormal. University of Pennsylvania Press, Philadelphia, 1990

18. Horsfield K: Morphometry of the small pulmonary arteries in man. Circ Res 42:593, 1978

19. Weibel ER, Gomez EM: Architecture of the human lung. Science 137:577, 1962

20. Weibel ER: Morphometry of the Human Lung. Academic Press, New York, 1963

21. Gil J, Bachofen H, Gehr P, Weibel ER: Alveolar to surface area relationships in air and saline filled lungs fixed by vascular perfusion. J Appl Physiol 47:990, 1979

22. Howell JBL, Permutt S, Proctor D, Riley RL: Effects of inflation of the lung on different parts of the pulmonary bed. J Appl Physiol 16:712, 1961

23. Permutt S, Howell JBL, Proctor D, Riley RL: Effects of lung inflation on static pressure-volume characteristics of pulmonary vessels. J Appl Physiol 16:64, 1961

24. Whittenberger JL, McGregor M, Berglund E, Borst MC: Influence of state of inflation of the lung on pulmonary vascular resistance. J Appl Physiol 15:878, 1960

25. Scharf SM, Brown R: Influence of the right ventricle on canine left ventricular function with PEEP. J Appl Physiol 52:254, 1982

26. Schulman DS, Biondi JW, Zohgbi S et al: Left ventricular diastolic function during positive end-expiratory pressure. Impact of right ventricular ischemia and ventricular interaction. Am Rev Respir Dis 145:515, 1992

27. Dhainaut JF, Aouate P, Brunet FP: Circulatory effects of positive end-expiratory pressure in patients with acute lung injury. p. 809. In Scharf SM, Cassidy SS (eds): Heart-lung Interactions in Health and Disease. Marcel Dekker, New York, 1989

28. Permutt S: Relation between pulmonary arterial pressure and pleural pressure during the acute asthmatic attack. Chest 63 (suppl.):25S, 1973

29. Scharf SM: Mechanical cardiopulmonary interactions with asthma. Clin Rev Allergy 3:487, 1985

30. West JB, Dollery CT: Distribution of blood flow and the pressure-flow relations in the whole lung. J Appl Physiol 20:175, 1965

31. Cournand A, Riley RL, Himmelstein A, Austrian R: Pulmonary circulation and alveolar ventilation-perfusion relationships after pneumonectomy. J Thorac Surg 19:80, 1950

32. Prewitt RM, Ducas J: Hemodynamic management of acute respiratory failure. p. 879. In Scharf SM, Cassidy SS (eds): Heart-lung Interactions in Health and Disease. Marcel Dekker, New York, 1989

33. McGregor M, Sniderman A: On pulmonary vascular resistance: the need for more precise definition. Am J Cardiol 55:217, 1985

34. D'Orio V, Fatemi M, Marnette J-M et al: Pressure-flow relationships of the pulmonary circulation during endotoxin infusion in intact dogs. Crit Care Med 20:1005, 1992

35. McDonald DA: Blood Flow in Arteries. Williams & Wilkins, Baltimore, 1974

36. Milnor WR: Pulsatile blood flow. N Engl J Med 287:27, 1972

37. Calvin JE, Baer RW, Glantz SA: Pulmonary artery constriction produces a greater right ventricular dynamic afterload than lung microvascular injury in the open chest dog. Circ Res 56:40, 1985

38. Aviado DM: The Lung Circulation. Vol. I. Pergamon Press, London, 1965

39. Stecenko AA, Lefferts P, Mitchell J et al: Vasodilatory effect of aerosoal histamine during pulmonary vasoconstriction in the unanesthetized sheep. Pediatr Pulmonol 3:94, 1987

40. Palmer RMJ, Ferrige AG, Moncada S: Nitric oxide release accounts for the biological activity of endothelium derived relaxing factor. Nature 327:524, 1987.

41. Furchgott RF, Zawdzki JV: The obligatory role of endothelial cells in the relaxation of arterial smooth muscle by acetylcholine. Nature 288:373, 1980

42. Ingarro LJ, Harbison RG, Wood KS, Kadowitz PJ: Activation of purified soluble guanylate cyclase by endothelium-derived relaxing factor from intrapulmonary artery and vein. Stimulation by acetylcholine, bradykinin and arachidonic acid. J Pharmacol Exp Ther 237:893, 1987

43. Brigham KL: Mediators in the pulmonary circulation. p. 91. In Fishman AP (ed): The Pulmonary Circulation: Normal and Abnormal. University of Pennsylvania Press, Philadelphia, 1990

44. Malik AB, Johnson A: Role of humoral mediators in the pulmonary vascular response to pulmonary embolism. p. 445. In Weir EK, Reeves JT (eds): Pulmonary Vascular Physiology and Pathophysiology. Marcel Dekker, New York, 1988

45. Rubin LJ, Mendoza J, Houd M et al: Treatment of primary pulmonary hypertension with continuous intravenous prostacyclin (Epoprostenol): results of a randomized trial. Ann Intern Med 112:485, 1990

46. Long WA, Brown DL: Central neural regulation of the pulmonary circulation. p. 131. In Fishman AP (ed): The Pulmonary Circulation, Normal and Abnormal. University of Pennsylvania Press, Philadelphia, 1990

47. Kotlikoff MI, Fishman AP: Endothelin: mediator of hypoxic vasoconstriction? p. 85. In Fishman AP (ed): The Pulmonary Circulation, Normal and Abnormal. University of Pennsylvania Press, Philadelphia, 1990

48. Weir EK, Reeves JT: Pulmonary Vascular Physiology and Pathophysiology. Marcel Dekker, New York, 1989

49. Barer GR, Howard P, Shaw JW: Stimulus-response curves for the pulmonary vascular bed to hypoxia and hypercapnia. J Physiol (Lond) 211:139, 1970

50. Heath DA, Edwards JE: The pathology of hypertensive pulmonary vascular disease. Circulation 18:533, 1958

51. Hales CA, Kraden RL, Brandstetter RD, Zho YJ: Impairment of pulmonary hypoxic remodeling by heparin in mice. Am Rev Respir Dis 128:747, 1983

52. Riley DJ: Vascular remodeling. In Crystal RG, West JB (eds): The Lung: Scientific Foundations. Raven Press, New York, 1991

53. Harvey RM, Enson Y, Ferrer MI: A reconsideration of the origins of pulmonary hypertension. Chest 59:82, 1971

54. Fulton RM: The heart in chronic pulmonary disease. Q J Med 22:43, 1953

55. Flint RJ: Cor pulmonale. Lancet 2:51, 1954

56. Robin ED, Gaudio R: Cor Pulmonale. Disease-a-Month. Year Book, Chicago, 1970

57. Behnke RH, Bristow JD, Carrieri V et al: Resource for the optimal care of acute respiratory failure. Circulation 43:A185, 1971

58. Enson Y: The influence of hydrogen ion concentration and hypoxia on the pulmonary circulation. J Clin Invest 43:1146, 1964

59. Fishman AP, McClement J, Himmelstein A, Cournand A: Effects of acute hy-

poxia on the circulation and respiration in patients with chronic pulmonary disease studied during the steady state. J Clin Invest 31:770, 1952

60. Oswald-Mommosser M, Apprill M, Bachez P et al: Pulmonary hemodynamics in chronic obstructive pulmonary disease of the emphysematous type. Respiration 58:304, 1991

61. Jamal K, Fleetham JA, Thurlbeck WM: Cor pulmonale: correlation with central airway lesions, peripheral airway lesions, emphysema, and control of breathing. Am Rev Respir Dis 141:1172, 1990

62. Harris P, Sagel N, Green K, Housley E: The influence of airways resistance and alveolar pressure on the pulmonary vascular resistance in chronic bronchitis. Cardiovasc Dis 2:84, 1968

63. Emergil C, Sobol BJ, Herbert WH et al: Routine pulmonary function studies as a key to the status of the lesser circulation in chronic obstructive pulmonary disease. Am J Med 50:191, 1971

64. Trulock EP, Cooper JD, Kaiser L et al: The Washington University-Barnes Hospital experience with lung transplantation. JAMA 266:225, 1991

65. Fayemi AO: Pulmonary vascular disease in systemic lupus erythematosus. Am J Clin Pathol 65:284, 1976

66. Sackner MA, Akgrin N, Kimbel P, Lewis DH: Pathophysiology of scleroderma involving the heart and respiratory system. Ann Intern Med 60:611, 1964

67. Pronk LL, Swaak AJ: Pulmonary hypertension in connective tissue disease. Report of three cases and review of the literature. Rheumatol Int 11:83, 1991

68. Zapol WM, Snider MJ: Pulmonary hypertension in severe acute respiratory failure. N Engl J Med 296:476, 1976

69. Lavie P: Incidence of sleep apnea in a presumably healthy working population: a significant relationship with excessive daytime sleepiness. Sleep 6:312, 1983

70. Podzus T, Bauer W, Mayer J: Sleep apnea and pulmonary hypertension. Klin Wochenschir 64:131, 1986

71. Podzus T, Greenberg H, Scharf SM: The influence of sleep state and sleep-disordered breathing on cardiovascular function. p. 257. In Saunders N, Sullivan C (eds): Sleep and Breathing II. Marcel Dekker, New York, 1993

72. Bradley TD, Rutherford R, Grossman R et al: Role of daytime hypoxemia in the pathogenesis of right heart failure in the obstructive sleep apnea syndrome. Am Rev Respir Dis 137:835, 1985

73. Rapaport DM, Garay SM, Epsteen H, Goldring RM: Hypercapnia in the obstructive sleep apnea syndrome: a reevaluation of the pickwickian syndrome. Chest 89:627, 1986

74. McIntyre KM, Sasahara AA: The hemodynamic response to pulmonary embolism in patients without prior cardiopulmonary disease. Am J Cardiol 28:288, 1971

75. Dantzker DR: Pulmonary embolism. p. 1198. In Crystal RG, West JB (eds): The Lung Scientific Foundations. Raven Press, New York, 1991

76. McIntyre KM, Sasahara AA, Sharma GVRK: Pulmonary thromboembolism: current concepts. Ann Intern Med 18:192, 1972

77. Urokinase pulmonary embolism trial: a national cooperative study. Circulation 47 (suppl. II):1, 1973

78. Sharma GVRK, Burleson VA, Sasahara AA: Effect of thrombolytic therapy on pulmonary capillary blood volume in patients with pulmonary embolism. N Engl J Med 303:842, 1980

79. Dalen JE, Alpert JS: Natural history of pulmonary embolism. Prog Cardiovasc Dis 17:259, 1975

80. Weir EK, Archer SI, Edwards JE: Chronic primary and secondary thromboembolic pulmonary hypertension. Chest 93 (suppl. 3):49s, 1988

81. Rich S, Levitsky S, Brundage BH: Pulmonary hypertension from chronic pulmonary thromboembolism. Ann Intern Med 108:425, 1988

82. Sabiston DC Jr, Wolfe WG, Oldham HN, Jr et al: Surgical management of chronic pulmonary embolism. Ann Surg 185:699, 1977

83. D'Alonzo GE, Barst RJ, Ayres SM et al:

Survival in patients with primary pulmonary hypertension: results from a national prospective registry. Ann Intern Med 115:343, 1991

84. Palevsky H, Schlov BL, Petra G et al: Primary pulmonary hypertension: vascular structure, morphometry and responsiveness to vasodilator agents. Circulation 80:1207, 1989

85. Eisenberg PR, Lucore C, Kaufman L: Fibrinopeptide-A levels indicative of pulmonary vascular thrombosis in patients with primary pulmonary hypertension. Circulation 82:841, 1990

86. Cohen M, Edwards WD, Fuster V: Regression in thromboembolic type of primary pulmonary hypertension during 2 1/2 years of antithrombotic therapy. J Am Coll Cardiol 7:172, 1986

87. Rich S, Kaufman E, Levy PS: The effect of high dose calcium-channel blockers on survival in primary pulmonary hypertension. N Engl J Med 327:76, 1992

88. Nicholas WJ, Liebson PR: ECG changes in COPD: what do they mean? Part I: Atrial and ventricular abnormalities. J Respir Dis 8:13, 1987

89. Nicholas WJ, Liebsom PR: ECG changes in COPD: what do they mean? Part II: Right ventricular and biventricular hypertrophy and low voltage. J Respir Dis 8:103, 1987

90. Phillips RW: The electrocardiogram in cor pulmonale secondary to pulmonary emphysema: A study of 18 cases proved by autopsy. Am Heart J 56:352, 1958

91. Ikeda K, Kubota I, Takahashi R, Yasui S: P-wave changes in obstructive and restrictive lung diseases. J Electrocardiol 18:233, 1985

92. Lehtonen J, Sutinen S, Ikaheimo M, Paakko P: Electrocardiographic criteria for the diagnosis of right ventricular hypertrophy verified at autopsy. Chest 93:839, 1988

93. Mittal SR, Jain SC, Sharma SK, Sethi AK: The role of oesophageal electrocardiography in the diagnosis of right ventricular hypertrophy in chronic obstructive pulmonary disease. Int J Cardiol 11:165, 1986

94. Behar JV, Howe CM, Wagner NB et al: Performance of new criteria for right ventricular hypertrophy and myocardial infarction in patients with pulmonary hypertension due to cor pulmonale and mitral stenosis. J Electrocardiol 24:231, 1991

95. Murphy ML, Dinh H, Nichelson D: Chronic cor pulmonale. Dis Monthly. 35:657, 1989

96. Shih HT, Webb CR, Conway WA: Frequency and significance of cardiac arrhythmias in chronic obstructive lung disease. Chest 94:44, 1988

97. Kanemoto N, Sasamoto H: Arrhythmias in primary pulmonary hypertension. Jpn Heart J 20:765, 1979

98. Rich S, Dantzker DR, Ayres SM et al: Primary pulmonary hypertension: a national prospective study. Ann Intern Med 107:216, 1987

99. Matthay RA, Niederman MS, Weidemann HP: Cardiovascular-pulmonary interaction in chronic obstructive pulmonary disease with special reference to the pathogenesis and management of cor pulmonale. Med Clin North Am 74:571, 1990

100. Feigenbaum H: Echocardiography 4th Ed. p. 157. Lea & Febiger, Philadelphia, 1986

101. Niederman MS, Matthay RA: Cardiovascular function in secondary pulmonary hypertension. Heart Lung 15:341, 1986

102. Bommer W, Weinert L, Neumann A et al: Determination of right atrial and right ventricular size by two-dimensional echocardiography. Circulation 60:91, 1979

103. Danchin N, Cornette A, Henriquez A et al: Two-dimensional echocardiographic assessment of the right ventricle in patients with chronic obstructive lung disease. Chest 92:229, 1987

104. Zenker G, Forche G, Harnoncourt K: Two-dimensional echocardiography using a subcostal approach in patients with COPD. Chest 88:722, 1985

105. Yock PG, Naasz C, Schnittger I et al: Doppler tricuspid and pulmonic regur-

gitation in normals: is it real? abstracted. Circulation 70 (suppl. II):II-40, 1984

106. Skjaerpe T, Hatle L: Noninvasive estimation of pulmonary artery pressure by Doppler ultrasound in tricuspid regurgitation. p. 247. In Spencer MP (ed): Cardiac Doppler Diagnosis. Martinus Nijhoff Publishing, Boston, 1983

107. Currie PJ, Seward JB, Chan KL et al: Continuous wave Doppler: determination of right ventricular pressure: a simultaneous Doppler catheterization study in 127 patients. J Am Coll Cardiol 6:750, 1985

108. Himelman RB, Struve SN, Brown JK et al: Improved recognition of cor pulmonale in patients with severe chronic obstructive pulmonary disease. Am J Med 84:891, 1988

109. Chow LC, Dittrich HCX, Hoit BD et al: Doppler assessment of changes in right-sided cardiac hemodynamics after pulmonary thromboendarterectomy. Am J Cardiol 61:1092, 1988

110. Marchandise B, DeBruyne B, Delaunois I et al: Noninvasive prediction of pulmonary hypertension in chronic obstructive pulmonary disease by Doppler echocardiography. Chest 91:361, 1987

111. Janicki JS, Weber KT: The pericardium and ventricular interaction, distensibility and function. Am J Physiol 238:H494, 1980

112. Weyman AE, Wann S, Feigenbaum H, Dillon JC: Mechanism of abnormal septal motion in patients with right ventricular volume overload. Circulation 54:179, 1976

113. Popp RL, Wolfe SB, Hirata T, Feigenbaum H: Estimation of right and left ventricular size by ultrasound. A study of echos from the interventricular septum. Am J Cardiol 24:523, 1969

114. Diamond MA, Dillon JC, Haine CL et al: Echocardiographic features of atrial septal defect. Circulation 43:129, 1971

115. Klinger JR, Hill NS: Right ventricular dysfunction in chronic obstructive pulmonary disease. Chest 99:715, 1991

116. Matthay RA, Berger HJ, Davies RA et al: Right and left ventricular exercise performance in chronic obstructive pulmonary disease: radionuclide assessment. Ann Intern Med 93:234, 1980

117. Biernacki W, Flenley DC, Muir AL, MacNee W: Pulmonary hypertension and right ventricular function in patients with COPD. Chest 94:1169, 1988

118. Matthay RA, Berger HJ: Cardiovascular function in cor pulmonale. Clin Chest Med 4:269, 1983

119. Weitzenblum E, Sautegeau A, Ehrhart M et al: Long-term oxygen therapy can reverse the progression of pulmonary hypertension in patients with chronic obstructive pulmonary disease. Am Rev Respir Dis 131:493, 1985

120. Pattynama PMT, Willems LNA, Smit AH et al: Early diagnosis of cor pulmonale with MR imaging of the right ventricle. Radiology 182:375, 1992

121. Turnbull LW, Ridgway JP, Biernacki W et al: Assessment of the right ventricle by magnetic resonance imaging in chronic obstructive lung disease. Thorax 147, 371, 1990

122. Cooper N, Brazier J, Buckley G: Effects of systemic-pulmonary shunts on regional blood flow in experimental pulmonary stenosis. J Thorac Cardiovasc Surg 70:166, 1975

123. Fixler DE, Archie JP, Ulloyot DJ et al: Effects of acute right ventricular systolic hypertension on regional myocardial blood flow in anesthetized dogs. Am Heart J 85:491, 1973

124. Vlahakes GJ, Turley K, Hoffman JIE: The pathophysiology of failure in acute right ventricular hypertension: hemodynamic and biochemical correlations. Circulation 63:87, 1981

125. Weidemann HP, Matthay RA: The management of acute and chronic cor pulmonale. p. 656. In Scharf SM, Cassidy SS (eds): Heart-Lung Interactions in Health and Disease. Marcel Dekker, New York, 1989

126. Calvin JE, Ascah KJ: Impact of leftward septal shift and potential role of ischemia in its production during experimental right ventricular pressure overload. J Crit Care 7:106, 1992

127. Ghignone M, Girling L, Prewitt RM: Volume expansion versus norepinephrine in treatment of a low cardiac output complicating an acute increase in right ventricular afterload in dogs. Anesthesiology 60:132, 1984

128. Molloy WD, Lee KY, Girling L et al: Treatment of shock in a canine model of pulmonary embolism. Am Rev Respir Dis 130:870, 1984

129. Urokinase-streptokinase pulmonary embolism trial: phase II results. JAMA 229:1606, 1974

130. Meywerwitz MF, Galdhaber SZ, Reagan K et al: Recombinant tissue-type plasminogen activator versus urokinase in peripheral and graft occlusions: a randomized trial. Radiology 175:75, 1990

131. Brenner O: Pathology of the vessels of the pulmonary circulation. Arch Intern Med 56:211, 1935

132. Laks MM, Morady F, Swan HJC: Canine right and left ventricular sarcomere lengths after banding of the pulmonary artery. Circ Res 24:705, 1969

133. Wyse RKH, Jones M, Welhan KC, deLeval MR: Cardiac performance and myocardial blood flow in pigs with compensated right ventricular hypertrophy. Cardiovasc Res 18:733, 1985

134. Kawakami Y, Kishi Y, Yammamoto H, Miyamoto K: Relations of oxygen delivery, mixed venous oxygenation and pulmonary hemodynamics to prognosis in chronic obstructive pulmonary disease. N Engl J Med 308:1045, 1983

135. Weitzenblum E, Sautegeau A, Ehrhart M et al: Long-term course of pulmonary arterial pressure in chronic obstructive pulmonary disease. Am Rev Respir Dis 130:993, 1984

136. Boushy SF, North LB: Hemodynamic changes in chronic obstructive pulmonary disease. Chest 72:565, 1977

137. Mahler DA, Brent BN, Loke J et al: Right ventricular performance and central circulatory hemodynamics during upright exercise in patients with chronic obstructive pulmonary disease. Am Rev Respir Dis 130:722, 1984

138. Schrijen F, Uffholtz H, Olee JM, Poincelot F: Pulmonary and systemic hemodynamic evolution in chronic bronchitis. Am Rev Respir Dis 117:25, 1978

139. Burrows B, Kettel LJ, Niden AH, Rabinowitz M, Diener CF: Patterns of cardiovascular dysfunction in chronic obstructive lung disease. N Engl J Med 286:912, 1972

140. Weitzenblum E, Loiseau A, Hirth C et al: Course of pulmonary hemodynamics in patients with chronic obstructive pulmonary disease. Chest 75:656, 1979

141. Stein PD, Sabbah HN, Anbe DT, Marzilli M: Performance of the failing and nonfailing right ventricle of patients with pulmonary hypertension. Am J Cardiol 44:1050, 1979

142. Bove AA, Santamore WP: Ventricular interdependence. Prog Cardiovasc Dis 23:365, 1981

143. Krayenbuehl HP, Turina J, Hess O: Left ventricular function in chronic pulmonary hypertension. Am J Cardiol 41:1150, 1978

144. Rao BS, Cohn KE, Eldridge FL, Hancock HW: Left ventricular failure secondary chronic pulmonary disease. Am J Med 45:229, 1968

145. Hooper RG, Whitecomb ME: Systolic time intervals in chronic obstructive pulmonary disease. Circulation 50:1205, 1974

146. Chipps BE, Alderson PO, Roland JA et al: Noninvasive evaluation of left ventricular function in chronic obstructive pulmonary disease. J Pediatr 95:379, 1979

147. Jardin F, Gueret P, Prost J-F: Two-dimensional echocardiographic assessment of left ventricular function in chronic obstructive pulmonary disease. Am Rev Respir Dis 129:135, 1984

148. Caldwell EN: The left ventricle in chronic obstructive lung diseases. p. 247. In Rubin LJ (ed): Pulmonary Heart Disease. Martinus Nijhoff Publishing, The Hague, 1984

149. Fishman AP: The left ventricle in chronic bronchitis and emphysema (editorial). N Engl J Med 285:402, 1971

150. Kachel RG: Left ventricular function in chronic obstructive pulmonary disease. Chest 74:266, 1978

151. Weisse AB: Contralateral effects of cardiac disease affecting either the left or right changers of the heart. Am Heart J 87:654, 1974

152. Kohama A, Tanouchi J, Hori M et al: Pathologic involvement of the left ventricular in chronic cor pulmonale. Chest 98:794, 1990

153. Jardin F, Farcot JC, Boisante L et al: Mechanism of paradoxic pulse in bronchial asthma. Circulation 66:887, 1982

154. Gomez A, Mink S: Increased left ventricular stiffness impairs filling in dogs with pulmonary emphysema in respiratory failure. J Clin Invest 78:228, 1986

155. Guz A: Regulation of respiration in man. Annu Rev Physiol 37:303, 1975

156. Viar WN, Harrison TR: Chest pain in association with pulmonary hypertension. Circulation 5:1, 1953

157. Ross RS: Right ventricular hypertension as a cause of precordial pain. Am Heart J 61:134, 1961

158. Zimmerman D, Parker BM: The pain of pulmonary hypertension. Fact or fancy? JAMA 246:2345, 1981

159. Fanta CH, Wright TC, McFadden ER: Differentiation of recurrent pulmonary emboli from chronic obstructive pulmonary disease as a cause of cor pulmonale. Chest 79:92, 1981

160. Rubin LJ: Clinical evaluation. p. 113. In Rubin LJ (ed): Pulmonary Heart Disease. Martinus Nijhoff Publishing, Boston, 1984

161. Reihman DH, Farber MO, Weinberger MH et al: Effect of hypoxemia on sodium and water excretion in chronic obstructive lung disease. Am J Med 78:87, 1985

162. Campbell EJM, Short DS: The cause of edema in 'cor pulmonale.' Lancet 1:1184, 1960

163. Degaute JP, Domenighetti G, Naeije R et al: Oxygen delivery in acute exacerbation of chronic obstructive pulmonary disease. Am Rev Respir Dis 124:26, 1981

164. MacNee W, Wathen CG, Flenley DC, Muir AD: The effects of controlled oxygen therapy on ventricular function in patients with stable and decompensated cor pulmonale. Am Rev Respir Dis 137:1289, 1988

165. Stuart-Harris C, Flenley DC, Bishop JH: British Medical Research Council Working Party: Long-term domiciliary oxygen therapy in chronic hypoxic cor pulmonale complicating bronchitis and emphysema. Lancet 1:681, 1981

166. Cooper CB, Howard P: An analysis of sequential physiologic changes in hypoxic cor pulmonale during long-term oxygen therapy. Chest 100:76, 1991

167. Wilkinson M, Langhorne CA, Heath D et al: A pathologic study of 10 cases of hypoxic cor pulmonale. Q J Med 66:65, 1988

168. Weitzenblum E, Hirth C, Ducolone A et al: Prognostic value of pulmonary artery pressure in chronic obstructive pulmonary disease. Thorax 36:752, 1981

169. Anthonisen NR: Long-term oxygen therapy. Ann Intern Med 99:519, 1983

170. Continuous nocturnal oxygen therapy in hypoxemic chronic obstructive pulmonary disease. Nocturnal oxygen therapy trial. Ann Intern Med 93:391, 1980

171. Timms RM, Khaja FU, Williams GW, the Nocturnal Oxygen Therapy Trial Group: hemodynamic response to oxygen therapy in chronic obstructive pulmonary disease. Ann Intern Med 102:29, 1985

172. MacNee W: Predictors of survival in patients treated with long-term oxygen therapy. Respiration 59 (suppl. 2):5, 1992

173. Ashutosh K, Mead G, Dunsky M: Early effects of oxygen administration and prognosis in chronic obstructive pulmonary disease and cor pulmonale. Am Rev Respir Dis 127:399, 1983

174. Olvey SK, Reduto LA, Stevens PM et al: First-pass radionuclide assessment of right and left ventricular ejection fraction in chronic obstructive pulmonary disease: effect of oxygen upon exercise response. Chest 78:4, 1980

175. Further recommendations for presenting and supplying long-term oxygen therapy. Conference report. Am Rev Respir Dis 138:745, 1988

176. Rich S, Brundage BH: High dose cal-

cium channel blocking therapy for primary pulmonary hypertension: evidence for long term reduction in pulmonary artery pressure and regression of right ventricular hypertrophy. Circulation 76:135, 1987

177. Weir EK, Rubin LJ, Hyers JM: The acute administration of vasodilators in primary pulmonary hypertension. Am Rev Respir Dis 140:1623, 1989

178. Packer M: Is it ethical to administer vasodilator drugs to patients with primary pulmonary hypertension? Chest 95:1173, 1989

179. Dantzker DR, D'Alonzo GE, Gianotti L et al: Vasodilators and primary pulmonary hypertension: variability of long-term response. Chest 95:1185, 1989

180. Matthay RA, Berger HJ, Davies R et al: Improvement in cardiac performance by oral long-acting theophyllin in chronic obstructive pulmonary disease. Am Heart J 104:1022, 1982

181. Matthay RA: Favorable cardiovascular effects of theophylline in COPD. Chest 92:22S, 1987

182. Winter RJD, Langford JA, George RJD et al: The effects of theophylline and salbutamol on right and left ventricular function in chronic bronchitis and emphysema. Br J Dis Chest 78:358, 1984

183. Whyte KF, Flenley DC: Can pulmonary vasodilators improve survival in cor pulmonale due to hypoxic chronic bronchitis and emphysema? Thorax. 43:1, 1988

184. MacNee W, Wathen CG, Hannan WJ et al: Effects of pirbuterol and sodium nitroprusside on pulmonary haemodynamics in hypoxic cor pulmonale. Br Med J 287:1169, 1983

185. Brown SE, Linden GS, King RR et al: Effects of verapamil on pulmonary haemodynamics during hypoxia, at rest, and during exercise in patients with chronic obstructive pulmonary disease. Thorax 38:840, 1983

186. Clozel JP, Delorme N, Battistella P et al: Hemodynamic effects of intravenous diltiazem in hypoxic pulmonary hypertension secondary to chronic obstructive lung disease. Cardiology 74:196, 1987

187. Saadjian AY, Philip-Joet FF, Arnaud AG: Hemodynamic and oxygen delivery responses to nifedipine in pulmonary hypertension secondary to chronic obstructive lung disease. Cardiology 74:196, 1987

188. Rubin LJ, Moser K: Long-term effects of nitrendipine on hemodynamics and oxygen transport in patients with cor pulmonale. Chest 89:141, 1986

189. Agostoni P, Doria E, Galli C et al: Nifedipine reduces pulmonary pressure and vascular tone during short but not long-term treatment of pulmonary hypertension in patients with chronic obstructive pulmonary disease. Am Rev Respir Dis 139:120, 1989

190. Saadjian AY, Philip-Joet FF, Vestri R, Arnoud AG: Long-term treatment of chronic obstructive lung disease by nifedipine: an eighteen-month hemodynamic study. Eur Respir J 1:716, 1988

191. Keller CA, Shepard JW, Chun DS et al: Effects of hydralazine on hemodynamics, ventilation, and gas exchange in patients with chronic obstructive pulmonary disease and pulmonary hypertension. Am Rev Respir Dis 130:606, 1984

192. Lupi-Herrera E, Seoane M, Verdejo J et al: Hemodynamic effect of hydralazine in interstitial lung disease patients with cor pulmonale. Chest 87:564, 1985

193. Miller MJ, Chappell TR, Cook W et al: Effects of oral hydralazine on gas exchange in patients with cor pulmonale. Am J Med 75:937, 1983

194. Morely TF, Zappasodi SJ, Belli A, Giudice JC: Pulmonary vasodilator therapy for chronic obstructive pulmonary disease and cor pulmonale. Chest 92:71, 1987

195. Vik-Mo H, Walde N, Jentoft H, Halvosen FJ: Improved haemodynamics but reduced arterial blood oxygenation at rest and during exercise after long-term oral prazosin therapy in chronic cor pulmonale. Eur Heart J 6:1047, 1985

196. Adnot S, Andrivet P, Brun-Buisson C et al: The effects of urapidil therapy on hemodynamics and gas exchange in exercising patients with chronic obstruc-

tive pulmonary disease and pulmonary hypertension. Am Rev Respir Dis 137:1068, 1988

197. Zielinski J, Hawrylkiewicz I, Gorecka D et al: Captopril effects on pulmonary and systemic hemodynamics in chronic cor pulmonale. Chest 90:562, 1986

198. Burke CM, Harte M, Duncan J et al: Captopril and domiciliary oxygen in chronic airflow obstruction. Br Med J 290:1251, 1985

199. Peier RH, Rubin LJ: The pharmacologic control of the pulmonary circulation in pulmonary hypertension. Adv Intern Med 29:495, 1984

200. Packer M: Vasodilator therapy for primary pulmonary hypertension: limitations and hazards. Ann Intern Med 103:258, 1985

201. McGoon MD, Vlietstra RE: Vasodilator therapy for primary pulmonary hypertension. Mayo Clin Proc 59:672, 1984

202. Rubin LJ, Peter RH: Oral hydralazine therapy for primary pulmonary hypertension. N Engl J Med 302:69, 1980

203. Lupi-Herrera E, Sandoval J, Seoane M et al: The role of hydralazine therapy for pulmonary arterial hypertension of unknown cause. Circulation 65:645, 1982

204. Fisher J, Borer JS, Moses et al: Hemodynamic effects of nifedipine versus hydralazine in primary pulmonary hypertension. Am J Cardiol 54:646, 1984

205. Groves BM, Rubin LJ, Fiosolono ME et al: Comparison of the acute hemodynamic effects of prostacyclin and hydralazine in primary pulmonary hypertension. Am Heart J 110:1200, 1985

206. Brown SE, Pakron FJ, Milnen N et al: Effects of digoxin on exercise capacity and right ventricular function during exercise in chronic airflow obstruction. Chest 85:187, 1984

207. Mathur PN, Prowles ACP, Pugstey SO: Effect of digoxin on right ventricular function in severe chronic airflow obstruction. Ann Intern Med 95:2843, 1981

208. Green LH, Smith TW: The use of digitalis in patients with pulmonary disease. Ann Intern Med 87:459, 1977

209. Torino GM, Edelman NH, Senior RM et al: Extravascular lung water in cor pulmonale. Aspen Emphysema Conf 11:139, 1968

210. Pare PD, Brooks LA, Baile EM: Effect of systemic venous hypertension on pulmonary function and lung water. J Appl Physiol 51:592, 1981

211. Chetty KG, Brown SE, Light RW: Improved exercise tolerance of the polycythemic lung patient following phlebotomy. Am J Med 74:415, 1983

212. Reitz BA, Wallwork JL, Hunt SA et al: Heart-lung transplantation: successful therapy for patients with pulmonary vascular disease. N Engl J Med 306:557, 1982

213. Bolman RM, Shumway SJ, Estrin JA, Hertz MI: Lung and heart-lung transplantation. Evolution and new applications. Ann Surg 214:456, 1991

214. Pasque MK, Trulock EP, Kaiser LR, Cooper JD: Single lung transplantation for pulmonary hypertension. Three month hemodynamic follow-up. Circulation 84:2275, 1991

215. Hutter JA, Despins P, Higenbottom T, Stewart S, Wallwork J: Heart-lung transplantation: Better use of resources. Am J Med 85:4, 1988

216. McCarthy PM, Staines VA, Theordore J et al: Improved survival after heart-lung transplantation. J Cardiovasc Surg 99:54, 1990

217. Calhoun JH, Grover FL, Biggons WJ et al: Single-lung transplantation: alternative indications and techniques. J Thorac Cardiovasc Surg 101:816, 1991

218. Harris P, Heath D: The Human Pulmonary Circulation. p. 353. Churchill Livingstone, London, 1977

219. Lupi-Herrera E, Sandoval J, Seoane M, Bialostozky D: Behavior of the pulmonary circulation in chronic obstructive pulmonary disease. Am Rev Respir Dis 126:509, 1982

3

Neurologic Disease*

Joseph K. Perloff

The interplay between cardiac disease and neurologic disease is varied and complex.[1–3] Heredofamilial neuromuscular disorders are commonly accompanied by cardiac involvement, and diseases of the heart and circulation can express themselves as cerebral disorders. The central concerns of this chapter are the major heredofamilial neuromuscular diseases accompanied by heart disease as well as the cerebral disorders—acquired and congenital—associated with cardiovascular abnormalities.

Involvement of the heart is an inherent feature of three major groups of heredofamilial neuromyopathic diseases[1–3]: the progressive muscular dystrophies, the myotonic muscular dystrophies, and Friedreich's ataxia. The major nonmyotonic progressive muscular dystrophies include classic, early-onset, rapidly progressive Duchenne's dystrophy,[1,3,4–8] late-onset, slowly progressive Becker's muscular dystrophy,[1,3,9–11] facioscapulohumeral muscular dystrophy,[1,3,12] and limb-girdle dystrophy.[1,3,13]

EARLY-ONSET, RAPIDLY PROGRESSIVE X-LINKED DUCHENNE'S MUSCULAR DYSTROPHY

Duchenne's muscular dystrophy is an X-linked recessive neuromuscular disorder that involves striated muscle fibers (skeletal, cardiac), specialized cardiac tissues, smooth muscle fibers (vasculature, including intramural coronary arteries), and nervous system (neurons of central brain and cortex) (Fig. 3-1).[14–20] The Duchenne's dystrophy gene has been identified on the Xp21 locus of the short arm of the X chromosome.[14,18] Dystrophin, the protein product of the gene, is normally present on and limited to myogenic cells in every tissue tested except the central nervous system, and is absent or nearly so in Duchenne's dystrophy.[14–20] Because Duchenne's dystrophy is sex-linked, the disorder is transmitted by the mother to one-half of her sons as overt disease and to one-half of her daughters as a carrier state.[1,3] Approximately one-third of cases represent new mutations in either the patient or his mother. The incidence of Duchenne's dystrophy in the general popu-

* Portions of this chapter adapted from Perloff,[1] with permission.

53

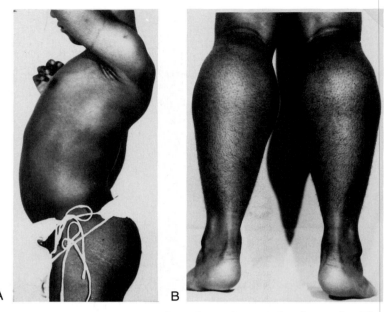

Fig. 3-1. (A & B) Boy with classic X-linked Duchenne's muscular dystrophy. There is lumbar lordosis (**A**) and striking calf "pseudohypertrophy" (**B**). The patient stands with heels elevated because of shortening of the Achilles tendons. (From Perloff,[1] with permission.)

lation is estimated at 1/3,000 to 1/5,000 male births, making it the commonest lethal X-linked neuromuscular disorder.[1,3]

Overt clinical manifestations typically begin in the second year of life, although there is histologic and enzymatic evidence that the disease exists from birth and therefore in utero. Patients are likely to succumb to pulmonary complications in the second decade, although cardiac disease is an important and sometimes dramatic cause of death.[1,2,21] Rapidly progressive preterminal heart failure, sometimes triggered by atrial flutter,[22,23] may follow years of circulatory stability during which the chief, if not only, indicator of cardiac involvement is an abnormal electrocardiogram.[4,5,7,8,24,25] The standard scalar electrocardiogram is the simplest and most reliable tool for detecting cardiac involvement in Duchenne's dystro-phy[4,5,7,8,24,25] (Fig. 3-2). Abnormal electrocardiograms are present even in early childhood and are typically represented by tall right precordial R waves and increased R/S amplitude ratios together with deep but narrow Q waves in leads 1, aVL, and $V_{5,6}$. There is convincing morphologic (gross, histologic, ultrastructural) (Figs. 3-3 and 3-4) and metabolic evidence (positron emission tomography) (Fig. 3-5) that myocardial involvement initially targets the posterobasal left ventricular wall (cardiac phenotype)[4,5,21,24] (Fig. 3-4). This regional localization of myocardial dystrophy is believed to account for the distinctive 12-lead electrocardiogram described above (Fig. 3-2). There is relative sparing of the ventricular septum and comparatively little involvement of right ventricular and atrial myocardium.

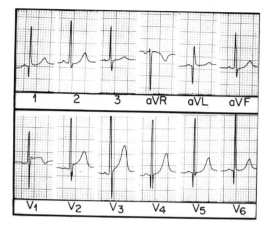

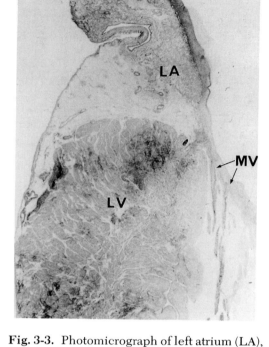

Fig. 3-2. Typical electrocardiogram from a 12-year-old boy with classic Duchenne's muscular dystrophy. Posterobasal myocardial dystrophy (scarring) with lateral extension (documented at necropsy) was believed to account for the anterior shift of the QRS—tall R wave in lead V_1—and the deep Q waves in leads 1, aVL, and $V_{5,6}$. The PR interval is 0.12 s. (From Perloff,[22] with permission.)

Fig. 3-3. Photomicrograph of left atrium (LA), mitral valve (MV), and infra-atrial (posterobasal) wall of the left ventricle (LV) showing extensive fibrosis of the posterobasal left ventricle with foci of myocardial fibers. Verhoeff van Gieson elastic tissue stains, original magnification ×4. (From Perloff et al.,[4] with permission.)

In addition, abnormalities of cardiac rhythm (Table 3-1) and conduction (Table 3-2) have been reported in Duchenne's muscular dystrophy, but the pathogenesis of the electrophysiologic disturbances remains to be estab-

Table 3-1. Abnormalities in Rhythm

Sinus node
    Sinus tachycardia
        Labile (gradual or abrupt)
        Persistent
    Sinus arrhythmia—marked
    Shifting atrial pacemaker
Atrial ectopic rhythms
    Flutter
    Fibrillation
    Supraventricular tachycardia
    Junctional
Ventricular ectopic rhythms
    Premature ventricular beats—uniform,
        multiform, single, couplets
    Nonsustained ventricular tachycardia

Table 3-2. Abnormalities in Conduction

Prolonged intra-atrial conduction (AV conduction)
    Accelerated (short PR interval)
    Prolonged (long PR interval)
Infranodal
    Right ventricular conduction delay
    Right bundle branch block
    Left anterior fascicular block
    Left posterior fascicular block
    Complete heart block

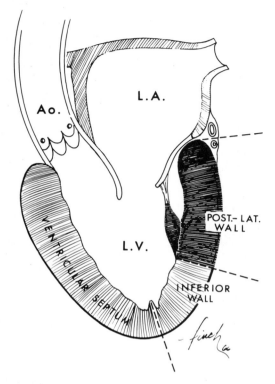

Fig. 3-4. Schematic illustration of the typical localization of myocardial dystrophy in classic X-linked Duchenne's muscular dystrophy. Ao, aorta; LA, left atrium, LV, left ventricle. (From Perloff,[5] with permission.)

lished.[22,23] Two variables are relevant to cardiac electrophysiologic involvement—the small vessel coronary arteriopathy (medial hypertrophy, luminal narrowing) and abnormalities that might originate in the specialized cardiac tissues.[23] The role of coronary arteriopathy is speculative, and it is not currently known whether dystrophin is normally present on the cell membrane of normal cardiac specialized tissues and, if so, whether these tissues are dystrophin deficient in Duchenne's dystrophy.[23] Because of the abnormality of plasma cell membrane of skeletal muscle, enzymes are copiously released into the plasma in Duchenne's dystrophy, and calcium enters the cell.[14,16,19] The determinants of

calcium homeostasis in dystrophin-deficient myogenic cells (skeletal or cardiac) is unclear, and the relationships among dystrophin deficiency, calcium homeostasis, cellular response, and phenotypic expression in skeletal muscle and myocardium are imperfectly understood.[23]

Rhythm Abnormalities

The most common rhythm disturbance (Table 3-1) is inappropriate sinus tachycardia (rate acceleration without discernible cause).[22,23] The sinus tachycardia is represented by persistent sinus acceleration or labile sinus tachycardia, the latter

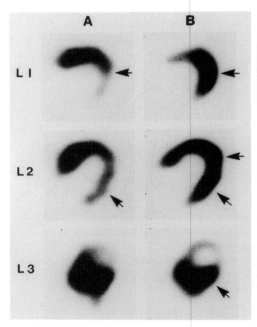

Fig. 3-5. Regional myocardial $^{13}NH_3$ **(A)** and ^{18}F 2-fluoro-2-deoxyglucose (FDG) uptake **(B)** visualized in three contiguous positron-CT images of the left ventricular myocardium in a patient with classic Duchenne's muscular dystrophy. There is a segmental decrease in ^{13}N activity in the posterolateral wall (*arrows*) with a discordant increase in FDG concentrations in the same segment (*arrows*). (From Perloff et al.,[5] with permission.)

so designated when a relatively sudden acceleration in cardiac rate occurs without a change in P-wave morphology, and is unprovoked by a definable circumstantial cause.[22,23,26] The most important disturbance in atrial rhythm is atrial flutter, a rare tachyarrhythmia in children, but a relatively common preterminal tachyarrhythmia in Duchenne's muscular dystrophy.[4,21,23] Ventricular ectopic rhythms take the form of premature ventricular beats, couplets, and nonsustained ventricular tachycardia.[22,23] The incidence of ventricular electrical instability appears to be greater than normal, especially in older patients with depressed left ventricular function. Put differently, the clinical substrate for an increased incidence of ventricular ectopic rhythms is apparently disease duration and depressed left ventricular performance.[23] Late potentials recorded by signal-averaged electrocardiograms in patients with Duchenne's muscular dystrophy were found to be closely coupled to left ventricular wall motion abnormalities and left ventricular dysfunction in older patients.[27] However, the significance of late potentials in Duchenne's dystrophy remains unclear. A correlation with malignant ventricular tachycardia or sudden death has not been established.

A word of caution is in order regarding pharmacologic management of disturbances in rhythm in Duchenne's muscular dystrophy.[1,28] Certain antiarrhythmic drugs have undesirable neuromuscular effects. Procainamide and phenytoin may reinforce muscular weakness in Duchenne's muscular dystrophy, and intravenous verapamil has resulted in fatal respiratory arrest.[28]

Conduction Abnormalities

Abnormalities of conduction (Table 3-2) are clinically less important than disturbances in rhythm and include prolonged intra-atrial conduction and short PR intervals early in the natural history, indicating accelerated atrioventricular conduction, but increased PR intervals in the late stages of the disease.[22,23] Infranodal conduction defects are manifested by minor right ventricular conduction delay, left posterior fascicular block, left anterior fascicular block, right bundle branch block, and exceptionally bifascicular block.[22,23]

Treatment

Prednisone administration in Duchenne's muscular dystrophy is reportedly accompanied by significant improvement in muscle strength, pulmonary function, and urinary creatinine excretion, the latter suggesting an increase in muscle mass accompanying the increase in muscle strength.[29] However, important aspects of the disease remained unchanged. Patients in wheelchairs were still unable to walk after treatment with prednisone, and changes in serum creatinine kinase concentrations were minimal calling into question a salutary effect on plasma cell membrane.[29] Relevant to this chapter is the lack of data regarding the effect (if any) of prednisone on cardiac involvement in Duchenne's dystrophy, either myocardial or in specialized tissues. Potential side effects of prednisone remain a major barrier to its widespread use in the treatment of Duchenne's muscular dystrophy.

LATE-ONSET, SLOWLY PROGRESSIVE X-LINKED BECKER'S MUSCULAR DYSTROPHY

Becker's muscular dystrophy is later in onset and slower in progression than Duchenne's dystrophy, with most patients remaining ambulant into adulthood.[1,3] Because the diagnosis of Becker's dystrophy was less than secure before the advent of dystrophin assays,[17,30] reports of the incidence and type of associated heart disease are open to question. Becker's dystrophy can now be confidently distinguished from Duchenne's dystrophy by dystrophin assays of skeletal muscle biopsies.[17,30] The protein product of the gene is present but is abnormal in molecular weight, contrary to Duchenne's dystrophy, in which the protein product is absent or nearly so but is of normal molecular weight.[17,30] The Becker's and Duchenne's muscular dystrophy genes are in close proximity on the short arm of the X chromosome. There is evidence that the frequency of cardiac involvement in the former disorder increases after adolescence. Adults with Becker's dystrophy not only have cardiomyopathy but may die of it[1,2,9–11] (Fig. 3-6). Cardiac involvement expresses itself differently from that of Duchenne's dystrophy. All four chambers are in-

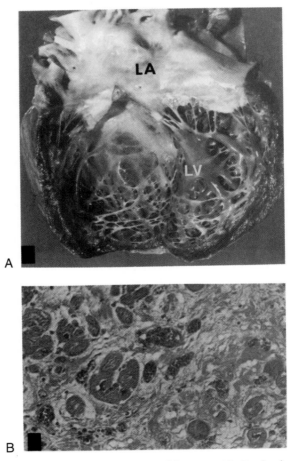

Fig. 3-6. (A) Necropsy specimen from a 40-year-old man with Becker's muscular dystrophy. The left ventricle (LV) is dilated. LA, left atrium. **(B)** Histologic section of LV showing extensive connective tissue replacement of myocardium. (From Perloff,[2] with permission.)

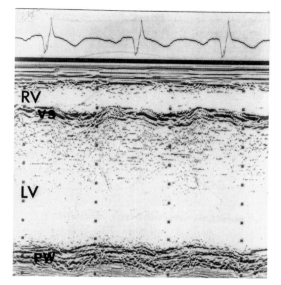

volved, with dilatation and failure of the ventricles (Fig. 3-7), in addition to abnormalities of the His-bundle and of infranodal conduction that express themselves as fascicular block and complete heart block.

Fig. 3-7. M-mode echocardiogram from a 28-year-old man with Becker's muscular dystrophy. The left ventricle (LV) is markedly dilated and hypokinetic. RV, right ventricle; VS, ventricular septum; PW, posterior wall.

FACIOSCAPULOHUMERAL MUSCULAR DYSTROPHY

Facioscapulohumeral dystrophy is an autosomal dominant disorder with strong penetrance and an incidence estimated at 3 to 10 cases/million.[1,3,12] The disease typically becomes overt in late childhood or adolescence, is slowly progressive but variable in expression even within a single family, and is characterized in part by facial (facio) and shoulder/arm (scapulohumeral) weakness and atrophy (Fig. 3-8). Infrequently, the disease expresses

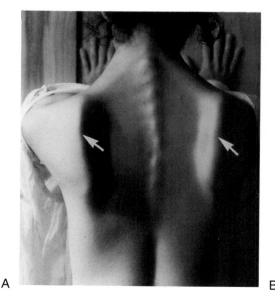
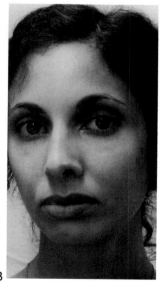

A   B

Fig. 3-8. Patient with facioscapulohumeral muscular dystrophy. **(A)** Winging of the scapulae. **(B)** Myopathic facies with dimpling at corners of the mouth. (From Stevenson et al.,[12] with permission.)

itself in infancy and runs a rapid course that leads to death in adolescence. Asymptomatic or minimally affected parents may have severely affected offspring with the infantile form of the disease.[31] Facial weakness in the adult form may be signaled initially by no more than an inability to whistle or drink through a straw. More distinctive and troublesome is the inability to close the eyes, even during sleep. The face becomes smooth and the forehead unlined, loss of the normal upward curvature of the lower lip creates a pouting appearance, and the only marks on an otherwise expressionless face are the dimples on either side of the angles of the mouth (enigmatic smile)[1,3] (Fig. 3-8B). Muscles of the arms and shoulders become weak and atrophic, and typical winging of the scapulae develops (Fig. 3-8A).

Permanent atrial paralysis, a unique electrophysiologic abnormality, has been reported in a small number of patients believed to have facioscapulohumeral muscular dystrophy.[32–34] Criteria for the diagnosis of atrial paralysis include absence of P waves on scalar, esophageal, and intracardiac electrocardiograms; lack of response to direct (intracardiac) electrical or mechanical stimuli to the atria; absence of A waves in the jugular venous and right atrial pressure pulses; a supraventricular QRS; and immobility of the atria on two-dimensional echocardiography or fluoroscopy.[12,35]

Although the presence of atrial standstill was convincingly established in the above reports, the diagnoses of facioscapulohumeral muscular dystrophy are open to question. Those patients are now believed to have had a phenotypically similar but genetically different disorder—Emery-Dreifuss muscular dystrophy, an X-linked disorder.[36–39] Permanent atrial paralysis, ectopic atrial rhythms, atrial fibrillation, and abnormalities of infranodal conduction have been firmly linked to Emery-Dreifuss dystrophy, but not to facioscapulohumeral muscular dystrophy.[12]

The electrophysiologic abnormalities in facioscapulohumeral dystrophy are represented by a high susceptibility to inducible atrial arrhythmias (atrial fibrillation or atrial flutter) and sinus node dysfunction in patients with no clinically overt cardiac disorders, apart from occasional and often subtle evidence in the surface electrocardiogram.[12] P-wave abnormalities are relatively common on the surface electrocardiogram and are unrelated to atrial size on echocardiography. Broad bifid P waves or prolonged P-terminal components in lead V_1 (left atrial) or increased amplitude of the initial component of the P wave in lead II (right atrial) imply abnormalities of intra-atrial conduction. Electrophysiologic abnormalities outside of the atria are less common. Evidence for atrioventricular node or infranodal conduction disturbances are represented by PR interval prolongation, complete right bundle branch block, prolonged right bundle branch refractory period during atrial pacing, and (rarely) left anterior fascicular block or left posterior fascicular block. Each of these AV nodal or infranodal abnormalities is relatively infrequent, if not sporadic. Electrocardiographic evidence of alterations in infranodal and AV nodal conduction, together with the high incidence of induced atrial fibrillation or flutter during electrophysiologic study, supports the hypothesis that cardiac involvement in facioscapulohumeral muscular dystrophy may represent an analogous but relatively benign form of the cardiac involvement found in Emery-Dreifuss dystrophy and its genetic variants.[12] Why the genetic markers in this group of systemic neuromuscular diseases target specific cardiac electrophysiologic properties is unknown.

ERB'S LIMB-GIRDLE DYSTROPHY

Neuromuscular disorders designated as Erb's limb-girdle dystrophy are heterogeneous and represent perhaps the most poorly defined group within the major muscular dystrophies.[1,3] Within this category, there is variation in the mode of inheritance, age of onset, and progression of illness, as well as in the distribution of muscle weakness. What may be a dominant theme is onset in late childhood or adolescence of difficulty in walking, involvement chiefly of the pelvic girdle with less involvement of upper limbs and shoulder girdle, and sparing of the face.[3] Calf pseudohypertrophy occurs but is relatively late in onset and usually mild to moderate in degree. Because limb-girdle dystrophy has been poorly defined, conclusions regarding the type and prevalence of co-existing heart disease cannot be drawn with confidence.[13] It is likely that a number of patients diagnosed as having limb-girdle dystrophy with calf pseudohypertrophy represent examples of Becker's muscular dystrophy (see earlier).

MYOTONIC MUSCULAR DYSTROPHY (STEINERT'S DISEASE

Myotonic muscular dystrophy is a multisystem disorder inherited as an autosomal dominant (locus on chromosome 19) with an estimated incidence of 13/100,000, making it a relatively common neuromuscular disease.[3,40,41] The phenotype of the adult with myotonic dystrophy is characteristic[1,3] (Fig. 3-9A). A consistent and early feature is weakness of the flexor muscles of the neck with atrophy of the sternocleidomastoid muscles that often progresses to virtual disappearance. Myotonia (delayed relaxation after contraction) is provoked by voluntary, mechanical, or electrical stimulation of

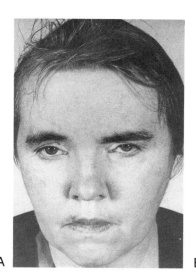 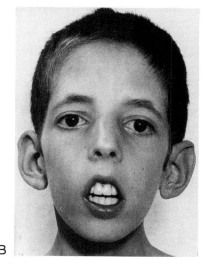

A   B

Fig. 3-9. (A) Expressionless facies of a 50-year-old woman with myotonic muscular dystrophy. There is thinning and graying of hair. The patient had cataracts. (B) Facial appearance of the infantile form of congenital myotonic distrophy. Note the "cupid's bow" upper lip. (From Perloff,[108] with permission.)

muscles of the hands, forearms, tongue, and jaw.[3] The electromyogram is characteristic. A myotonic response is best elicited by tapping the thenar eminence with a percussion hammer (percussion myotonia), especially after patients rapidly open and close their fists. Myotonic dystrophy is a systemic disease with important nonmyotonic/nonmyopathic features, including disorders of smooth muscle (esophagus, colon, uterus), central nervous system (mental retardation, mental deterioration), endocrine system (testicular tubular atrophy), eyes (cataract, retinal degeneration), and skin (premature balding).[3]

Cardiac involvement, which is often the major extraskeletal muscle expression of myotonic dystrophy, manifests chiefly by abnormalities of specialized tissues, less frequently of myocardium.[42–51] Involvement is relatively specific, primarily assigned to the His-Purkinje system. The most frequent histopathologic lesions are fibrosis, fatty infiltration, and atrophy of the sinus node, atrioventricular node, His bundle, and bundle branches.[46,48] The most common electrocardiographic abnormalities—prolongation of the PR interval, left anterior fascicular block (Fig. 3-10)—reflect His-Purkinje disease that can progress rapidly, although neither the scalar electrocardiogram nor a single HV internal predicts the rate of progression.[42,51] The His-Purkinje involvement can culminate in fatal Stokes-Adams episodes unless anticipated and treated by placement of a pacemaker. Sudden death caused by atrioventricular block is relatively rare, but remains the gravest cardiac threat to patients with myotonic dystrophy.[42,51] Ventricular tachycardia has also been held responsible for sudden death.[47,50]

The myocardium is seldom involved extensively enough to cause clinically overt signs or symptoms.[42,43] Involve-

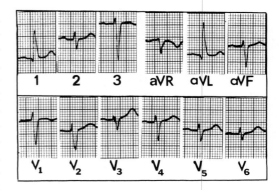

Fig. 3-10. Typical electrocardiogram from a patient with myotonic muscular dystrophy. The PR interval is 0.20 s, and there is left anterior fascicular block.

ment of cardiac muscle is not selective, appearing with approximately equal distribution in all four chambers. Fewer than 10 percent of patients have clinical evidence of heart failure. The electrocardiogram is a sensitive reflection of involvement of specialized cardiac tissues but not of the myocardium, although Q waves with normal coronary arteries indicate regional myocardial dystrophy.[42] Apart from abnormalities of the initial forces in the electrocardiogram, occult involvement of the myocardium can be assessed by radionuclide angiography during exercise.[42,43] In addition, myocardial dystrophy may be responsible for atrial and ventricle arrhythmias including premature atrial beats, atrial flutter, atrial fibrillation, premature ventricular beats, and ventricular tachycardia.[42,45,47,50]

Abnormal ventricular function has been ascribed chiefly if not exclusively to depressed contraction (systolic dysfunction). However, recent studies disclose that patients with myotonic dystrophy may have abnormally slow relaxation rates of the posterior left ventricular wall (myocardial myotonia) using a two-dimensionally targeted M-mode echocardiographic cursor, whereas fewer had evidence of abnormal left ventricular diastolic function by Doppler spectral recordings of mitral inflow profiles.[52] The presence of slow ventricular relaxation was unrelated to patient age or to the degree of skeletal muscle expression of myotonic dystrophy. Studies of hereditary myotonia in the goat have led to the hypothesis that myotonia results from a decreased conductance of chloride ions, and subsequent experimental studies support the conclusion that reduced chloride conductance is sufficient to cause the membrane instability necessary for myotonia.[40,53–58] It has also been postulated that a defect in calcium transport might be responsible for myotonia.[40]

Could either of these hypotheses apply to the myocardium and provide a potential substrate for impaired relaxation (myocardial myotonia)? The calcium hypothesis finds little support, at least in skeletal muscle, from observations in Duchenne's muscular dystrophy in which calcium copiously enters the cytosol without known impairment of relaxation.[23] Studies in isolated heart cells disclose that stimulation of β-adrenergic receptors activates adenylate cyclase, resulting in the production of cyclic adenosine monophosphate (cAMP) and subsequent protein kinase action, a pathway involved in the regulation of several ions including Ca^{++}, K^+, and Cl^-. Single Cl^- channels were observed in planar lipid bilayers into which cardiac sarcolemmal proteins had been incorporated, but the function of these channels is unknown. A Cl^- current has been demonstrated in cardiac myocytes and is regulated by β-adrenergic and muscarinic receptors. When activated, Cl^- current can modulate the duration of cardiac action potentials.

An important variation from the above pattern is seen in the offspring of mothers with myotonic dystrophy.[40,59] The disorder expresses itself in infants as hypoto-

nia and facial paralysis rather than myotonia, at least initially.[40] Respiratory distress is largely responsible for neonatal death from congenital myotonic dystrophy. Affected children have characteristic faces, with the upper lip forming a cupid's bow (Fig. 3-9B). Observations of cardiac involvement in congenital myotonic dystrophy are limited but tentatively indicate atrioventricular and interventricular conduction defects and less commonly reduced left ventricular systolic function.[40,59] Apart from genetic transmission from the mother (probably cytoplasmic inheritance), pregnancy is hazardous to the gravida with myotonic dystrophy.[40]

FRIEDREICH'S ATAXIA

The hereditary ataxias are divided into (1) the hereditary spinocerebellar ataxia of Friedreich, (2) hereditary ataxia with muscle atrophy (Roussy-Lévy syndrome), (3) hereditary spinocerebellar ataxia, and (4) olivopontocerebellar atrophy.[60,61] Despite a century of lively interest, there is still disagreement about where Friedreich's disease fits into the complex framework of the hereditary ataxias.[60,61] Disorders that are phenotypically similar to Friedreich's ataxia are seldom if ever associated with heart disease, but when strict neurologic and genetic criteria were used to identify what appeared to be a homogeneous group of patients with Friedreich's ataxia, cardiac involvement was found in more than 90 percent of the subjects; with longitudinal follow-up the incidence was 100 percent.[62–67] Friedreich's ataxia is a neurologic rather than myopathic disorder and is inherited as an autosomal recessive trait characterized by ataxia of the limbs and trunk, absence of tendon reflexes, extensor plantar responses, and loss of proprioceptive sensations in the limbs. Remissions are unknown, and ataxia of gait together with muscle weakness progress relentlessly, affecting first the lower limbs and then all four extremities. Pes cavus (Friedreich's foot) and kyphoscoliosis, often severe (Fig. 3-11A), develop within a few years of onset. Progressively severe ataxia occurs long before clinically overt heart disease, although occasionally the reverse is true. There is no apparent relationship between the degrees of neurologic and cardiac involvement.[62–67]

There is reason to believe that phenotypically identical Friedreich's patients are not biochemically homogeneous because the cardiac expressions differ.[62] The most common echocardiographic finding is concentric (symmetrical) left ventricular hypertrophy (Fig. 3-12), with asymmetrical septal thickening found less frequently.[62–67] Left ventricular outflow gradients have been reported in occasional patients with disproportionate septal thickness. Importantly, septal cellular disarray—the histologic hallmark of genetic hypertrophic cardiomyopathy—has been absent or only focal in necropsy studies of Friedreich's ataxia, an observation that may in part explain why the potentially malignant ventricular arrhythmias common in genetic hypertrophic cardiomyopathy are essentially unknown in Friedreich's ataxia.[62] In the hypertrophic cardiomyopathy of Friedreich's ataxia, systolic ventricular function is normal, not supernormal, and diastolic function is not deranged as in genetic hypertrophic cardiomyopathy.

A second and much less common type of cardiac involvement in Friedreich's ataxia takes the form of dilated cardiomyopathy (Fig. 3-11B and C) that may be initially expressed as global hypokinesis with normal left ventricular internal dimensions.[62–67] Patients with Friedreich's ataxia and dilated cardiomyopathy experience progressive cardiac deterioration

(poor prognosis), in contrast to the favorable prognosis of Friedreich's ataxia with hypertrophic cardiomyopathy. There is convincing evidence that the dilated form of cardiomyopathy in Friedreich's ataxia is distinct from the hypertrophic form (not a transition from one to the other) and, therefore, represents a fundamentally different type of cardiac disease that has been designated dystrophic.[62]

Initial force deformities on electrocardiograms are believed to represent areas of regional myocardial dystrophy that, if sufficiently widespread, might result in depressed systolic function. Atrial flutter or fibrillation and ventricular arrhythmias are features of the dilated cardiomyopathy of Friedreich's disease but not of the hypertrophic form. Accordingly, there appear to be two distinct types of cardiac involvement in Friedreich's ataxia: (1) hypertrophic cardiomyopathy represented by symmetrical (less commonly asymmetrical) left ventricular hypertrophy with normal cavity size, and normal systolic and diastolic function; and (2) relatively uncommon dilated cardiomyopathy represented by depressed systolic function with normal or increased ventricular cavity size. It is possible that the frequently observed initial force abnormalities on the scalar electrocardiogram represent regional "dystrophic" disease that anticipates dilated cardiomyopathy, but that contention remains to be proven.

Why a nonmyopathic spinocerebellar-corticospinal disorder is accompanied by two widely different types of cardiac disease is unknown. Phenotypically indistinguishable patients with Friedreich's ataxia appear to be genetically different, at least in terms of cardiac expression. The mechanism governing the relationship between the spinocerebellar-corticospinal disorder and an increase in ventricular mass—hypertrophic cardiomyopathy—is also unknown, but a unify-

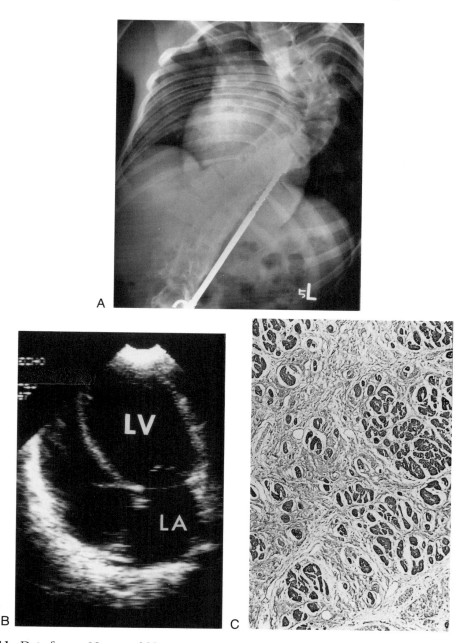

Fig. 3-11. Data from a 13-year-old boy with Friedreich's ataxia. (**A**) X-ray shows striking scoliosis. Note the Harrington rod. (**B**) Two-dimensional echocardiogram showing the thin-walled dilated left ventricle (LV). LA, left atrium. (**C**) Necropsy section showing extensive fibrous replacement of left ventricular myocardium. (Fig. B from Child et al.,[62] with permission.)

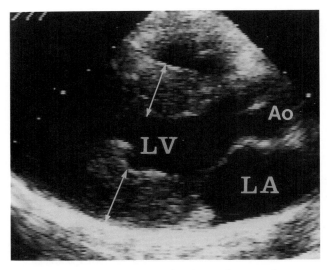

Fig. 3-12. Parasternal long axis two-dimensional echocardiogram from a 14-year-old girl with Friedreich's ataxia and concentric left ventricular (LV) hypertrophy. LA, left atrium; Ao, aorta.

ing concept may lie in the "catecholamine hypothesis."[68] This hypothesis has been a focus of interest in the pathogenesis of genetic hypertrophic cardiomyopathy, and plasma catecholamine levels are sometimes increased in patients with Friedreich's ataxia.[69,70]

CARDIOVASCULAR ABNORMALITIES AND ACUTE CEREBRAL DISORDERS

Abnormalities of the heart can set the stage for acute cerebral injury, and acute cerebral injury can provoke cardiovascular abnormalities. Approximately 90 percent of patients with acute cerebral accidents due to intracerebral or subarachnoid hemorrhage or acute cerebral trauma exhibit electrocardiographic abnormalities of cardiac rhythm, conduction, and repolarization.[71–81] Rhythm disturbances include sinus bradycardia, sinus tachycardia, atrial fibrillation, atrial flutter or supraventricular tachycardia, junctional rhythms, ectopic ventricular beats, and ventricular tachycardia or fibrillation. Conduction disturbances include first, second, or atrioventricular block. Repolarization abnormalities are similar if not identical to those of ischemic heart disease and are manifested by ST segment elevations and by T-wave inversions that may be striking in their degree[82] (Fig. 3-13). Acute cerebral trauma is sometimes accompanied by what has been called the "catecholamine storm."[83,84] Copious release of norepinephrine is held responsible for myocardial damage manifested by a rise in serum cardiac enzymes, left ventricular wall motion abnormalities, and myofiber degeneration.[83,84] Neurogenic pulmonary edema has been reported with a number of central nervous system disorders and with brain stem hemorrhage.[85]

Acute cerebral accidents originating from a cardiac source are typically represented by cerebral emboli, generally systemic, less commonly paradoxic[86] (see

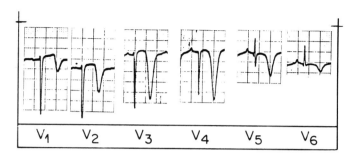

Fig. 3-13. Grant T-wave negativity in a patient who sustained a cerebral hemorrhage. (Courtesy of John H. Phillips, M.D., Tulane University Medical Center, New Orleans, LA.)

below). The principle cardiac sources of embolic stroke are "nonvalvular" atrial fibrillation (thrombus in left atrial appendage), ischemic heart disease (cardiac infarction, ventricular aneurysm with thrombus), and prosthetic cardiac valves, generally rigid, in the aortic or mitral position.[87,88] Important but less frequent cardiac sources of embolic stroke are rheumatic mitral stenosis especially with atrial fibrillation (now uncommon in developed countries), idiopathic dilated cardiomyopathy (thrombus attached to left ventricular endocardium), infective endocarditis, noninfectious "marantic" endocarditis, mitral valve prolapse, and left atrial myxoma.[86] Paradoxical embolization and emboli from an atrial septal aneurysm are discussed below.

Nonvalvular atrial fibrillation (normal mitral valve) is the commonest cardiac disorder associated with cerebral emboli.[81,87,88] Treatment remains controversial, with opinions differing regarding the inherent risk of cerebral embolization from atrial fibrillation unassociated with structural heart disease. There is, however, a growing tendency to recommend aspirin or Coumadin for the prevention of systemic embolization from this source.[81,87,88]

The relationship between mitral valve prolapse and cerebral events has been attributed to noninfectious thromboembo-lism (fibrin/platelet thrombi) originating from the cul-de-sac between the atrial surface of the base of the posterior leaflet and the contiguous endocardium of the posterior wall of the left atrium, or from the apex of the atrial surface of a prolapsed leaflet at sites of endothelial discontinuity or rupture of subendothelial connective tissue.[89] Irrespective of the pattern taken by cerebral events, patients typically recover completely or nearly so. Nevertheless, there is a general consensus that transient ischemic attacks believed to be due to fibrin/platelet emboli from mitral valve prolapse should be treated with aspirin at least in the short term.

CEREBRAL DISORDERS ASSOCIATED WITH CONGENITAL HEART DISEASE

Brain Abscess

When patients present with headache, focal neurologic signs, seizures, and fever, brain abscess should be suspected.[90,91] A recent brain abscess can be diagnosed by computed axial tomography, which establishes the presence not only of the lesion but also the distinctive ring enhancement typical of a recent abscess[91] (Fig. 3-14A). A fresh abscess may be accompanied by seizures, and the seizures may persist or recur years later because of focal brain injury caused by the healed lesion (Fig. 3-14B).

Susceptibility to abscess formation, irrespective of patient age, appears to be related to three variables: bacteremia, venoarterial mixing intrinsic to cyanotic congenital heart disease, and cerebral vulnerability because of focal brain injury.[91] Blood-borne bacteria are normally filtered by the pulmonary circulation and the reticuloendothelial system. Right-to-left shunts in cyanotic congenital heart disease circumvent the pulmonary filter, permitting bacteria to enter the systemic and therefore cerebral circulations. Encephalomalacia caused by a paradoxic or systemic embolus can provide the focal zone of cerebral vulnerability that appears to be necessary for abscess formation.

Cerebral Emboli

Bland or infected cerebral emboli can originate either in the systemic circulation or from peripheral or pelvic veins (paradoxical embolization in cyanotic congenital heart disease).[92-97] Systemic emboli from left-sided prosthetic cardiac valves, left atrial appendage (atrial fibrillation), left-sided infective endocarditis, and left ventricular endocardium were commented on earlier. Somewhat more unique to congenital heart disease, usually but not necessarily cyanotic, are paradoxical emboli that form in lower extremity or pelvic veins and reach the

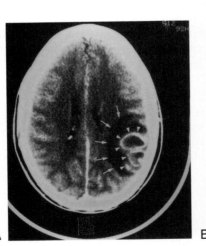
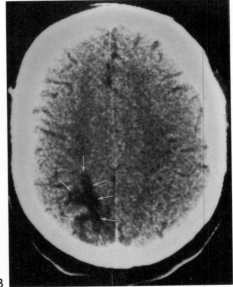

Fig. 3-14. (A) Computed axial tomograph from a 34-year-old cyanotic woman in whom a brain abscess followed oral surgery and announced itself as a seizure. The tomographic scan shows ring enhancement (*arrowheads*) and surrounding edema (*arrows*) characteristic of a recent abscess. **(B)** Computed axial tomograph from a 28-year-old man with cyanotic congenital heart disease. As a child he had a brain abscess (represented here in the healed state [*arrows*]) and that was manifested overtly as a seizure disorder requiring Dilantin.

brain because peripheral venous blood has direct access to the systemic circulation via a right-to-left shunt. In adults with cyanotic congenital heart disease, anticoagulants should be used with caution because these drugs reinforce the intrinsic hemostatic defects of cyanotic patients and increase the risk of hemorrhage, possibly cerebral.[98–100] The injudicious use of intravenous lines for infusions or medications represents a potential source of paradoxical embolization in hospitalized cyanotic patients. Introduction of air or particles into peripheral veins risks delivery into the systemic circulation via the right-to-left shunt. Insertion of an air/particle filter into the intravenous line circumvents the risk.[100]

An interatrial communication—ostium secundum atrial septal defect or patent foramen ovale—permits inferior vena caval blood to stream across the atrial septum into the left atrium and systemic circulation.[93,94] Accordingly, emboli from pelvic or leg veins pose risks in this setting. A pregnant woman with an ostium secundum atrial septal defect is at risk, especially during the puerperium, so meticulous leg care and early ambulation are recommended.[97]

Recent interest has focused on young adults with embolic stroke ascribed to paradoxic emboli through a patent foramen ovale[93] (Fig. 3-15). Straining or vigorous cough is often necessary to initiate transient venoarterial mixing that provides the physiologic substrate for a paradoxical embolus through a patent foramen ovale.[91] The Valsalva maneuver is also important diagnostically and is used to provoke a right-to-left shunt through a foramen ovale during contrast echocardiography or transcranial contrast ultrasound.

An atrial septal aneurysm at the site of a foramen ovale (patent or not) (Fig. 3-16) may provide the substrate for fibrin/

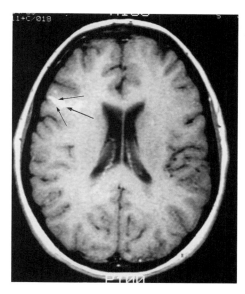

Fig. 3-15. Computed axial tomograph from a 39-year-old woman who sustained a paradoxical cerebral embolus (*arrows*) via a patent foramen ovale.

platelet thrombi that express themselves as embolic strokes, generally manifested by transient ischemic attacks in clinically well acyanotic young patients.[95] Thrombotic material can lodge on the systemic surface of an aneurysm that may be either convex or concave toward the left atrium, but is often quite mobile. The diagnosis of an atrial septal aneurysm is best established by transesophageal echocardiography,[95] although the lesion can sometimes be suspected in a transthoracic echocardiogram.

In otherwise normal young adults with strokes believed to be caused by paradoxic emboli via a patent foramen ovale, or by emboli from an atrial septal aneurysm, therapeutic options include antiplatelet agents, anticoagulants, closure of the patent foramen ovale with a catheter-delivered umbrella device, or surgical repair of the atrial septal aneurysm.[91] If a single mild transient ischemic attack is provoked by straining or cough, and if a

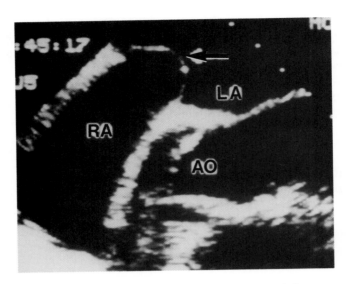

Fig. 3-16. Transesophageal echocardiogram showing a large, mobile aneurysm of the atrial septum (*arrow*) in a 28-year-old woman with transient ischemic attacks believed to originate from platelet/fibrin emboli from the left atrial (LA) surface of the aneurysm. RA, right atrium; Ao, aorta. (From Schneider et al.,[95] with permission.)

right-to-left shunt through a patent foramen ovale is detected only after a Valsalva maneuver in a patient without a detectable source of embolization, the current recommendation is to reduce the inciting stimulus by avoiding vigorous cough and straining.

In the same setting, a peripheral venous source of an embolus requires the use of anticoagulants (Coumadin). If the transient ischemic attack recurs, if either the initial or subsequent transient ischemic attack is more than mild, and if the right-to-left shunt via the foramen ovale is detected by echocardiography without provocation by a Valsalva maneuver or cough, closure with a catheter-delivered umbrella device is recommended. When cerebral emboli are believed to originate from an atrial septal aneurysm without a patent foramen ovale, antiplatelet agents are recommended. If the transesophageal echocardiogram identifies a large mobile septal aneurysm with a patent foramen

ovale and a right-to-left shunt, surgical correction is preferable to umbrella closure.

Cerebral Thrombosis

Older children and adults with cyanotic congenital heart disease and elevated hematocrit levels are often phlebotomized and occasionally anticoagulated because of an assumed risk of cerebral arterial thrombotic stroke.[98,99] However, the risk of thrombotic stroke in cyanotic patients is confined to those under 4 years of age with iron deficiency and microcytosis. Cerebral infarction in these young patients results from thromboses of intracranial veins and sinuses, not of cerebral arteries.[101–103] Adults with cyanotic congenital heart disease have not been found to be at risk of cerebral arterial or venous thrombosis and infarction despite wide ranges of hematocrit levels, irrespective of the frequency and degree of hyperviscosity symptoms, and whether or not iron deficiency is present or absent.[99,100] Erythrocytosis per se is not a risk factor for strokes in adults with cyanotic congenital heart disease even when the hematocrit level exceeds 65 percent, whether or not the erythrocytosis is iron replete and normocytic or iron deficient and microcytic. Because a risk of stroke due to cerebral thrombosis has not been demonstrated, because the circulatory effects of phlebotomy are transient, and because of the untoward sequelae of phlebotomy-induced iron deficiency, phlebotomy is recommended for temporary relief of significant, intrusive hyperviscosity symptoms but not because of the hematocrit level per se.[100] Phlebotomy is not warranted to reduce an assumed risk of stroke.

It is important to underscore that symptomatic hyperviscosity seldom occurs in an iron-replete state with hematocrit levels less than 65 percent. When hyperviscosity symptoms are present with hematocrit levels less than 65 percent, iron deficiency should be suspected. Phlebotomy aggravates rather than alleviates the symptoms, reinforcing the iron depletion. When hematocrit levels are above 65 percent, it is important to be certain that dehydration is not the cause. Treatment for dehydration is volume repletion, not phlebotomy.

Cerebral Hemorrhage

Rupture of an aneurysm of the circle of Willis is one of the major (albeit uncommon) complications of coarctation of the aorta, operated or unoperated.[91,104] Hypertension is not a precondition, because the rupture can occur in normotensive patients years after successful coarctation repair. The majority of patients who succumb to cerebral hemorrhage in this setting do so in their second or third decade.[104]

A second cause of cerebral hemorrhage, the injudicious use of anticoagulants in patients with cyanotic congenital heart disease, is largely preventable.[99,100] Defects in hemostasis that accompany the erythrocytosis of cyanotic congenital heart disease warn against incurring the additional risks of anticoagulants that are sometimes given to reduce an assumed cerebral arterial thrombotic predisposition, which has been found to be negligible if not absent. Because the probability of cerebral arterial thrombosis is low in adults with cyanotic congenital heart disease (see earlier), anticoagulants or aspirin should be used cautiously if at all.

Hypoxic Spells

In infants with Fallot's tetralogy, hypoxic spells typically begin with a progressive increase in the rate and depth of respiration and culminate in paroxysmal hyperpnea, deepening cyanosis, limpness, syncope and occasionally convulsions, cerebrovascular accidents, or death.[91,104,105] Cerebral injury in infancy may result in late neurologic sequelae.[91]

The Blalock-Taussig shunt was originally applied to cyanotic patients with Fallot's tetralogy. An occasional neurologic complication of a classic Blalock-Taussig anastomosis is the subclavian steal.[106] The anastomosis may create an anatomic and physiologic substrate identical to that of the subclavian steal caused by atheromatous obstruction of the proximal subclavian artery. Symptoms of the steal may first appear decades after the Blalock-Taussig shunt, depending upon the development of cervical and intrathoracic collateral circulation. The anatomy of the shunt and the physiology of the subclavian steal are not necessarily reversed by intracardiac repair, even though the Blalock-Taussig anastomosis is ligated.

Syncope Followed by Sudden Death

Syncope is a feared sequela of discrete aortic stenosis, but the risk in young patients with congenital aortic valve stenosis and normal coronary arterial circulations is small compared with that in older adults with co-existing coronary artery disease.[91,104] Syncope in aortic valve stenosis is prompted by an exaggerated, prolonged, and poorly regulated exercise-induced fall in systemic vascular resistance mediated by left ventricular baroreceptors triggered during the increase in venous return associated with exercise.[107] Malignant ventricular arrhythmias seldom initiate syncope but are the principal cause of death *after* a faint. The hypotension accompanying syncope is much more likely to provoke electrical ventricular instability and sudden death in older adults with acquired calcific aortic stenosis and co-existing atherosclerotic coronary artery disease than in young patients with hemodynamically equivalent congenital aortic valve stenosis and normal coronary arteries.[104]

REFERENCES

1. Perloff JK: Neurological disorders and heart disease. p. 1810. In Braunwald E, (ed): Heart Disease: A Textbook of Cardiovascular Medicine. 4th Ed. WB Saunders, Philadelphia, 1992

2. Perloff JK, de Leon AC, O'Doherty D: The cardiomyopathy of progressive muscular dystrophy. Circulation 33:625, 1966

3. Brooke MH: A Clinician's View of Neuromuscular Disease. 2nd Ed. Williams & Wilkins, Baltimore, 1986

4. Perloff JK, Roberts WC, de Leon AC Jr et al: The distinctive electrocardiogram of Duchenne progressive muscular dystrophy: an electrocardiographic-pathologic correlative study. Am J Med 42:179, 1967

5. Perloff JK, Henze E, Schelbert HR: Alterations in regional myocardial metabolism, perfusion, and wall motion in Duchenne muscular dystrophy studied by radionuclide imaging. Circulation 69:33, 1984

6. Sanyal SK, Johnson WW: Cardiac conduction abnormalities in children with Duchenne progressive muscular dystrophy: electrocardiographic features and morphologic correlates. Circulation 66:853, 1982

7. Skyring A, McKusick VA: Clinical, genetic and electrocardiographic studies in childhood muscular dystrophy. Am J Med Sci 242:534, 1961

8. Slucka C: The electrocardiogram in Duchenne's progressive muscular dystrophy. Circulation 38:933, 1968

9. Vrints C, Mercelis R, Vanagt E et al: Cardiac manifestations of Becker-type muscular dystrophy. Acta Cardiol 38:479, 1983

10. Yazawa M, Ikeda S, Owa M et al: A family of Becker's progressive muscular dystrophy with severe cardiomyopathy. Eur Neurol 27:13, 1987

11. Lazzeroni E, Favaro L, Botti G: Dilated cardiomyopathy with regional myocardial hypoperfusion in Becker's muscular dystrophy. Int J Cardiol 22:126, 1989

12. Stevenson WG, Perloff JK, Weiss JN, Anderson TL. Facioscapulohumeral muscular dystrophy: evidence for selective, genetic electrophysiologic cardiac involvement. J Am Coll Cardiol 15:292, 1990

13. Kawashima S, Ueno M, Kondo T et al. Marked cardiac involvement in limb girdle muscular dystrophy. Am J Med Sci 299:411, 1990

14. Rojas CV, Hoffman EP: Recent advances in dystrophin research. Curr Opin Neurobiol 1:420, 1991

15. Hoffman EP, Hudecki MS, Rosenberg PA et al: Cell and figure-type distribution of dystrophin. Neuron 1:411, 1988

16. Lansman JB, Franco A: What does dystrophin do in normal muscle? J Muscle Res Cell Motil 12:409, 1991

17. Hoffman EP, Kunkel LM: Dystrophin abnormalities in Duchenne/Becker muscular dystrophy. Neuron 2:1019, 1989

18. Zubrzycka-Gaarn EE, Bulman DE, Karpati G et al: The Duchenne muscular dystrophy gene product is localized in sarcolemma of human skeletal muscle. Nature 333:466, 1988

19. Hoffman EP, Brown RH, Jr, Kunkel LM: Dystrophin: the protein product of the Duchenne muscular dystrophy locus. Cell 51:919, 1987

20. Bonilla E, Samitt CE, Miranda AF et al: Duchenne muscular dystrophy: deficiency of dystrophin at the muscle cell surface. Cell 54:447, 1988

21. Rubler S, Perloff JK, Roberts WC: Duchenne muscular dystrophy. Clinical pathological conference. Am Heart J 94:776, 1977

22. Perloff JK: Cardiac rhythm and conduction in Duchenne muscular dystrophy: a prospective study of 20 patients. J Am Coll Cardiol 3:1263, 1984

23. Perloff JK, Moise S, Stevenson WG et al: Cardiac electrophysiology in Duchenne muscular dystrophy—from basic science to clinical expression. J Cardiovasc Electrophysiol 3:394, 1992

24. Sanyal SK, Johnson WW, Thapar MK et al: An ultrastructural basis for the electrocardiographic alterations associated with Duchenne progressive muscular dystrophy. Circulation 57:1122, 1978

25. Ronan JA, Jr, Perloff JK, Bowen PJ et al: The vector-cardiogram in Duchenne progressive muscular dystrophy. Am Heart J 84:588, 1972

26. Miller G, D'Orsogna L, O'Shea JP: Autonomic function and the sinus tachycardia of Duchenne muscular dystrophy. Brain Dev 11:247, 1989

27. Yotsukura M, Ishizuka T, Shimada T et al: Late potentials in progressive muscular dystrophy of the Duchenne type. Am Heart J 121:1137, 1991

28. Zalman F, Perloff JK, Durant NN et al: Acute respiratory failure following intravenous verapamil in Duchenne's muscular dystrophy. Am Heart J 105:510, 1983

29. Mendell JR, Moxley RT, Griggs RC et al: Randomized, double-blind 6-month trial of prednisone in Duchenne's muscular dystrophy. N Engl J Med 320:1592, 1989

30. Kunkel LM: Analysis of deletions in DNA from patients with Becker and Duchenne muscular dystrophy. Nature 322:73, 1986

31. Bailey RO, Marzulo DC, Hans MB: Infantile facioscapulohumeral muscular dystrophy: new observations. Acta Neurol Scand 74:51, 1986

32. Bloomfield DA, Sinclair-Smith BC: Persistent atrial standstill. Am J Med 39:335, 1965

33. Caponnetto S, Patorini C, Tirelli G: Persistent atrial standstill in a patient affected with facioscapulohumeral dystrophy. Cardiologia 53:341, 1968

34. Baldwin BJ, Talley RC, Johnson C, Nutter O: Permanent paralysis of the atrium in a patient with facioscapulohumeral muscular dystrophy. Am J Cardiol 31:649, 1973

35. Woolliscroft J, Tuna N: Permanent atrial standstill: the clinical spectrum. Am J Med 49:2037, 1982

36. Emery AEH: X-linked muscular dystrophy with early contractures and cardiomyopathy (Emery-Dreifuss type). Clin Genet 32:360, 1987

37. Hopkins LC, Jackson JA, Elsas LJ: Emery-Dreifuss humeroperoneal muscular dystrophy: an X-linked myopathy with unusual contractures and bradycardia. Ann Neurol 10:230, 1981

38. Emery AEH, Dreifuss FE: Unusual type of benign X-linked muscular dystrophy. J Neurol Neurosurg Psychiatry 29:338, 1966

39. Takamoto K, Hirose K, Nonaka I: A genetic variant of Emery-Dreifuss disease. Arch Neurol 41:1292, 1984

40. Harper PS: Myotonic Dystrophy, 2nd Ed. WB Saunders, Philadelphia, 1989

41. Wieringa B, Brunner H, Hulsebos T et al: Genetic and physical demarcation of the locus for dystrophia myotonica. Adv Neurol 48:47, 1988

42. Perloff JK, Stevenson WG, Roberts NK

et al: Cardiac involvement in myotonic muscular dystrophy (Steinert's disease): a prospective study of 25 patients. Am J Cardiol 54:1074, 1984

43. Moorman JR, Coleman RE, Packer DL et al: Cardiac involvement in myotonic muscular dystrophy. Medicine 64:371, 1985

44. Hiromasa S, Ikeda T, Kubota K et al: Myotonic dystrophy: ambulatory electrocardiogram, electrophysiology study, and echocardiographic evaluation. Am Heart J 113:1482, 1987

45. Milner MR, Hawley RJ, Jachim M et al: Ventricular late potentials in myotonic dystrophy. Ann Intern Med 115:607, 1991

46. Bharati S, Bump FT, Bauernfeind R et al: Dystrophica myotonia. Correlative electrocardiographic, electrophysiologic and conduction system study. Chest 86:444, 1984

47. Hiromasa S, Ikeda T, Kubota K et al: Ventricular tachycardia and sudden death in myotonic dystrophy. Am Heart J 115:914, 1988

48. Nguyen HH, Wolfe JT, III, Holmes DR, Jr et al: Pathology of the cardiac conduction system in myotonic dystrophy: a study of 12 cases. J Am Coll Cardiol 11:662, 1988

49. Olofsson BO, Forsberg H, Andersson S et al: Electrocardio-graphic findings in myotonic dystrophy. Br Heart J 59:47, 1988

50. Grigg LE, Chan W, Mond HG et al: Ventricular tachycardia and sudden death in myotonic dystrophy: clinical electrophysiologic and pathologic features. Am J Cardiol 6:254, 1985

51. Prystowski EN, Pritchett ELC, Roses AD et al: The natural history conduction system disease in myotonic muscular dystrophy as determined by serial electrophysiologic studies. Circulation 60:1360, 1979

52. Child JS, Perloff JK: Myocardial myotonia in myotonic muscular dystrophy. In preparation.

53. Rüdel R, Lohmann-Horn F: Membrane changes in cells from myotonic patients. Physiol Rev 65:310, 1985

54. Renaud JF: Involvement of cation transporting systems in myotonic disease. Biochemie 69:407, 1987

55. Bryant SH, Morales-Aguilera A: Chloride conductance in normal and myotonic muscle fibers and the action potential of monocarboxylic aromatic acids. J Physiol 219:367, 1971

56. Barchi RL: Myotonia. An evaluation of the chloride hypothesis. Arch Neurol 32:175, 1975

57. Harvey RD, Hume JR: Autonomic regulation of a chloride current in heart. Science 244:983, 1989

58. Plishker GA, Gitelman JT, Appel SH: Myotonic muscular dystrophy: altered calcium transport in erythrocytes. Science 200:323, 1978

59. Forsberg H, Olofsson BO, Eriksson A, Andersson S: Cardiac involvement in congenital myotonic dystrophy. Br Heart J 63:119, 1990

60. Barbeau A: Friedreich's ataxia 1980. Our overview of the pathophysiology. J Can Sci Neurol 7:455, 1980

61. Harding AE: Friedreich's ataxia: a clinical and genetic study of 90 families with analysis of early diagnostic criteria and intrafamilial clustering of clinical features. Brain 104:589, 1981

62. Child JS, Perloff JK, Bach PM et al: Cardiac involvement in Friedreich's ataxia. J Am Coll Cardiol 7:1370, 1986

63. Brumback RA, Panner BJ, Kingston WJ: The heart in Friedreich's ataxia. Arch Neurol 43:189, 1986

64. Grenadier E, Goldberg SJ, Stern LZ, Feldman J: M-mode and two-dimensional echocardiographic examination of patients with Friedreich's ataxia. J Cardiovasc Ultrasonogr 3:5, 1984

65. Harding AE, Hewer RL: The heart disease of Friedreich's ataxia: a clinical and electrocardiographic study of 115 patients with an analysis of serial electrocardiographic changes in 30 cases. Q J Med 28:489, 1983

66. Unverferth DV, Schmidt WR, Baker PB, Wooley CF: Morphologic and functional characteristics of the heart in Friedreich's ataxia. Am J Med 82:5, 1987

67. Hawley RJ, Gottdiener JS: 5-Year fol-

low-up of Friedreich's ataxia cardiomy-opathy. Arch Intern Med 146:483, 1986

68. Perloff JK: Pathogenesis of hypertrophic cardiomyopathy. In Goodwin JF (ed): Heart Muscle Disease. MTP Press Ltd, Lancaster, 1985

69. Pasternac A, Wagniart P, Olivenstein R et al: Increased plasma catecholamines in patients with Friedreich's ataxia. Can J Neurol 9:195, 1982

70. Merkel AD, Barbeau A: Plasma cate-cholamines in Friedreich's ataxia as-sayed using high performance liquid chromatography with electrochemical detection. Can J Neurol 9:205, 1982

71. Yamour BJ, Sridharan MR, Rice JF, Flowers NC: Electrocardiographic changes in cerebrovascular hemorrhage. Am Heart J 99:294, 1980

72. Clifton GL, Robertson CS, Kyper K et al: Cerebrovascular response to severe head injury. J Neurosurg 59:447, 1983

73. McLoed AA, Neil-Dwyer G, Meyer CHA et al: Cardiac sequelae of acute head injury. Br Heart J 47:221, 1982

74. Tobias SL, Bookatz BJ, Diamond TH: Myocardial damage and electrocardio-graphic changes in acute cerebrovascu-lar hemorrhage: a report of three cases and review. Heart Lung 16:521, 1987

75. Pollick C, Cujec B, Parker S, Tator C: Left ventricular wall motion abnormali-ties in subarachnoid hemorrhage: an echocardiographic study. J Am Coll Car-diol 12:600, 1988

76. Mikolich JR, Jacobs WC, Fletcher GF: Cardiac arrhythmias in patients with acute cerebrovascular accidents. JAMA 246:1314, 1981

77. Myers MG, Norris JW, Hachinski VC et al: Cardiac sequelae of acute stroke. Stroke 13:838, 1982

78. Stober T, Anstätt T, Sen S et al: Cardiac arrhythmias in subarachnoid haemor-rhage. Acta Neurochir 93:37, 1988

79. Rudehill A, Olsson GL, Sundqvist K, Gordon E: ECG abnormalities in pa-tients with subarachnoid haemorrhage and intracranial tumours. J Neurol Neurosurg Psychiatry 50:1375, 1987

80. Melin J, Fogelhohm R: Electrocardio-graphic findings in subarachnoid hemor-rhage. Acta Med Scand 213:5, 1983

81. Oppenheimer SM, Cechetto DF, Ha-chinski VC: Cerebrogenic cardiac ar-rhythmias. Arch Neurol 47:513, 1990

82. Gascon P, Ley TJ, Toltzis RJ, Bonow RO: Spontaneous subarachnoid hemor-rhage simulating acute transmural myocardial infarction. Am Heart J 105:511, 1983

83. Chen HI, Liao JF, Ho ST: Centrogenic pulmonary hemorrhagic edema induced by cerebral compression in rats. Circ Res 47:366, 1980

84. Brunninkhuis LGH: Electrocardio-graphic abnormalities suggesting myo-cardial infarction in a patient with se-vere cranial trauma. PACE 6:1336, 1983

85. Schell AR, Shenoy MM, Friedman SA, Patel AR: Pulmonary edema associated with subarachnoid hemorrhage. Arch In-tern Med 147:591, 1987

86. Cerebral Embolism Task Force: Car-diogenic brain embolism. Arch Neurol 43:71, 1986

87. Kopecky SL, Gersh BJ, McGoon MD et al: The natural history of lone atrial fibrillation. N Engl J Med 317:669, 1987

88. Stroke Prevention in Atrial Fibrillation Study Group Investigators: Preliminary report of the stroke prevention in atrial fibrillation study. N Engl J Med 322:863, 1990

89. Perloff JK, Child JS: Clinical and epide-miologic issues in mitral valve prolapse. Am Heart J 113:1324, 1987

90. Shaher RM, Deuchar DC: Hematoge-nous brain abscess in cyanotic congeni-tal heart disease. Am J Med 52:349, 1972

91. Perloff JK, Marelli A, Miner P: Neuro-logical and psychosocial disorders in adults with congenital heart disease. Heart Disease Stroke 1:218, 1992

92. Biller J, Johnson MR, Adams HP Jr et al: Further observations on cerebral or reti-nal ischemia in patients with right-left intracardiac shunts. Arch Neurol 44:740, 1987

93. Lechat P, Mas JL, Lascault G et al: Prev-alence of patent foramen ovale in pa-tients with stroke. N Engl J Med 318:1148, 1988

94. Harvey JR, Teague SM, Anderson JL et al: Clinically silent atrial septal defects with evidence of cerebral embolization. Ann Intern Med 105:695, 1986

95. Schneider B, Hanrath P, Vogel P, Meinertz T: Improved morphologic characterization of atrial septal aneurysm by transesophageal echocardiography: relation to cerebrovascular events. J Am Coll Cardiol 16:1000, 1990

96. Pearson AC, Nagelhout D, Castello R et al: Atrial septal aneurysm and stroke: a transesophageal echocardiographic study. J Am Coll Cardiol 18:1223, 1991

97. Pitkin RM, Perloff JK, Koos BJ, Beall MH: Pregnancy and congenital heart disease. Ann Intern Med 112:445, 1990

98. Perloff JK, Rosove MH, Child JS, Wright GB: Adults with cyanotic congenital heart disease: hematologic management. Ann Intern Med 109:406, 1988

99. Rosove MH, Perloff JK, Hocking WG et al: Chronic hypoxaemia and decompensated erythrocytosis in cyanotic congenital heart disease. Lancet 2:313, 1986

100. Territo M, Rosove MH, Perloff JK: Cyanotic congenital heart disease: hematologic management, renal function and urate metabolism. p. 93. In Perloff JK, Child JS (eds): Congenital Heart Disease in Adults. WB Saunders, Philadelphia, 1991

101. Cottrill CM, Kaplan S: Cerebral vascular accidents in cyanotic congenital heart disease. Am J Dis Child 125:484, 1973

102. Lindercamp O, Klose HJ, Betke K et al: Increased blood viscosity in patients with cyanotic congenital heart disease and iron deficiency. J Pediatr 95:567, 1979

103. Phornphutkul C, Rosenthal A, Nadas AS, Berenberg W: Cerebrovascular accidents in infants and children with cyanotic congenital heart disease. Am J Cardiol 32:329, 1973

104. Perloff JK: Clinical Recognition of Congenital Heart Disease. p. 84. WB Saunders, Philadelphia, 1987

105. Morgan BC, Guntheroth WG, Bloom RS, Flyer DC: A clinical profile of paroxysmal hyperpnea in cyanotic congenital heart disease. Circulation 31:66, 1965

106. Kurlan R, Krall RL, Deweese JA: Vertebrobasilar ischemia after total repair of tetralogy of Fallot: significance of subclavian steal created by Blalock-Taussig anastomosis. Stroke 15:359, 1984

107. Mark AL, Kioschos JM, Abboud FM et al: Abnormal vascular responses to exercise in patients with aortic stenosis. J Clin Invest 52:1138, 1973

108. Perloff JK: Neurological disorders and heart disease. In Braunwald E (ed): Heart Disease: A Textbook of Cardiovascular Medicine. 3rd Ed. WB Saunders, Philadelphia, 1988

4

Liver Disease

Elliot Rapaport

Approximately 25 percent of the cardiac output courses through the liver. It is therefore understandable that diseases of the liver may impact significantly on the cardiovascular system.

PORTAL HYPERTENSION

Portal hypertension arises from a variety of causes. First, portal pressure, which is normally less than 5 mmHg, may be high as a passive response to increases in inferior vena caval pressure secondary to constrictive pericarditis, tricuspid stenosis, or chronic dilated congestive cardiomyopathy. Any increase in central venous pressure produces a comparable rise in hepatic vein pressure. Portal vein pressure, which normally is 1 to 2 mmHg higher than hepatic vein pressure, rises correspondingly. If these pressures become significantly and persistently elevated, particularly if there is some degree of hypoalbuminemia, ascites as well as peripheral edema may result. The term "cardiac cirrhosis" has sometimes been used to describe the resultant clinical picture.

If massive ascites develops suddenly, particularly if it is associated with hepatomegaly and abdominal pain, one should suspect the possibility of Budd-Chiari syndrome resulting from occlusion or obstruction of hepatic venous outflow. This may arise from several causes, ranging from disseminated intravascular coagulation to the classic hepatic venous endophlebitis described by Chiari. It should be appreciated that the response of the liver and hepatic circulation proximal to the occluded hepatic veins will be essentially the same as if the hepatic sinusoids were facing a high pressure from severe heart failure or constrictive pericarditis.

Portal hypertension may be seen transiently early in the course of acute alcoholic hepatitis. Such hypertension results from hepatocyte enlargement, which can increase the resistance to hepatic blood flow, but is reversible as alcohol use is curtailed. A similar transient rise in portal vein pressure can be seen in patients with acute viral hepatitis when it is related to the severity of liver damage.[1] With subsidence of the inflammatory response, the pressure will return to normal levels.

Cirrhosis, particularly Laennec's cirrhosis, is the most common cause of portal hypertension. Nodular regeneration and fibrosis around the sinusoidal and postsinusoidal hepatic venules result in an increased resistance to flow, leading to a decreased hepatic blood flow and an increase in presinusoidal and portal vein pressures. There is evidence that increased sympathetic activity may also contribute to the increased resistance to blood flow through the presinusoidal area, since plasma norepinephrine concentrations are elevated in cirrhotics,[2] and β-adrenergic blockade with propranolol appears to increase the proportion of the cardiac output delivered to the liver as well as to reduce portal pressure.[3] Among the changes in the cardiovascular system that may be seen in relationship to portal hypertension are the development of collaterals linking the portal and systemic circulations, an expanded blood volume, a decreased arterial oxygen saturation, a decrease in arterial pressure, systemic vasodilatation, and an increase in cardiac output.

The presence of portal hypertension will eventually result in esophageal varices, and this in turn increases the pressure within the azygos and hemiazygos veins. As a consequence, communications between the pulmonary venous and azygos systems, which normally result in a small physiologic left-to-right shunt across the lungs, may reverse, and blood may be shunted from right to left into the pulmonary veins. Additionally, right-to-left shunts may occur from mediastinal and periesophageal-pulmonary venous communication.[4] This will be reflected by a mild degree of arterial hypoxemia. A rise in arterial saturation can be demonstrated in some patients with bleeding esophageal varices following surgical ligation of the varices and interruption of this shunting mechanism.

Several other mechanisms may also contribute to hypoxemia. The first is the result of shunting across small pulmonary arteriovenous connections, bypassing portions of the capillary bed of the lung. Patients with Laennec's cirrhosis frequently have small star-like lesions in the lung fields (seen post mortem) similar to spider angiomata seen on the skin.[5] Such lesions result in small communications between distal branches of the pulmonary artery and the pulmonary venous systems; pulmonary capillary flow is bypassed, and therefore a small right-to-left shunt across the pulmonary bed results. Secondly, ascites can elevate the diaphragm, which might restrict alveolar ventilation, contributing to arterial hypoxemia; however, hypoxemia may be seen in patients without significant ascites.[6] Finally, a shift to the right occurs in the oxyhemoglobin-dissociation curve in cirrhosis, reducing the affinity of hemoglobin for oxygen.[7] Whatever the mechanisms, patients with established esophageal varices and portal hypertension will frequently have a mild degree of arterial hypoxemia. This is likely to be accentuated if tense ascites is present, since the increase in intra-abdominal pressure is transmitted to the portal vein, resulting in a greater peripheral to central venous pressure gradient encouraging variceal flow.

Pulmonary Hypertension

Pulmonary arterial hypertension occurs on rare occasions in patients with portal hypertension. Although idiopathic pulmonary hypertension is an uncommon entity, it nevertheless occurs more frequently in patients with portal hypertension than one would expect from the overall incidence in the general population. It has been estimated that the incidence of pulmonary hypertension in patients with portal hypertension is approximately six times that seen in its absence. In a prospective study of 507 patients hospitalized with portal hypertension who underwent cardiac catheterization, 2 percent had pulmonary hypertension.[8] In most cases, the underlying etiology of the portal hypertension is Laennec's cirrhosis. The risk of pulmonary hypertension appears to be directly related to the duration of portal hypertension. Thus, paradoxically, those patients who have varices successfully controlled by either sclerotherapy or through the use of surgery are at an increased risk for the development of pulmonary artery hypertension. The pathogenesis is obscure. One proposed explanation is the likelihood that patients suffer from recurrent small venous thromboemboli, which can bypass the liver and be carried directly to the lung through portopulmonary communications. Eventually sufficient obliteration of the pulmonary vascular bed from silent pulmonary emboli may result in pulmonary hypertension. Another favored explanation is that the cirrhotic liver fails to remove or detoxify vasoconstrictive or other substances absorbed from the bowel that can produce pulmonary vascular damage.

It is known that pulmonary hypertension in humans can be produced by substances absorbed from the bowel. Adulterated rapeseed oil and the antiobesity drug Aminorex resulted in past outbreaks of pulmonary hypertension.[9,10] Pulmonary hypertension accompanying hepatic cirrhosis is a fixed obstructive type of pulmonary vascular disease and is not reversible with the chronic use of pulmonary arterial vasodilators. Consequently, such patients cannot be expected to be candidates for liver transplantation since the pulmonary vascular disease is irreversible.

One of the postulates related to the possible etiology of pulmonary hypertension in patients with portal hypertension has been the presence of an increase in pulmonary blood flow or high cardiac output, which is commonly seen in patients with decompensated Laennec's cirrhosis.[11,12] The high-output state is a reflection, in part, of the generalized vasodilation. It may also reflect an increase in left ventricular (LV) volumes

that will increase stroke output if cardiac function is adequate.[13] The increased LV volume reflects an expanded blood volume. It is, of course, possible that a chronic high-output state, along with the presence of some degree of hypoxemia, may contribute to the development of pulmonary hypertension, although the fact that it appears to be irreversible after liver transplantation makes this explanation unlikely.[14] Furthermore, cardiac index actually varies inversely with pulmonary arterial pressure, making this explanation even more unlikely.[8]

The presence of exertional dyspnea, exertional syncope, excessive fatigue, and atypical chest pain should raise one's threshold of suspicion that pulmonary hypertension may be present. Accentuation of the pulmonic component of the second sound will be present with or without an associated soft systolic ejection murmur in the second left interspace on physical examination. The electrocardiogram will generally show frank right ventricular (RV) hypertrophy, and chest x-ray will demonstrate the presence of disproportionate enlargement of the main and major proximal branches of the pulmonary artery. Relative avascularity of the peripheral lung fields is seen.

In general, one does not see a patient with pulmonary hypertension develop portal hypertension. Rather, a patient with portal hypertension may either be discovered to have co-existing pulmonary hypertension or develop pulmonary hypertension at a later date. Echocardiography may demonstrate evidence of right ventricular free-wall hypertrophy often associated with some degree of right ventricular dilatation; Doppler echo interrogation, if there is some degree of tricuspid insufficiency present, as there often is, may permit estimation of the degree of pulmonary hypertension present.

If evidence of RV hypertrophy is present electrocardiographically, or pul-

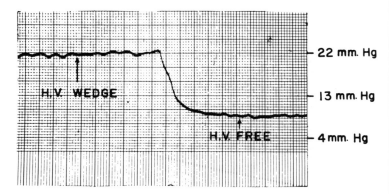

Fig. 4-1. Hepatic vein (HV) wedge pressure in cirrhosis; continuous withdrawal of a catheter from the wedged hepatic vein to the free position. A very high initial pressure, an indication of portal hypertension, is seen that falls to the level of the central venous pressure as the catheter is withdrawn to lie freely in a hepatic vein. The pressure gradient reflects the increased sinusoidal and postsinusoidal resistance to hepatic blood flow resulting from cirrhosis.

monary hypertension is suspected by echo Doppler, right heart catheterization can be performed with a Swan-Ganz catheter in order to document that the wedge pressure is normal and that there is increased pulmonary vascular resistance causing pulmonary arterial hypertension. One can at the same time use the opportunity to wedge the catheter into a branch of the hepatic vein: the wedged hepatic vein pressure accurately estimates portal vein pressure. Normally, the pressure is 1 to 2 mmHg higher than free hepatic vein pressure. However, in cirrhosis a significant pressure gradient can usually be demonstrated as the catheter is pulled from the wedged to the free position, establishing the presence of sinusoidal or postsinusoidal obstruction to hepatic flow (i.e., cirrhosis) (Fig. 4-1). We have recorded pressures as high as 39 mmHg in patients with decompensated cirrhosis and tense ascites.[15]

CIRRHOSIS

The hyperkinetic circulatory state in many patients with cirrhosis has been a subject of interest for several decades. Not only may the systemic output be elevated at rest, but the increase with exercise may exceed that seen in normals exercising to a comparable degree.[16] It is clear that a generalized increase in various regional blood flows is present.[17] For example, antecubital vein blood is frequently brighter than usual, reflecting the fact that venous saturation in the forearm is increased. This implies an increased upper extremity blood flow. An increase in blood flow has also been documented using plethysmography of the lower extremities in patients with cirrhosis. Although most vascular beds will be vasodilated and regional blood flow increased, estimated hepatic blood is decreased.[18] Such a decrease reflects the increased sinusoidal and postsinusoidal resistance to hepatic blood flow produced by the cirrhotic process. It should be noted that total portal vein flow may actually be increased, since portohepatic vein shunts, as well as portal collateral flow to gastric and esophageal varices, would not be measured by the techniques usually employed to estimate hepatic blood flow.

The presence of systemic vasodilatation has traditionally been explained by the inability of the cirrhotic liver to detoxify circulating vasodilators. More recently, however, the role of endothelial-derived relaxing factor (EDRF; what appears to be chemically the same as nitric oxide) has been highlighted. It has been suggested that increased nitrous oxide synthase production in the vascular endothelium occurs in cirrhosis, with subsequent sustained nitric oxide release and resultant reduced vascular tone.[19]

The chronic arterial vasodilatation observed in cirrhotics has been generally considered to be the causative factor in the genesis off the high cardiac output state that is seen in many patients with Laennec's cirrhosis. Recently, however, this view has been challenged.[13] In an echocardiographic study of 24 patients with cirrhosis, elevated LV end-diastolic and end-systolic diameters were demonstrated in comparison with a group of age- and sex-matched controls. The finding of an increase in end-diastolic diameter suggests that diminished afterload is not the major explanation for the high-output state. Increased emptying related to the increase in end-diastolic volume may be responsible, since LV end-systolic diameter would be expected to be decreased if decreased afterload were the principal operating mechanism. The increase in ventricular volume apparently results from the presence in many of these patients of an expanded blood volume.

Catecholamines

Circulating catecholamine levels are also increased in patients with cirrhosis, which may contribute to the hyperkinetic circulation.[2] However, chronic elevations in serum norepinephrine concentrations lead to β-adrenergic receptor downregulation within the myocardium, which can depress myocardial contractility. Myocardial hyporesponsiveness to catecholamines has been observed in cirrhotics.[20]

A significant correlation has been demonstrated between pulmonary artery plasma epinephrine concentration and cardiac index in patients with presinusoidal portal hypertension, as well as in patients with Laennec's cirrhosis.[2] Thus, increased adrenal medullary activity with liberation of epinephrine may also be a contributing mechanism to the development of the hyperkinetic circulatory state. The observation that patients with presinusoidal portal hypertension also have a high-output state, with a cardiac index similar to that seen in a comparable group of cirrhotic patients, suggests that liver function per se is not a determining factor, and gives further evidence to the role of sympathetic nerve stimulation and catecholamine release. It is important to appreciate, however, that catecholamine levels in portal hypertension associated with normal liver function and sinusoidal pressures are normal, and sympathetic nerve activity does not appear to be increased.

Thus, it appears that there is chronic increased sympathetic nerve activity when liver disease or increased sinusoidal pressure is present. In contrast to presinusoidal portal hypertension, there is no correlation between serum epinephrine levels and the elevated cardiac index. The lack of correlation between epinephrine concentration and cardiac index in cirrhotics may result from increased sympathetic nerve traffic, leading to chronic elevations of plasma norepinephrine. Such elevations may in turn cause downregulation or desensitization of β-adrenergic receptors altering the myocardial response.

Drug Use in Portal Hypertension

Several of the drugs used to treat bleeding esophageal varices may have an effect on the heart or circulatory system. β-Adrenergic blocking agents such as propranolol produce a significant decrease in directly measured variceal pressure,[21] and have been demonstrated to decrease portal vein pressure by the hepatic vein wedge technique.[22] Presumably, the mechanism is a significant reduction in portal blood flow coursing through the liver and decreasing collateral flow, as reflected in measurements of azygos blood flow as well. This mechanism has been the basis of its use in managing patients with varices. Vasodilators such as isosorbide-5-mononitrate and molsidomine have also been used to lower portal vein pressure.[23,24] Combined nitrate and propranolol use appears to be additive in the ability to reduce portal hypertension.[23]

Patients with bleeding esophageal varices are often treated with intravenous vasopressin. However, this drug is a vasoconstrictor that can result in coronary vasoconstriction, which in turn may cause myocardial ischemia. Additionally, there may be hypertension and bradycardia. These untoward side effects may be offset by the simultaneous infusion of either nitroprusside or nitroglycerin.[25] Occasionally, torsade de pointes has been reported in patients receiving vasopressin.[26] Bradycardia may also result from a vagal reflex secondary to the systemic arterial vasoconstriction. How often cardiac complications occur from IV vasopressin is not well documented. However, one should, when infusing vasopressin in the treatment of esophageal bleeding, be sensitive to the possibility, particularly in the older patient, of increased arrhythmias, aggravation of preexisting conges-

tive heart failure, or the development of myocardial ischemia.

Ascites

The marked increase in intra-abdominal pressure accompanying tense ascites results in pronounced elevation of the diaphragm. This in turn makes intrapleural pressure less negative by approximately 2 to 3 mmHg. The net effect will be a corresponding rise in central venous pressure, which is the sum of the intravascular and intrapleural pressures.

Ascites is generally managed by the judicious use of diuretics. Excessive diuretics resulting in a negative balance of a liter or more in a nonedematous patient is likely to result in a significant contraction of the vascular volume. Additionally, one may encounter hyponatremia, hypokalemia, and azotemia as well as encephalopathy. When tense ascites develops despite diuretic use, abdominal paracentesis may be necessary. One must limit the amount of fluid withdrawn at any setting, however, since there will be a rapid transfer of albumin from plasma into the abdominal cavity. This can cause a marked contraction of vascular volume and result in peripheral vascular collapse. Paracentesis will also result in a drop in right atrial pressure as intra-abdominal pressure is reduced.

Echocardiographic studies of patients with decompensated hepatic cirrhosis and ascites document a high prevalence of pericardial effusion.[27] In a group of 27 consecutively hospitalized patients with alcoholic cirrhosis and ascites, 17 showed a pericardial effusion, whereas only 23 of 28 control subjects were found to have detectable pericardial effusion by echocardiography. It was further noted that the pericardial effusion either diminished or disappeared in four of six patients following resolution of ascites. This finding suggests that increased sodium and water retention, which contribute to the presence of ascites and a small hydrothorax also frequently seen in cirrhotics, may contribute to the formation of a pericardial effusion.

Lipid Alterations

At San Francisco General Hospital, we examined postmortem 105 patients with Laennec's cirrhosis together with 105 age and sex-matched controls.[15] The patients with cirrhosis demonstrated a lesser incidence in the severity of underlying coronary atherosclerosis. The interpretation of this observation, however, is clouded by the fact that our postmortem control groups probably included an excess of patients with systemic hypertension and hypercholesterolemia, and in that sense were not really true controls. It should be noted that most similar studies in the literature appear to confirm a lower likelihood of coronary atherosclerosis and myocardial infarction among cirrhotics. A variety of factors may contribute to this observation.

First, there is a bias when one studies at necropsy two diseases such as cirrhosis and coronary atherosclerosis, both of which can cause premature death, since there will be a negative correlation under these circumstances. Nevertheless, other factors probably contribute significantly to this observation, including the generalized vasodilatation with resultant lower levels of systemic blood pressure seen in cirrhotics compared with controls; the presence of hyperestrogenemia in cirrhotics; the increase in fibrinolytic activity; and the fact that high-density lipoprotein (HDL) cholesterol is significantly raised in alcoholics. In addition, liver disease decreases production of very-low-density lipoprotein (VLDL) by the liver and thus lowers the amount of circulating atherogenic lipoproteins.

Primary biliary cirrhosis, an autoimmune disorder leading to chronic destruction of the intrahepatic bile ducts, results in significant serum lipid abnormalities in most patients. Serum cholesterol levels in particular are likely to be elevated, although triglycerides are often normal or only mildly increased.[28] Large increases in LDL cholesterol are seen, but HDL cholesterol also rises. Xanthomatous skin lesions may be observed; in fact, this chronic progressive cholestatic disease of the liver was originally referred to as "xanthomatous biliary cirrhosis." It is of interest to note, however, that mortality from coronary heart disease among patients with primary biliary cirrhosis is similar to that seen in age- and sex-matched control populations.

ALCOHOL AND THE HEART

Chronic alcohol ingestion can have multiple effects on the cardiovascular system. Epidemiologic studies suggest that low to moderate alcohol intake, in the neighborhood of two drinks daily, can over time actually exert a protective effect against the subsequent development of coronary heart disease.[29] It is likely that the mechanism involved relates to the fact that alcohol can result in a significant increase in HDL cholesterol levels.

At the same time, alcohol has the potential of producing damaging effects on the cardiovascular system. Alcohol has been associated with worsening of arterial hypertension and should be cut back significantly in those patients who present with systemic hypertension.[29] Even more important is the potential damage that alcohol can directly produce on the heart. Myocardial damage can result from chronic excessive alcohol use, leading to the syndrome of chronic dilated congestive cardiomyopathy. Alcoholic cardiomyopathy is a low-output type of heart failure, characterized by physical and laboratory findings similar to those seen in other cases of dilated congestive cardiomyopathy. Of note, however, is the fact that patients who are seen early in the course of alcoholic congestive cardiomyopathy can get significant improvement in cardiac contractility and restoration of competency upon the discontinuance of alcohol. Although abstinence from alcohol consumption is often difficult to accomplish, when achieved, it can produce dramatic changes in the patient's clinical course. We have followed a number of such patients in whom global contractility was moderately to severely depressed as a result of alcoholic cardiopathy; 1 to 2 years later patients may exhibit normal ventricular function by echo-Doppler examination (Fig. 4-2).

Alcohol, along with nutritional factors, is the most common cause of cirrhosis in the United States. Patients with heavy alcoholic intake in whom nutrition has been poorly maintained may demonstrate cirrhotic changes in the liver without apparent myocardial damage clinically. Such patients are likely to present with a hyperkinetic circulatory state, reflecting the generalized vasodilatation accompanying the cirrhotic state. The clinical manifestations of a hyperkinetic circulation in the patient with cirrhosis include palmar erythema, warm extremities, bounding peripheral pulses, and clubbing of the nails. It is of interest that the high-output state seen in patients with Laennec's cirrhosis can usually be reversed, with cardiac output returning into the normal range over time, if the patient stops alcohol intake (Fig. 4-3).

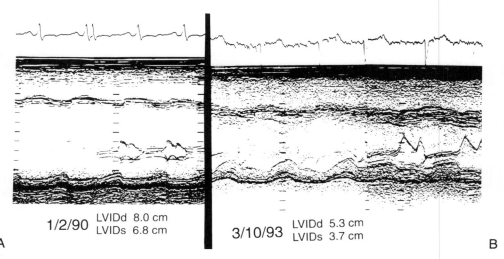

1/2/90   LVIDd 8.0 cm
          LVIDs 6.8 cm

3/10/93   LVIDd 5.3 cm
          LVIDs 3.7 cm

A   B

Fig. 4-2. (**A**) Marked left ventricular dilatation is seen with severely decreased myocardial contractility in a patient with alcoholic cardiomyopathy. The small stroke output is reflected in the poor excursion of the mitral valve. (**B**) The same patient 3 years after cessation of alcohol consumption. The first three beats are below the mitral valve and show the decrease in left ventricular volume and the restoration of normal myocardial contractility. The last two beats are at the mitral valve level and show a normal valve excursion pattern.

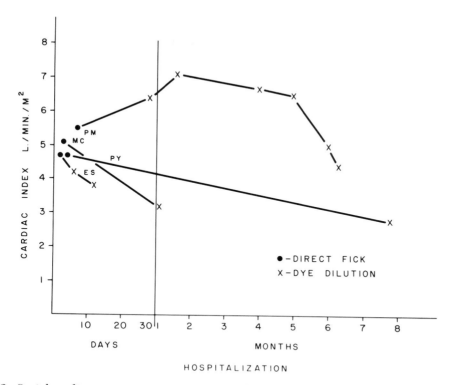

Fig. 4-3. Serial cardiac output measurements are plotted against time on four patients hospitalized with decompensated Laennec's cirrhosis. As compensation was restored, cardiac output fell from initial elevated levels to normal.

A number of patients presenting with alcoholic cirrhosis who do not show evidence of a high-output state probably have a latent cardiomyopathy. It is likely that some degree of impaired myocardial function is masking the otherwise high-output state that would be present. Evidence for this theory is supported by the observation that the infusion of a vasoconstrictor that increases afterload into such patients will result in evidence of impaired left ventricular function, particularly with exercise, even though preinfusion function may be normal.[30] The classic picture of a low-output congestive heart failure state secondary to alcoholic cardiomyopathy is seldom seen in patients who have clinical manifestations of Laennec's cirrhosis. In some, overt fail-

ure may be masked due to chronic afterload reduction resulting from the systemic vasodilatation, which chronically unloads the left ventricle.

Alcoholic cardiomyopathy requires many years of heavy alcohol consumption to develop. If the patient maintains a poor overall nutritional status during years of heavy alcohol consumption, cirrhosis may ensue before sufficient time has elapsed to produce myocardial failure; contrariwise, heavy alcohol intake in a patient with good nutrition over the years may result in an alcoholic cardiomyopathy without detectable clinical or laboratory findings of Laennec's cirrhosis. Most of the patients we see at San Francisco General Hospital have poor dietary habits associated with their heavy alcohol consumption and develop cirrhosis prior to the expected time interval required to develop full-blown and cardiomyopathy. Nevertheless, despite the absence of clinical manifestations of cardiac failure, there will be some amount of damage to the left ventricle that tends to be masked by the vasodilator circulatory state; clinical evidence of LV failure is then not apparent. It must also be noted that the failure to observe more frequent evidence of clinical alcoholic cardiomyopathy in patients with cirrhosis can reflect the fact that when two diseases co-exist (each of which may result in premature death), a negative correlation in their co-existence may be found.

The presence of a hyperkinetic circulatory state, together with evidence of ascites, hydrothorax, and a pericardial effusion, as well as dependent edema, may lead to the erroneous conclusion that one is dealing with high-output heart failure in a patient with alcoholic cirrhosis. The key to the correct interpretation of these findings lies in careful observation of the central venous pressure. Central venous and pulmonary wedge pressures may be minimally elevated, but this will inevitably be modest and reflect the fact that tense ascites with elevation of the diaphragm has increased intrapleural pressure. This leads to a modest 2.0 or 3.0 cm increase in central venous and pulmonary wedge pressures. Central venous pressure never approaches the high levels one sees when a patient presents with ascites due to cardiomyopathy or constrictive pericarditis. Paracentesis and reduction of intra-abdominal pressure will result in a comparable fall in central venous pressure as intrapleural pressure is reduced with descent of the diaphragm.[15] Additional evidence that one is not dealing with heart failure under these circumstances is provided by the failure to hear an S_3 gallop, the absence of pulsus alternans, the lack of pulmonary rales,

and the normal contractility that is generally demonstrated on a resting echocardiographic examination.

Another clinical manifestation of excessive alcohol intake on the heart is the so-called holiday heart syndrome.[31] Patients develop cardiac arrhythmias, most commonly atrial fibrillation (but other atrial and ventricular arrhythmias as well) at the time of, or immediately after, heavy binge drinking. It is likely to occur in patients over a weekend or during the holiday seasons, hence the name "holiday heart." Such patients generally respond to the usual management of atrial fibrillation and do not require chronic suppressive antiarrhythmic therapy or chronic anticoagulant use. The obvious management is a reduction in alcohol intake.

Sudden death accounts for a significant proportion of deaths in alcoholic cirrhosis. It has recently been shown that QT prolongation occurs more frequently in alcoholic cirrhotic patients than in age- and sex-matched controls. When pronounced prolongation of the QT interval is present, it identifies those at risk of sudden death, if excess alcohol consumption continues.[32]

REFERENCES

1. Valla D, Flejou JF, Lebrec D et al: Portal hypertension and ascites in acute hepatitis: clinical hemodynamic and histological correlations. Hepatology 10:482, 1989
2. Gaudin C, Braillon A, Poo JL et al: Plasma catecholamines in patients with presinusoidal portal hypertension: comparison with cirrhotic patients and nonportal hypertensive subjects. Hepatology 13:913, 1991
3. Mastai R, Bosch J, Bruix J et al: Beta-blockade with propranolol and hepatic artery blood flow in patients with cirrhosis. Hepatology 10:269, 1989 or 11:1102, 1990

4. Calabresi P, Abelmann WH: Porto-caval and porto-pulmonary anastomoses in Laennec's cirrhosis and in heart failure. J Clin Invest 36:1257, 1957

5. Berthelot P, Walker JG, Sherlock S et al: Arterial changes in lungs in cirrhosis of the liver—lung spider nevi. N Engl J Med 74:291, 1966

6. Rodman T, Sobel M, Close HP: Arterial oxygen saturation and the ventilation-perfusion of Laennec's cirrhosis. N Engl J Med 73:263, 1960

7. Keys A, Snell A: Respiratory properties of the arterial blood in normal man and in patients with disease of the liver: portion of the oxygen dissociation curve. J Clin Invest 17:59, 1938

8. Hadengue A, Benhayoun MK, Lebrec D, Benhamou JP: Pulmonary hypertension complicating portal hypertension: prevalence and relation to splanchnic hemodynamics. Gastroenterology 100:320, 1991

9. Garcia-Dorado D, Miller DD, Garcia E et al: An epidemic of pulmonary hypertension after toxic rapeseed oil ingestion in Spain. J Am Coll Cardiol 5:1216, 1983

10. Saner J, Gurtner HP, Preisig R, Kupfer A: Polymorphic debrisoquine and mephenytoin hydroxylation in patients with pulmonary hypertension of vascular origin after aminorex fumarate. Eur J Clin Pharmacol 31:437, 1986

11. Kowalski HJ, Abelmann WH: The cardiac output at rest in Laennec's cirrhosis. J Clin Invest 32:1025, 1953

12. Kobayashi A, Katsuta Y, Aramaki T, Hidemasa O: Interrelation between esophageal varices and systemic and hepatic hemodynamics in male patients with compensated cirrhosis. Jpn J Med 30:318, 1991

13. Lewis FW, Adair O, Rector WG, Jr: Arterial vasodilation is not the cause of increased cardiac output in cirrhosis. Gastroenterology 102:1024, 1992

14. Prager MC, Cauldwell CA, Ascher NL et al: Pulmonary hypertension associated with liver disease is not reversible after transplantation. Anesthesiology 77:375, 1992

15. Rapaport E: Cardiopulmonary complications of liver disease. p. 529. In Zakin D, Boyer TD (eds): Hepatology—A Textbook of Liver Disease. WB Saunders, Philadelphia, 1982

16. Abelmann WN, Kowalski HJ, McNeely WF: Hemodynamic responses to exercises in patients with Laennec's cirrhosis. J Clin Invest 34:890, 1955

17. Fernandez-Seara J, Prieto J, Quiroga J et al: System and regional hemodynamics in patients with liver cirrhosis and ascites with and without functional renal failure. Gastroenterology 97:1304, 1989

18. Bradley SE, Ingelfinger TJ, Bradley GP: Hepatic circulation in cirrhosis of the liver. Circulation 5:419, 1952

19. Vallance P, Moncada S: Hyperdynamic circulation in cirrhosis: a role for nitric oxide? Lancet 337:776, 1991

20. Lee SS, Marky J, Mantz J et al: Desensitization of myocardial beta-adrenergic receptors in cirrhotic rats. Hepatology 12:481, 1990

21. Feu F, Bordas JM, Garcia-Pagan JC et al: Double-blind investigation of the effects of propranolol and placebo on the pressure of esophageal varices in patients with portal hypertension. Hepatology 13:917, 1991

22. Garcia-Pagan JC, Navasa M, Bosch J et al: Enhancement of portal pressure reduction by the association of isosorbide-5-mononitrate to propranolol administration in patients with cirrhosis. Hepatology 11:230, 1990

23. Garcia-Pagan JC, Feu F, Bosch J, Rodes J: Propranolol compared with propranolol plus isosorbide-5-mononitrate for portal hypertension in cirrhosis. A randomized controlled study. Ann Intern Med 114:869, 1991

24. del Arbol LR, Garcia-Pagan JC, Feu F et al: Effects of molsidomine, a long acting venous dilator, on portal hypertension: a hemodynamic study in patients with cirrhosis. J Hepatol 13:179, 1991

25. Sirinek KR, Adcock DK, Levine BA: Simultaneous infusion of nitroglycerin and nitroprusside to offset adverse effects of vasopressin during portosystemic shunting. Am J Surg 157:33, 1989

26. Jacoby AG, Weigman MV: Cardiovascular complications of intravenous vaso-

pressin therapy. Focus Crit Care 17:63, 1990

27. Shah A, Variyam E: Pericardial effusion and left ventricular dysfunction associated with ascites secondary to hepatic cirrhosis. Arch Intern Med 148:565, 1988

28. Crippin JS, Lindor KD, Jorgensen R et al: Hypercholesterolemia and atherosclerosis in primary biliary cirrhosis. Hepatology 15:858, 1992

29. Suh I, Shaten BJ, Cutler JA, Kuller LH: Alcohol use and mortality from coronary heart disease: the role of high-density lipoprotein cholesterol. Ann Intern Med 116:881, 1992

30. Limas CJ, Guiha NH, Lekagul O et al: Impaired left ventricular function in alcoholic cirrhosis with ascites. Circulation 49:755, 1974

31. Ettinger PO, Wu CF, De La Cruz C, Jr et al: Arrhythmias and the "holiday heart": alcohol-associated cardiac rhythm disorders. Am Heart J 95:555, 1978

32. Day CP, James OF, Butler T, Campbell RW: QT prolongation and sudden death in patients with alcoholic liver disease. Lancet 341:1423, 1993

5

Endocrine Disorders

Thomas P. Bersot

THYROTOXICOSIS AND CARDIAC DISEASE

Clinical Presentation

Thyrotoxicosis is associated with cardiac manifestations in about 25 to 30 percent of patients. The common cardiac effects include atrial fibrillation, angina pectoris, and congestive heart failure, but mitral valve prolapse and pericarditis are other less common conditions that are also induced by the hyperthyroid state. The diagnosis of thyrotoxicosis in patients with one of these cardiac conditions is usually not difficult, as most patients present with Graves' disease (thyromegaly and exophthalmos). However, in elderly patients these two physical findings may be absent and the usual physical findings may also not be readily apparent (Table 5-1). For this reason, thyrotoxicosis should be excluded in every patient with new onset atrial fibrillation in the absence of any other readily apparent etiology.

Establishing the Diagnosis

A sensitive assay should be employed to determine the serum level of thyroid stimulating hormone (TSH) or thyrotropin.[1] A low value indicating suppression

of TSH secretion should be followed by determination of the serum free thyroxine (FT_4) and triiodothyronine (T_3) levels, which will be elevated in most thyrotoxic patients. However, in a few patients the FT_4 level may be normal and the thyrotoxicity occurs in association with an elevated T_3 concentration alone.

At this point, the evaluation of thyroid disease should turn to identifying the specific cause of hyperthyroidism so that it can be appropriately managed. A convenient way to sort through the diagnostic possibilities is to carry out a study of radioiodine uptake by the thyroid gland. The causes of hyperthyroidism can be categorized according to whether the thyroidal uptake of iodine is increased, as is seen in most hyperthyroid patients, or if it is suppressed. The various causes of thyrotoxicosis, catalogued according to this scheme, are listed in Table 5-2.

Treatment

Hyperthyroidism
In patients with increased values of radioiodine uptake, treatment is designed to inhibit excess thyroid hormone synthesis, in addition to inhibiting peripheral T_4 conversion to T_3 and the peripheral effects of thyroid hormone. First, the patient is started on an antithyroid drug—

Table 5-1. Symptoms and Signs of Hyperthyroidism

Cardiac
  Rhythm (atrial fibrillation, sinus tachycardia, supraventricular tachycardia)
  Blood pressure (widened pulse pressure, systolic hypertension)
  Cardiomegaly
  P_2 enhancement
  Midsystolic click and murmur
  S_3 present
  Pericarditis
  Congestive heart failure
  Dyspnea
Other:
  Heat intolerance
  Fatigue
  Weight loss
  Irritability to psychosis
  Tremor
  Periodic
  Paralysis in Asians
  Hyperphagia
  Increased bowel motility
  Anemia
  Menstrual irregularity
  Thinning of hair
  Hair loss
  Sweating
  Ophthalmopathy in Graves' disease (lid lag, exophthalmos)
  Pretibial myxdema (Graves' disease)

methimazole, 10 mg t.i.d., or propylthiouracil (PTU), 100 mg t.i.d. The use of PTU may be preferred because, unlike methimazole, PTU inhibits the peripheral conversion of T_4 to T_3. If the patient is severely hyperthyroid, inorganic iodine given as supersaturated potassium iodide (SSKI), 5 drops every 6 hours, can be added but should not be started until at least 1 hour after administering the first dose of antithyroid agent. Iodine will enrich glandular thyroid hormone stores unless PTU or methimazole use prevents glandular uptake of iodine. The desired effect of iodide in the hyperthyroid patient is to inhibit the release of T_4 from the gland. Sodium ipodate, 1.0 g daily, in addition to providing iodide, also reduces peripheral conversion of T_4 to T_3. Iodide or sodium ipodate administration should be continued for 3 to 5 days, and can then be stopped. Antithyroid therapy with PTU or methimazole should be continued until the patient is euthyroid, which usually requires 4 to 8 weeks. Most patients relapse if definitive therapy by radioiodine ablation is not undertaken. In many cases, especially patients with cardiac disease, it is advisable to ablate the thyroid after the first course of antithyroid therapy, to prevent redevelopment of the hyperthyroid state. When the patient is euthyroid, the antithyroid drug is stopped, and after 3 to 5 days, a test dose of radioiodine is administered to assess the glandular uptake of iodine. A therapeutic dose can then be calculated and administered with resumption of antithyroid medication after 1 week to maintain the euthyroid status, until radioiodine ablation is effective. Several weeks later, the antithyroid medication can be stopped as well, but the patient should be observed to ensure that the gland was ablated. Agranulocytosis is a rare but serious complication of PTU and methimazole. Patients should be advised to report symptoms of infection immediately. Severe liver toxicity is another rare side effect for which patients

Table 5-2. Causes of Thyrotoxicosis

Radioiodine Uptake Enhanced
  Graves' disease
  Toxic adenoma
  Multimodular toxic goiter
  TSH overproduction (by pituitary or other tumors)
Radioiodine Uptake Reduced
  Thyroiditis
  Excessive thyroid hormone ingestion
  Excessive iodine ingestion
  Metastatic thyroid follicular cancer and struma ovarii

should be monitored. Many patients become hypothyroid after radioiodine therapy. They should be informed of the likelihood of this possibility, and the TSH should be monitored periodically for this development.

Patients who develop thyrotoxicosis from causes associated with reduced radioiodine uptake should be questioned to ascertain whether ingestion of excess thyroid hormone or iodide has occurred. Hyperthyroidism associated with thyroiditis is usually not severe and is not a cause of significant cardiac disease.

Cardiac Conditions

Angina pectoris precipitated or aggravated by thyrotoxicosis requires treatment to restore the euthyroid state as rapidly as possible.[2] Propranolol, an antithyroid drug, and inorganic iodide should be instituted as described above to afford the maximal treatment benefit. Atrial fibrillation is associated with a rapid ventricular response in hyperthyroidism. The ventricular rate can be managed with a nonspecific β-blocking agent such as propranolol or with a calcium channel blocker. Propanolol has an additional advantage in that it reduces conversion of T_4 to T_3 in peripheral tissues, but its use may be contraindicated in patients with bronchospastic disease, or congestive heart failure that antedated the onset of thyrotoxicosis. Control of the hyperthyroidism is essential before attempting cardioversion of patients in atrial fibrillation. Those without a prior history of heart disease often revert to sinus rhythm spontaneously within 2 months of achieving euthyroid status. Patients with thyrotoxic congestive heart failure require rate control by a β-blocker, or a calcium channel blocker, and diuresis since they are volume overloaded. Those patients in atrial fibrillation are at increased risk of thromboembolization and should be considered for warfarin therapy if there are no contraindications.

HYPOTHYROIDISM

Clinical Presentation

The development of clinically significant heart disease in hypothyroidism lags behind the onset of the other symptoms and signs of hypothyroidism (Table 5-3). The predominant cardiac abnormality is congestive heart failure, and it tends to occur more commonly in patients with underlying heart disease.[3] The physical findings may include bradycardia, and also hypertension that is associated with increased peripheral resistance. However, in the patient with congestive heart failure, hypotension is more likely. Pleural effusions may be present and cardiac enlargement occurs due to true cardiomegaly or to pericardial effusion. The heart sounds may be distant on auscultation.

The electrocardiogram may demonstrate bradycardia and QT interval prolongation. Conduction defects have also been described. There is often low voltage in all leads, as well as diffuse T-wave flattening. The T-wave effects may be due to the presence of a pericardial effu-

Table 5-3. Symptoms and Signs of Hypothyroidism

Symptoms	Signs
Fatigue	Bradycardia
Cold intolerance	Hoarseness
Dry skin	Dry skin
Constipation	Myxedema
Irregular menses	Delayed relaxation of
Depression	reflexes
Weight gain	Goiter
Hoarseness	

sion and may improve following pericardiocentesis. Removal of this proteinaceous fluid is rarely required, however, because it accumulates slowly and usually is not associated with any hemodynamic compromise. After thyroxine replacement is adequate, the effusion requires months to resolve.

There is a matched decrease in cardiac output and peripheral tissue oxygen demand that usually does not cause cardiac symptoms unless there is severe myxedema or additional preexisting cardiac pathology. Unlike left-sided congestive heart failure, the pulmonary artery wedge and pulmonary artery pressures are normal in congestive heart failure associated with hypothyroidism. Furthermore, there is no response to cardiac glycosides and diuretics in hypothyroid-induced congestive heart failure. It is also worth noting that creatine kinase concentrations may be increased in hypothyroid patients, and this increase may be associated with slight MB band increments that are unrelated to ischemic heart disease.

Diagnosis

The causes of hypothyroidism may be separated according to whether there is primary failure of the thyroid gland (due to glandular destruction [most common] or defects in thyroxine synthesis), or secondary failure due to hypothalamic or pituitary disease.[4] In the case of primary failure, TSH values are high, whereas secondary failure is associated with low TSH values. Glandular destruction occurs most commonly as a consequence of autoimmune thyroiditis, which may result in a goitrous or atrophic gland. A small proportion of patients with autoimmune thyroiditis have other endocrine autoimmune disorders that should be considered whenever a patient presents with hypothyroidism, including diabetes

mellitus and adrenal insufficiency. Parathyroid gland and ovarian failure have also been reported. Pernicious anemia may also occur in association with hypothyroidism.

Treatment

Congestive heart failure in the myxedematous patient can be treated effectively only by thyroid hormone replacement. To preclude precipitation of a coronary event, a thyroxine dose of 25 μg/day should be the initial dose, and 12.5 μg/day increments in the total dose may be made at 4- to 6-week intervals. Although rare, precipitation of angina pectoris has been reported even in the setting of gradual thyroxine replacement. Propranolol and calcium entry blockers may be used, but caution should be exercised in the hypothyroid patient with congestive heart failure who develops angina pectoris.

ACROMEGALY

Acromegaly was first described and associated with pituitary adenomas in the late nineteenth century. It is due to excess growth hormone (GH) production by pituitary adenomas in almost all cases, although a few cases of tumors producing growth hormone-releasing hormone (GHRH) and a single case of ectopic GH production by a pancreatic islet cell tumor have been described. The incidence of acromegaly has been estimated to be 3 cases per 1 million individuals per year. The mutation(s) that account for acromegaly are being defined, and their occurrence appears to be primarily sporadic, but there are also rare familial syndromes of dominantly inherited acromegaly occurring alone or as part of multiple endocrine tumor syndromes.[5,6] The most common of these syndromes is multiple endocrine neoplasia (MEN) type 1. A rarer syndrome of which cardiologists should be aware includes cardiac and cutaneous myxomas, spotty pigmentation, and acromegaly or other endocrine tumors.[7]

Clinical Features

The primary features of acromegaly can be divided into those that are due to pituitary mass effects and those that are a consequence of unregulated GH hypersecretion. Mass lesion effects include headache and visual abnormalities such as field defects or diplopia. Pituitary compression may also compromise secretion of gonadotropins, thyroid stimulating hormone, or ACTH, thus causing secondary failure of the target organs of these trophic hormones. The hypersecretion of GH increases the production of the insulin-like growth factor known as *somatomedin C*. It is somatomedin C that causes the cartilage and bone changes that are typically seen in acromegalics. Most cases occur in adults after cessation of growth. In adult-onset patients there is more thickening of bones and soft tissues than longitudinal bone growth. This results in thickened and coarsened features (enlarged fingers so that rings and gloves no longer fit, enlarged feet requiring larger shoe sizes, and enlarged skulls).

Presenting Symptoms

Discovery of acromegaly occurs most frequently by chance (about 40 percent of all cases) when a physician or dentist becomes suspicious on the basis of physical or x-ray signs of the disease. The most common presenting complaints include menstrual irregularity in women (13 percent), appearance and/or growth changes (11 percent), headaches (8 percent), carpal tunnel syndrome or paresthesias (6 percent), and diabetes mellitus (5 percent). Cardiovascular disease is the cause of presentation in about 4 percent.[8]

Mortality

Mortality is increased from two- to fivefold in acromegalics. Causes include cardiovascular disease in men, cerebrovascular disease in women, respiratory disease, and malignancy. Overt diabetes mellitus has also been observed to be associated with a substantial increase in mortality. Available evidence suggests that treatment by irradiation and/or transsphenoidal surgery reduces mortality. Observations regarding the prevalence of respiratory disease have not been reported consistently. When they are, upper respiratory obstruction is common due to enlargement of the tongue, jaw, and epiglottis. The obstructed airway causes sleep apnea, but sleep apnea is also associated with central nervous system dysfunction that appears to correlate directly with somatostatin concentrations. Treatment of acromegaly improves sleep apnea in most patients.

Carcinoma of the colon and adenematous polyps are neoplasms that have been clearly documented to occur more frequently in acromegalics than in the general population.[9] There is a three- to eight-fold excess risk, and the risk is especially great in male acromegalics who are over age 50, have three or more skin tags, or have a family history of colon cancer.

Related Cardiovascular Disease

Hypertension occurs in one-third of patients with acromegaly, and is reported to improve following eradication of the pituitary tumor. Octreotide, an antagonist of somatomedin C, also has been reported to reduce blood pressure. Plasma renin activity and aldosterone concentrations are low, but total body sodium content is increased. The increased sodium content is thought to be due to GH-mediated enhancement of renal tubular sodium reabsorption.

Clinically recognizable heart disease syndromes commonly found in acromegalics include coronary heart disease, congestive heart failure, and arrhythmias. About 20 percent of acromegalics are affected. The pathogenesis of these syndromes is complex, since risk factors such as diabetes mellitus and dyslipidemia occur more frequently, but it is likely that there is a fundamental effect of the acromegalic state upon cardiac muscle itself. Cardiac hypertrophy has been observed in the hearts of patients at autopsy, and echocardiographic studies suggest that hypertrophy and increased ventricular mass are common. Diastolic dysfunction has been noted in acromegalics who were free of hypertension and coronary heart disease, suggesting that the acromegalic state itself causes cardiac pathology.[10] In addition to hypertrophy noted at autopsy, mononuclear cell infiltrates and interstitial fibrosis also have been noted. However, the precise pathophysiology of acromegalic cardiac disease requires further delineation.

Diagnosis

Morning Blood Growth Hormone Concentration

Secretion of GH is pulsatile throughout the day and single measurements in confirmed acromegalics may give results in the normal range.[11] In most assays, the basal value for normal individuals is below 2 μg/L, a value of 2 to 5 μg/L is likely to be normal, a value of 5 to 10 μg/L is suspicious for acromegaly, and a value that exceeds 10 μg/L is highly suggestive of acromegaly. However a variety of stresses (emotional and physical) can increase GH secretion, and these circumstances should be considered when evaluating GH levels.

Oral Glucose Loading

Due to the difficulties associated with interpreting basal values, the preferred method is to measure GH following the ingestion of a glucose load. The patient fasts overnight, and an indwelling cannula is inserted 1 hour before a basal sample is obtained at −30 minutes. After 30 minutes, the glucose is consumed and blood samples to measure GH and glucose levels are obtained at 30, 60, 90, 120, and 180 minutes after glucose ingestion. Reduction of GH concentration below 20 μg/L does not occur in patients with acromegaly as it does in patients without this condition.

Somatomedin C

The measurement of somatomedin C (SmC) is more reliable than single measurements of basal GH. The synthesis and secretion of SmC is under the control of GH, and the SmC level is indicative of the amount of GH secreted in the preceding 24 hours. There are several kits commercially available, and normal ranges vary depending on the kit and the standards employed. The SmC level is elevated only in active disease, and so it can be used to monitor treated patients for recurrences.

Growth Hormone Releasing Hormone

Since only a handful of acromegalic patients have been reported with GHRH-producing neoplasms, routine GHRH determination does not appear to be warranted. However, in the acromegalic who has no demonstrable pituitary pathology, it is useful to measure the GHRH level. If the GHRH producing tumor is outside of the central nervous system (CNS), then elevated blood GHRH levels can be detected. However, tumors producing GHRH within the CNS do not release GHRH into the blood, so that peripheral blood concentrations are not affected.

Other Tests
A variety of other tests exist that can be used to support the diagnosis of acromegaly when the results of the tests described above are equivocal. These include determination of the GH response to thyrotropin-releasing hormone, l-dopamine, bromocriptine, l-arginine, somatostatin, luteinizing hormone, and insulin-induced hypoglycemia.[11]

Cardiovascular Evaluation
Since CHD, hypertension, congestive heart failure, and arrhythmias are the most common causes of heart disease in acromegalics, each patient should be specifically evaluated to exclude these problems. If an acromegalic patient has a heart murmur, cutaneous myxoma(s), lentigines, or blue nevi, then echocardiographic evaluation should be done to exclude a cardiac myxoma. Treatment of the underlying acromegaly ameliorates the cardiac pathology in most cases.

HYPERLIPIDEMIA AND ATHEROSCLEROSIS

Atherogenic Lipoproteins

There are four dyslipidemic states that account for most lipid, related atherosclerosis. Of these four, two (elevated low density lipoprotein and reduced high-density lipoprotein concentrations) are readily identifiable. The other two are not because there are no reliable tests to measure the concentrations of remnant lipoproteins and lipoprotein (a), or Lp(a).

Elevations of Low-Density Lipoprotein
Low-density lipoprotein (LDL) is the most cholesterol-enriched lipoprotein in the plasma, and high concentrations of LDL are associated with the development of atherosclerosis.[12] Certain dietary saturated fats, dietary cholesterol, and inherited disorders of LDL metabolism cause LDL concentrations to be elevated by a variety of mechanisms. Furthermore, it is likely that LDL must undergo modification in the arterial wall for this lipoprotein to stimulate atherogenesis. One of the modifications may be oxidation, but others have also been suggested.

Elevations of Very Low-Density Lipoprotein and Remnant Lipoproteins
Very low-density lipoproteins (VLDLs) are triglyceride-rich lipoproteins, but also contain a complement of cholesterol. The ratio of triglyceride to cholesterol in VLDL is approximately 5 : 1. Remnant lipoproteins are the catabolites of VLDL and of chylomicrons from which much of the triglyceride has been removed. As a consequence, the relative content of cholesterol in the remnants is much greater than that in native chylomicrons or native VLDL. Remnants occur in the plasma of all individuals during the normal course of the metabolism of chylomicrons and VLDL. If there is arterial wall damage such as that which occurs in smokers, hypertensive individuals, or diabetics, then there is an increased flux of remnant lipoproteins into the arterial wall. Remnant lipoproteins, unlike LDL, do not have to undergo modification in the arterial wall

to stimulate atherogenesis.[13] This is because the macrophage, the key cell involved in atherogenesis, has cell surface receptors that recognize and initiate uptake of remnant lipoproteins. On the other hand, the macrophage has few functioning receptors that recognize unmodified LDL. Remnant lipoproteins also accumulate in the plasma of patients who are homozygous for mutations of apolipoprotein E, which leads to retarded clearance of remnant lipoproteins. Normally, remnant lipoproteins are produced in peripheral tissues as lipoprotein lipase removes triglycerides from chylomicrons and VLDL. The remnant lipoproteins then detach from the capillary endothelial surface following the removal of the triglyceride and circulate back to the liver. There apolipoprotein E serves as the ligand that modulates the uptake of remnant lipoproteins by liver lipoprotein receptors. Patients with mutations in apoprotein E that affect the binding of apo E to hepatic receptors develop increased concentrations of remnant lipoproteins due to their reduced clearance. These high concentrations of remnant lipoproteins cause accelerated atherosclerosis.

Reduced High-Density Lipoprotein Concentrations

The concentration of high-density lipoproteins (HDL) is inversely correlated with atherosclerosis risk.[14] There are two groups of patients who develop premature atherosclerosis associated with low HDL concentrations. The first has isolated low HDL concentrations, usually in the range of 10 to 30 mg/dl of HDL cholesterol, and a normal or only slightly elevated total cholesterol concentration. The second includes those patients who are hypertriglyceridemic. There is an inverse relationship between plasma triglyceride concentrations and HDL concentrations. Most patients with low HDL and high triglycerides are at risk of developing premature atherosclerosis. The risk is most likely not related to the hypertriglyceridemia, but to the low HDL concentrations. The mechanism of accelerated atherogenesis in patients with low HDL concentrations is not well understood. This is because the precise mechanism by which HDL normally functions is poorly understood. It is hypothesized that HDL removes cholesterol from tissues and that individuals with low HDL concentrations have an impaired ability to affect this so-called reverse cholesterol transport. Confounding the HDL and atherosclerosis story are the rare patients who have mutations of the major HDL apoprotein, apolipoprotein A-I. Patients who are homozygous for mutations of the A-I apoprotein gene usually have very low levels of HDL cholesterol (below 10 mg/dl), but surprisingly are not at risk of developing premature atherosclerosis.

Elevated Lp(a) Concentrations

Lipoprotein (a) was discovered approximately 30 years ago, but only in the last 8 years have we begun to understand its role in atherogenesis.[15] Some studies suggest that high concentrations of Lp(a) are associated with increased risk of developing coronary artery disease. By and large, this risk occurs only in those patients with additional coronary disease risk factors.[15a] The Lp(a) molecule is identical to LDL except for an additional protein component that is designated as apoprotein (a). This apoprotein is linked to the apo B-100 apoprotein of LDL by a single disulfide bond. The apo(a) does not interact with the lipid of LDL. It is exposed entirely to the aqueous plasma environment in which the Lp(a) circulates. The atherogenic nature of apo(a) is due to the fact that it bears structural similarity to plasminogen and competes with plasminogen for binding at sites where thrombus formation occurs. In essence, apo(a) appears to be a competitive inhibitor of plasmin-mediated thrombolysis.

Classifying Hyperlipidemia

A simple system of classifying hyperlipidemia for the purposes of diagnosing familial disorders and treatment is based on the fasting triglyceride concentration and cholesterol concentrations. Patients who have elevated cholesterol levels only, or who have elevations of both cholesterol and triglycerides but in whom the cholesterol value exceeds the triglyceride value, may be considered as having a "cholesterol problem." Conversely, those with hypertriglyceridemia alone, or those in whom an elevated fasting triglyceride concentration exceeds the cholesterol concentration, may be considered as having a "triglyceride problem." Listed in Table 5-4 are the inherited disorders associated with both cholesterol and triglyceride problems.

DISORDERS ASSOCIATED WITH HYPERCHOLESTEROLEMIA

Familial Hypercholesterolemia

Familial hypercholesterolemia is one of the more common genetic disorders occurring in humans. The prevalence of individuals who are heterozygous is approximately 1 in 500. Mutations in the gene for the LDL receptor protein account for this disorder. About 150 separate mutations have been described, but the patients are phenotypically similar.[16]

The disorder is inherited as an autosomal dominant trait.

The patients with the heterozygous form have cholesterol concentrations that are two- to three-fold elevated (usually 300 to 400 mg/dl), and they are hypercholesterolemic at the time of birth. In fact, a cord blood cholesterol that exceeds 93 mg/dl identifies affected infants at birth.[17]

Patients who are heterozygous develop tendon xanthomas. These are first noted as Achilles' tendon thickening and subsequently as tendon xanthomas of the extensor tendons of the hands. Tendon xanthomas are specific for patients who have familial hypercholesterolemia or familial defective apo B-100. Corneal arcus that develops under the age of 40 years is often associated with hypercholesterolemia, but does not indicate any particular specific inherited disorder. Coronary heart disease is common in heterozygous familial hypercholesterolemia patients. The disorder accounts for 5 percent of patients with coronary heart disease who present below the age of 60.

Those patients who are homozygous occur with a prevalence of 1 in 1,000,000. These patients have few, if any, functioning LDL receptors because there are mutations of both alleles of the LDL receptor protein gene. The children are born with cholesterol levels that approach 1,000 mg/dl, often develop coronary artery disease before the age of 10, and are usually dead before the age of 20, unless their diagnosis is recognized early and they are treated appropriately. The patients benefit little, if at all, from drugs that lower cholesterol concentrations, because most of these drugs depend on the upregulation of at least one allele of a normal LDL receptor gene. As a consequence, these patients must be treated by either chronic plasma exchange or a liver transplant that supplies them with a sufficient number of normally

Table 5-4. Inherited Disorders of Plasma Lipid Metabolism

Disorders	Mutation	Cholesterol Level	Triglyceride Level	Premature Vascular Disease	Xanthomas
Cholesterol Disorders					
Familial hypercholesterolemia	LDL receptor	250–500	<200	Yes	T
Familial defective apolipoprotein B-100	Apo B-100	250–400	<200	Yes	T
Familial combined hyperlipidemia	Unknown	250–350	Normal to slightly increased	Yes	
Familial low HDL	Unknown	170–250	<200	Yes	
Triglyceride Disorders:					
Familial hypertriglyceridemia	Unknown	200–300	300–500	Yes	
Familial combined hyperlipidemia	Unknown	200–300	300–1000	Yes	
Familial type III hyperlipoproteinemia (primary dysbetalipoproteinemia)	Apo E	300–500	300–500	Yes	P,TE
Chylomicronemia syndrome					
Lipoprotein lipase mutations	LPL	300–600	>1,000	No	E
Apolipoprotein C-II mutations	Apo C-II	300–600	>1,000	No	E

Abbreviations: T, tendon; P, planar; TE, tuberoeruptive; E, eruptive.

functioning LDL receptors to nearly normalize their blood cholesterol concentrations.

Familial Defective Apolipoprotein B-100

Patients with familial defective apolipoprotein B-100 have normally functioning LDL receptors but have a mutation in the apo B-100 gene, which creates an apo B-100 protein that fails to bind to the LDL receptor.[18] To date, only heterozygous individuals have been identified. The prevalence of familial defective apo B-100 is approximately 1 in 700 in Caucasian individuals.[19] These patients are also hypercholesterolemic at birth, but the cholesterol concentrations in childhood are not as severely elevated as in individuals with familial hypercholesterolemia. Tendon xanthomas occur, but usually develop later in life than in patients with familial hypercholesterolemia. There is also a predilection for the development of premature coronary artery disease.

Treatment of patients with familial defective apo B-100 can be done with reductase inhibitors and bile acid sequestrants that increase the hepatic expression of LDL receptors. However, there is speculation that increasing the number of LDL receptors in these heterozygous patients increases clearance of only their normal LDL. As a consequence, it may be that the total cholesterol diminishes due to a decrease in normal LDL, and there is only minimal if any reduction in the concentration of LDL with the defective apo B-100. Further study of these patients is required to determine the optimal drug treatment regimen for this type of hypercholesterolemia.

Familial Combined Hyperlipidemia

Patients with familial combined hyperlipidemia may have elevated levels of LDL, elevated levels of VLDL and LDL, or elevation in the concentrations of chylomicrons and VLDL.[20] Familial combined hyperlipidemia is one of the more common lipid disorders in patients with premature coronary heart disease. Approximately 10 percent of patients with premature coronary heart disease are affected.[21] Patients who have elevated LDL levels in association with familial combined hyperlipidemia do not have tendon xanthomas, which discriminates them from patients with familial hypercholesterolemia or familial defective apo B-100. Usually the hypercholesterolemia is not as severe as in familial hypercholesterolemia or familial defective apo B-100, and patients do not actually develop hypercholesterolemia until the third decade of life. Making a diagnosis of familial combined hyperlipidemia requires plasma sampling of a large number of family members in a kindred. Identifying the various lipoprotein abnormalities in different individuals within the same kindred establishes the diagnosis of this disorder. However, establishing the diagnosis is not a prerequisite for successfully treating these patients. They can be treated with the same diet and drug regimens used in treating patients with familial hypercholesterolemia.

Polygenic Hypercholesterolemia

Patients with polygenic hypercholesterolemia are hyperlipidemic because of the combined effects of several different genes that impact upon blood cholesterol concentrations.[20] Not all of these genetic factors have been identified, but responsiveness to dietary saturated fat and cholesterol is probably one of the genetic factors involved. Since the disorder is polygenic in nature, there is no bimodal distribution of blood cholesterol concentrations within family members and less than 10 percent of first-degree relatives have elevated LDL levels. There are no characteristic physical findings that allow one to assign this diagnosis either. Treatment of these patients is similar to that of patients with familial hypercholesterolemia.

DISORDERS ASSOCIATED WITH HYPERTRIGLYCERIDEMIA

Familial Hypertriglyceridemia

Patients with familial hypertriglyceridemia have triglyceride concentrations that rarely exceed 500 mg/dl; in their kindred, the only lipoprotein abnormality is elevation of VLDL concentrations. Although hypertriglyceridemia characterizes this disorder, it is the hypercholesterolemia and usually associated low HDL concentrations that place familial hypertriglyceridemia patients at risk of developing coronary artery disease.[21] The disorder is inherited as an autosomal dominant trait, but the underlying pathophysiology is not understood.

Familial Combined Hyperlipidemia

As described in the section on cholesterol disorders, familial combined hyperlipidemia patients may present with elevations of VLDL alone or with elevated chylomicron and VLDL concentrations, both of which produce hypertriglyceridemia. As in familial hypertriglyceridemia, patients are at risk of developing accelerated coronary artery disease due to elevated cholesterol levels and reduced HDL levels. Hypertriglyceridemia can be detected in affected patients during childhood, although the degree of hypertriglyceridemia is not striking.[22] Diabetes mellitus and gout occur in association with this disorder, but the pathophysiology of the relationship between blood lipids, glucose metabolism, and uric acid metabolism is not understood.

Chylomicronemia Syndrome

Patients with chylomicronemia syndrome are a heterogeneous group. There are rare individuals who are homozygous for mutations of the lipoprotein lipase gene or the apolipoprotein C-II gene. These patients develop severe hypertriglyceridemia in childhood and pancreatitis. There is no risk of developing accelerated atherosclerosis, although pancreatitis in these patients is often life-threatening. Treatment requires restriction of fat in the diet, often to 20 g/day or less.

Severe hypertriglyceridemia in association with chylomicronemia occurs more commonly in patients who are affected by familial combined hyperlipidemia or familial hypertriglyceridemia in association with a secondary cause of hypertriglyceridemia. These secondary conditions include obesity, diabetes mellitus, hypothyroidism, nephrotic syndrome, and other less common disorders.[23] These individuals should also be treated with fat restriction, but weight reduction and management of diabetes mellitus is also useful. Treatment of the cause of secondary hypertriglyceridemia is mandatory.

Type III Hyperlipoproteinemia

Type III hyperlipoproteinemia is due to one of several mutations in the gene for apolipoprotein E.[24] Type III patients with the most common mutation of apo E must be homozygous for the hyperlipidemia to develop. This mutation is characterized by a substitution of cysteine for arginine at position 158 of the apo E molecule, which contains 299 amino acids. Approximately 1 percent of the population is homozygous for this mutation although only one-tenth of 1 percent actually develop hyperlipidemia. Thus, additional factors are required for patients to develop type III hyperlipoproteinemia in addition to the mutation of apoprotein E. These additional factors include the development of obesity, diabetes mellitus, menopause, and hypothyroidism. Patients usually do not become hyperlipidemic until adulthood. The mutation in apo E affects the clearance of remnants of VLDL and chylomicrons, and is associated with nearly equal elevations of the triglyceride and cholesterol concentrations in the range of 400 to 600 mg/dl. These patients often have unusual xanthomas that are pathognomonic of type III hyperlipoproteinemia. These include planar xanthomas of the palmar creases and tuberoeruptive xanthomas of the extensor surfaces of the forearm near the elbow or of the knees. The diagnosis is established by determining the apoprotein E genotype and quantitating the amount of cholesterol in the VLDL fraction directly by ultracentrifugation. Patients are easily treated if they can maintain a normal weight and avoid alcohol. Niacin and gemfibrozil are also effective in normalizing the lipids of these patients

who are at increased risk of developing premature atherosclerosis.

Evaluation of Patients for Hyperlipidemia

For screening purposes, a nonfasting blood sample can be obtained and the total cholesterol concentration and HDL cholesterol concentration determined. At the same time, the patient's risk factor profile should be assessed (Table 5-5). Further testing including assessment of the LDL cholesterol concentration should be carried out under three circumstances: (1) if the screening HDL cholesterol is below 35 mg/dl, (2) if the total cholesterol exceeds 240 mg/dl, or (3) if the total cholesterol is between 200 and 240 mg/dl and the patient has two additional coronary artery disease risk factors (Table 5-6). Values for normal plasma, total cholesterol, and triglycerides are shown in Table 5-6. At this point, secondary causes of hyperlipidemia should be excluded as well (Table 5-7). Treatment recommendations based on LDL choles-

Table 5-5. Risk Factors for Coronary Heart Disease

Positive
  Hypercholesterolemia
  Reduced high-density lipoprotein cholesterol (HDL) level (<35 mg/dl)
  Hypertension
  Age (men ≥45; women ≥55 or premature menopause without hormone replacement)
  Cigarette smoking
  Diabetes mellitus
  Family history of coronary artery disease (CHD)—MI, sudden death, or other ischemic vascular disease in a male parent or sib <55 years old, or in a female parent or sib <65 years old
Negative
  High HDL cholesterol level (≥60 mg/dl)

Table 5-6. Recommended Values for Plasma Lipid Concentrations

Age (yr)	Lipid	Desirable (% tile) (mg/dl)	Borderline (mg/dl)	High (% tile) (mg/dl)
2–19	Cholesterol	<170 (75th)	170–199	>200 (95th)
All adults	Cholesterol	<200 (50th)	200–239	>240 (80th)
All adults	Triglycerides	<200	200–400	>400

terol levels are shown in Table 5-8. It is important to emphasize that the treatment goal for patients with established ischemic vascular disease of any sort is to reduce the LDL cholesterol below 100 mg/dl.

Dietary Treatment of Hyperlipidemia

For all patients, diet therapy is essential, and there are two diets recommended for this purpose. The less stringent Step 1 diet is described in Table 5-9. Further degrees of total and saturated fat restriction require the involvement of a dietitian. If the treatment goals are not met with diet therapy alone, then drug treat- ment is initiated according to the scheme shown in Table 5-8. For patients who are hypertriglyceridemic, alcohol restriction, total fat restriction, and calorie restriction are also important.

Drug Treatment of Hyperlipidemia

Drugs for patients with hypercholesterolemia include niacin, bile acid sequestrants (resins), and reductase inhibitors (statins).

Niacin
Niacin reduces LDL concentrations because of an inhibition of VLDL synthesis in the liver. It is the most effective drug

Table 5-7. Causes of Secondary Forms of Hyperlipidemia Listed in Terms of the Predominant Lipoprotein Abnormality

Elevated Plasma Lipoprotein	Underlying Disorders
Chylomicrons	Systemic lupus erythematosus, multiple myeloma, and other dysglobulinemias
LDL	Hypothyroidism, nephrotic syndrome, hepatoma, Cushing's syndrome, acute intermittent porphyria, dysglobulinemias
LDL + VLDL	Nephrotic syndrome, contraceptive steroids, dysglobulinemias
β-VLDL	Hypothyroidism, systemic lupus erythematosus, multiple myeloma
VLDL	Uremia, renal transplantation, renal dialysis, alcoholic hyperlipidemia lipodystrophy, hypopituitarism, glycogen storage disease (type I), contraceptive steroids, dysglobulinemias, nephrotic syndrome
VLDL + Chylomicrons	Insulin-dependent diabetes mellitus, contraceptive steroids, alcoholic hyperlipidemia, glycogen storage disease (type I), nephrotic syndrome
Lipoprotein X	Biliary cirrhosis, other causes of obstructive jaundice

Table 5-8. Treatment in Adults Based on LDL Cholesterol

Treatment	Initiation Level (mg/dl)	Goal (mg/dl)
Diet		
Without CHD or 2 other risk factors	>160	<160
Without CHD plus 2 other risk factors	>130	<130
With CHD, PVD or CVD	>100	<100
Drugs		
Men below 35 and women, premenopausal		
No CHD, 1 or less risk factors	190–220	<160
No CHD, 2 or more risk factors	>190	<160
Men over 35 and women, postmenopausal		
No CHD, 1 or less risk factors	>190	<160
No CHD, 2 or more risk factors	>160	<130
Ischemic Vascular Disease	>130	<100

available for reducing the synthesis of VLDL, and hence LDL.

Niacin is a highly effective drug for both hypercholesterolemia and hypertriglyceridemia. In addition, it is the most effective drug available for raising HDL concentrations and reducing the

Table 5-9. Step 1 Dietary Therapy of High Blood Cholesterol

1. Calorie restriction depending on the degree of obesity
2. Alcohol restriction is usually necessary in patients with elevated triglyceride concentrations
3. Distribution of calories:
   20% Protein
   30% Fat:
   Saturated, <10% of total calories
   Monounsaturated, 10–15% of total calories
   Polyunsaturated, up to 10% of total calories
   50% Carbohydrate (complex carbohydrate preferred)
4. Cholesterol content: 250 mg/day or less
5. Salt restriction: as needed for co-existing conditions

concentration of Lp(a). Due to side effects, compliance with niacin use by patients requires extra effort on the part of physicians or their staff persons. These side effects include flushing with a sensation of intense warmth over the blush areas of the body. There can be associated pruritis, nausea, and dyspeptic symptoms as well. It is important to reassure patients, who develop any of these side effects, that these symptoms do not indicate a medically serious problem. The side effects can be lessened if patients are started on a low dose (100 mg b.i.d.), with each dose being taken prior to a meal. Each dose is then increased by 100 mg every 4 to 5 days until the desired therapeutic level is reached. If patients experience the side effects described above, despite a gradual increase in the dose, then an aspirin administered 30 minutes prior to each dose helps diminish or eliminate them. Patients also should be reassured that after they reach their final dose the incidence and severity of side effects lessen and that after 4 to 8 weeks they will rarely experience any of these problems. Medically significant side effects include elevation of the blood glucose concentration, hyperuricemia, and elevated hepatic transaminases. It is often necessary for patients to stop drinking alcohol if transaminases increase. There have been reports of liver failure in patients using sustained release preparations of niacin and, for this reason, this type of niacin is not recommended.

Resins

Bile acid sequestrants (resins) are nonabsorbable and therefore quite safe agents that reduce blood cholesterol concentrations by interrupting the enterohepatic circulation of bile acids. The decreased reabsorption of bile acids causes an increased demand for cholesterol within the liver that is met by enhancement of LDL receptor expression and increased clearance of LDL from the blood. Full doses of bile acid sequestrants are difficult for patients to comply with. However, reduced dosages (up to two-thirds of the maximum dose) are well tolerated, and when used in combination with niacin or reductase inhibitors, the resins are quite effective in reducing blood cholesterol concentrations. In fact, reductions of 50 percent can be achieved by the dual use of either niacin plus sequestrant or reductase inhibitors plus sequestrant. There are few clinically significant side effects associated with bile acid-sequestrant use other than the absorption of other drugs by the resins in the gut. As a consequence, patients should be instructed to take their other medications 1 hour before or 3 hours after taking a dose of bile acid sequestrant.

Statins

Reductase inhibitors (statins) are the most effective single agents for reducing blood cholesterol concentrations. These drugs inhibit cholesterol biosynthesis and cause an increased expression of LDL receptors on the cell surface. This effect is particularly notable in the liver, which is responsible for the clearance of two-thirds of the LDL from the blood. Up to 40 percent reduction in blood LDL concentrations can be achieved with maximal doses of reductase inhibitors. However, about two-thirds of the cholesterol-lowering effect of these drugs can be seen when employing doses that are no more than 25 percent of the maximally prescribed dosages. Based on cost considerations alone, it then makes sense to use low-dose statin in combination with a resin that easily achieves a 50 percent reduction in blood cholesterol levels. Up to 60 to 70 percent reductions in LDL cholesterol can be achieved by the combination of low dose niacin (1 to 2 g daily) plus resin and statin. Caution with regard to the reductase inhibitors primarily relates to the development of a myopathy that has been reported to cause myoglobinuria and renal failure. However, this myopathy occurs most commonly in association with the concomitant treatment with cyclosporine, niacin, gemfibrozil, or certain antibiotics in seriously ill patients. In patients with normal renal function, limiting the dose of reductase inhibitor to 25 percent of the maximum dose or less allows the statins to be used safely in patients taking cyclosporine.

There are three available reductase inhibitors: lovastatin, simvastatin, and pravastatin. Lovastatin and pravastatin are equal in cholesterol-lowering potency. Simvastatin is twice as potent as the other two. Choice of a particular agent should be governed by cost and efficacy considerations.

Drugs for Hypertriglyceridemia

One of the drugs for hypertriglyceridemia is niacin, its use is described above. Patients with hypertriglyceridemia are more likely to have diabetes mellitus or hyperuricemia, and therefore blood glucose and uric acid concentrations should be followed carefully in patients with hypertriglyceridemia who are treated with niacin. Gemfibrozil is also an effective drug for lowering triglycerides. However, gemfibrozil may be associated with an increase in LDL concentration as the triglyceride concentration declines. If this occurs, the addition of a small amount of niacin or a small amount of a statin to gemfibrozil may be indicated, although there is the added risk of myopathy when these combinations are used. If statin plus niacin, or statin plus gemfibrozil, is employed, the statin dose should be limited to no more than 25 percent of the maximum for the particular statin. Renal function should also be normal when employing this combination, and patients should be warned about the symptoms of the myopathy syndrome and advised to discontinue the drugs if symptoms develop.

REFERENCES

1. Bayer MF: Effective laboratory evaluation of thyroid status. Med Clin North Am 75:1, 1991
2. Woeber KA: Thyrotoxicosis and cardiac disease. Heart Dis Stroke 2:415, 1993
3. Nicoloff JT, LoPresti JS: Myxedema coma. Endocrinol Metab Clin North Am 22:279, 1993
4. Singer PA: Thyroiditis. Med Clin North Am 76:61, 1991
5. Melmed S: Etiology of pituitary acromegaly. Endocrinol Metab Clin North Am 21:539, 1992
6. Pestell RG, Alford FP, Best JD: Familial acromegaly. Acta Endocrinol (Copenh) 121:286, 1989
7. Carney JA, Hruska LS, Beauchamp GD, Gordon H: Dominant inheritance of the complex of myxomas, spotty pigmentation, and endocrine overactivity. Mayo Clin Proc 61:165, 1986
8. Molitch ME: Clinical manifestations of acromegaly. Endocrinol Metab Clin North Am 21:597, 1992
9. Brunner JE, Johnson CC, Zafar S et al: Colon cancer and polyps in acromegaly: increased risk associated with family history of colon cancer. Clin Endocrinol 32:65, 1990
10. Rodrigues EA, Caruana MP, Lahiri A et al: Subclinical cardiac dysfunction in acromegaly: evidence for a specific disease of heart muscle. Brit Heart J 62:185, 1989
11. Chang-DeMoranville BM, Jackson IMD: Diagnostics and endocrine testing in acromegaly. Endocrinol Metab Clin North Am 21:649, 1992
12. Castelli WP, Garrison RJ, Wilson P et al: Incidence of coronary heart disease and lipoprotein cholesterol levels: The Framingham Study. J Am Med Assoc 256:2835, 1986
13. Mahley RW, Weisgraber KH, Innerarity TL, Rall SC Jr: Genetic defects in lipoprotein metabolism: elevation of atherogenic lipoproteins caused by impaired catabolism. J Am Med Assoc 265:78, 1991
14. Wilson PWF, Abbott RD, Castelli WP: High density lipoprotein cholesterol and mortality: The Framingham Study. Arteriosclerosis 8:737, 1988
15. Scanu AM, Fless GM: Lipoprotein (a). Heterogeneity and biological relevance. J Clin Invest 85:1709, 1990
15a. Ridker PM, Hennekens CH, Stampfer MJ: A prospective study of lipoprotein (a) and the risk of myocardial infarction. JAMA 270:2195, 1993
16. Hobbs HH, Brown MS, Goldstein JL: Molecular genetics of the LDL receptor gene in familial hypercholesterolemia. Hum Mutat 1:445, 1992
17. Kwiterovich PO Jr, Levy RI, Fredrickson DS: Neonatal diagnosis of familial type-II hyperlipoproteinaemia. Lancet 1:118, 1973
18. Innerarity TL, Weisgraber KH, Arnold KS et al.: Familial defective apolipoprotein B-100: low density lipoproteins with abnormal receptor binding. Proc Natl Acad Sci USA 84:6919, 1987

19. Bersot TP, Russell SJ, Thatcher SR et al: A unique haplotype of the apolipoprotein B-100 allele associated with familial defective apolipoprotein B-100 in a Chinese man discovered during a study of the prevalence of this disorder. J Lipid Res 34:1149, 1993

20. Goldstein JL, Schrott HG, Hazzard WR et al.: Hyperlipidemia in coronary heart disease. II. Genetic analysis of lipid levels in 176 families and delineation of a new inherited disorder, combined hyperlipidemia. J Clin Invest 52:1544, 1973

21. Goldstein JL, Hazzard WR, Schrott HG et al: Hyperlipidemia in coronary heart disease. I. Lipid levels in 500 survivors of myocardial infarction. J Clin Invest 52:1533, 1973

22. Cortner JA, Coates PM, Gallagher PR: Prevalence and expression of familial combined hyperlipidemia in childhood. J Pediatr 116:514, 1990

23. Chait A, Brunzell JD: Chylomicronemia syndrome. Adv Intern Med 37:249, 1992

24. Mahley RW, Rall SC Jr: Type III hyperlipoproteinemia (dysbetalipoproteinemia): the role of apolipoprotein E in normal and abnormal lipoprotein metabolism. p. 1195. In Scriver CR, Beaudet AL, Sly WS, Valle D (ed): The Metabolic Basis of Inherited Disease. McGraw-Hill, New York, 1989

6

Diabetes Mellitus

Mohammed F. Saad
Julio F. Tubau
Willa A. Hsueh

Diabetes mellitus is a major health problem, affecting approximately 14 million Americans.[1] It causes significant morbidity and mortality and currently is the seventh leading cause of death in the United States.[2] Most of the morbidity and mortality of diabetes is caused by its long-term complications. In the United States, diabetes is the most common cause of blindness[3] and the second leading cause of renal disease.[4] It is also associated with a two- to sixfold increase in the risk of cardiovascular disease.[5–7] Diabetes imposes a substantial socioeconomic burden because of its complications and the large number of affected individuals. Recent estimates indicate that the economic cost of diabetes exceeds $20 billion annually.[8,9] The socioeconomic burden of diabetes is expected to escalate with the increase in its prevalence due to aging of the American society[10] and the rapid growth of minority populations at high risk for the disease (e.g., Mexican Americans).[11]

Diabetes has a multifaceted effect on the cardiovascular system. It is associated with several metabolic and hemostatic abnormalities that accelerate the development and increase the severity of atherosclerosis. Diabetic patients have,

therefore, higher rates of myocardial infarction (MI), stroke, and peripheral vascular disease (PVD). Diabetes also leads to a specific myocardial dysfunction that increases susceptibility to heart failure and contributes to increased mortality after MI. Hypertension occurs with increased frequency in diabetic patients and in turn aggravates the micro- and macrovascular complications of diabetes. Cardiovascular autonomic neuropathy interferes with heart rate and blood pressure regulation and appears to predispose diabetic patients to silent ischemia and sudden death. Cardiovascular involvement is, therefore, the major cause of morbidity and mortality in diabetic patients.

DEFINITIONS

According to the World Health Organization (WHO) criteria[12] (Table 6-1), diabetes is diagnosed if fasting plasma glucose concentration is 140 mg/dl (7.8 mmol) or more, 2-hour postload (75 g) plasma glucose, is 200 mg/dl (11.1 mmol) or more, or random plasma glucose is 200 mg/dl or more on two separate occasions. Normal

Table 6-1. Classification of Glucose Tolerance According to the World Health Organization Criteria

Category	Plasma Glucose (mg/dl)		
	Fasting		2-h[a]
Normal glucose tolerance	<140	and	<140
Impaired glucose tolerance	<140	and	140–199
Diabetes mellitus	≥140	or	≥200

[a] After a 75-g glucose load.

glucose tolerance is present when fasting and 2-hour postload plasma glucose concentrations are less than 140 mg/dl. Impaired glucose tolerance (IGT) is defined by a normal fasting plasma glucose concentration (less than 140 mg/dl), and a 2-hour postload glucose 140 mg/dl or more and less than 200 mg/dl. This latter category was introduced by the National Diabetes Data Group[13] in 1979, and was subsequently adopted by the WHO[14] to replace the old nomenclatures of chemical, borderline, or latent diabetes since subjects with IGT do not develop the microangiopathic complications of diabetes. IGT is a common disorder affecting approximately 11 percent of the population; the prevalence is particularly high in older subjects.[1] Although IGT is not a clinical entity, it is of considerable importance. It is a precursor of diabetes as 30 to 50 percent of subjects with IGT develop diabetes in 5 to 10 years.[15–21] However, many subjects with IGT revert back to normal glucose tolerance or continue to have this abnormality. In addition, IGT is associated with increased prevalence of hypertension, dyslipidemia, and doubling of the risk of atherosclerosis.[22–24] Subjects with IGT could, therefore, be a target for intervention for the prevention of both diabetes and atherosclerosis.[25]

CLASSIFICATION AND PATHOGENESIS

Diabetes mellitus is a syndrome that includes a heterogenous group of disorders (Table 6-2), all of which are characterized by hyperglycemia and absolute or relative insulin deficiency.[13] In the Western world, the great majority of cases of diabetes are attributed to insulin-dependent diabetes mellitus (IDDM) or noninsulin-dependent diabetes mellitus (NIDDM). Malnutrition-related diabetes is common in parts of Africa, Asia, and the Caribbean. Diabetes secondary to pancreatic disease (e.g., chronic pancreatitis, cystic fibrosis); other endocrinopathies (e.g., Cushing syndrome, pheochromocytoma,

Table 6-2. Classification of Diabetes Mellitus

I. Insulin-dependent diabetes (IDDM, type I)

II. Noninsulin-dependent diabetes (NIDDM, type II)
   a. Nonobese
   b. Obese
   c. MODY (maturity-onset diabetes in the young)

III. Malnutrition-related diabetes
   a. Fibrocalculous pancreatic diabetes
   b. Protein-deficient diabetes

IV. Other types
   a. Pancreatic disease
   b. Endocrine disease (pheochromocytoma, Cushing syndrome, acromegaly, etc.)
   c. Drug- or chemically-induced
   d. Abnormal insulin or insulin-receptor
   e. Certain genetic syndromes

(Modified from WHO Study Group,[12] with permission.)

acromegaly, etc); drugs; certain genetic syndromes (e.g., lipoatrophic diabetes, lipodystrophy, muscular dystrophies, etc.); and abnormal insulin (e.g., familial hyperproinsulinemia) or insulin-receptor abnormalities (e.g., leprechaunism, Rabson-Mendenhall syndrome) are uncommon or rare.

Insulin-Dependent Diabetes Mellitus

IDDM accounts for 10 to 15 percent of diabetes in the Western world. It usually starts in childhood or adolescence with a peak onset during the second decade. IDDM is characterized by absolute insulin deficiency due to autoimmune destruction of the β-cells. Genetic factors play an important role in the predisposition to IDDM. In whites, IDDM is strongly associated with the histocompatibility antigens HLA-DR3 and DR4 that are located on chromosome 6.[26,27] DR3 is also associated with IDDM in Chinese, Asian Indians, and some black populations, but not in Japanese. DR4 is associated with the disease in blacks and in most Asian populations except the Chinese. Other antigens are associated with IDDM in other ethnic groups (e.g., DR7 in blacks and DR9 in blacks, Japanese, and Chinese).[28] It appears, however, that DQ antigens exert a greater influence in determining the susceptibility for IDDM. Specifically, the substitution of an amino acid for the normally present aspartic acid at position 57 of the DQ β-chain (DQβ 57 Asp-) results in a remarkably increased susceptibility for the disease. In addition, the presence of arginine at position 52 on the DQ α-chain (DQα Arg+) increases the risk of IDDM.[29] These genetic factors are necessary but not sufficient for the development of IDDM. Environmental factors such as certain viruses (e.g., retrovirus, rubella, cytomegalovirus), dietary proteins (e.g., cow's milk), or toxic agents trigger the immune response that leads to the destruction of β-cells.[30,31] Thus, an inflammatory destructive process, mediated by humoral and cellular factors, takes place and is associated with the appearance of islet cell and insulin antibodies in the circulation. This process can be acute, leading to overt diabetes within days or weeks. More commonly, it follows a slow progressive course with clinical disease occurring months or years later.[32]

NonInsulin-Dependent Diabetes Mellitus

NIDDM accounts for 85 to 90 percent of cases of diabetes in the western world. It occurs in older subjects, usually after the age of 40. Among whites, the incidence of NIDDM increases progressively with age until the seventh decade. Among some ethnic groups with an unusually high prevalence of the disease, such as American Indians and Mexican-Americans, NIDDM occurs at a younger age and the incidence peaks in the 5th or 6th decade.[33] NIDDM is a disease of affluent societies and is more common in obese subjects, of whom 15 to 20 percent develop the disease. The incidence of NIDDM is increasing in many populations because of the adoption of a Western life-style.

Both insulin resistance and β-cell dysfunction contribute to the pathogenesis of NIDDM, but controversy exists about which disorder is primary.[34–37] Current evidence suggests a two-step process for the development of NIDDM.[38] The first step is the transition from normal to impaired glucose tolerance, for which insulin resistance is the main determinant. The second step is worsening from IGT to diabetes, in which β-cell dysfunction plays a critical role.

Insulin resistance precedes the development of NIDDM. Hyperinsulinemia, which reflects insulin resistance, especially in the presence of normoglycemia, is common in populations with a high prevalence of NIDDM.[39–42] It is also an early abnormality that is characteristic of subjects who subsequently develop IGT or NIDDM.[15–19,43,44] High fasting and/or 2-hour postglucose load insulin or fasting C-peptide levels are major predictors of development of IGT or NIDDM in whites,[19,43] Nauruans,[16] Mexican-Americans,[17] Japanese-Americans,[18] and Pima Indians[15] with normal glucose tolerance. Diminished insulin sensitivity is found in normoglycemic white offspring of two noninsulin-dependent diabetic parents, and is a major indicator of their predisposition to the subsequent development of NIDDM.[45] Decreased insulin-mediated glucose disposal is common in Pima Indians with normal glucose tolerance and is a predictor of subsequent development of both IGT and NIDDM.[46] Insulin resistance is also found in nonobese, nondiabetic Mexican-Americans, another population with a high risk for developing NIDDM.[47] The mechanism of insulin resistance in NIDDM is unknown, but is caused mainly by a postreceptor defect(s) which is genetically determined.[48–50] Other factors such as obesity, aging, and physical inactivity can, however, worsen insulin resistance.

Whereas insulin resistance is the main factor that leads to a progression from normal to impaired glucose tolerance, β-cell dysfunction plays an essential role in the progression from IGT to NIDDM. Among subjects with IGT, a lower 2-hour postload insulin concentration predicts NIDDM among Mexican-Americans,[17] Pima Indians,[15] and Nauruans.[16] Whether this β-cell dysfunction is primary or secondary is controversial. Warram et al.[43]

found normal β-cell function in response to intravenous glucose in the normoglycemic white offspring of two non insulin-dependent diabetic parents who subsequently developed diabetes. Studies in Pima Indians showed no apparent deficit in insulin secretion prior to development of IGT.[51] Impaired β-cell function may result from long-term exposure to insulin resistance and prolonged increased demand for insulin secretion that eventually exceeds β-cell capacity (exhaustion). Alternatively, or in addition, the minimal chronic postprandial hyperglycemia associated with IGT may injure the signalling response to glucose (glucose toxicity).[52,53] However, not all people with insulin resistance or IGT develop NIDDM. Some subjects can maintain high levels of insulin secretion for prolonged periods. Others may have acquired or inherited abnormalities that make β-cells susceptible to exhaustion or glucose toxicity. Such defects might include reduced islet-cell mass, limited replicative capacity and more rapid age-related demise, or intrinsic functional or structural abnormalities.[54–56]

ATHEROSCLEROSIS

Diabetes mellitus is associated with accelerated atherogenesis and premature development of atherosclerotic cardiovascular disease (ASCVD).[57,58] Atherosclerotic lesions of coronary,[59–61] carotid,[62,63] and peripheral[64–66] arteries are more extensive and more severe in diabetic than in nondiabetic individuals. ASCVD, therefore, accounts for more than 75 percent of hospital admissions attributable to diabetic complications[8] and is a major cause of death in diabetic patients.[9] The magnitude and the determinants of ASCVD differ in the two main types of diabetes.[58,67] ASCVD is nearly as common in patients with newly diagnosed NIDDM as in those with several years of the disease.[68,69] Subjects with IGT, a precursor of NIDDM, also have a high risk for ASCVD.[58,70,71] Moreover, several ASCVD risk factors such as obesity, central fat distribution, dyslipidemia, and high blood pressure and glucose concentrations cluster in prediabetic individuals who still have normal glucose tolerance.[72,73] Conversely, ASCVD affects predominantly IDDM patients with long-standing disease who have nephropathy.[74] It appears, therefore, that the increased risk of ASCVD in IDDM is mainly secondary to the metabolic and hemostatic derangements of diabetes,[67] whereas ASCVD and NIDDM may share common genetic or metabolic antecedents.[75] The following sections will highlight the differences in the relation between the two types of diabetes and ASCVD.

Epidemiology

Coronary Artery Disease

IDDM increases the risk of death from coronary artery disease (CAD) approximately 11-fold.[67,76] CAD is rarely manifest, however, before the age of 30 years. Subsequently, the morbidity and mortality from CAD increases progressively (Fig. 6-1). Krolewski et al.[77] found that by the age of 55 years, one-half of their IDDM patients had some clinical manifestation of CAD or had already died of it. IDDM patients who develop clinical nephropathy (persistent albuminuria more than 300 mg/24 h or proteinuria more than 500 mg/24 h), are particularly susceptible to CAD.[77–80] In a case-control

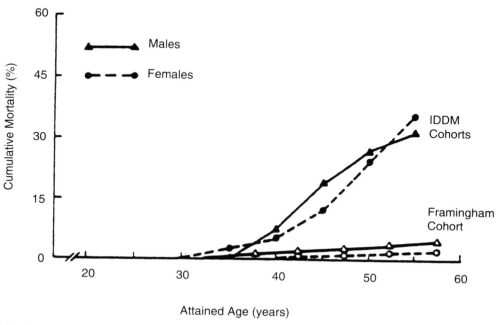

Fig. 6-1. Cumulative mortality due to coronary heart disease up to age 55 years in patients with insulin-dependent diabetes compared with the population of the Framingham Heart Study. (From Krolewski et al.,[77] with permission.)

study, Jensen et al.[79] followed 59 pairs of IDDM patients with and without clinical nephropathy, who were matched for age, sex, and diabetes duration, for 10 years. The cumulative incidence of CAD was 40 percent within 6 years from the onset of clinical nephropathy compared with 5 percent for those without nephropathy (Fig. 6–2). It is to be emphasized, however, that even in the absence of nephropathy, IDDM patients still have four times the risk of CAD as the general population.[78]

NIDDM patients have also increased risk for CAD. Several studies showed that NIDDM patients have 2 to 9 times the incidence of fatal and nonfatal CAD as nondiabetic individuals.[6,58,81–88] In fact, CAD is the cause of death of more than 50 percent of subjects with NIDDM.[81] The Multiple Risk Factor Intervention Trial, which included 5,163 diabetic and 342,815 nondiabetic men, showed that NIDDM increased the risk of death from CAD 3.2 times.[85] When the presence of other risk factors such as serum cholesterol, blood pressure, and smoking was taken into consideration, diabetic men still had a three- to fivefold higher CAD mortality rate (Fig. 6-3). Similar data were reported for women from the Nurses's Health Study; NIDDM was associated with 6.7 times increased risk for fatal and nonfatal CAD.[86] After

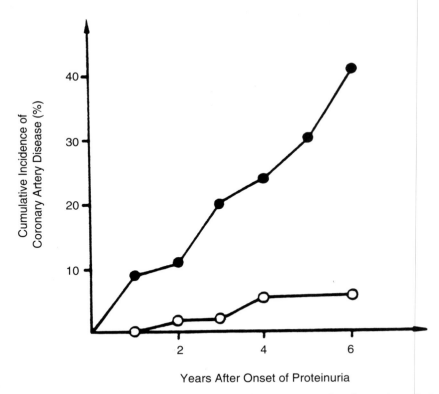

Years After Onset of Proteinuria

Fig. 6-2. Cumulative incidence of coronary artery disease in insulin-dependent diabetes with clinical nephropathy (solid circles, n = 59) and without nephropathy (open circles, n = 59). The two groups were matched in age, sex, and duration of diabetes. (From Jensen et al.,[79] with permission.)

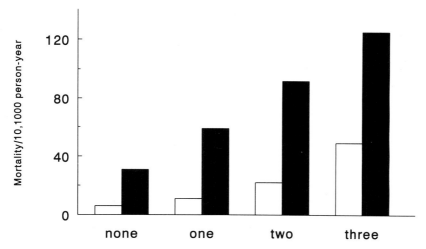

Fig. 6-3. Age-adjusted cardiovascular mortality by the presence of number of risk factors (hypertension, high serum cholesterol, and smoking) in diabetic (solid bars) and nondiabetic (open bars) men who participated in the Multiple Risk Factor Intervention Trial (Modified from Stamler et al.,[85] with permission.)

controlling for hypertension, cholesterol level, cigarette smoking, and obesity, diabetic women exhibited 3.1 times higher rates of CAD than nondiabetic ones. These two studies also demonstrated that the adverse effect of diabetes was amplified in the presence of other ASCVD risk factors.

Cerebrovascular Disease

Diabetes confers increased risk of cerebrovascular disease independent of the effect of other risk factors such as age, hypertension, and hypercholesterolemia.[89] Mortality rate from stroke is 1.6 to 2.4 times higher in IDDM patients than in the general population.[58] In NIDDM, the risk of fatal and nonfatal stroke is increased two- to five-fold. The Multiple Risk Factor Intervention Trial showed that diabetic men had a 2.8 higher stroke mortality rate than nondiabetic men.[85] In the Nurses' Health Study, diabetic women had 5.4 times the incidence of stroke as nondiabetic women.[86]

Peripheral Vascular Disease

The prevalence of PVD increases with age and duration of disease in IDDM patients. After 30 years of IDDM, approximately 20 percent of patients have PVD as defined by ankle-arm blood pressure ratio.[67] PVD occurs in 22 percent of patients with NIDDM compared with 3 percent of controls.[90] PVD not uncommonly leads to lower limb amputations in diabetic patients resulting in significant disability. It is estimated that the lifetime risk of lower extremity amputation is 5 to 15 percent among diabetic patients, which is 15 times higher than the lifetime risk for nondiabetic individuals.[91,92]

Risk Factors

The traditional risk factors for atherosclerosis are more prevalent among diabetic patients. Nevertheless, their contribution accounts for no more than 25 percent of the excess risk of ASCVD in diabetes. It appears that certain factors unique to the diabetic process confer increased susceptibility and contribute to atherogenesis in diabetes. The risk factors for atherosclerosis in diabetes (Table 6-3) are discussed briefly. The interested reader is referred to two recent comprehensive reviews of the subject.[93,94]

Sex

Several studies have demonstrated that diabetes imposes a greater risk of ASCVD in women than in men and eliminates the female advantage of decreased ASCVD risk.[76,84,95–97] In the Rancho Bernardo Study, the risk of fatal CAD in diabetics versus nondiabetics was 1.9 in men and 3.3 in women.[96] Similar findings were reported in patients with IDDM from the Wisconsin Epidemiologic Study of Diabetic Retinopathy; CAD mortality was 9 and 14 times higher in men and women, respectively, than in the general population.[76]

Duration of Diabetes

Controversy exists regarding the impact of the duration of diabetes on the risk of ASCVD. In IDDM, it is difficult to differentiate between the effect of its duration and that of the age of the patient since the disease often starts during childhood. Krolewski et al.[77] found no effect of duration on the incidence of CAD in 292 IDDM patients followed for up to 40

Table 6-3. Risk Factors for Atherosclerosis in Diabetes

Sex
Duration of diabetes
Hyperglycemia
Hypertension
Dyslipidemia
Hypercoagulability
Advanced glycation endproducts
Insulin resistance and hyperinsulinemia
Albuminuria
Smoking

years. Studies including larger numbers of subjects suggest, however, that diabetes duration may increase the incidence of ASCVD independent of other risk factors.[58,98,99] In NIDDM, several studies demonstrated that the incidence of ASCVD was nearly as high in subjects with newly diagnosed diabetes as in those with previously known disease.[71,75,100] It has been argued, therefore, that NIDDM is not a cause of ASCVD, but rather both diseases share common genetic or metabolic antecedents.[75] Nevertheless, the inability to demonstrate a relation between the duration of NIDDM and ASCVD can be attributable to the difficulty in ascertaining the onset of hyperglycemia. Harris[101] suggested that undiagnosed NIDDM may exist for as long as 12 years before clinical diagnosis. For example, the duration of NIDDM has been shown to be related to the incidence of fatal CAD in the Pima Indians, in whom the onset of NIDDM is more accurately determined through biennial oral glucose tolerance testing.[102]

Glycemic Control

The role of hyperglycemia per se in increasing the risk of ASCVD is unclear. Several studies have demonstrated no relation between the severity of hyperglycemia and the risk of ASCVD in IDDM or NIDDM.[102–104] Conversely, evidence exists that elevated glucose levels, while still within the nondiabetic range, significantly increase the risk of atherosclerosis in nondiabetic subjects.[57,70,105–107] It is possible, therefore, that glycemia has a threshold effect on the predisposition to ASCVD. The Diabetes Control and Complications Trial has recently shown that intensive insulin therapy and better glycemic control reduced, albeit not significantly, the risk of ASCVD in IDDM patients by 41 percent (95 percent confidence interval, 10 to 68 percent)[108] This reduction cannot be attributed completely to improved glycemia, however, since intensive insulin therapy led to improvement in the lipid profile and decreased the incidence of proteinuria. Chronic hyperglycemia may accelerate atherogenesis through excessive glycation of various proteins in the plasma and in the arterial wall (see below).[109]

Dyslipidemia

Abnormalities in plasma lipid and lipoproteins that increase the risk of ASCVD are common in diabetic patients.[110–113] In IDDM patients with poor metabolic control, hypertriglyceridemia, and increased low-density lipoprotein (LDL) cholesterol concentrations are the main abnormalities. These changes improve with insulin treatment; patients with well- and moderately-controlled glycemia have normal or even subnormal concentrations of total cholesterol, triglycerides, very-low-density lipoproteins (VLDL), and LDL and normal or elevated high-density lipoprotein (HDL) concentrations. In patients with incipient or clinical nephropathy, the concentrations of total cholesterol, triglycerides, VLDL and LDL are elevated, whereas those of HDL are reduced. In NIDDM, the most frequent abnormalities are hypertriglyceridemia, and increased VLDL and reduced HDL cholesterol concentrations. LDL cholesterol levels are often normal. Data on the level of lipoprotein(a) (Lp[a]), a strong independent risk factor for ASCVD in the general population, are discrepant, with some studies reporting increased[114–117] and others normal[118–120] concentrations. So far, there is no conclusive evidence that Lp(a) is related to the risk of ASCVD in either type of diabetes.[120–122]

Hypertriglyceridemia, which occurs in both IDDM and NIDDM, has been shown to be an independent risk factor for ASCVD in diabetes.[123] Relative or absolute insulin deficiency causes acceler-ated lipolysis and excessive delivery of free fatty acids to the liver, resulting in increased very-low-density lipoprotein (VLDL) production and hence the hypertriglyceridemia. In addition, decreased activity of the insulin-dependent lipoprotein lipase reduces plasma triglycerides clearance and contributes to the increase in the concentrations of VLDL.[124] The accumulation of VLDL in the circulation leads to increased production of intermediate-density lipoproteins (IDL), which are particularly atherogenic.[113]

In addition, several qualitative changes in lipoproteins, which make them more atherogenic have been observed. Increased concentrations of free cholesterol on lipoprotein particles have been described, and are perhaps related to abnormalities in cholesteryl ester transfer. Diabetic patients have a high free cholesterol-to-lecithin ratio (an index of CAD risk) in plasma and in both LDL and VLDL. There is also reduction in the phospholipid content of HDL. Lipoprotein fractions from persons with NIDDM may show a broad diffuse LDL band (termed *polydisperse LDL*) that represents an increase in IDL concentration and a loss of normal LDL peak. These compositional changes may affect lipoprotein interaction with artery wall cells by either enhancing delivery of free cholesterol to cells or altering reverse cholesterol transport.[125–130] There is also an increase in the number of small, dense LDL particles (termed *LDL pattern B*) that are more atherogenic, possibly because they more readily undergo oxidative modification (see below).[131–134]

Furthermore, glycation (nonenzymatic glycosylation) of apolipoproteins occurs in diabetic patients, and its extent is related to the severity of hyperglycemia.[135,136] Glycated LDL has a decreased affinity to bind to LDL receptors and thereby accumulates in the circulation contributing to hyperlipidemia. In the meantime, the uptake of glycated LDL by monocyte-macrophages is increased, through a high-capacity, low-affinity pathway, and thereby their transformation into foam cells, the major component of fatty streaks, is enhanced.[137] Diabetes is also associated with increased lipid peroxidation and lipoprotein oxidation.[138,139] Oxidized LDL is thought to play a major role in atherogenesis. It is chemotactic for monocytes and induces their transformation into foam cells; is cytotoxic to vascular endothelial and smooth muscle cells; inhibits the ability of macrophages to egress from the vessel wall; alters gene expression of arterial cells inducing leukocyte adhesion molecules, monocyte chemotactic protein-1 and colony stimulating factors; and interferes with endothelium-derived relaxing factor-mediated vasodilation of coronary arteries.[140] Oxidation and glycation are thought to be interrelated, as the presence of nonenzymatically bound glucose on lipoproteins increases the likelihood of oxidative damage. When lipoproteins are extravasated and sequestered for prolonged periods in the vessel wall, the processes of glycation, oxidation, and glycoxidation may affect both lipoproteins and vascular connective tissue proteins, leading to a vicious cycle of vascular injury.[137]

Modified lipoproteins may also promote atherogenesis through triggering an immune response leading to the formation of antibodies and subsequently to the formation of immune complexes. LDL-containing immune complexes are taken avidly by macrophages through their F_c receptors, and induce not only massive intracellular accumulation of cholesteryl esters, but also a paradoxical increase in LDL-receptor expression, with subsequent increase in LDL uptake. The end result of these effects is an increase in foam-cell formation. In addition, these immune complexes activate macrophages resulting in the release of different cytokines such as interleukin 1β and tumor necrosis factor-α, which can cause endothelial damage and induce smooth muscle proliferation.[141] It appears, therefore, that qualitative rather than quantitative abnormalities in lipoproteins play a major role in the acceleration of atherosclerosis in diabetic patients.

Hypertension

Raised blood pressure is a major risk factor for ASCVD in diabetic patients.[85,142–144] In the Multiple Risk Factor Intervention Trial, a linear relation between systolic blood pressure and cardiovascular mortality was present among men with NIDDM.[85] In the WHO Multinational Study of Vascular Disease in Diabetics, the risk of cardiovascular mortality was 2.2 and 3.7 times higher in hypertensive men and women with NIDDM, respectively, than in normotensive ones.[144] In IDDM, the relative risk of cardiovascular mortality of hypertensive subjects was 3.5 for men and 2.5 for women compared with normotensive patients, and the relationship of blood pressure to mortality was independent of the effect of proteinuria.[144]

Hypercoagulability

Diabetes is a procoagulant state that is thought to contribute to the increased risk of atherosclerosis and thrombosis.[93] Abnormalities in coagulation factors, fibrinolysis, and platelet function have all been reported in diabetic patients.[145–151] Changes in the coagulation system include increased plasma levels of fibrinogen[152–154] (a risk factor for ASCVD in the general population) and von Willebrand factor,[155] decreased protein C (a physiologic inhibitor of coagulation factors V and VIII),[156] and depressed activity of antithrombin III.[157] Fibrinolysis is impaired possibly due to increased levels of plasminogen activator inhibitor-1 as well as glycation of fibrin and plasminogen.[145,147,153,158–160] In addition, the increased levels of Lp(a), which occurs in some diabetic patients (especially those with nephropathy), may play a role.[116,117,122] A component of this lipoprotein, apo(a), is homologous to plasminogen, but lacks its fibrinolytic activity. Moreover, it can compete with plasminogen in binding with fibrin and the endothelial plasminogen receptors, interfering with its fibrinolytic activity.[122]

Several platelet abnormalities contribute to the procoagulant state in diabetes. Platelets from diabetic patients with and without vascular disease are hypersensitive to aggregating agents and exhibit increased adhesiveness.[148–151,161–165] Several studies have demonstrated increased plasma levels of the platelet-specific proteins (β-thromboglobulin, and platelet factor 4) that reflect in vivo platelet activation and release of the contents of their α-granules.[166,167] The increased functional properties of diabetic platelets are thought to result from the primary release of larger platelets with enhanced thromboxane formation capacity and increased numbers of functional glycoprotein receptors GPIb and GPIIb/IIIa (the platelet receptors for cytoadhesive plasma proteins [e.g., fibrinogen and von Willebrand factor antigen]).[151,168] In addition, decreased fluidity of platelet membranes, possibly due to glycation of their proteins, may have a role in platelet hypersensitivity and enhanced activation.[169,170]

According to the endothelial injury theory for atherogenesis,[171] platelets adhere to the subendothelial constituents at the site of vessel injury, releasing the contents of their granules. Released materials include mitogenic factors such as platelet-derived growth factor and transforming growth factor α that stimulate vascular smooth muscle cell proliferation and migration into the intima. Adenosine diphosphate and serotonin, which can cause platelet aggregation and thus recruit other platelets to the site of injury, are also released. Platelet adherence to collagen also leads to the release of thromboxane A_2, which causes aggregation and release of granule contents from platelets not directly adherent to the collagen. Activation of coagulation factors can occur at the site of injury with subsequent formation of platelet-fibrin thrombi. If these mural thrombi persist and become organized, they can become incorporated into the vessel wall and further contribute to the atherosclerotic process. Thus, the hyperactive platelets in diabetes can promote atherogenesis in several ways.[148]

Endothelial Dysfunction

Vascular endothelium contributes to the regulation of vascular tone, hemostasis, fibrinolysis, and synthesis of growth factors and subendothelial matrix components.[172] Endothelial injury is a critical initiating event in atherogenesis (see above)[171] and appears to have a role in the increased risk of ASCVD in diabetic patients.[94,173] The plasma levels of several markers of endothelial damage such as von Willebrand factor,[154,173] angiotensin-converting enzyme,[174] and thrombomodulin[175] are elevated in diabetic patients. Other features of endothelial dysfunction include impaired prostacyclin[176] and plasminogen activator release,[177] decreased lipoprotein lipase activity,[124] and increased transcapillary albumin escape[178] in diabetic patients. In addition, several[179–181] but not all[182] studies have demonstrated reduced endothelium-dependent vasodilatation in IDDM and NIDDM patients. Plasma levels of endothelin, a vasoconstrictor hormone produced by the endothelium, are elevated in some diabetic patients, but it is not clear whether this elevation has functional significance or simply represents endothelial damage.[183,184] These abnormalities can promote platelet aggregation and adherence to the endothelium, and thus create an environment conducive to acceleration of atherogenesis. Advanced glycation end products, dyslipidemia, and hypertension are thought to contribute to the endothelial damage observed in diabetes.[185]

Advanced Glycation End Products

Nonenzymatic binding of glucose to the amino groups of proteins is called *nonenzymatic glycosylation* or *glycation*. This reaction, which results in the formation of Schiff bases, occurs at a rate proportional to the glucose concentration and is reversible. Schiff bases undergo a slow chemical rearrangement that lasts several weeks to form more stable early glycation products (named *Amadori products* after the chemist who first described this type of rearrangement). Amadori products are still chemically reversible; their amount increases when blood glucose levels are high and returns to normal when glycemia decreases. This phenomenon is the basis for the use of glycated hemoglobin or proteins (the fructosamine test) to assess glycemic control in diabetic patients over the preceding months or weeks respectively.[109,186–188]

Amadori products may undergo a series of dehydrations and rearrangements to form a heterogeneous group of brown or fluorescent protein-bound moieties, termed advanced glycation end products (AGEs). The formation of AGEs is irreversible and, therefore, they continue to accumulate indefinitely, mainly in long-lived proteins such as the extracellular matrix, basal membranes, collagen, and the lens.[109,186–188] The rate of AGE forma-

tion is approximately of second order with respect to glucose concentration (i.e., proportional to the square of the glucose concentration). Thus, even modestly elevated levels of blood glucose can significantly increase the accumulation of AGEs.[109]

AGEs are, perhaps, the link between hyperglycemia and the chronic complications of diabetes, including atherosclerosis. Vlassara et al.[189] have recently demonstrated that administration of AGEs to nondiabetic rats and rabbits induced several vascular alterations resembling those seen in diabetes. In the vessel wall, formation of AGE cross-links on collagen and laminin leads to distorted ultrastructural assembly of the basement membrane components and decreases their susceptibility to proteolytic degradation. These changes result also in trapping and deposition of plasma proteins that enter the vessel wall, such as LDL, fibrinogen, and immune complexes. Once immobilized, these cross-linked proteins provide additional sites for AGE formation. Accumulation of glycated LDL in the vessel wall increases its susceptibility to oxidation and enhances atherogenesis[137,190] (see above). Furthermore, formation of AGEs on collagen leads to stiffening of matrix proteins with increased vascular rigidity.[191] The resulting increase in shear stresses may lead to endothelial injury and the loss of arterial elasticity could adversely affect cardiovascular hemodynamics.[190,191] In addition, AGEs can rapidly inactivate nitric oxide (endothelium-derived relaxing factor) which is produced tonically by endothelial cells and appears to be an important modulator of vascular tone.[192] Impairment of the vasodilator effect of nitric oxide may play a role in the development of hypertension and in the acceleration of vascular occlusion in diabetic patients.[109,192] Inactivation of nitric oxide also eliminates its cytostatic activity with subsequent stimulation of myointimal proliferation, an integral part of the atherogenic process.[193]

Subendothelial AGEs are chemotactic to monocytes, facilitating their migration into the vessel wall and conversion to macrophages.[194] Monocytes and macrophages also have specific high affinity receptors for AGEs. When in the vessel wall, they engulf AGEs as well as subendothelial lipoproteins with subsequent foam cell formation. Furthermore, when monocytes and macrophages interact with AGE-modified proteins, they secrete tumor necrosis factor, interleukin 1, insulin-like growth factor-I, and platelet-derived growth factor. These growth promoters contribute to accelerated atherogenesis by stimulating endothelial and smooth muscle cell proliferation.[195] Endothelial cells also express AGE-specific receptors. Binding of AGEs to endothelial cells has a procoagulant effect through suppression of thrombomodulin activity, which prevents activation of the anticoagulant protein C pathway; and augmentation of tissue factor activity, thus activating coagulation factors IX and X. The factor Xa generated along with thrombin stimulates endothelial cell release of mitogenic platelet-derived growth factor.[195] Thus, AGEs appear to promote the development of atherosclerosis through a wide array of actions. Blocking the effects of AGEs with pharmacologic agents may offer a new approach for preventing diabetes complications.[109]

Insulin Resistance and Hyperinsulinemia

The role of insulin resistance and hyperinsulinemia in the pathogenesis of ASCVD is controversial.[196–200] Several risk factors for atherosclerosis, such as glucose intolerance, dyslipidemia, hypertension and central obesity, cluster in some individuals.[72,73,201,202] In 1988, Reaven postulated that insulin resistance and concomitant compensatory hyperinsulinemia underlie this clustering. He coined the term "syndrome X" (or the "insulin resistance syndrome") to describe the association among insulin resistance, hyperinsulinemia, and these risk factors, speculating that this syndrome may be an important cause of ASCVD in affluent societies.[34] Since insulin resistance and hyperinsulinemia often precede and play a key role in the development of IGT and NIDDM, they may also contribute to the increased risk of ASCVD observed in these two conditions.[34,196,197] Moreover, they may take part in promoting atherogenesis in patients with IDDM, in whom hyperinsulinemia and insulin resistance often result from exogenous insulin administration and from the associated metabolic derangements (hyperglycemia and increased free fatty acid levels), respectively.[203]

Several mechanisms have been proposed for the association of insulin with ASCVD risk factor abnormalities. Insulin may contribute to the pathogenesis of hypertension by stimulating the sympathetic nervous system, promoting renal sodium retention, modulating cellular cation transport, and/or stimulating vascular smooth muscle hypertrophy.[196,197] Insulin also may induce dyslipidemia by stimulating hepatic synthesis of VLDL, leading to raised serum concentrations of triglycerides and depressed concentration of HDL cholesterol.[34]

Indeed, hyperinsulinemia is common in some populations with high rates of ASCVD such as in Edinburgh men[204] and immigrant Asian Indians.[205] Three prospective population studies—the Helsinki Policemen Study,[206] the Paris Prospective Study,[105] and the Busselton Study[207]—have associated high insulin concentrations with an increased risk of ASCVD in men, but not in women (only the Busselton study included women). These studies have some limitations: HDL cholesterol was not measured and the findings were not consistent regarding a relation between ASCVD and fasting or postglucose challenge insulin concentrations. In addition, a follow-up of the Busselton study found that insulinemia was an independent risk factor for total mortality in men, but not for cardiovascular mortality in either men or women.[208] Insulin was not a risk factor for ASCVD in Edinburgh[209] or Gothenburg[210] men. Pima Indians, who are markedly hyperinsulinemic, have a low prevalence rate of ASCVD, and insulinemia is not a predictor of ischemic electrocardiographic abnormalities.[211] Thus, insulinemia is not consistently associated with ASCVD.

The failure to find a consistent association between insulinemia and ASCVD and some of its risk factors suggests that the relation is not causal or that the effects of insulin are primarily permissive. Insulin may act to accelerate atherogenesis only in the presence of other risk factors, such as hyperlipidemia or hypertension.[199] Modan et al.[212] reported that the excess risk of ASCVD found in hyperinsulinemic men was confined to those who had at least one of three conditions: obesity, glucose intolerance, or hypertension. The Pima Indians, who are markedly hyperinsulinemic but have low total cholesterol concentration and a low prevalence of hypertension, have a low prevalence of ASCVD despite a considerably increased prevalence of NIDDM.[211] Limited evidence from clinical trials suggests that inducing hyperinsulinemia may not have adverse effects on rates for ASCVD. The Coronary Drug Project showed that the hypolipidemic drug nicotinic acid decreased total and cardiovascular mortality in men with previous MI,[213] although it

causes insulin resistance and hyperinsulinemia.[214] The University Group Diabetes Program did not show any adverse effects of insulin treatment on cardiovascular complications.[215] The Diabetes Control and Complications Trial has recently shown that intensive insulin therapy (which was most likely associated with hyperinsulinemia) reduced, albeit not significantly, the risk of ASCVD in IDDM patients by 41 percent (95 percent confidence interval, 10 to 68 percent).[108]

These observations and the stronger associations of insulin resistance than insulinemia with blood pressure and lipid abnormalities in several studies[216–218] suggest that insulin resistance rather than insulin may be the key factor, with insulin as an innocent bystander merely reflecting insulin resistance. Several mechanisms have been proposed. Decreased insulin sensitivity in adipose tissue, especially visceral fat, can cause accelerated lipolysis and excessive delivery of free fatty acids to the liver, resulting in increased VLDL production and hypertriglyceridemia. Insulin resistance may reduce plasma triglyceride clearance (because of an associated reduction in lipoprotein lipase activity within the vasculature), further amplifying the increase in the concentration of triglyceride-rich lipoproteins. When the plasma residence time of these lipoproteins is increased, they become cholesterol enriched and presumably more atherogenic, with reduction in HDL-cholesterol concentration.[219] In addition, the levels of the more atherogenic small dense LDL are increased.[220] Insulin resistance could lead to the development of hypertension through blunting of insulin-induced vasodilatation.[221] Insulin resistance also is associated with increased concentrations of plasminogen activator inhibitor-1 that inhibits fibrinolysis.[222] These changes could accelerate the development of atherosclerosis and predispose to thrombosis, leading to an increased risk of ASCVD.

Alternatively, the association between hyperinsulinemia or insulin resistance and ASCVD may not be causal but merely linked through common underlying factors. Both insulinemia and insulin resistance are strongly correlated with adiposity, and much of the impact of insulin on the risk of ASCVD could be related to amounts of body fat and its distribution. Increased sensitivity to glucocorticoids could produce an association.[223] Glucocorticoids favor deposition of central fat and can induce insulin resistance, hypertension, and hyperlipidemia. Increased activity of the sympathetic nervous system could lead to hypertension, insulin resistance, and hyperlipidemia.

Hyperinsulinemia and insulin resistance are related to ASCVD and to the clustering of its risk factors in some individuals. Their role as independent ASCVD risk factors is, however, less certain. At present, it can be concluded that neither hyperinsulinemia nor insulin resistance is a major risk factor for the development of ASCVD in the absence of other risk factors. Further laboratory research and prospective population studies of insulin resistance are needed to determine whether the observed relations are part of a causal chain for the development of atherosclerosis.

Albuminuria

Several studies have demonstrated that albuminuria is associated with increased risk of ASCVD and cardiovascular mortality in both IDDM[77–79,224–226] and NIDDM.[227–230] The presence of albuminuria is more ominous in patients with IDDM, in whom it increases the risk of ASCVD at least 15-fold.[77–79] In NIDDM, there is approximately a twofold increase in the incidence of cardiovascular mortality in patients with albuminuria.[227–230] Diabetic patients with albuminuria tend to have higher blood pressure, increased prevalence of hypertension,[228,231,232] and a more atherogenic lipoprotein profile.[233,234] Albuminuria is also associated with hyperfibrinogenemia and increased activity of factory VII and plasminogen activator inhibitor-1.[233,235] However, the presence of these risk factors cannot fully explain the increased cardiovascular morbidity and mortality observed in these patients. Deckert et al.[236] suggested that albuminuria reflects a more generalized vasculopathy, that affects the glomeruli, the retina, and the intima of large vessels simultaneously. They postulated that loss of anionic heparan sulfate proteoglycan, the main glycosaminoglycan component of the basement membrane, underlies the presence of albuminuria and the associated complications. Absence of heparan sulfate proteoglycan from the basement membrane in diabetes is due to formation of AGEs on collagen, which interferes with its binding sites. Heparan sulfate proteoglycan has multiple functions; it maintains the integrity of the basement membrane, inhibits cell proliferation, stimulates lipoprotein lipase, and accelerates thrombin-antithrombin complex formation. Thus, loss of the anionic heparan sulfate proteoglycan in the glomeruli permits leakage of albumin and in vascular endothelium allows lipoproteins to leak into the vascular wall. In addition, its absence promotes smooth muscle cell proliferation, contributes to development of dyslipidemia, and increases the risk of thrombosis. Thus, the presence of albuminuria heralds widespread vascular damage affecting both small and large blood vessels.

Smoking

Several prospective studies have shown that smoking is an independent risk factor for cardiovascular morbidity and mortality in IDDM[237] and NIDDM.[85,238] The mechanism of the adverse effect of smoking is poorly understood. Smoking induces changes in aortic endothelial cell turnover and ultrastructure, and inhibits the interaction of some prostaglandins with smooth muscle cells. Diabetes can also affect vascular endothelial and smooth muscle cells (see above). Diabetes and smoking may, therefore, have a synergistic hazardous effect on vessel wall components.[239]

Clinical Manifestations

The clinical features, diagnosis, and investigations of ASCVD in diabetic patients are generally similar to those seen in nondiabetics. Special features that are more common in diabetes are discussed in some detail now.

Coronary Artery Disease

Silent Ischemia.   Diabetic patients are more prone to silent exertional ischemia (electrocardiographic [ECG] ST-segment depression in the absence of angina).[240–243] Koistinen[243] found evidence of silent ischemia by exercise ECG, 24-hour Holter monitoring, or thallium tomographic imaging in 40 (29 percent) of 140 asymptomatic diabetic patients compared with 5 percent of controls. Thirty percent of those with positive findings had angiographic evidence of significant coronary artery stenosis. Thus, 9 percent of diabetic patients had asymptomatic CAD with active myocardial ischemia compared with 2 to 3 percent of the general population. In a similar study, Naka et al.[244] reported that the prevalence of angiographically confirmed silent ischemia was 2.2 times higher in diabetic than that in nondiabetic individuals. Silent MI is also more common in diabetic patients, occurring in approximately 25 percent of

cases compared with 12 percent in the general population.[245,246]

Silent ischemia occurs more frequently in diabetic patients with autonomic neuropathy, perhaps due to involvement of the sensory innervation of the heart.[247,248] A heightened somatic pain threshold, possibly due to peripheral neuropathy, may also blunt the perception of angina in some diabetic patients.[249,250] Ranjadayalan et al.[251] speculated that silent ischemia and decreased perception of angina could be hazardous as they deprive patients of the warning sign of anginal pain and thereby allow ischemia to intensify. Thus, patients become exposed to an exaggerated ischemic burden with the attendant risk of arrhythmias and myofibrillar damage. Noninvasive screening of diabetic patients for silent ischemia, however, is not warranted because of the high incidence of false-positive results.[243,244]

Acute Myocardial Infarction.   Diabetic patients with MI may present with unclassical manifestations. Chest pain may be absent in up to one-third of cases[252–255] and when present it is not uncommonly of mild or moderate intensity.[252] Patients may, however, present with nausea, vomiting, dyspnea, heart failure, confusion, collapse, uncontrolled diabetes, or ketoacidosis.[253] These atypical manifestations can lead to a delay in seeking medical care, in making the diagnosis, in admitting the patient to the coronary care unit, and/or in starting the proper treatment.[256] Solar et al.[254] reported that 35 percent of diabetic patients with MI were admitted to a general medical ward rather than to a coronary care unit. Approximately 75 percent of those admitted to the ward lacked chest pain, and the majority presented with heart failure, uncontrolled diabetes, or vomiting. These atypical presentations and the resulting delay in diagnosis may contribute to the increased morbidity and mortality of MI in diabetic patients.

Diabetic patients are more prone to develop certain complications of MI. Congestive heart failure occurs in 30 to 40 percent of cases (i.e., twice as common as in nondiabetic patients).[255-258] Latent diabetic cardiomyopathy is the most likely cause of the increased incidence of heart failure. Echocardiographic[259] and radionuclide angiocardiographic[260,261] studies showed that myocardial contractility was impaired to a greater extent in diabetic than in nondiabetic patients after sustaining MI of similar size, extent, and location. Other factors, however, may contribute to myocardial dysfunction in diabetic patients, including small vessel disease, impaired reflex adaptation to hemodynamic stress due to autonomic neuropathy, increased incidence of antecedent hypertension, and previously unrecognized infarction. Other complications such as infarct extension, cardiogenic shock, atrioventricular and bundle branch block, and ventricular arrhythmias occur more frequently in diabetic patients.[262,263] A high rate of recurrent infarction has also been described;[264,265] up to one-fourth of diabetic patients with MI may have reinfarction within 1 year.[265]

Not only do diabetic patients experience a high incidence of complications, but also they have a poor short- and long-term mortality after MI.[265-269] The in-hospital mortality rate is as high as 30 percent compared with 15 percent in the general population. In-hospital mortality appears to be declining, however, with the improvement in coronary care units and the use of newer methods of treatment.[270,271] The 5-year mortality of MI is approximately 50 percent, compared with 30 percent in nondiabetics. Both short- and long-term mortality are higher in diabetic women than in men for some unknown reasons.[272,273] Factors associated with increased mortality after MI in diabetic patients include an ejection fraction less than 40 percent, pulmonary congestion at the time of infarction, frequent ventricular premature beats (more than 10/h), and functional class II to IV before the infarction.[267] Diabetes *per se* still confers an independent risk of increased mortality even in the absence of these prognostic factors.

Cerebrovascular Disease

Transient Ischemic Attacks. Transient ischemic attacks (TIAs) are three times more frequent in diabetic patients than in the general population.[274] TIAs are an important warning sign; several studies have demonstrated that diabetic patients with TIAs have an approximately twofold increased risk of vascular death, stroke or MI within 5 years.[275-277] Cerebral infarctions are, however, more likely to occur without prior warning TIAs in diabetics.[278,279]

Cerebral Infarctions. A large proportion of strokes in diabetic patients is due to occlusion of the small paramedian penetrating arteries resulting in lacunar infarctions.[280-282] The increased risk of small vessel occlusion is possibly due to the associated impaired vasodilation and/or increased coagulability. Autonomic neuropathy also increases the risk of stroke by causing postural hypotension. Dobkin[283] found that 8 of 13 patients with cerebral ischemic episodes induced by hypotension were diabetic. Lacunar infarctions can present with pure motor hemiparesis, pure sensory stroke, sensorimotor stroke, ataxic-hemiparesis, and the dysarthria-clumsy-hand syndrome.[284]

Diabetes affects adversely the outcome of stroke. Diabetic patients usually have more severe neurologic deficits and are more likely to require institutional care after stroke.[285] The mechanism of increased brain damage is not known. It is possibly attributable to the presence of more severe atherosclerosis in diabetic patients, who thereby develop more extensive brain infarctions after ischemic episodes.[286] In addition, hyperglycemia has been shown to be associated with pronounced cerebral edema and ischemic damage both in humans[287–289] and experimental animals.[286] Diabetic patients also have a higher rate of stroke recurrence[290–292] and increased short and long-term mortality.[285,291,292] Asplund et al.[285] reported that one-half of the diabetic patients died within 1 year after the index stroke, and only 20 percent were alive after 5 years.

Hypoglycemia, hyperosmolar nonketotic diabetic coma, and ketoacidosis should be considered in any diabetic patient presenting with a cerebral event of sudden onset. Focal neurologic deficits, such as transient hemiplegia or aphasia with preservation of alertness, can be a manifestation of hypoglycemia.[293,294] These attacks can be recurrent in some patients and are caused by overdosage with oral hypoglycemic drugs or insulin, skipping meals, and alcohol consumption. Neurologic deficits associated with hypoglycemia usually resolve dramatically following glucose administration. Focal neurologic findings that disappear with correction of dehydration and hyperglycemia are features of hyperosmolar nonketotic diabetic coma. Therefore, this condition should be ruled out in any diabetic patient presenting with a stroke-like syndrome.[295] Finally, stroke could occur as a complication of diabetic ketoacidosis or hyperosmolar nonketotic coma. Either condition could, however, be precipitated by stroke in a diabetic patient.[284]

Peripheral Vascular Disease

Although smaller vessels below the knee, such as the tibial and peroneal arteries, are more severely affected in diabetics,

the femoropopliteal segment is still the most common site of arterial occlusion.[296,297] PVD carries a significantly higher risk for the development of gangrene in diabetic patients because of the associated peripheral neuropathy, microangiopathy, bone deformities, and increased susceptibility to infection. Therefore, palpation of peripheral pulses should be an integral part of examination of any diabetic patient. Despite its limited sensitivity, a significant number of cases of PVD will be identified by detection of a weak or absent pulse. Ankle-brachial index measurement by Doppler ultrasound is recommended in all diabetic patients with decreased pulses, femoral bruits, foot ulcer, or leg pain of unknown etiology and in the initial evaluation of IDDM patients 35 years of age or older; in patients with 20 years or more duration of diabetes, and in NIDDM patients 40 years of age or older.[298] However, the ankle-brachial pressure index may be misleadingly high, despite the presence of ischemic disease, due to medial arterial calcification. It has been suggested, therefore, that toe systolic pressure measurements could be more informative in diabetic patients.[299]

Management

Prevention

The Diabetes Control and Complications Trial[108] demonstrated that glycemic control may reduce the risk of ASCVD in IDDM. In addition, recent data showed that the incidence of ASCVD in NIDDM patients increases progressively with worsening of traditional risk factors such as dyslipidemia, hypertension, and smoking.[85,86] These findings underscore the importance and potential for prevention of ASCVD in diabetic individuals through sustained control of glycemia and control of the major risk factors for ASCVD. The management of diabetes and dyslipidemia will be discussed briefly here. Treatment of hypertension will be discussed in a subsequent section.

Diet. Proper diet can improve both glycemic control and dyslipidemia. Caloric restriction is indicated in obese patients to promote weight loss. A high carbohydrate intake (55 to 60 percent of total caloric intake), especially of complex carbohydrates such as starches and cereals, is recommended. Simple sugars are better avoided. Fat intake should be limited to 30 to 35 percent of total calories; saturated animal fats should be restricted and replaced by mono- and polyunsaturated fats. In patients with dyslipidemia, total fat intake is reduced to less than 30 percent of total calories. Saturated fat intake should be restricted to less than 10 percent of total calories; reduction to less than 7 percent of total calories may provide greater reduction in total and LDL-cholesterol. Cholesterol intake should be reduced to less than 300 mg/day; further reduction to less than 200 mg/day is indicated in patients with hypercholesterolemia. A high fiber content is encouraged. Limitation of protein intake to 0.8 g/kg/day is advocated to avoid any adverse effect on kidney function. Alcohol intake should be limited to below 20 and 14 units for men and women, respectively.[300–302]

Life-Style Modification

Regular physical exercise is recommended. It can increase insulin sensitivity, lower plasma glucose concentration, promote weight loss, improve the lipid profile with an increase in HDL cholesterol and a decrease in total and LDL cholesterol, lower blood pressure, and increase physical working capacity. However, patients should be carefully evaluated and the exercise program should be individualized to fit the patient's life-style and physical condition. Patients

with CAD are at a higher risk of developing angina pectoris, MI, and arrhythmias during unusual physical activity. Peripheral neuropathy may increase the risk of traumatic lesions, and autonomic neuropathy may limit physical performance. Poorly controlled diabetes, proliferative retinopathy, and overt diabetic nephropathy are contraindications to strenuous physical exercise. Mild to moderate physical activity, such as brisk walking for 30 to 45 minutes for 3 to 5 days per week, is adequate. Patients on insulin or sulfonylureas should be educated about the different strategies of avoiding hypo- or hyperglycemia during exercise.[303] Smokers should be encouraged to stop smoking. Yudkin[304] has estimated that stopping diabetic patients from smoking would save more lives than antihypertensive or lipid-lowering drugs.

Hypoglycemic Agents. In view of recent data documenting the effectiveness of stringent glycemic control in preventing or delaying the development of diabetic complications, intensive insulin therapy is recommended for all patients with IDDM.[108,305] The conventional twice daily insulin therapy should be discouraged and treatment should be tailored for each patient. Combinations of different types of insulin can be given 3 to 4 times a day to achieve around-the-clock optimal glycemic control. Several options are available. Long-acting insulin (e.g., ultralente) can be given once in the morning before breakfast with supplemental regular insulin administered before each meal. Alternatively, intermediate acting insulin can be given before breakfast and dinner with additional doses of regular insulin before each meal. A third approach is to give intermediate insulin before breakfast and at bedtime with supplemental regular insulin before meals.[306] The latter approach aims at preventing morning hyperglycemia. Intensive insulin therapy requires, however, proper patient education and home glucose monitoring especially as the risk of hypoglycemia is significantly increased. Intensive insulin therapy is not recommended in patients with autonomic neuropathy, hypoglycemia unawareness, severe retinopathy or nephropathy, recurrent severe hypoglycemic attacks, or preexisting CAD or cerebrovascular disease.

Fifty percent of patients with NIDDM can be managed effectively with diet, life-style changes, and weight loss. If these measures fail, oral hypoglycemic drugs or insulin are indicated. Sulfonylureas are the only oral hypoglycemic drugs available in the United States. They act mainly by stimulating insulin secretion by the β-cells. They may have also some extrapancreatic effects, such as improving insulin sensitivity and glucose transport.[307] Second-generation sulfonylureas (e.g., glibenclamide, glipizide, gliclazide) are more powerful insulin secretagogues and less protein-bound than older drugs (e.g., tolbutamide, tolazomide, acetohexamide, chlorpropamide). Hypoglycemia is the major side effect of sulfonylureas. It can be particularly prolonged and more serious with glibenclamide and chlorpropamide. Therefore, these two drugs should be avoided in the elderly and in patients with impaired renal function. The sulfonylureas were thought to have an adverse effect on cardiovascular mortality because of the results of The University Group Diabetes Program study in the 1960s. These results could not be substantiated and are currently attributable to statistical flaws.[308] Chlorpropamide can cause water retention and is not recommended in cardiac patients.

The biguanide metformin is also available in many other countries and may be approved by the Food and Drug Administration for use in the United States in the near future.[309,310] Biguanides have no effect on insulin secretion, but act through increasing peripheral glucose utilization and inhibiting hepatic glucose production. They inhibit also intestinal glucose absorption and have a mild anorexigenic effect. The side effects of metformin are mainly gastrointestinal (anorexia, nausea, abdominal discomfort, and diarrhea). They are usually transient, dose-dependent, and are minimized by taking the drug with meals. Biguanides can also precipitate lactic acidosis. Metformin is, however, much safer than the earlier compound phenformin, which has been abandoned. The reported incidence of lactic acidosis during metformin therapy is 0.027 to 0.084 cases/1,000 patient-year. Metformin is therefore contraindicated in conditions that predispose to lactic acidosis, such as renal insufficiency, hepatic disease, congestive heart failure, and hypoxic respiratory disease.

When diet fails in controlling blood glucose in diabetic patients, an oral hypoglycemic is indicated. It is preferable to start with metformin (if available) in obese patients and with a sulfonylurea in lean ones. The dose of the drug is gradually increased until optimal glycemic control is achieved or the maximum therapeutic dose is reached. If the target glycemia is not achieved, a drug of the other group is added (i.e., a sulfonylurea is combined with metformin or vice versa). If oral drugs fail they can be combined with or replaced by insulin.

Hypolipidemic Agents. Fasting total cholesterol, triglycerides, HDL cholesterol, and calculated LDL cholesterol levels should be determined annually in diabetic adults and biennially in children. If LDL cholesterol is 130 mg/dl or higher, triglycerides 200 mg/dl or higher, or HDL cholesterol less than 35 mg/dl, treatment should be started by optimization of diabetes control with diet, exercise, and hypoglycemic drugs. Lipid-lowering drugs are indicated when the response to these measures is unsatisfactory. The acceptable levels of lipids in diabetic patients as recommended by the American Diabetes Association are a total cholesterol lower than 200 mg/dl and LDL cholesterol lower than 130 mg/dl (Table 6-4).[302] These recommendations are more strict than those of the National Cholesterol Education Program[311] because of the increased risk of ASCVD in diabetic patients. In addition, triglyceride levels should be kept under 200 mg/dl since they have been shown to be an independent risk factor for ASCVD in diabetics.[123]

Most diabetic patients have both hypercholesterolemia and hypertriglyceridemia. Treatment can be started in these patients with a fibric acid derivative (e.g., gemfibrozil, clofibrate, bezafibrate). This group of drugs activates lipoprotein lipase, reduces VLDL, IDL, triglyceride, and to a lesser extent LDL cholesterol levels and increase HDL cholesterol levels. Gemfibrozil was shown in the Helsinki Heart Study to be effective in improving the lipid profile and reducing coronary events in NIDDM patients.[312] Garg and Grundy[313] have shown, however, that the LDL cholesterol lowering effect of gemfibrozil was observed only in NIDDM patients with marked hypertriglyceridemia. Therefore, if the LDL cholesterol level continues to be elevated, gemfibrozil can be combined with a bile acid sequestrant. The combi-nation of gemfibrozil and lovastatin is also effective, but it carries a significant risk of myositis and should be avoided.[314] The main side effects of gemfibrozil include mild gastrointestinal upset, elevation of liver enzymes, and increased incidence of cholelithiasis.

Hydroxymethylglutaryl coenzyme A (HMG-CoA) reductase inhibitors (e.g., lovastatin, pravastatin, simvastatin) are the drugs of choice for treatment of diabetic patients with elevated LDL cholesterol levels. This group of drugs inhibits the rate-limiting enzyme for cholesterol biosynthesis. Thus, hepatic cholesterol synthesis decreases and cellular LDL receptors increase with subsequent increase in the clearance of LDL and IDL from the plasma. Administration of lovastatin results in an approximately 25 percent reduction in total and LDL cholesterol levels in NIDDM patients.[315] Pravastatin has been shown also to be effective in hypercholesterolemic diabetic patients.[316] If the response to a drug of this group is inadequate, a bile acid sequestrant can be added. Lovastatin has been shown also to lower triglyceride levels in NIDDM patients,[315] but it should not be used singly for that purpose.

Elevation of serum creatine phosphokinase level and clinically significant myositis may occur in patients treated with large doses of lovastatin. The risk of myositis increases if lovastatin is combined with gemfibrozil, nicotinic acid, cyclo-

Table 6-4. Lipid Levels for Diabetic Patients

	Cholesterol (mg/dl)	LDL (mg/dl)	HDL (mg/dl)	Triglycerides (mg/dl)
Acceptable	<200	<130	—	<200
Borderline	200–239	130–160	—	200–239
High	≥240	>160	<35	≥400

(From American Diabetes Association,[302] with permission.)

sporin, or erythromycin. No such interaction between these drugs and second-generation agents (e.g., pravastatin) has been reported. Mild reversible elevation of liver enzymes may also occur. This group of drugs should be avoided, therefore, in patients with a history of liver disease.[317]

Nicotinic acid (niacin) inhibits lipolysis and decreases VLDL production by the liver. Subsequently, the levels of VLDL and its products IDL and LDL are decreased. The net effect is reduction in total and LDL cholesterol and triglyceride levels. In addition, the level of HDL-cholesterol increases. Nicotinic acid is not recommended, however, in diabetic patients because it worsens insulin resistance[318] and could impair glycemic control.[319] Conversely, the nicotinic acid derivative acipimox (not available yet in the United States) has been reported to increase insulin sensitivity and improve glycemia in addition to lowering cholesterol and triglyceride levels.[320,321] It may be useful, therefore, in the management of combined hyperlipidemia in diabetic patients.

Bile acid sequestrants (colestipol and cholestyramine) are ion-exchange resins that bind bile acids in the gastrointestinal tract, preventing their reabsorption and thereby interrupting their enterohepatic recirculation. Hepatic conversion of cholesterol to bile acids subsequently increases, thus reducing serum total and LDL cholesterol levels. Bile acid sequestrants should not be used as first-line drugs in diabetic patients because they can increase VLDL levels and worsen the hypertriglyceridemia which is common in diabetic patients. Small doses can be used, however, in combination with gemfibrozil in the management of combined hyperlipidemia or with HMG-CoA reductase inhibitors in the management of hypercholesterolemia. Bile acid sequestrants should be used cautiously in

the elderly and in patients with autonomic neuropathy since they can cause constipation or even fecal impaction.[302]

Treatment

Management of diabetes and hyperlipidemia in diabetic patients with ASCVD follows the same lines described above under Prevention. Care should be taken, however, to avoid hypoglycemic attacks in patients with CAD since they can provoke arrhythmias and trigger silent ischemic episodes.[322] Treatment of diabetic patients with ASCVD is similar, in general, to that of nondiabetics. The following section addresses only the therapeutic problems specific to the diabetic state.

Angina Pectoris. There are no restrictions on the use of nitrates in diabetic patients. If β-adrenergic blockers are to be used, only cardioselective drugs should be used. Nonselective β-blockers can mask the symptoms of and impede the recovery from hypoglycemia. Calcium channel blockers have no effect on the manifestations of or the recovery from hypoglycemia and can be used safely as antianginal agents in diabetic patients. If medical therapy fails, the options are percutaneous transluminal coronary angioplasty (PTCA) or coronary artery bypass grafting. PTCA is less suitable in diabetic patients because of the higher incidence of more severe and widespread disease involving multiple vessels or segments of the same vessel. In addition, long-term results are less favorable because of the higher rate of restenosis.[323,324] Diabetic patients have also a significantly higher rate of restenosis after coronary artery stenting.[325] Coronary artery bypass grafting is of proven benefit and improves anginal symptoms and long-term survival.[326,327] However, diabetic patients still have a higher failure rate and a lower 5-year survival than nondiabetics. Morris et al.[326] found that the probability of 5-year survival was 80 percent in diabetic patients compared with 91 percent for nondiabetics.

Acute Myocardial Infarction. Thrombolytic therapy is recommended in diabetic patients, since it improves both survival and left ventricular function. Several studies have demonstrated that thrombolytic therapy reduces mortality to a similar extent in both diabetic and nondiabetic patients.[271,328–331] However, diabetic patients still have a higher mortality than nondiabetics even after thrombolytic therapy.[330] The risk of bleeding or stroke is not higher in diabetic patients than in controls.[329,330] A high incidence of hemorrhagic complications associated with increased mortality has been observed only, however, in elderly diabetic patients (older than 75 years).[332] Thrombolysis in such patients should be limited to those with life-threatening MI until further data are available.[256] The presence of proliferative retinopathy should not preclude thrombolytic therapy. However, patients should be examined regularly by an ophthalmologist during the thrombolytic therapy. Myocardial revascularization is indicated in patients who do not respond to thrombolytic therapy. Coronary artery bypass grafting or PTCA can be used. PTCA may be less successful because of the more extensive atherosclerotic lesions that occur in diabetes.

After the acute phase of MI, cardioselective blockers can be used for secondary prevention. Several studies have demonstrated significant reduction in mortality and reinfarction rates in diabetic patients who received timolol[333] or metoprolol[334] after acute MI. In fact, diabetic patients benefited more from β-adrenoceptor blocker administration than nondiabetics.[333,334] Aspirin in small doses can be added to inhibit platelet activity, which is usually heightened in diabetic patients. Although no data on secondary prevention are available, aspirin was shown to reduce the risk of MI in diabetic patients in a primary prevention trial.[335]

Transient Ischemic Attacks. Antiplatelet agents could decrease the risk of stroke in diabetic patients with TIA. Several studies that included both diabetic and nondiabetic individuals have demonstrated that aspirin reduced the risk of stroke equally in both groups.[336–338] In addition, ticlopidine, a potent inhibitor of platelet aggregation, has been recently shown to be more effective than aspirin in preventing stroke, especially in diabetic patients.[339] Carotid endarterectomy is highly beneficial in patients with 70 percent or more ipsilateral internal carotid artery stenosis.[340–342] Surgery was not effective in patients with less than 30 percent stenosis.[340] An ongoing study is evaluating surgical treatment with intermediate degrees of stenosis.[341] Thus, carotid endarterectomy combined with antiplatelet therapy is indicated in patients with TIA and 70 percent or more ipsilateral internal carotid artery stenosis. Patients with lesser degrees of stenosis should be treated medically with no surgical intervention until more data become available.

Stroke. Treatment of stroke is the same as in nondiabetic patients. Glycemic control is important to decrease the risk of cerebral edema and brain damage.[343] In addition, stroke can precipitate diabetic ketoacidosis. An insulin drip is the best approach to glycemic control. Careful monitoring of blood glucose is of paramount importance to avoid any hypoglycemic attacks that can cause further brain damage. Early ambulation and active rehabilitation are essential, especially as stroke leads to more severe neurological deficits in diabetic patients. The presence of peripheral neuropathy, muscle wasting, neuropathic joints, or preexisting lower limb amputation can complicate rehabilitation. Aspirin or the antiplatelet agent ticlopidine are recommended for secondary prevention after a stroke.[344]

Peripheral Vascular Disease. All diabetic patients, especially those with PVD or peripheral neuropathy, should be instructed on how to examine and take care of their feet. If the patient's eyesight is affected, a family member should be instructed on how to examine the feet. Patient education has been proven to be successful in reducing the incidence of amputation in diabetics.[345] Drugs that could worsen blood flow (e.g., β-adrenergic receptor blockers) should be discontinued. Smoking cessation and regular exercise often improve blood flow and relieve intermittent claudication. If ischemic ulcers are present, debridement and prompt antibiotic therapy to eradicate any infection are critical. Vasodilators and antiplatelet agents can be also helpful. Pentoxifylline, a xanthine derivative that can improve blood flow by decreasing erythrocyte rigidity and blood viscosity, is effective in approximately 30 percent of cases. It has been shown to improve walking distance, skin temperature, and promote the healing of foot ulcers.[346] The antiplatelet agent cilostazol has been shown recently to improve blood flow in diabetic patients with PVD.[347]

Surgical revascularization is indicated in patients with intractable claudication, night pain, or rest pain not responding to medical therapy, and in those with non-healing ulcers. Revascularization may also be attempted before amputating gangrenous toes or a foot to increase blood flow and thereby the chances of healing. However, earlier surgical intervention has been recently advocated to reduce the incidence of amputation from isch-

emia in diabetic patients.[348] Arterial reconstruction with bypass grafting has been shown to have a high success rate in diabetic patients with 1- and 5-year patency rates of approximately 90 percent and 75 percent, which are no different from those of nondiabetics.[349] Alternatively, percutaneous transluminal angioplasty can be used especially if the symptoms are not disabling enough to warrant surgery or if the patient is a high operative risk.[350] Amputation should be the last resort. Single toe amputation is indicated to treat severe necrotic ulceration of the distal third of the toe. Amputation of a toe together with a metatarsal head ("ray" amputation) is usually unsuccessful in the ischemic foot. Below-the-knee amputation is indicated for rampant infection, extensive tissue destruction, or intractable rest pain in a limb in which revascularization is not possible or has failed.[351]

DIABETIC CARDIOMYOPATHY

In 1972, Rubler et al.[352] described four patients with cardiomegaly and congestive heart failure due to diffuse myocardial fibrosis without significant CAD and suggested the existence of a cardiomyopathy specific for diabetes. This postulate was supported by data from the Framingham study[353] showing that congestive heart failure (CHF) was two and five times as common in diabetic as in nondiabetic men and women, respectively, independent of known CAD or hypertension. In addition, Hamby et al.[354] reported a twofold increase in the prevalence of diabetes among patients with idiopathic cardiomyopathy. Subsequent human[355–359] and experimental[360,361] studies brought evidence that diabetes *per se* can adversely affect the myocardium.

Thus, diabetic cardiomyopathy gained acceptance as a separate pathologic entity in which histologic and functional myocardial abnormalities occur in the absence of CAD, hypertension, autonomic neuropathy, or other etiologic factors (e.g., alcoholism, valvular disease, etc.).[362–364]

Pathogenesis

Both abnormal myocardial metabolism and structural changes appear to contribute to the development of diabetic cardiomyopathy. The diabetic state is associated with alteration in both glucose and lipid metabolism in the myocardium as well as in the whole body. A major metabolic abnormality is impaired myocardial glucose uptake due to suppression of glucose transporter 4 (GLUT 4) gene expression and reduction of its activity.[365] Intracellular glucose phosphorylation is also decreased because of inhibition of certain key enzymes (namely, phosphofructokinase and pyruvate dehydrogenase). Thus, despite hyperglycemia, glucose is actually unavailable for energy production. The heart, therefore, preferentially utilizes free fatty acids as an energy source, especially as they are readily available due to the excessive lipolysis characteristic of uncontrolled diabetes. When compared with glucose, free fatty acid utilization has an oxygen wasting effect that results in increased myocardial oxygen consumption at any given level of cardiac work. Thus, under conditions of increased work load or ischemia, diminished glucose availability culminates in impaired cardiac performance.[366]

High concentrations of free fatty acids can also exert a cardiodepressant and an arrhythmogenic effect. The intracellular accumulation of potentially toxic intermediates of fatty acid metabolism can modify the structure of sarcolemmal and other subcellular membranes, alter membrane fluidity and molecular dynamics, inhibit critical enzymes such as Ca^{++}-ATPase of sarcoplasmic reticulum and Na^+/K^+-ATPase, and subsequently inhibit Na^+/Ca^{++} exchange, suppress the adenine nucleotide translocator in mitochondria leading to a reduction in the myocardial level of ATP, and directly interfere with voltage dependent Ca^{++} channels. Alteration in handling of Ca^{++} leads to its intracellular accumulation with increased myocardial stiffness and delayed relaxation.[366,367]

Microangiopathic changes could be involved in the pathogenesis of diabetic cardiomyopathy. Saccular and fusiform microaneurysms and thickening of capillary basement membranes have been reported in the diabetic heart.[368,369] Endomyocardial biopsy demonstrated microangiopathic changes in diabetic patients with abnormal left ventricular (LV) ejection fraction during exercise.[370] An association between diabetic retinopathy and left ventricular dysfunction has been demonstrated in some[371,372] but not all studies.[373,374] Increased myocardial fibrosis can also contribute to LV systolic and diastolic abnormalities. Perivascular and interstitial infiltration with periodic acid-Schiff (PAS) positive material and fibrosis, along with degeneration and fragmentation of myocytes, have been reported in the diabetic myocardium.[357]

Pathophysiology

Left Ventricular Systolic Function

Most echocardiographic and radionuclide cineangiographic studies indicate that resting LV ejection fraction is normal in diabetic patients with no evidence of CAD or autonomic neuropathy.[372–374]

Conversely, some studies have reported decreased fractional shortening in children and young adults with IDDM.[375,376] A third group of studies, however, described increased resting LV ejection fractions in diabetic patients free of CAD compared with controls.[377–379] Thuesen[380] has recently demonstrated a positive correlation between the ejection fraction and urinary albumin excretion (up to 200 μg/min) in IDDM patients without clinical signs of heart disease. The ejection fraction decreased progressively at higher degrees of urinary albumin excretion (i.e., in patients with clinical nephropathy). He postulated that the increased ejection fraction in patients with microalbuminuria was a manifestation of transient generalized organ hyperperfusion that precedes the development of the microvascular complications of diabetes. It is possible, therefore, that the discrepancy in the results was due to differences in the characteristics of patients included. Most agree, however, that the LV ejection fraction is reduced in up to 50 percent of diabetic patients during exercise in the absence of clinical heart disease.[372–374,377]

Left Ventricular Diastolic Function

Several noninvasive studies have examined diastolic function in diabetic patients using either echocardiography or radionuclide ventriculography. LV diastolic dysfunction has been described in up to 70 percent of diabetic patients with no evidence of clinical heart disease. Such abnormalities include prolonged isovolumic relaxation time (and/or the time from minimum LV dimension to mitral valve opening), prolonged rapid filling period, slowing in the thinning of the LV wall, and increased atrial contribution to LV filling.[381–388] Abnormal diastolic function in diabetes is thought to reflect both abnormal myocardial relaxation

and diminished ventricular compliance.[364] The former can occur in the absence of structural myocardial abnormality and is attributed to myocyte dysfunction.[389] Conversely, diminished ventricular relaxation implies increased chamber stiffness due to increased myocardial collagen content. Recently, an echocardiographic study employing ultrasound tissue characterization demonstrated abnormal myocardial acoustic properties in diabetic patients that was attributed to increased collagen deposition in the heart.[390] In addition, decreased preload may contribute to diastolic function abnormalities. Diabetic patients with microvascular complications manifest increased capillary permeability to albumin with subsequent decrease in intravascular volume.[391] The resulting decrease in LV preload causes prolongation of isovolumic relaxation period and diminution of early rapid filling velocity, the main features of diastolic dysfunction.[364]

Clinical Implications

Diabetic cardiomyopathy is mostly a subclinical entity. Some patients present with anginal chest pain or heart failure in the absence of significant CAD or hypertension.[354,357,358,392] Conduction and rhythm disturbances and abnormal P waves are common manifestations of diabetic cardiomyopathy and have been reported in 50 percent of 89 normotensive diabetic patients with no manifestations of heart involvement. Intra-atrial conduction disturbances were present in approximately 20 percent of these patients in the absence of atrial enlargement.[393,394]

Cardiomyopathy appears to account for the increased incidence of CHF and the more adverse outcome of MI in diabetic patients. The presence of LV diastolic dysfunction may increase the susceptibility to CHF after MI even in the presence of normal resting systolic function. The detrimental effect of diabetes on the myocardium is often made worse by the frequent concomitant occurrence of hypertension. Both diseases can cause similar abnormalities in LV function, and their coexistence increases the risk of LV hypertrophy and cardiac failure to a significantly greater extent than either alone.[395,396]

Management

Correction of the metabolic abnormalities associated with diabetes (namely, hyperglycemia and hyperlipidemia), may improve at least in part some of the manifestations of diabetic cardiomyopathy.[397–399] Shapiro et al.[398] have demonstrated that the improvement was limited to patients with mild but not severe abnormalities in LV function. Tight glycemic control and correction of the hyperlipidemia according to the lines described earlier are therefore recommended.

Management of CHF is similar to that in nondiabetic individuals, using a combination of diuretics and vasodilators. Diuretics may impair glucose tolerance and adjustment of the hypoglycemic drugs may be needed. Loop diuretics are preferred since they are more potent and may have a milder effect on glycemic control than thiazides. For vasodilator therapy, angiotensin-converting enzyme (ACE) inhibitors are preferred; they improve symptoms of heart failure and long-term survival[400] and may improve glycemic control through increasing insulin sensitivity.[401] Careful monitoring of renal function and serum potassium level is required after starting ACE inhibitors since diabetic patients are more prone to renovascular disease and hyporenninemic hypoaldosteronism. Combining ACE inhibitors with a diuretic decreases the risk of hyperkalemia. ACE inhibitors should be discontinued, however, if deterioration of renal function occurs. A combination of hydralazine and isosorbide dinitrate has also been shown to improve symptoms of heart failure and can be used in patients who cannot tolerate ACE inhibitors because of side effects or deterioration of renal function. Digoxin is indicated in patients with atrial fibrillation with rapid ventricular response.

HYPERTENSION

The increased prevalence of hypertension in diabetic patients was recognized more than 70 years ago.[402] While diabetic nephropathy accounts for the great majority of cases in IDDM, essential hypertension is more commonly seen in NIDDM. Regardless of its cause, hypertension impacts seriously on the course and outcome of diabetes by accelerating the development and/or the progression of its micro- and macrovascular complications. The recognition and treatment of hypertension ranks next in line to glycemic control in the overall management of the diabetic patient.

Epidemiology

The prevalence of hypertension is 2 to 3 times higher in diabetic patients compared with the general population.[403] In the majority of patients with IDDM, hypertension develops in conjunction with the appearance of persistent proteinuria. By the age of 55, approximately one-half of IDDM patients have both hypertension and diabetic nephropathy.[404] The prevalence of hypertension among IDDM patients who do not have significant nephropathy is similar to that observed in nondiabetic individuals (Fig. 6-4).[232] In NIDDM, hypertension

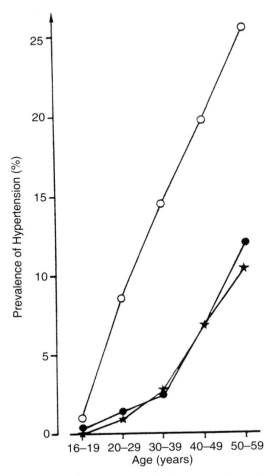

Fig. 6-4. Prevalence of hypertension in IDDM patients with (open circles) and without (closed circles) nephropathy compared with the general Danish population (stars). (From Norgaard et al.,[232] with permission.)

commonly develops several years before or is discovered at the time of diagnosis of diabetes. Data from the U.S. Second National Health and Nutrition Examination Survey demonstrated that hypertension was present in 61 percent of subjects aged 40 to 69 years with previously undiagnosed NIDDM compared with 69 percent in those with previously known diabetes and with 36 percent in nondiabetic individuals.[101] In the United Kingdom

Prospective Diabetes Study, hypertension was present in 39 percent of the patients with newly diagnosed NIDDM.[405] Hypertension is also more common in subjects with IGT who are at a higher risk for subsequent development of NIDDM. In a study among 2,233 subjects ages 50 to 89 years in Rancho Bernardo, California,[406] the age-adjusted prevalence of hypertension was 31.9 percent in healthy men, 45.3 percent in subjects with IGT, 57.4 percent in those with newly diagnosed NIDDM, and 60.9 percent in those with known NIDDM. The corresponding figures for women were 36.4, 44.7, 49.0, and 59.5 percent, respectively (Fig. 6-5). It has been suggested, therefore, that hypertension and NIDDM may share common antecedents or pathogenic mechanisms (see below).

Pathogenesis

A distinction should be made between the pathogenesis of hypertension in the two types of diabetes. IDDM occurs mainly in younger individuals with a peak incidence in the second decade of life. Thus, hypertension is usually a consequence of IDDM and is predominantly due to diabetic nephropathy. Conversely, NIDDM develops after the age of 40 in the majority of patients. Essential hypertension is more commonly seen in these older patients in whom it may even precede the development of NIDDM or be discovered at the time of diagnosis.

Hypertension in IDDM
Diabetic nephropathy plays an important role in the pathogenesis of hypertension in IDDM. Norgaard et al.[232] have demonstrated that the increased occurrence of hypertension in IDDM patients was completely accounted for by the presence of the disease in those with nephropathy and that the prevalence of hy-

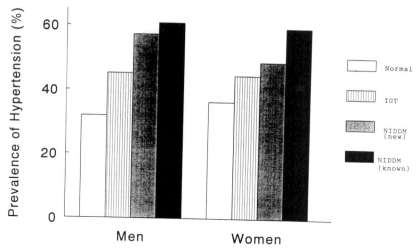

Fig. 6-5. Age-adjusted prevalence of hypertension among men and women aged 50 to 89 years by the different categories of glucose tolerance (Data from Reaven et al.[406])

pertension among those with no evidence of renal disease was not different from that observed in the general population (Fig. 6-4). Diabetic nephropathy develops slowly, in several stages that have been characterized by Mogensen et al.[407] The earliest abnormality is *glomerular hyperfunction* and *hypertrophy* (stage I) which is often present at the time of diagnosis of IDDM. This stage is characterized by renal enlargement and an increase in both the glomerular filtration rate and creatinine clearance. These changes regress with improved metabolic control and pass into a *silent phase* (stage II) that usually lasts for 7 to 15 years. During this stage, structural changes in the form of mesangial expansion and thickening of basement membrane develop. The third stage is known as *incipient nephropathy* and is characterized by persistent and increasing microalbuminuria (urinary albumin 30 to 300 mg/24 h or albumin excretion rate 20 to 200 µg/min). Blood pressure starts to rise slowly and, although still in the normal range, is slightly higher than in nondiabetic individuals and in diabetic patients with normal urinary albumin excretion rate. The glomerular filtration rate may also start to decline. In the majority of patients, the incipient phase progresses over 5 to 10 years to *overt* or *clinical nephropathy* (stage IV) in which proteinuria (urinary protein more than 0.5 g/24 h or urinary albumin excretion rate more than 200 µg/min) and hypertension are the main features. In addition, the glomerular filtration rate deteriorates progressively at an average rate of 1.0 ml/min/month and *end-stage renal disease* (stage V) eventually ensues.

The development of clinical nephropathy increases with the duration of diabetes. In addition, poor metabolic control and higher blood pressure accelerate the progression of diabetic nephropathy. Nevertheless, more than 50 percent of IDDM patients never develop severe diabetic renal disease regardless of the duration of diabetes or the degree of metabolic derangement. Diabetic nephropathy has been shown to cluster in families, suggesting that genetic factors may underlie the susceptibility to renal disease in patients with IDDM.[408,409] A familial influence in the development of nephropathy has also been described in Pima Indians with NIDDM.[410] It has been postulated that a genetic factor may be linked to hereditary predisposition to essential hypertension. Viberti et al.[141] showed that IDDM patients with proteinuria were more likely to have hypertensive parents than those without evidence of renal disease. Krolewski et al.[412] and Barzilay et al.[413] reported similar data, and suggested that increased red blood cell sodium/lithium countertransport could be a genetic marker for increased predisposition to both hypertension and diabetic nephropathy. However, a relationship between parental history of hypertension or red blood cell sodium lithium countertransport and diabetic ne-

phropathy could not be confirmed by Jensen et al.[414]

The mechanism of the association between diabetic nephropathy and hypertension in IDDM is unknown. IDDM patients with or without nephropathy have increased extracellular fluid volume and exchangeable sodium.[415,416] Sodium retention is more pronounced, however, in patients with incipient or overt nephropathy.[417] A significant correlation has been demonstrated between body exchangeable sodium and blood pressure (Fig. 6-6). Sodium retention is due in part to increased glomerular filtration of glucose and ketones that are actively reabsorbed along with sodium at the level of the proximal renal tubules. Thus, a tendency for sodium retention is present in all sub-

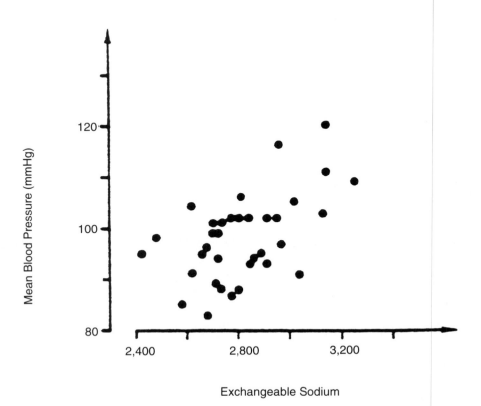

Fig. 6-6. Relation between exchangeable sodium and mean blood pressure in IDDM patients with microalbuminuria. (From Feldt-Rasmussen et al.,[416] with permission.)

jects with hyperglycemia except in poorly controlled patients in whom the associated osmotic diuresis leads to dehydration and sodium depletion. Other factors that contribute to sodium retention include iatrogenically-induced hyperinsulinemia (see below), impaired tubular response to atrial naturitic hormone,[418] and increased capillary permeability.[178] Sodium retention possibly leads to increased intracellular sodium with subsequent elevation of intracellular calcium. Increased vascular smooth muscle intracellular calcium enhances contractility resulting in increased peripheral resistance.[419] In addition, vascular, hyperreactivity to norepinephrine[420] and angiotensin II[421] has been described in early uncomplicated stages of diabetes. This hypersensitivity to pressor stimuli is perhaps due to increased intracellular sodium and/or calcium.

Essential hypertension can also occur in patients with IDDM. Its prevalence, however, is not different from that observed in the general population.[232] Christensen et al.[422] have demonstrated that diabetic patients with essential hypertension have a normal or a relatively moderate increase in urinary albumin excretion that is disproportionate to the degree of elevation of blood pressure.

Hypertension in NIDDM

Contrary to IDDM, diabetic nephropathy contributes to the pathogenesis of hypertension in only a small proportion of patients with NIDDM. The great majority of cases are due to coexisting essential hypertension or are obesity-related, especially as 80 percent of NIDDM patients are overweight. Hypertension can precede the development of NIDDM and is also frequent in prediabetic persons with normal or impaired glucose tolerance.[405,406] It is thought, therefore, that hypertension and NIDDM share common determinants or antecedents such as insulin resistance and/or the concomitant compensatory hyperinsulinemia.[34] Insulin resistance often precedes and plays a crucial role in the development of IGT and NIDDM.[46] Obesity is also associated with insulin resistance and hyperinsulinemia.[423] In addition, recent data indicate that some hypertensive patients are insulin resistant and hyperinsulinemic.[216]

Hyperinsulinemia and insulin resistance can impact on a number of mechanisms that affect the development of hypertension (Fig. 6-7). Insulin can promote sodium retention through a direct effect on the renal tubules without causing a change in the glomerular filtra-

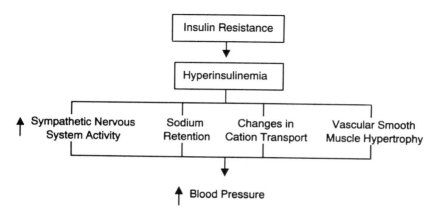

Fig. 6-7. The insulin resistance-hyperinsulinemia-hypertension hypothesis.

tion rate.[424] It can also enhance sympathetic nervous system activity.[425] In addition, insulin stimulates the activity of the Na^+/H^+ antiport, a cell membrane system involved in the control of intracellular Na^+ concentration and pH, in cell growth, and in proximal rental tubular sodium reabsorption.[426] Overactivity of this system, as a result of hyperinsulinemia, can lead to increased intracellular Na^+ in vascular smooth muscle making them more sensitive to the pressor effects of catecholamines and angiotensin II. Increased intracellular Na^+ is usually associated with elevated intracellular Ca^{++} resulting in heightened vascular tone. Finally, insulin can cause proliferation of vascular smooth muscle cells with subsequent narrowing of the lumen of resistant vessels.[427]

The role of insulin and insulin resistance in the pathogenesis of hypertension is, however, controversial.[428] The relation between insulinemia and blood pressure is not consistent or universal. Hyperinsulinemia is not always associated with hypertension and vice versa. Plasma insulin concentrations are correlated with blood pressure in some but not all ethnic groups or individuals.[217] Moreover, the strength of the correlation, when significant, varies markedly, and correlations, at any rate, do not prove causality.

In addition, there is no solid experimental evidence that insulin causes hypertension. Acute insulin infusion in humans raises blood pressure only when supraphysiologic plasma insulin concentrations are achieved.[425] On the contrary, infusion of low doses of insulin causes vasodilatation and tends to lower blood pressure.[429,430] Animal experiments have also been inconclusive. In dogs, insulin infusions for 28 days caused only transient sodium retention followed by a renal escape without any increase in blood pressure.[431] In rats, however, similar

infusions caused elevation of blood pressure.[432] The animal data that can be extrapolated to humans is difficult to determine.

Although compelling evidence for the insulin-hypertension hypothesis is lacking, insulin cannot be completely exonerated. The discrepancy in the data on the relation between insulinemia and blood pressure might be attributable to differences in the sensitivity to the postulated effects of insulin among different individuals or ethnic groups. Haffner[433] suggested that insulin might contribute to the pathogenesis of hypertension in lean but not in obese subjects. Furthermore, regulation of blood pressure and pathogenesis of hypertension are complicated processes in which myocardial, hemodynamic, renal, neural, humoral, and myogenic factors interact. The role of insulin in the pathogenesis of hypertension should be considered in the context of its interaction with these factors.

Alternatively, insulin resistance and hypertension may not be causally related, but linked through shared functional or structural mechanisms of an inherited or acquired nature. A possible link is the sympathetic nervous systems (Fig. 6-8). Enhanced adrenergic tone leads to an increase in insulin resistance[434] on one hand and a rise in blood pressure through inotropic, chronotropic, and peripheral vasoconstrictor effects[435] on the other. Ethnic differences in sympathetic nervous system activity appear to exist and could create differences in the relationship of insulin resistance to blood pressure. In support of this possibility is the ethnic difference in the relationship between blood pressure and the resting metabolic rate, which is in part sympathetically mediated.[436] Twenty-four hour energy expenditure has been shown to be related to sympathetic nervous system activity in whites but not in Pima Indians.[437] In addition, Bogardus et

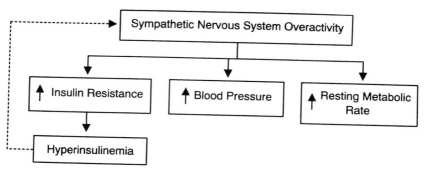

Fig. 6-8. The sympathetic nervous system may be the link between insulin resistance and hypertension.

al.[438] demonstrated a reduced thermic effect of insulin and glucose infusions in Pima Indians, and suggested that this might have been a result of blunted activation of the sympathetic nervous system. Blacks, also, have lower basal cardiac sympathetic responses compared with whites.[439]

A variety of cellular defects may constitute the link between insulin resistance and blood pressure. Reduced activity of sodium-potassium ATPase is found in hypertension[440] and insulin-resistant states.[441,442] This reduction leads to increased intracellular sodium with a concomitant increase in intracellular calcium which increases vascular smooth muscle contractility. Ferrannini et al.[443] demonstrated, however, that stimulation of glucose metabolism and sodium-potassium exchange by insulin were independent of each other. Doria and colleagues[444] suggested that red blood cell sodium-lithium countertransport was the link between insulin resistance and hypertension. Resnick and co-workers[445] reported negative associations between intracellular free magnesium concentration and both blood pressure and plasma insulin concentration, and found that the positive relationship between insulinemia and blood pressure became insignificant when adjusted for intracellular magnesium. They

postulated that decreased availability of intracellular magnesium would enhance calcium-mediated vasoconstriction and decrease cellular glucose utilization. Racial differences in ion regulation have been described[446] and could account for the observed variation in the relationship of insulin resistance to blood pressure.

A further possibility is that the relationship of blood pressure to insulin resistance results from constitutional differences in muscle fiber composition.[447] In the vastus lateralis muscle, the percentage of type I fibers (which have elevated oxidative capacity) is reduced in hypertensive patients and correlates inversely with intra-arterial blood pressure and leg vascular resistance.[448] Because insulin-mediated glucose disposal correlates positively with percent type I fibers,[449] Ferrannini and DeFronzo[447] postulated that the association of insulin resistance and blood pressure could be a genetic trait related to muscle fiber type.

Finally, since insulin resistance and high blood pressure[450,451] each show a cluster-effect in families, both conditions may be more likely to occur together in some individuals or ethnic groups. Ferrari et al.[452] reported that normotensive offspring of essential hypertensive parents tended to be more insulin resistant than those of normotensive parents. Furthermore, Berntorp and Lindgärde[453] found normoglycemic nonobese middle-aged men with a strong family history of NIDDM to have significantly higher blood pressure than controls. Haffner et al.[454] reported that normoglycemic subjects with parental history of NIDDM had higher blood pressures than those whose parents did not have diabetes. Thus, it is possible that genes contributing to insulin resistance and high blood pressure are linked. Recently, Ying et al.[455] demonstrated an association of a restriction fragment length polymorphism of the insulin receptor gene with essential hypertension.

Other Causes of Hypertension in Diabetes

Atherosclerotic renal artery stenosis appears to be more frequent in diabetic patients (mainly NIDDM), but it is uncommonly the cause of hypertension. A recent autopsy study has shown that atherosclerotic renal artery stenosis was 3.5 times as common in NIDDM patients as in nondiabetic individuals, being present in 10.1 percent of hypertensive diabetic patients.[456] However, Ritchie et al.[457] reported that 5 of 24 hypertensive NIDDM patients had angiographically demonstrable unilateral renal artery stenosis, but functional tests showed that it was not the cause of hypertension in any of them.

Nondiabetic renal disease can also cause hypertension in diabetic patients. Glomerulonephritis and diabetic nephropathy not uncommonly co-exist. Kincaid-Smith and Whitworth[458] reported that renal biopsy showed evidence of some type of glomerulonephritis in addition to diabetic nephropathy in 21 (18 percent) of 116 diabetic patients with renal disease. Finally, several endocrinologic disorders can cause both diabetes and hypertension including acromegaly,

Cushing syndrome, pheochromocytoma, and primary hyperaldosteronism.

Hypertension and Diabetic Complications

Hypertension has a grave impact on the development of diabetic complications. It accelerates the development of ASCVD and increases the risk of cardiovascular mortality in diabetic patients.[77,85,99] Most of the increased mortality is due to CAD with a smaller component from stroke. The incidence of CAD is increased six and threefold in hypertensive patients with IDDM and NIDDM, respectively, compared with normotensives.[77,459] Moreover, hypertension can aggravate symptomatic or silent ischemic attacks in diabetic patients with CAD by increasing LV wall stress. The combination of diabetes and hypertension, even in the absence of CAD, can lead to severe cardiomyopathy characterized by extensive myocardial fibrosis, focal or confluent scarring, and myocytolytic lesions.[395,396]

Hypertension is also significantly involved in the development and progression of diabetic microangiopathy. High blood pressure is a significant predictor of diabetic nephropathy and is closely associated with mesangial expansion and the decline of renal function in both IDDM and NIDDM.[460–463] A positive correlation between blood pressure and the rate of deterioration in the glomerular filtration rate has been demonstrated.[460,464,465] Walker[466] reported a progressive increase in serum creatinine in individuals whose systolic blood pressure remained above 140 mmHg despite therapy. Conversely, patients whose blood pressure was maintained below that level showed no significant deterioration in renal function. Thus, blood pressure appears to have a complex relation with diabetic nephropathy: nephropathy raises blood pressure and blood pressure accelerates the course of nephropathy. Hypertension also increases the risk of diabetic reinopathy.[467–469] Knowler et al.[467] described a higher incidence of retinopathy among diabetic Pima Indians with systolic blood pressure greater than 145 mmHg.

Clinical Evaluation of the Hypertensive Diabetic Patient

The purpose of the clinical evaluation is to rule out secondary causes of hypertension and/or diabetes; to evaluate the patient for the presence of diabetic complications (retinopathy, nephropathy, macrovascular disease) or other risk factors for ASCVD (e.g., hyperlipidemia); and to determine the type of therapy in the light of the clinical condition of the patient. A medical history should include (1) family history of hypertension, diabetes, renal disease, and ASCVD; (2) history of ASCVD, renal disease, and retinopathy; (3) known duration of diabetes and hypertension; (4) effect and side effects of previous hypoglycemic and antihypertensive medications; (5) use of drugs that may influence blood pressure or diabetes; (6) history of weight gain or loss, proteinuria, sodium intake, other dietary factors, exercise habits, and alcohol use; and (7) other ASCVD risk factors such, as smoking, hyperlipidemia, and obesity.

The physical examination should include (1) careful measurement of blood pressure on at least two different occasions in all three positions using a cuff appropriate for the size of the patient; (2) determination of height and weight; (3) fundoscopic examination for signs of hypertension and diabetic retinopathy; (4)

examination for signs of atherosclerosis and heart failure; (5) neurologic assessment especially for peripheral neuropathy. Laboratory tests should include fasting plasma glucose, lipids, liproproteins, glycated hemoglobin, serum blood urea nitrogen, creatinine, and electrolytes and a urine test for proteinuria or microalbuminuria. These laboratory measurements should be determined before and 6 to 12 weeks after starting treatment to assess the effect of the antihypertensive drugs on glycemic control and the lipid profile and the need to treat hyperlipidemia if present. Plasma glucose and glycated hemoglobin should be determined every 3 months and the other investigations should be repeated at least once a year, unless deemed necessary for the management of the patient.

Treatment

Aggressive management of hypertension is recommended. Control of blood pressure has been shown to reduce the risk of fatal or nonfatal stroke, CAD death or nonfatal MI, all major cardiovascular events, and total mortality in both diabetics and nondiabetics.[70,71] In addition, it is effective in decreasing albuminuria, improving the glomerular filtration rate, and delaying the progression of retinopathy.[472–474] The aim of antihypertensive therapy is to maintain blood pressure at 130/85 mmHg or less.[475] This is particularly the case in younger patients who are free from diabetic complications. Older patients, especially those with cardiovascular or renal complications, should be treated more cautiously to avoid precipitating further end-organ damage, and a target blood pressure of 140/90 mmHg is more prudent. Proper management of diabetes is essential; recent data from the Diabetes Control and Complications

Trial[108] demonstrated a significant decrease in the development and progression of diabetic complications with strict glycemic control. Hyperlipidemia, if present, should also be treated. Since some antihypertensive drugs can increase glucose and lipid concentration, it is advisable to choose an antihypertensive regimen that does not adversely affect metabolic control.

An attempt to control blood pressure with nonpharmacologic measures (weight loss, exercise, salt restriction, etc.) should be tried for 3 months before initiating drug therapy in patients with mild hypertension (stage 1). Antihypertensive drugs are indicated in patients with more severe hypertension (blood pressure 160/100 mmHg or higher) and in those whose blood pressures continue to be higher than 140/90 mmHg after behaviour modification. Weight loss, diet, and exercise should continue, however, to be part of the treatment regimen. Figure 6-9 shows the approach recommended by the National High Blood Pressure Education Program Working Group.[475]

Life-Style Modification
Dietary intervention is important for the management of both diabetes and hypertension. Diet should follow the same lines described under management of atherosclerosis (see above). Caloric restriction and weight loss are associated with improvement in glycemic control and decrease in blood pressure in obese patients. Modest weight loss (i.e., 10 percent of body weight) improves blood pressure, and some patients can achieve a normal blood pressure without attaining "ideal" body weight.[476] In addition, salt restriction (6 g sodium chloride/day) and maintaining an adequate dietary potassium, calcium, and magnesium intake can be useful in the management of hypertension in patients with both IDDM and NIDDM.[475,477] Dietary protein restriction should be considered in patients with diabetic nephropathy as it may slow the deterioration of renal function. Reduction of alcohol consumption has been shown to decrease blood pressure and should be encouraged. Finally, smoking should be discouraged since it increases the risk of atherosclerosis as well as diabetic microangiopathy.

Physical exercise can also reduce blood pressure. Patients should be carefully evaluated and the exercise program should be individualized to fit the patient's life-style and physical condition. Patients with CAD are at a higher risk of developing angina pectoris, MI, and arrhythmias during unusual physical activity. Autonomic neuropathy may limit physical performance. Patients with peripheral neuropathy should take more precautions with foot care since exercise can increase the risk of traumatic lesions. Poorly controlled diabetes, proliferative retinopathy, and overt diabetic nephropathy are contraindications to strenuous physical exercise. Mild to moderate physical activity is preferred since some diabetic patients may develop an excessive rise in blood pressure even after moderate exertion.[478] Brisk walking for 30 to 45 minutes for 3 to 5 days per week is adequate.[479] Patients on insulin or sulfonylureas should be educated about the different strategies of avoiding hypo- or hyperglycemia during exercise.[303]

Drug Therapy
None of the antihypertensive drugs is specifically contraindicated in diabetes, but caution is needed with most. The major classes of antihypertensive agents are listed in Table 6-5 along with their advantages and drawbacks in the treatment of hypertensive diabetic patients.[480] Simplicity of the overall drug regimen is of utmost importance because many patients may need several other medications.

Treatment Goal <130/85 mm Hg

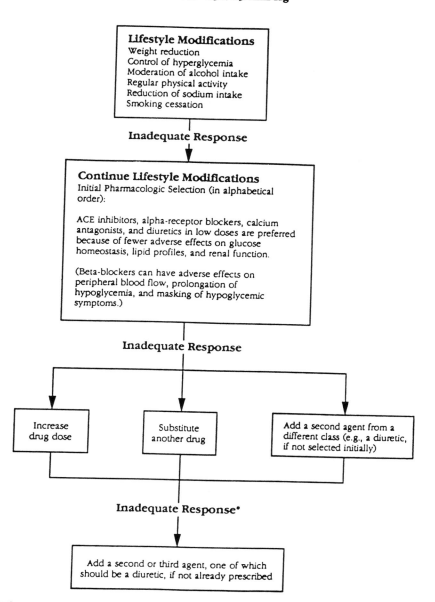

Fig. 6-9. The approach recommended by the National High Blood Pressure Education Program Working Group for management of hypertension in diabetes.[475] Response means achieved goal blood pressure or considerable progress towards this goal.

Table 6-5. Advantages and Drawbacks of the Main Groups of Antihypertensive Drugs in the Treatment of Hypertension with Diabetes

Advantages	Drawbacks	Recommendations
ACE inhibitors Monotherapy lowers high blood pressure effectively Once-daily regimen possible Nephroprotection Effective in heart failure Metabolic "neutrality" (glucose, lipid, potassium) Cardioprotection Antiatherosclerotic(?) Relative rarity of orthostatic and impotence problems(?)	Proteinuria (rare) Dose adjustment with declining renal function Renal failure (reversible) in renal artery stenosis Hyperkalemia in hyporeninemic hypoaldosteronism (rare)	Low to moderate dose Control: renal function; proteinuria; plasma potassium
Calcium antagonists Monotherapy lowers high blood pressure effectively Once-daily regimen possible Antianginal effects Antiarrhythmic properties (verapamil, diltiazem) Metabolic "neutrality" (glucose, lipids, potassium) Nephroprotection(?) Cardioprotection (?) Antiatherosclerotic(?) Relative rarity of orthostatic and impotence problems (?)	Impair insulin secretion in vitro; in high doses in vivo (?) Headache (often transient) Flushing, ankle edema Constipation (verapamil)	Low to moderate dose Control: AV conduction (verapamil, diltiazem); glucose (at higher dosages)
α-Adrenergic receptor blockers Improve insulin sensitivity Improve lipid profile Improve blood flow in peripheral vascular disease	Postural hypotension Salt and water retention Nasal congestion Headache	Use carefully in patients with autonomic neuropathy
Diuretics Monotherapy lowers high blood pressure effectively Once-daily regimen Inexpensive Pathophysiologically sound (lower elevated exchangeable sodium and reduce exaggerated noradrenaline reactivity)	Impair glucose homeostasis Hypokalemia Serum lipid alterations Hyperuricemia Hyperosmolar coma Erectile impotence Orthostatic hypotension	Low dose Control: potassium; glucose; lipids Potassium substitution if needed (diet, KCl, combination with potassium-sparing diuretic)
β-Adrenergic receptor blockers Monotherapy lowers high blood pressure effectively Once daily regimen Cardioprotection Antiangial/antiarrythmic properties	β_2-Blockade impairs insulin output Hypoglycaemia: prolonged by β_2-blockers; altered perception of the symptoms; hypertensive crisis (β_2-blockers) Serum lipid alterations Decrease physical exercise performance	Cardioselective (β_1-)blocker (i.e., atenolol, metoprolol, acebutolol) Low (-moderate) dose Instruction: hypoglycemia problems Control: cardiac performance; AV conduction; serum lipoproteins

(Modified from Trost,[480] with permission.)

Monotherapy with a long-acting preparation is preferred to assure compliance. In case of inadequate response, substitution with another drug is preferable to using a combination of two or more drugs. Such combinations should be used only when a single-drug regimen fails to control blood pressure or causes unacceptable side effects. It is recommended to start treatment with a low dose of an ACE inhibitor, a calcium channel antagonist, or an α_1-adrenergic blocker because of their metabolic neutrality and possible renoprotective effects. A low-dose thiazide diuretic can be used also as a first-line agent. The dose of the antihypertensive drug can be increased gradually until the optimal effect is obtained, or the maximum dose is reached. If one group of drugs is ineffective, it can be substituted by one of the others. If all first-line drugs fail, a cardioselective β-adrenergic blocker or a low-dose diuretic (if not already prescribed) can be tried. If monotherapy fails, a combination therapy of a calcium channel antagonist with an ACE inhibitor, or one of the first-line drugs with a thiazide diuretic or a cardioselective β-blocker, can be used.

Angiotensin-Coverting Enzyme Inhibitors. ACE inhibitors are an attractive choice for the treatment of hypertension in diabetic patients. They are metabolically neutral and may improve insulin sensitivity and glycemic control.[401,481-484] They may also lead to a decrease in LDL and triglyceride with an increase in HDL concentrations.[483,484] ACE inhibitors appear to have a specific renal protective effect by decreasing intraglomerular capillary hydraulic pressure and/or interfering with a possible trophic effect of angiotensin II on mesangial cells.[485] In addition, they may have a specific effect on the glomerular basement membrane that leads to a decrease in glomerular pore size and permeability.[486] Adminis-

tration of ACE inhibitors has been shown to decrease urinary protein excretion in patients with microalbuminuria as well as in those with more advanced degrees of nephropathy. In addition, they prevent or retard the decline in the glomerular filtration rate in patients with established diabetic nephropathy.[487-489] These effects are independent of the salutary result of reduction in blood pressure. A meta-analysis of 100 published studies showed that blood pressure reduction from ACE inhibitor therapy caused a significantly greater improvement in glomerular filtration rate than did a comparable blood pressure reduction from other antihypertensive agents.[474] A recent multicenter study has demonstrated that captopril led to substantial decrease in mortality and the need for dialysis or transplantation in IDDM patients with nephropathy who were followed for up to 5 years.[489] Furthermore, ACE inhibitors may cause regression of LV hypertrophy, a risk factor for CAD mortality, CHF, and sudden death.[490] They may also have a beneficial effect in preventing or delaying the progression of atherosclerosis.[491,492] ACE inhibitors are, therefore, recommended as first-line drugs in the management of hypertensive diabetic patients. They should be used cautiously, however, in patients with declining renal function since they can induce hyperkalemia. This is particularly the case in patients with hyporeninemic hypoaldosteronism. ACE inhibitors can also cause deterioration of renal function in patients with renal artery stenosis.[493]

Calcium Channel Antagonists. Certain calcium channel antagonists (e.g., verapamil, diltiazem, nitrendipine) appear to have a renoprotective effect similar to that of ACE inhibitors, and are therefore recommended as first-line drugs in hypertensive diabetic patients.[494-497] Several studies have demonstrated that these calcium channel antagonists can reduce urinary albumin excretion and slow the decline in renal function to a degree exceeding that expected from blood pressure reduction alone.[495–497] This renoprotective effect is ascribed to lowering of glomerular capillary pressure, inhibition of mesangial cell and matrix proliferation, and modulation of mesangial traffic of macromolecules.[498] These effects are not shared, however, by all calcium channel antagonists. Nifedipine, a first-generation dihydropyridine, has been shown to have no effect on or to cause an increase in urinary albumin excretion and worsening of renal function despite effective reduction of blood pressure.[499,500] Other studies reported, however, that nifedipine caused a modest improvement in albuminuria as well as renal function in diabetic hypertensive subjects.[501,502] In view of these conflicting results, it seems appropriate to avoid using nifedipine in diabetic patients. Nitrendipine, a second-generation dihydropyridine, has been reported, however, to exert a renoprotective effect in diabetic hypertensive patients.[497] Calcium channel antagonists have other beneficial effects, including promoting the regression of LV hypertrophy[503] and retarding the development and progression of atherosclerosis.[504] In addition, they have no adverse affect on glucose homeostasis or lipid profile.[505–506] However, some reports indicate that nifedipine in large doses may cause deterioration of glycemic control in diabetic patients.[505] Most calcium channel antagonists are generally contraindicated in the presence of CHF. Second-generation dihydropyridines, however, have a more favorable side-effect profile and are less cardiodepressant.

α_1-Adrenergic Receptor Blockers. α_1-Adrenergic receptor blockers are another useful class of agents that can be used as first-line drugs to treat hypertension in diabetic patients.[507] They can lower blood pressure to the same extent as ACE inhibitors and calcium channel antagonists. In addition, they have favorable metabolic effects. Prazosin and doxazosin have been shown to improve insulin sensitivity and lower plasma glucose and insulin concentrations in diabetic and nondiabetic individuals.[508–511] α_1-adrenergic receptor blockers also improve the lipid profile. Prazosin, doxazosin, and terazosin could decrease fasting triglycerides and total cholesterol concentrations, increase HDL cholesterol, and decrease apolipoprotein B levels. These results are due to the effect of α_1-adrenergic receptor blockade, which increases serum lipoprotein lipase activity, enhances hydrolysis of triglyceride-rich lipoproteins, improves receptor-mediated clearance of LDL, and inhibits hepatic cholesterol and triglycerides synthesis.[507,510,511] Treatment with α_1-adrenergic receptor blockers could also induce regression of LV hypertrophy[512] and might inhibit atherogenesis.[513] There are no data, however, on the effect of this group of drugs on diabetic nephropathy, but doxazosin had no adverse effect on kidney function in nondiabetic hypertensive subjects with mild to moderate renal insufficiency.[514] α_1-Adrenergic receptor blockers are contraindicated in diabetic patients with autonomic neuropathy and postural hypotension.

Diuretics. Efficacy, simplicity, and low cost are factors which favor the use of a low dose of a thiazide diuretic (12.5 to 25 mg of hydrochlorothiazide or chlorthalidone) in the management of hypertension as long as kidney function is normal.[515] If serum creatinine exceeds 2 mg/dl, a loop-diuretic such as furosemide should be used. However, these agents, especially at higher doses, can cause deterioration of glucose tolerance because of worsening of insulin resistance and/or secretion.[401,516] These effects are partially caused by potassium depletion. Other problems of diuretic therapy include elevation of LDL cholesterol. The combination of worsening glycemia and increasing dyslipidemia may nullify the cardiovascular benefits of lowering blood pressure.[517] Warram et al.[518] have reported that mortality from CAD was 3.8 times higher in diabetic hypertensive patients receiving diuretics as the sole therapy than in those receiving other antihypertensive agents (with and without a diuretic) or no treatment at all. However, results of the Systolic Hypertension in the Elderly Program showed reduced incidence of stroke and CAD when hypertension was treated with thiazides in diabetics and nondiabetics alike.[471] Low-dose diuretic therapy can still be used cautiously as a first-line therapy in diabetic patients especially in the presence of heart failure or edema.

β-Adrenergic Receptor Blockers.   β-Adrenergic receptor blockers can be useful in hypertensive diabetic patients with concomitant CAD because of their antianginal and cardioprotective effects.[519] They have, however, several drawbacks. They could increase insulin resistance and decrease insulin secretion and therefore may worsen glycemic control.[520,521] They can also induce a mild increase in triglyceride and a decrease in HDL cholesterol concentrations, which might increase the risk of atherosclerosis. β-Adrenergic blockers can also blunt the perception of hypoglycemia by blocking its adrenergic manifestations, such as tachycardia, apprehension, and sweating. Furthermore, β_2-blockade can delay the recovery from hypoglycemia by decreasing glycogenolysis and lipolysis and thereby decreasing the substrates available for gluconeogenesis.[522] β_2-Blockade may also decrease exercise performance, which

can be problematic for physically active patients. For all these reasons, β-adrenergic blockers should not be used as first-line drugs in hypertensive diabetic patients and should be avoided in those on insulin pump or intensive insulin therapy. In addition, only cardioselective β-adrenergic blockers should be employed and in low to moderate dosage (e.g., not more than 50 mg/day of atenolol, 150 mg/day of metoprolol, or 600 mg/day of acebutolol), because cardioselectivity is lost at higher doses.

Management of Hypertension In Diabetic Patients With Specific Problems

1. *Orthostatic Hypotension:* In patients with supine hypertension and orthostatic hypotension, normalization of supine hypertension does not have first priority. Elevation of blood pressure during the day, to allow the patient to lead a normal life, is essential. Therefore, blood pressure in the standing position should be considered the therapeutic endpoint. ACE inhibitors and calcium channel antagonists are preferred, whereas α_1-adrenoceptor blockers are contraindicated. In severe cases, 9-α-fluorohydrocortisone can be given in small doses to increase the intravascular volume. This drug should be used carefully to avoid precipitating heart failure or aggravating hypertension.

2. *Renal Impairment:* ACE inhibitors and some calcium antagonists may prevent or retard further deterioration of renal function. Loop diuretics can be helpful in patients with serum creatinine higher than 2 mg/dl, but they should be used cautiously to avoid in-

travascular volume contraction and reduction of renal blood flow. Impairment of the naturally occurring nocturnal decrease in arterial blood pressure is common in diabetic patients with nephropathy and autonomic neuropathy. The lack of the nocturnal dip in blood pressure increases cardiac strain and may thus contribute to the enhanced cardiovascular mortality found in patients with diabetic renal disease.[523] Night-time antihypertensive coverage is essential in these patients.

3. *Isolated Systolic Hypertension:* Reduction of isolated systolic elevation of blood pressure has been shown to decrease ASCVD mortality.[524] Thiazides can be useful in small doses. Initially, patients should be seen frequently and evaluated for volume depletion and postural hypotension. If a second drug is needed, ACE inhibitors or calcium channel antagonists can be added.

4. *Ischemic Heart Disease:* If angina is present or the patient already has an infarction, calcium antagonists are recommended. Cardioselective β-adrenergic receptor blocking agents should also be considered because of their cardioprotective effect.

5. *Heart Failure:* Diuretics and/or ACE inhibitors are the preferred line of therapy in patients with cardiomegaly or congestive heart failure.

6. *Peripheral Vascular Disease:* β-adrenergic receptor blocking agents are contraindicated since they can reduce peripheral blood flow and decrease exercise tolerance. ACE inhibitors, calcium antagonists, and α1-adrenoceptor blockers can be used in this situation.

7. *Hyporeninemic Hypoaldosteronism:* ACE inhibitors can cause hyperkalemia in patients with hyporeninemic hypoaldosteronism. If ACE inhibitors are used, serum potassium should be monitored carefully and it is appropriate to combine them with diuretics.

8. *Impotence:* β-blockers and diuretics should be avoided in patients with impotence. ACE inhibitors, calcium antagonists and α1-adrenoceptor blockers are preferred.

CARDIOVASCULAR AUTONOMIC NEUROPATHY

Cardiovascular autonomic neuropathy is present in 20 to 40 percent of diabetic patients as shown by different autonomic tests (e.g., R-R variation, valsalva maneuver, sustained hand grip, etc[524] [for details on these tests see Ch. 10]). Patients more commonly present with symptoms pertaining to other organs such as impotence or diarrhea. However, cardiovascular involvement is of utmost importance since it carries a high risk of mortality.[526,527] The different features of cardiovascular involvement include resting tachycardia, the denervated heart syndrome, exercise intolerance, postural hypotension, sudden death, and the long Q-T interval syndrome. These different manifestations will be discussed briefly as follows:

1. *Resting Tachycardia:* Patients manifest with resting tachycardia when parasympathetic damage predominates. The heart rate tends to decrease as the sympathetic system becomes affected. However, diabetic patients in general are reported to have increased heart rate of about 10 beats/min above controls.

2. *The Denervated Heart Syndrome:* In patients with severe autonomic neuropathy, a fixed heart rate of 80 to 90 bpm with loss of the normal minute-to-minute and second-to-second varia-

tion is present. There is no response to stimuli that would normally alter the heart rate, such as exercise, stress, or sleep. Heart rate is not completely "fixed," however, since mild variations still occur in response to non-neuronal factors; a similar situation is observed in patients with transplanted hearts. The denervated heart syndrome is rare; Ewing et al.[528] found only one patient out of 61 with a truly "fixed" heart rate using 24-hour ambulatory electrocardiographic monitoring.

3. *Exercise Intolerance:* Autonomic neuropathy diminishes cardiac performance during exercise even in the absence of CAD. Roy et al.[529] studied a group of diabetic patients with no evidence of CAD or cardiomyopathy. They found that patients with autonomic neuropathy did more cardiovascular work at rest in order to achieve the same cardiac output than did those without neuropathy. This was caused by an increase in both the resting heart rate and systolic blood pressure. In addition, the increase in cardiac output in response to exercise was attenuated. Thus, autonomic neuropathy affects physical performance and can result in easy fatigability. The presence of autonomic neuropathy should be taken in consideration in designing exercise programs for diabetic patients.

4. *Postural Hypotension:* Postural hypotension is defined as a fall in systolic blood pressure of 30 mmHg or more or diastolic blood pressure of 10 mmHg or more within 2 minutes of standing-up from the lying position. Postural hypotension is mainly due to failure to increase systemic vascular resistance by reflex vasoconstriction, particularly in the splanchnic area, as a consequence of damage to the sympathetic postganglionic innervation of resistance vessels. The failure of compen-satory tachycardia on standing and diminished catecholamine responsiveness contribute also to the pathogenesis of this condition.

A large proportion of patients are asymptomatic and the condition is discovered only during routine examination. Symptoms can be incapacitating, however, and include postural weakness, faintness, visual impairment, and syncope. The symptoms are more severe in the elderly, especially if they have also diabetic diarrhea that could cause volume depletion. In addition, postural hypotension can be aggravated by some commonly prescribed drugs such as diuretics, vasodilator, tricyclic antidepressants, phenothiazines, and glyceryl trinitrate. Moreover, insulin may aggravate postural hypotension, possibly by direct vasodilatory action on peripheral blood vessels.

Treatment of postural hypotension is only indicated in symptomatic patients. Management includes mechanical measures such as sleeping with the head of the bed elevated 8 to 12 inches to moderate the sudden pooling of blood on standing up and wearing an elasticized support hose (e.g., waist-high Jobst stocking). If these measures fail, 9-α-fluorohydrocortisone can be given to expand vascular volume. Treatment should start with a small dose (e.g., 0.05 mg every day or two) and be increased gradually since that drug can cause hypertension and precipitate heart failure. If this drug fails, vasoconstrictor drugs such as nasal neosynephrine (10 percent ophthalmic solution, 1 to 3 drops every 4 hours while upright) or miodrine could be helpful. β-adrenergic receptor blockers such as pindolol may be also beneficial through inhibiting peripheral vasodilation.[530]

5. *Sudden Death and the Long Q-T Interval Syndrome:* Diabetic patients

with autonomic neuropathy have a 5-year mortality in excess of 50 percent.[525] Approximately one-half of the deaths are cardiac and the majority are sudden and unexplained. A long Q-T interval is associated with autonomic neuropathy in some diabetic patients, and has been thought to explain sudden death in these patients[531-533] Recently, Ong et al.[534] have demonstrated that decreased heart rate variability, which reflects cardiac autonomic neuropathy, was associated with higher heart rate and shorter Q-T intervals. They suggested that these manifestations were caused by sympathovagal imbalance toward sympathetic augmentation or parasympathetic denervation. In the setting of the inhomogeneous diabetic myocardium secondary to micro- or macroangiopathy and the increased sensitivity to catecholamines, life-threatening ventricular arrhythmias and sudden death could occur. A prospective study is needed to resolve this issue. However, until more information is available, diabetic patients with autonomic neuropathy should be monitored carefully while under anesthesia and should not be given drugs that might cause prolongation of the QT interval (e.g., quinidine). In addition, they may benefit from drugs that decrease sympathetic stimulation (e.g., β-adrenergic receptor, or augment parasympathetic activity (e.g., cholinergic agonists).

REFERENCES

1. Harris MI, Hadden WC, Knowler WC et al: Prevalence of diabetes and impaired glucose tolerance and plasma glucose levels in U.S. population aged 20–74 yr. Diabetes 36:523, 1987

2. Wetterhall SF, Olson DR, DeStefano F et al: Trends in diabetes and diabetic complications, 1980–1987. Diabetes Care 15:960, 1992

3. National Society to Prevent Blindness: Vision Problems in the U.S. New York, 1980

4. Herman WH, Teutsch SM, Geiss LH: Diabetes mellitus. In Almar RW, Dull PH (eds): Closing the Gap: The Burden of Unnecessary Illness. Oxford New York, 1987

5. Pan WH, Cedres LB, Liu K et al: Relationship of clinical diabetes and asymptomatic hyperglycemia to risk of coronary heart disease mortality in men and women. Am J Epidemiol 123:504, 1986

6. Uusitupa MI, Niskanen LK, Siitonen O et al: 5-Year incidence of atherosclerotic vascular disease in relation to general risk factors, insulin level, and abnormalities in lipoprotein composition in non-insulin-dependent diabetic and nondiabetic subjects. Circulation 82:27, 1990

7. Abbott RD, Brand FN, Kannel WB: Epidemiology of some peripheral arterial findings in diabetic men and women: experience from the Framingham Study. Am J Med 88:376, 1990

8. Fox NA, Jacobs J: Direct and Indirect Cost of Diabetes in the United States in 1987. American Diabetes Association, Alexandria, Virginia, 1988

9. Leese B: The costs of diabetes and its complications. Soc Sci Med 35:1303, 1992

10. Schneider EL, Guralnik JM: The aging of America. JAMA 263:2335, 1990

11. Stern MP: Primary prevention of type II diabetes mellitus. Diabetes Care 14:399, 1991

12. Report of a WHO Study Group: Diabetes mellitus. WHO Tech Rep Ser 727:9, 1985

13. National Diabetes Data Group: Classification and diagnosis of diabetes mellitus and other categories of glucose intolerance. Diabetes 28:1039, 1979

14. Report of a WHO study group. Diabetes mellitus. Tech Rep Ser 646:1, 1980

15. Saad MF, Knowler WC, Pettitt DJ et al:

The natural history of impaired glucose tolerance in the Pima Indians. N Engl J Med 319:1500, 1988

16. Sicree RA, Zimmet PZ, King HOM et al: Plasma insulin response among Nauruans: prediction of deterioration in glucose tolerance over 6 years. Diabetes 36:179, 1987

17. Haffner SM, Stern MP, Mitchell BD et al: Incidence of type II diabetes in MexicanAmericans predicted by fasting insulin and glucose levels, obesity, and body-fat distribution. Diabetes 39:283, 1990

18. Bergstrom RW, Newell-Morris LL, Leonetti DL et al: Association of elevated fasting C-peptide level and increased intra-abdominal fat distribution with development of NIDDM in Japanese-American men. Diabetes 39:104, 1990

19. Charles MA, Fontbonne A, Thibult N et al: Risk factors for NIDDM in white population. Paris Prospective Study. Diabetes 40:796, 1991

20. King H, Zimmet P, Raper LR et al: The natural history of impaired glucose tolerance in the Micronesian population of Nauru: a six-year follow-up study. Diabetologia 26:39, 1984

21. Motala AA, Omar MAK, Gouws E: High risk of progression to NIDDM in South-African Indians with impaired glucose tolerance. Diabetes 42:556, 1993

22. Jarrett RJ, McCartney P, Keen H: The Bedford Survey: ten year mortality rates in newly diagnosed diabetics, borderline diabetics and normoglycemic controls and risk indices for coronary heart disease in borderline diabetics. Diabetologia 22:79, 1982

23. Zavaroni I, Dall'Aglio E, Bonora E et al: Evidence that multiple risk factors for coronary artery disease exist in persons with abnormal glucose tolerance. Am J Med 83:609, 1987

24. Burchfiel CM, Shetterly SM, Baxter J et al: The roles of insulin, obesity, and fat distribution in the elevation of cardiovascular risk factors in impaired glucose tolerance. The San Luis Valley Diabetes Study. Am J Epidemiol 136:1101, 1992

25. Bennett PH: Impaired glucose tolerance: a target for intervention? Arteriosclerosis 5:315, 1985

26. MacDonald MJ, Gottschall J, Hunter JA, Winter KL: HLA-DR4 in insulin-dependent diabetic parents and their diabetic offspring: a clue to dominant inheritance. Proc Natl Acad Sci USA 83:7049, 1986

27. Ludvigsson J, Samuelsson U, Beauforts C et al: HLA-DR3 is associated with a more slowly progressive form of type I (insulin-dependent) diabetes. Diabetologia 29:207, 1986

28. Deschamps I, Beressi JP, Khalil I et al: The role of genetic predisposition to type I (insulin-dependent) diabetes mellitus. Ann Med 23:427, 1991

29. Khalil I, D'Auriol L, Gobet M et al: A combination of HLA-DQβ Asp 57 negative and HLA-DQα Arg 52 confers susceptibility to IDDM. J Clin Invest 85:1315, 1990

30. Yoon J-W: Role of viruses in the pathogenesis of IDDM. Ann Med 23:437, 1991

31. Martin TM, Trink B, Daneman D et al: Milk proteins in the etiology of insulin-dependent diabetes mellitus (IDDM). Ann Med 23:447, 1991

32. Eisenbarth GS: Type I diabetes mellitus: a chronic autoimmune disease. N Engl J Med 314:1360, 1986

33. Knowler WC, Pettitt DJ, Saad MF et al: Diabetes mellitus in the Pima Indians: incidence, risk factors and pathogenesis. Diabetes Metab Rev 6:1, 1990

34. Reaven GM: Role of insulin resistance in human disease. Diabetes 37:1595, 1988

35. DeFronzo RA: The triumvirate: β-cell, muscle, liver: a collusion responsible for NIDDM. Diabetes 37:667, 1988

36. Polonsky KS, Given BD, Hirsch LJ et al: Abnormal patterns of insulin secretion in non-insulin-dependent diabetes mellitus. N Engl J Med 318:1231, 1988

37. Bergman RN: Toward physiological understanding of glucose tolerance: minimal-model approach. Diabetes 38:1512, 1989

38. Saad MF, Knowler WC, Pettitt DJ et al:

A two-step model for development of non-insulin-dependent diabetes. Am J Med 90:229, 1991

39. Aronoff SL, Bennett PH, Gorden P et al: Unexplained hyperinsulinemia in normal and "prediabetic" Pima Indians compared with normal Caucasians: an example of racial differences in insulin secretion. Diabetes 26:827, 1979

40. Balkau B, King H, Zimmet P, Raper LR: Factors associated with the development of diabetes in the Micronesian population of Nauru. Am J Epidemiol 122:594, 1985

41. Haffner SM, Stern MP, Hazuda HP et al: Hyperinsulinemia in a population at high risk for non-insulin-dependent diabetes mellitus. N Engl J Med 315:220, 1986

42. Mohan V, Sharp PS, Cloke HR et al: Serum immunoreactive insulin responses to a glucose load in Asian Indian and European type 2 (non-insulin-dependent) diabetic patients and control subjects. Diabetologia 29:235, 1986

43. Warram JH, Martin BC, Krolewski AS et al: Slow glucose removal rate and hyperinsulinemia precede the development of type II diabetes in the offspring of diabetic parents. Ann Intern Med 113:909, 1990

44. Saad MF, Knowler WC, Pettitt DJ et al: Sequential changes in serum insulin concentration during development of non-insulin-dependent diabetes. Lancet 1:1356, 1989

45. Martin BC, Warram JH, Krolewski AS et al: Role of glucose and insulin resistance in development of type 2 diabetes mellitus: results of a 25-year follow-up study. Lancet 340:925, 1992

46. Lillioja S, Mott DM, Spraul M et al: Insulin resistance and insulin secretory dysfunction as precursors of non-insulin-dependent diabetes mellitus: prospective studies of Pima Indians. N Engl J Med 329:1988, 1993

47. Haffner SM, Stern MP, Dunn JF et al: Diminished insulin sensitivity and increased insulin response in nonobese, nondiabetic Mexican Americans. Metabolism 39:842, 1990

48. Gulli G, Ferrannini E, Stern M et al: The metabolic profile of NIDDM is fully established in glucose-tolerant offspring of two Mexican-American NIDDM parents. Diabetes 41:1575, 1992

49. Eriksson J, Fransilla-Kallunki A, Ekstrand A et al: Early metabolic defects in persons at increased risk for non-insulin-dependent diabetes mellitus. N Eng J Med 321:337, 1989

50. Bogardus C, Lillioja S, Nyomba BL et al: Distribution of in vivo insulin action in Pima Indians as mixture of three normal distributions. Diabetes 38:1423, 1989

51. Lillioja S, Nyomba BL, Saad MF et al: Exaggerated early insulin release and insulin resistance in a diabetic prone population: a metabolic comparison of Pima Indians and Caucasians. J Clin Endocrinol Metab 73:866, 1991

52. Unger RH, Grundy S: Hyperglycemia as an inducer as well as a consequence of impaired islet cell function and insulin resistance: implications for the management of diabetes. Diabetologia 28:119, 1985

53. Leahy JL, Bonner-Weir S, Weir GC: Minimal chronic hyperglycemia is a critical determinant of impaired insulin secretion after an incomplete pancreatectomy. J Clin Invest 81:1407, 1988

54. Weir GC, Bonner-Weir S, Leahy JL: Islet mass and function in diabetes and transplantation. Diabetes 39:401, 1990

55. O'Rahilly S, Turner RC, Matthews DR: Impaired pulsatile secretion of insulin in relatives of patients with non-insulin-dependent diabetes. N Engl J Med 318:1225, 1988

56. Porte D Jr, Kahn SE: Hyperproinsulinemia and amyloid in NIDDM: clues to etiology of islet β-cell dysfunction? Diabetes 38:1333, 1989

57. Kannel WB, McGee DL: Diabetes and cardiovascular disease. The Framingham Study. JAMA 241:2035, 1979

58. Jarrett RJ: Cardiovascular disease and hypertension in diabetes mellitus. Diabetes Metab Rev 5:547, 1989

59. Waller BF, Palumbo PJ, Lie T et al: Status of the coronary arteries at necropsy

in diabetes mellitus with onset after age 30 years. Am J Med 69:498, 1980

60. Robertson WB, Strong JP: Atherosclerosis in persons with hypertension and diabetes mellitus. Lab Invest 18:538, 1968

61. Vigorito C, Betocchi S, Bonzani G et al: Severity of coronary artery disease in patients with diabetes mellitus. Angiographic study of 34 diabetic and 120 nondiabetic patients. Am Heart J 100:782, 1980

62. Chan A, Beach KW, Martin DC, Strandness DE Jr: Carotid artery disease in NIDDM diabetes. Diabetes Care 6:562, 1983

63. Kawamori R, Yamasaki Y, Matsushima H et al: Prevalence of carotid atherosclerosis in diabetic patients. Diabetes Care 15:1290, 1992

64. Strandness DE, Priest RE, Gibbons GE: Combined clinical and pathologic study of diabetic and non-diabetic peripheral arterial disease. Diabetes 13:366, 1964

65. Kingsbury KJ: The relation between glucose tolerance and atherosclerotic vascular disease. Lancet 2:1374, 1966

66. Menzoian JO, LaMorte WW, Paniszyn CC et al: Symptomatology and anatomic patterns of peripheral vascular disease: differing impact of smoking and diabetes. Ann Vasc Surg 3:224, 1989

67. Donahue RP, Orchard TJ: Diabetes mellitus and macrovascular complications: an epidemiological perspective. Diabetes Care 15:1141, 1992

68. Keen H, Rose G, Pyke DA et al: Blood sugar and arterial disease. Lancet 2:505, 1965

69. Uusitupa M, Siitonen O, Aro A et al: Prevalence of coronary heart disease, left ventricular failure and hypertension in middle-aged, newly diagnosed Type 2 (non-insulin-dependent) diabetic subjects. Diabetologia 28:22, 1985

70. Fuller JH, Shipley MJ, Rose G et al: Mortality from coronary heart disease and stroke in relation to degree of glycaemia: the Whitehall Study. Br Med J 287:867, 1983

71. Eschwege E, Richard JL, Thibult N et al: Coronary heart disease mortality in relation with diabetes, blood glucose and plasma insulin levels: the Paris Prospective Study, ten years later. Horm Metab Res Suppl Ser 15:41, 1985

72. McPhillips JB, Barrett-Connor E, Wingard DL: Cardiovascular disease risk factors prior to the diagnosis of impaired glucose tolerance and non-insulin dependent diabetes mellitus in a community of older adults. Am J Epidemiol 131:443, 1990

73. Haffner SM, Stern MP, Hazuda HP et al: Cardiovascular risk factors in confirmed prediabetic individuals: Does the clock for coronary heart disease start ticking before the onset of clinical diabetes? JAMA 263:2893, 1990

74. Jensen T: Albuminuria—a marker of renal and generalized vascular disease in insulin-dependent diabetes mellitus. Dan Med J 38:134, 1991

75. Jarrett RJ, Shipley MJ: Type 2 (non-insulin-dependent) diabetes mellitus and cardiovascular disease—putative association via common antecedents, further evidence from the Whitehall Study. Diabetologia 31:737, 1988

76. Moss SE, Klein R, Klein BE: Cause-specific mortality in a population-based study of diabetes. Am J Public Health 81:1158, 1991

77. Krolewski AS, Kosinski EJ, Warram JH et al: Magnitude and determinants of coronary artery disease in juvenile-onset insulin-dependent diabetes mellitus. Am J Cardiol 59:750, 1987

78. Borch-Johnsen K, Kreiner S: Proteinuria: value as predictor of cardiovascular mortality in insulin dependent diabetes mellitus. Br Med J 294:1651, 1987

79. Jensen T, Borch-Johnsen K, Kofoed-Enevoldsen A et al: Coronary heart disease in young type I (insulin-dependent) diabetic patients with and without diabetic nephropathy: incidence and risk factors. Diabetologia 30:144, 1987

80. Manske CL, Wilson RF, Wang Y, Thomas W: Prevalence of, and risk factors for, angiographically determined coronary artery disease in type I-diabetic patients with nephropathy. Arch Intern Med 152:2450, 1992

81. Panzram G: Mortality and survival in type 2 (non-insulin-dependent) diabetes mellitus. Diabetologia 30:123, 1987

82. Kleinman JC, Donahue RP, Harris MI et al: Mortality among diabetics in a national sample. Am J Epidemiol 128:389, 1988

83. Rosengren A, Welin L, Tsipogianni A et al: Impact of cardiovascular risk factors on coronary heart disease and mortality among middle aged diabetic men: a general population study. BMJ 299:1127, 1989

84. Lapidus L, Bengtsson C, Blohme G et al: Blood glucose, glucose tolerance and manifest diabetes in relation to cardiovascular disease and death in women. Acta Med Scand 218:455, 1985

85. Stamler J, Vaccaro O, Neaton JD et al: Diabetes, other risk factors, and 12-year cardiovascular mortality for men screened in the Multiple Risk Factor Intervention Trial. Diabetes Care 16:434, 1992

86. Manson JE, Colditz GA, Stampfer MJ et al: A prospective study of maturity-onset diabetes mellitus and risk of coronary heart disease and stroke in women. Arch Intern Med 151:1141, 1991

87. Rewers M, Shetterly SM, Baxter J et al: Prevalence of coronary heart disease in subjects with normal and impaired glucose tolerance and non-insulin-dependent diabetes mellitus in a biethnic Colorado population: the San Luis Valley Diabetes Study. Am J Epidemiol 135:1321, 1992

88. Koskinen P, Mänttäri M, Manninen V et al: Coronary heart disease incidence in NIDDM patients in the Helsinki Heart Study. Diabetes Care 15:820, 1992

89. Barrett-Connor E, Khaw KT: Diabetes mellitus: An independent risk factor for stroke? Am J Epidemiol 128:116, 1988

90. Beach KW, Bedford GR, Bergelin RO et al: Progression of lower-extremity arterial occlusive disease in type II diabetes mellitus. Diabetes Care 11:464, 1988

91. Most RS, Sinnock P: The epidemiology of lower extremity amputation in diabetic individuals. Diabetes Care 6:87, 1983

92. Moss SE, Klein R, Klein BEK: The prevalence and incidence of lower extremity amputation in a diabetic population. Arch Intern Med 152:610, 1992

93. Bierman EL: Atherogenesis in diabetes. Arterioscler Thromb 12:647, 1992

94. Schwartz CJ, Valente AJ, Sprague EA et al: Pathogenesis of the atherosclerotic lesion: implications for diabetes mellitus. Diabetes Care 15:1156, 1992

95. Heyden S, Heiss G, Bartel AG et al: Sex differences in coronary heart disease among diabetics in Evans County, Georgia. J Chronic Dis 33:265, 1980

96. Barrett-Connor E, Wingard DL: Sex differential in ischemic heart disease mortality in diabetics: a prospective population-based study. Am J Epidemiol 118:489, 1983

97. Butler WJ, Ostrander LD, Carman WJ et al: Mortality from coronary heart disease in the Tecumseh Study: Long term effect of diabetes mellitus, glucose tolerance and other risk factors. Am J Epidemiol 121:541, 1985

98. Janka HU: Five-year incidence of major macrovascular complications in diabetes mellitus. Horm Metab Res 15(suppl):15, 1984

99. Morrish NJ, Stevens LK, Fuller JH et al: Risk factors for macrovascular disease in diabetes mellitus: The London follow-up to the WHO Multinational Study of Vascular Disease in Diabetics. Diabetologia 34:590, 1991

100. Herman JB, Medalie JH, Goldbourt U: Differences in cardiovascular morbidity and mortality between previously known and newly diagnosed adult diabetics. Diabetologia 13:229, 1977

101. Harris MI: Undiagnosed NIDDM: clinical and public health issues. Diabetes Care 16:642, 1993

102. Nelson RG, Sievers ML, Knowler WC et al: Low incidence of fatal coronary heart disease in Pima Indians despite high prevalence of non-insulin-dependent diabetes. Circulation 81:987, 1990

103. West KM, Ahuja MMS, Bennett PH et al: The role of circulating glucose and triglyceride concentrations and their interactions with other "risk factors" as de-

terminants of arterial disease in nine diabetic population samples from the WHO Multinational Study. Diabetes Care 6:361, 1983

104. Nielsen NV, Ditzel J: Prevalence of macro- and microvascular disease as related to glycosylated hemoglobin in type I and type II diabetic subjects: an epidemiologic study in Denmark. Horm Metab Res 15(suppl):19, 1985

105. Ducimetiere P, Eschwege E, Papoz JL et al: Relationship of plasma insulin levels to the incidence of myocardial infarction and coronary heart disease mortality in middle-aged population. Diabetologia 19:205, 1980

106. Donahue RP, Abbott RD, Reed DM, Yano K: Postchallenge glucose concentration and coronary heart disease in men of Japanese ancestry: Honolulu Heart Program. Diabetes 36:689, 1987

107. Singer DE, Nathan DM, Anderson KM et al: Association of HbA_{1c} with prevalent cardiovascular disease in the original cohort of the Framingham Heart Study. Diabetes 41:202, 1992

108. The Diabetes Control and Complications Trial Research Group: The effect of intensive treatment of diabetes on the development and progression of long-term complications in insulin-dependent diabetes mellitus. N Engl J Med 329:977, 1993

109. Brownlee M: Glycosylation products as toxic mediators of diabetic complications. Annu Rev Med 42:159, 1991

110. Howard BV: Lipoprotein metabolism in diabetes mellitus. J Lipid Res 28:613, 1987

111. Ginsberg HN: Lipoprotein physiology in nondiabetic and diabetic states: relationship to atherogenesis. Diabetes Care 14:839, 1991

112. Taskinen M-R: Quantitative and qualitative lipoprotein abnormalities in diabetes mellitus. Diabetes 41(suppl 2):12, 1992

113. Durrington PN: Diabetes, hypertension and hyperlipidemia. Postgrad Med J 69(suppl 1): S18, 1993

114. Haffner SM, Tuttle KR, Rainwater DL: Decrease of Lp(a) with improved glyce-

mic control in IDDM subjects. Diabetes Care 14:302, 1991

115. Ramirez C, Arauz-Pacheco C, Lackner C et al: Lipoprotein(a) levels in diabetes mellitus: relationship to metabolic control. Ann Intern Med 117:42, 1992

116. Jenkins AJ, Steele JS, Junus ED et al: Plasma apolipoprotein(a) is increased in type II (non-insulin-dependent) diabetic patients with microalbuminuria. Diabetologia 35:1055, 1992

117. Kapelrud H, Bangstad HJ, Dahl-Jorgensen K et al: Serum Lp(a) lipoprotein concentrations in insulin-dependent diabetic patients with microalbuminuria. BMJ 303:675, 1991

118. Császár A, Dieplinger H, Sandholzer C et al: Plasma lipoprotein(a) concentration and phenotypes in diabetes mellitus. Diabetologia 36:47, 1993

119. Ritter MM, Loscar M, Richter WO, Schwandt P: Lipoprotein(a) in diabetes mellitus. Clin Chim Acta 214:45, 1993

120. Nielsen FS, Voldsgaard AI, Gall MA et al: Apolipoprotein(a) and cardiovascular disease in type 2 (non-insulin-dependent) diabetic patients with and without diabetic nephropathy. Diabetologia 36:438, 1993

121. Haffner SM, Moss SE, Klein BEK, Klein R: Lack of association between lipoprotein(a) concentration and coronary heart disease mortality in diabetics: the Wisconsin Epidemiology Study of Diabetic Retinopathy. Metabolism 41:194, 1992

122. Haffner SM: Lipoprotein(a) and diabetes: an update. Diabetes Care 16:835, 1993

123. Fontbonne A, Eschwege E, Cambien F et al: Hypertriglyceridemia as a risk factor of coronary heart disease mortality in subjects with impaired glucose tolerance or diabetes: results from the 11-year follow-up of the Paris Prospective Study. Diabetologia 32:300, 1989

124. Taskinen MR. Lipoprotein lipase in diabetes. Diabetes Metab Rev 3:551, 1987

125. Fielding CJ, Reaven GM, Fielding PE: Human noninsulin-dependent diabetes: identification of a defect in plasma cholesterol transport normalized in vivo by insulin and in vitro by selective immu-

noabsorption of apolipoprotein E. Proc Natl Acad Sci USA 79:6365, 1982

126. Kuksis A, Myher JJ, Geher K et al: Decreased plasma phosphatidylcholine/free cholesterol ratio as an indicator of risk for ischemic vascular disease. Arteriosclerosis 2:296, 1982

127. Bagdade JD, Buchanan WE, Kuusi T, Taskinen M-R: Persistent abnormalities in lipoprotein composition in non-insulin dependent diabetes after intensive insulin therapy. Arteriosclerosis 10:232, 1990

128. Bagdade JD, Subbaiah PV: Whole-plasma and high-density lipoprotein subfraction surface lipid composition in IDDM men. Diabetes 38:1226, 1989

129. Slotte JP, Chait A, Bierman EL: Cholesterol accumulation in aortic smooth muscle cells exposed to low density lipoproteins: contribution of free cholesterol transfer. Arteriosclerosis 8:750, 1988

130. Fisher WR: Heterogeneity of plasma low density lipoproteins: manifestations of the physiologic phenomenon in man. Metabolism 32:283, 1983

131. James R, Pometta D. Differences in lipoprotein subfraction composition and distribution between type 1 diabetic men and control subjects. Diabetes 39:1158, 1990

132. James R, Pometta D: The distribution profiles of very low density and low density lipoproteins in poorly-controlled male, type 2 (non-insulin-dependent) diabetic patients. Diabetologia 34:246, 1991

133. Austin MA, Breslow JL, Hennekens CH et al: Low-density lipoprotein subclass patterns and risk of myocardial infarction. JAMA 260:1917, 1988

134. Ginsberg HN: Syndrome X: what's old, what's new, what's etiologic? J Clin Invest 92:3, 1993

135. Schleicher E, Deufel T, Wieland OH: Non-enzymatic glycosylation of human serum lipoproteins. FEBS Lett 129:1, 1981

136. Lyons TJ, Patrick JS, Baynes JW et al: Glycosylation of low density lipoprotein in patients with type 1 diabetes: correla-

tions with other parameters of glycemic control. Diabetologia 29:685, 1986

137. Lyons TJ: Lipoprotein glycation and its metabolic consequences. Diabetes 41(suppl 2):67, 1992

138. Baynes JW: Role of oxidative stress in development of complications in diabetes. Diabetes 40:405, 1991

139. Kawamura KM, Heinecke JW, Chait A: Glucose-dependent lipid peroxidation of low density lipoprotein. Clin Res 40:102A, 1992

140. Witztum JL: Role of oxidized low density lipoprotein in atherogenesis. Br Heart J 69 (suppl1):S12, 1993

141. Lopes-Virella MF, Virella G. Immune mechanisms of atherosclerosis in diabetes mellitus. Diabetes 41(suppl 2):86, 1992

142. Gottlieb MS: The natural history of diabetes: factors present at time of diagnosis which may be predictive of length of survival. J Chronic Dis 27:435,1974

143. Goodkin G: Mortality factors in diabetes: a 20-year mortality study. J Occup Med 17:716, 1975

144. Fuller JH, Head J, WHO Multinational Study Group: Blood pressure, proteinuria and their relationship with circulatory mortality: the WHO multinational study of vascular disease in diabetics. Diabete metab 15:273, 1989

145. Kwaan HC: Changes in blood coagulation, platelet function, and plasminogen-plasmin system in diabetes. Diabetes 41(suppl 2):32, 1992

146. Colwell JA: Vascular thrombosis in type II diabetes mellitus. Diabetes 42:8, 1993

147. Schneider DJ, Nordt TK, Sobel BE: Attenuated fibrinolysis and accelerated atherogenesis in type II diabetic patients. Diabetes 42:1, 1993

148. Winocour PD: Platelet abnormalities in diabetes mellitus. Diabetes 41(suppl 2):26, 1992

149. Nawata H, Umeda F, Ishii H: Platelet function in diabetes mellitus. Diabetes Metab Rev 8:53, 1992

150. Glassman AB: Platelet abnormalities in diabetes mellitus. Ann Clin Lab Sci 23:47, 1993

151. Tschoepe D, Rosen P, Schwippert B, Gries FA: Platelets in diabetes: the role in the hemostatic regulation in atherosclerosis. Semin Thromb Hemost 19:122, 1993

152. Kannel WB, D'Agostino RB, Wilson PW et al: Diabetes, fibrinogen and risk of cardiovascular disease: the Framingham experience. Am Heart J 120:672, 1990

153. Sharma SC: Platelet adhesiveness, plasma fibrinogen and fibrinolytic activity in juvenile onset and maturity onset diabetes mellitus. J Clin Pathol 34:501, 1981

154. Ceriello A, Taboga C, Giacomello R et al: Fibrinogen plasma levels as a marker of thrombin activation in diabetes. Diabetes 43:430, 1994

155. Lufkin EG, Fass DN, O'Fallon WM, Bowie EJW: Increased von Willebrand factor in diabetes mellitus. Metabolism 28:63, 1979

156. Ceriello A, Quatraro A, Dello Russo P et al: Protein C deficiency in insulin dependent diabetes: a hyperglycemia-related phenomenon. Thromb Haemost 64:104, 1990

157. Ceriello A, Giugliano D, Quattraro A et al: Daily rapid blood glucose variations may condition antithrombin III biologic activity but not its plasma concentration in insulin-dependent diabetes: a possible role for labile non-enzymatic glycation. Diabete Metab 13:16, 1987

158. Fearnly GR, Chakrabartti R, Avis PR: Blood fibrinolytic activity in diabetes mellitus and its bearing on ischaemic heart disease and obesity. Br Med J 1:921, 1963

159. Auwerx J, Bouillon R, Collen D, Geboers J: Tissue-type plasminogen activator antigen and plasminogen activator inhibitor in diabetes mellitus. Arteriosclerosis 8:68, 1988

160. Fears R, Standring R, Abraham R: Fibrinolytic activity in patients with diabetes mellitus: characterization of the effects of thrombolytic agents on plasma clot lysis in vitro. Semin Thromb Hemost 17:407, 1991

161. Kwaan HC, Colwell JA, Cruz S et al: Increased platelet aggregation in diabetes mellitus. J Lab Clin Med 80:236, 1972

162. Davi G, Catalano I, Averna M et al: Thromboxane biosynthesis and platelet function in type II diabetes mellitus. N Engl J Med 322:1769, 1990

163. Alessandrini P, McRae J, Feman S, FitzGerald GA: Thromboxane biosynthesis and platelet function in type I diabetes mellitus. N Engl J Med 319:208, 1988

164. Mandal S, Sarode R, Dash S, Dash RJ: Hyperaggregation of platelets detected by whole blood platelet aggregometry in newly diagnosed noninsulin-dependent diabetes mellitus. Am J Clin Pathol 100:103, 1993

165. Hendra TJ, Yudkin JS. 'Spontaneous' platelet aggregation in whole blood in diabetic patients with and without microvascular disease. Diabet Med 9:247, 1992

166. Campbell IW, Dawes J, Fraser DM et al: Plasma β-thromboglobulin in diabetes mellitus. Diabetes 26:1175, 1977

167. Betteridge DJ, Zahavi J, Jones NAG et al: Platelet function in diabetes mellitus in relationship to complications, glycosylated haemoglobin and serum lipoproteins. Eur J Clin Invest 11:273, 1981

168. Tschöpe D, Schwippert B, Schettler B et al: Increased GPIIB/IIIA expression and altered DNA-ploidy pattern in megakaryocytes of diabetic BB-rats. Euro J Clin Invest 22:591, 1992

169. Cohen I, Burk D, Fullerton RJ et al: Nonenzymatic glycation of human blood platelet proteins. Thromb Res 55:341, 1989

170. Winocour PD, Watala C, Kinlough-Rathbone RL: Membrane fluidity is related to the extent of glycation of proteins, but not to alterations in the cholesterol to phospholipid molar ratio in isolated platelet membranes from diabetic and control subjects. Thromb Haemost 67:567, 1992

171. Ross R. The pathogenesis of atherosclerosis—an update. N Engl J Med 314:488, 1986

172. Vane JR, Ånggärd EE, Botting RM: Regulatory functions of the vascular endothelium. N Engl J Med 323:27, 1990

173. Stehouwer CDA, Nauta JJP, Zeldenrust GC et al: Urinary albumin excretion, cardiovascular disease, and endothelial dysfunction in non-insulin-dependent diabetes mellitus. Lancet 340:319, 1992

174. Lieberman J, Sastre A: Serum angiotensin converting enzyme: elevation in diabetes mellitus. Ann Intern Med 93:825, 1980

175. Takahashi H, Ito S, Hanano M et al: Circulating thrombomodulin as a novel endothelial cell marker: comparison of its behavior with von Willebrand factor and tissue-type plasminogen activator. Am J Hematol 41:32, 1992

176. Koivisto VA, Jantunen M, Sane T et al: Stimulation of prostacyclin synthesis by physical exercise in type I diabetes. Diabetes Care 12:609, 1989

177. Jensen T, Bjerre-Knudsen J, Feldt-Rasmussen B, Deckert T: Features of endothelial dysfunction in early diabetic nephropathy. Lancet 1:461, 1989

178. Feldt-Rasmussen B: Increased transcapillary escape rate of albumin in type I (insulin-dependent) diabetic patients with microalbuminuria. Diabetologia 29:282, 1986

179. Calver A, Collier J, Vallance P: Inhibition and stimulation of nitric oxide synthesis in the human forearm arterial bed of patients with insulin-dependent diabetes. J Clin Invest 90:2548, 1992

180. McVeigh GE, Brennan GM, Johnston GD: Impaired endothelium-dependent and independent vasodilation in patients with Type 2 (non-insulin-dependent) diabetes mellitus. Diabetologia 35:771, 1992

181. Nitenberg A, Valensi P, Sachs R et al: Impairment of coronary vascular reserve and ACh-induced coronary vasodilation in diabetic patients with angiographically normal coronary arteries and normal left ventricular systolic function. Diabetes 42:1017, 1993

182. Smits P, Kapma J-A, Jacobs M-C et al: Endothelium-dependent vascular relaxation in patients with type I diabetes. Diabetes 42:148, 1993

183. Takahashi K, Ghatei MA, Lam HC et al: Elevated plasma endothelin in patients with diabetes mellitus. Diabetologia 33:306, 1990

184. Collier A, Leach JP, McLellan A et al: Plasma endothelinlike immunoreactivity levels in IDDM patients with microalbuminuria. Diabetes Care 15:1038, 1992

185. Vallance P, Calver A, Collier J: The vascular endothelium in diabetes and hypertension. J Hypertens 10(suppl 1):S25, 1992

186. Brownlee M, Cerami A, Vlassara H: Advanced glycosylation end products in tissue and the biochemical basis of diabetic complications. N Engl J Med 318:1315, 1988

187. Kennedy L, Lyons TJ. Non-enzymatic glycosylation. Br Med Bull 45:174, 1989

188. Pamplona R, Bellmunt MJ, Portero M, Prat J: Mechanisms of glycation in atherogenesis. Med Hypotheses 40:174, 1993

189. Vlassara H, Fuh H, Makita Z et al: Exogenous advanced glycosylation end products induce complex vascular dysfunction in normal animals: a model for diabetic and aging complications. Proc Nat Acad Sci USA 89:12043, 1992

190. Lyons TJ: Glycation and oxidation: a role in the pathogenesis of atherosclerosis. Am J Cardiol 71:26B, 1993

191. Huijberts MSP, Wolffenbuttel BHR, Boudier HAJS et al: Aminoguanidine treatment increases elasticity and decreases fluid filtration of large arteries from diabetic rats. J Clin Invest 92:1407, 1993

192. Bucala R, Tracey KJ, Cerami A: Advanced glycosylation products quench nitric oxide and mediate defective endothelium-dependent vasodilation in experimental diabetes. J Clin Invest 87:432, 1991

193. Hogan M, Cerami A, Bucala R: Advanced glycosylation endproducts block the antiproliferative effect of nitric oxide. Role in the vascular and renal com-

plications of diabetes mellitus. J Clin Invest 90:1110, 1992

194. Schmidt AM, Yan SD, Brett J et al: Regulation of human mononuclear phagocyte migration by cell surface-binding proteins for advanced glycation end products. J Clin Invest 91:2155, 1993

195. Vlassara H: Receptor-mediated interactions of advanced glycosylation end products with cellular components within diabetic tissues. Diabetes 41(suppl 2):52, 1992

196. Stout RW: Insulin and atheroma. 20-yr perspective. Diabetes Care 13:631, 1990

197. DeFronzo RA, Ferrannini E: Insulin resistance: a multifaceted syndrome responsible for NIDDM, obesity, hypertension, dyslipidemia, and atherosclerotic cardiovascular disease. Diabetes Care 14:173, 1991

198. Jarrett RJ: In defence of insulin: a critique of syndrome X. Lancet 340:469, 1992

199. Durrington PN: Is insulin atherogenic? Diabet Med 9:597, 1992

200. Savage PJ, Saad MF: Insulin and atherosclerosis: villain, accomplice, or innocent bystander? Br Heart J 69:473, 1993

201. Zavaroni I, Bonora E, Pagliara M et al: Risk factors for coronary artery disease in healthy persons with hyperinsulinemia and normal glucose tolerance. N Engl J Med 320:702, 1989

202. Haffner SM, Fong D, Hazuda HP et al: Hyperinsulinemia, upper body adiposity, and cardiovascular risk factors in non-diabetics. Metabolism 37:338, 1988

203. Martin FIR, Hopper JL: The relationship of acute insulin sensitivity to the progression of vascular disease in long-term type I (insulin-dependent) diabetes mellitus. Diabetologia 30:149, 1987

204. Logan RL, Reimesma RA, Thomson M et al: Risk factors for ischaemic heart-disease in normal men aged 40: Edinburgh-Stockholm Study. Lancet 1:949, 1978

205. McKeigue PM, Shah B, Marmot MG: Relation of central obesity and insulin resistance with high diabetes prevalence and cardiovascular risk in South Asians. Lancet 337:382, 1991

206. Pyorala K: Relationship of glucose tolerance and plasma insulin to the incidence of coronary heart disease: results from two population studies in Finland. Diabetes Care 2:131, 1979

207. Welborn TA, Wearne K: Coronary heart disease incidence and cardiovascular mortality in Busselton with reference to glucose and insulin concentrations. Diabetes Care 2:154, 1979

208. Cullen K, Stenhouse NS, Wearne KL Welborn TA: Multiple regression analysis of risk factors for cardiovascular disease and cancer mortality in Busselton, Western Australia—13 year study. J Chronic Dis 36:371, 1983

209. Hargreaves AD, Logan RL, Elton RA et al: Glucose tolerance, plasma insulin, HDL cholesterol and obesity: 12 year follow-up and development of coronary heart disease in Edinburgh men. Atherosclerosis 94:61, 1992

210. Welin L, Eriksson H, Larsson B et al: Hyperinsulinemia is not a major coronary risk factor in elderly men: the study of men born in 1913. Diabetologia 35:766, 1992

211. Liu QZ, Knowler WC, Nelson RG et al: Insulin treatment, endogenous insulin concentration, and ECG abnormalities in diabetic Pima Indians: cross-sectional and prospective analyses. Diabetes 41:1141, 1992

212. Modan M, Or J, Karasik A et al: Hyperinsulinemia, sex, and risk of atherosclerotic cardiovascular disease. Circulation 84:1165, 1991

213. Canner PL, Berge KG, Wenger NK et al: Fifteen year mortality in Coronary Drug Project patients: Long term benefit with niacin. J Am Coll Cardiol 8:1245, 1986

214. Kahn SE, Beard JC, Schwartz MW et al: Increased β-cell secretory capacity as mechanism for islet adaptation to nicotinic acid-induced insulin resistance. Diabetes 38:562, 1989

215. The University Group Diabetes Program: Effects of hypoglycemic agents on vascular complications in patients

with adult-onset diabetes. Diabetes 31 (suppl)5:1, 1982

216. Ferrannini E, Buzzigoli G, Bonadonna R et al: Insulin resistance in essential hypertension. N Engl J Med 317:350, 1987

217. Saad MF, Lillioja S, Nyomba BL et al: Racial differences in the relation between blood pressure and insulin resistance. N Engl J Med 324:733, 1991

218. Abbott WG, Lillioja S, Young AA et al: Relationships between plasma lipoprotein concentration and insulin action in an obese hyperinsulinemic population. Diabetes 36:897, 1987

219. Frayn KN, Coppack SW: Insulin resistance, adipose tissue and coronary heart disease. Clin Sci 82:1, 1992

220. Reaven GM, Chen Y-DI, Jeppesen J et al: Insulin resistance and hyperinsulinemia in individuals with small, dense, low-density lipoprotein particles. J Clin Invest 92:141, 1993

221. Laakso M, Edelman SV, Brechtel G et al: Decreased effect of insulin to stimulate skeletal muscle blood flow in obese men: a novel mechanism for insulin resistance. J Clin Invest 85:1844, 1990

222. Juhan-Vague I, Vague P: Hypofibrinolysis and insulin resistance. Diabete Metab 17:96, 1991

223. Brindley DN, Rolland Y: Possible connections between stress, diabetes, obesity, hypertension and altered lipoprotein metabolism that may result in atherosclerosis. Clin Sci 77:453, 1989

224. Messent JW, Elliott TG, Hill RD et al: Prognostic significance of microalbuminuria in insulin-dependent diabetes mellitus: a twenty-three year follow-up study. Kidney Int 41:386, 1992

225. Winocour PH, Durrington PN, Ishola M et al: Influence of proteinuria on vascular disease, blood pressure, and lipoproteins in insulin-dependent diabetes mellitus. Br Med J 294:1648, 1987

226. Mogensen CE. Microalbuminuria predicts clinical proteinuria and early mortality in maturity-onset diabetes. N Engl J Med 310:356, 1984

227. Jarrett RJ, Viberti GC, Argyropoulos A et al: Microalbuminuria in non-insulin-dependent diabetes. Diabet Med 1:17, 1984

228. Mattock MB, Keen H, Viberti GC et al: Coronary heart disease and urinary albumin excretion rate in type 2 (noninsulin-dependent) diabetic patients. Diabetologia 31:82, 1988

229. Schmitz A, Vaeth M: Microalbuminuria: a major risk factor in non-insulin-dependent diabetes: a 10-year follow-up study of 503 patients. Diabet Med 5:126, 1988

230. Neil A, Hawkins M, Potok M et al: A prospective population-based study of microalbuminuria as a predictor of mortality in NIDDM. Diabetes Care 16:996, 1993

231. Parving H-H, Hommel E, Mathiesen E et al: Prevalence of microalbuminuria, arterial hypertension, retinopathy and neuropathy in patients with insulin-dependent diabetes. Br Med J 296:156, 1988

232. Norgaard K, Feldt-Rasmussen B, Borch-Johnsen K et al: Prevalence of hypertension in type 1 (insulin dependent) diabetes mellitus. Diabetologia 33:407, 1990

233. Jones SL, Close CF, Mattock MB et al: Plasma lipid and coagulation factor concentrations in insulin dependent diabetics with microalbuminuria. BMJ 298:487, 1989

234. Reverter JL, Sentí M, Rubiés-Prat J et al: Relationship between lipoprotein profile and urinary albumin excretion in type II diabetic patients with stable metabolic control. Diabetes Care 17:189, 1994

235. Gruden G, Cavallo-Perin P, Bazzan M et al: PAI-1 and factor VII activity are higher in IDDM patients with microalbuminuria. Diabetes 43:426, 1994

236. Deckert T, Feldt-Rasmussen B, Borch-Johnsen K et al: Albuminuria reflects widespread vascular damage. The Steno hypothesis. Diabetologia 32:219, 1989

237. Moy CS, LaPorte RE, Dorman JS et al: Insulin-dependent diabetes mellitus mortality. The risk of cigarette smoking. Circulation 82:37, 1990

238. Suarez L, Barrett-Connor E: Interaction between cigarette smoking and diabetes

mellitus in the prediction of death attributed to cardiovascular disease. Am J Epidemiol 120:670, 1984

239. Howard BV, Howard Wm J: The compelling case for smoking cessation in diabetes. Circulation 82:299, 1990

240. Abenavoli T, Rubler S, Fisher VJ et al: Exercise testing with myocardial scintigraphy in asymptomatic diabetic males. Circulation 63:54, 1981

241. Chiariello M, Indolfi C, Cotecchia MR et al: Asymptomatic transient ST changes during ambulatory ECG monitoring in diabetic patients. Am Heart J 110:529, 1985

242. Nesto RW, Phillips RT, Kett KG et al: Angina and exertional myocardial ischemia in diabetic and non-diabetic patients: assessment by exercise thallium scintigraphy. Ann Intern Med 108:170, 1988

243. Koistinen MJ: Prevalence of asymptomatic myocardial ischaemia in diabetic subjects. BMJ 301:92, 1990

244. Naka M, Hiramatsu K, Aizawa T et al: Silent myocardial ischemia in patients with non-insulin-dependent diabetes mellitus as judged by treadmill exercise testing and coronary angiography. Am Heart J 123:46, 1992

245. Burchfiel CM, Reed DM, Marcus EB et al: Association of diabetes mellitus with coronary atherosclerosis and myocardial lesions. An autopsy study from the Honolulu Heart Program. Am J Epidemiol 137:1328, 1993

246. Kannel WB, Abbott RD. Incidence and prognosis of unrecognized myocardial infarction: an update on the Framingham study. N Engl J Med 311:1144, 1984

247. Langer A, Freeman MR, Josse RG et al: Detection of silent myocardial ischemia in diabetes mellitus. Am J Cardiol 67:1073, 1991

248. O'Sullivan JJ, Conroy RM, MacDonald K et al: Silent ischaemia in diabetic men with autonomic neuropathy. Br Heart J 66:313, 1991

249. Umachandran V, Ranjadayalan K, Ambepityia G et al: The perception of angina in diabetes: relation to somatic pain threshold and autonomic function. Am Heart J 121:1649, 1991

250. Ambepityia G, Kopelman PG, Ingram D et al: Exertional myocardial ischemia in diabetes: a quantitative analysis of anginal perceptual threshold and the influence of autonomic function. J Am Coll Cardiol 15:72, 1990

251. Ranjadayalan K, Umachandran V, Ambepityia G et al: Prolonged anginal perceptual threshold in diabetes: effects on exercise capacity and myocardial ischemia. J Am Coll Cardiol 16:1120, 1990

252. Bradley RF, Schonfeld A. Diminished pain in diabetic patients with acute myocardial infarction. Geriatrics 17:322, 1962

253. Partamian JO, Bradley RF: Acute myocardial infarction in 258 cases of diabetes. Immediate mortality and five-year survival. N Engl J Med 273:455, 1965

254. Soler NG, Bennett MA, Pentecost BL et al: Myocardial infarction in diabetics. Q J Med 44:125, 1975

255. Savage MP, Krolewski AS, Kenien GG et al: Acute myocardial infarction in diabetes mellitus and significance of congestive heart failure as a prognostic factor. Am J Cardiol 62:665, 1988

256. Jacoby RM, Nesto RW: Acute myocardial infarction in the diabetic patient: pathophysiology, clinical course and prognosis. J Am Coll Cardiol 20:736, 1992

257. Jaffe AS, Spadaro JJ, Schechtman K et al: Increased congestive heart failure after myocardial infarction of modest extent in patients with diabetes mellitus. Am Heart J 108:31, 1984

258. Stone PH, Muller JE, Hartwell T et al: The effect of diabetes mellitus on prognosis and serial left ventricular function after acute myocardial infarction: contribution of both coronary disease and diastolic left ventricular dysfunction to the adverse prognosis. J Am Coll Cardiol 14:49, 1989

259. Kouvaras G, Cokkinos D, Spyropoulou M: Increased mortality of diabetics after acute myocardial infarction attributed to diffusely impaired left ventricular per-

formance as assessed by echocardiography. Jpn Heart J 29:1, 1988

260. Lomuscio A, Bestetti A, Vergani D et al: Radionuclide assessment of left ventricular function in patients with myocardial infarction and diabetes mellitus. J Intern Med 231:73, 1992

261. Iwasaka T, Takahashi N, Nakamura S et al: Residual left ventricular pump function after acute myocardial infarction in NIDDM patients. Diabetes Care 15:1522, 1992

262. Czyzk A, Królewski AS, Szablowska A et al: Clinical course of myocardial infarction among diabetic patients. Diabetes Care 3:526, 1980

263. Kereiakes DJ: Myocardial infarction in the diabetic patient. Clin Cardiol 8:446, 1985

264. Gilpin E, Ricou F, Dittrich H et al: Factors associated with recurrent myocardial infarction within one year after acute myocardial infarction. Am Heart J 121:457, 1991

265. Karlson BW, Herlitz J, Hjalmarson Å: Prognosis of acute myocardial infarction in diabetic and non-diabetic patients. Diabet Med 10:449, 1993

266. Singer DE, Moulton AW, Nathan DM: Diabetic myocardial infarction. Interaction of diabetes with other preinfarction risk factors. Diabetes 38:350, 1989

267. Smith JW, Marcus FI, Serokman R: The Multicenter Postinfarction Research Group. Prognosis of patients with diabetes mellitus after acute myocardial infarction. Am J Cardiol 54:718, 1984

268. Wong ND, Cupples A, Ostfeld AM et al: Risk factors for long-term coronary prognosis after initial myocardial infarction: the Framingham Study. Am J Epidemiol 130:469, 1989

269. Herlitz J, Malmberg K, Karlson BW et al: Mortality and morbidity during a five-year follow-up of diabetics with myocardial infarction. Acta Med Scand 224:31, 1988

270. Sprafka JM, Burke GL, Folsom AR et al: Trends in prevalence of diabetes mellitus in patients with myocardial infarction and effect of diabetes on survival.

The Minnesota Heart Survey. Diabetes Care 14:537, 1991

271. Fibrinolytic Therapy Trials' (FTT) Collaborative Group. Indications for fibrinolytic therapy in suspected acute myocardial infarction: collaborative overview of early mortality and major morbidity results from all randomised trials of more than 1000 patients. Lancet 343:311, 1994

272. Liao Y, Cooper RS, Ghali JK et al: Sex differences in the impact of coexisting diabetes on survival in patients with coronary heart disease. Diabetes Care 16:708, 1993

273. Rytter L, Troelsen S, Beck-Nielsen H: Prevalence and mortality of acute myocardial infarction in patients with diabetes. Diabetes Care 8:230, 1985

274. Toole JF, Janeway R, Choi K et al: Transient ischemic attacks due to atherosclerosis. Arch Neurol 32:5, 1975

275. Howard G, Toole JF, Frye-Pierson J, Hinshelwood LC: Factors influencing the survival of 451 transient ischemic attack patients. Stroke 18:552, 1987

276. Hornig CR, Lammers C, Büttner T et al: Long-term prognosis of infratentorial transient ischemic attacks and minor strokes. Stroke 23:199, 1992

277. The Dutch TIA Trial Study Group: Predictors of major vascular events in patients with a transient ischemic attack or nondisabling stroke. Stroke 24:527, 1993

278. Fritz VU, Bilchik T, Levien LJ: Diabetes as risk factor for transient ischemic attacks as opposed to strokes. Eur J Vasc Surg 1:259, 1987

279. Weinberger J, Biscarra V, Weisberg MK, Jacobson JH: Factors contributing to stroke in patients with atherosclerotic disease of the great vessels: the role of diabetes. Stroke 14:709, 1983

280. Bell ET: A postmortem study of vascular disease in diabetes. Arch Pathol 53:444, 1952

281. Alex M, Baron EK, Goldenberg S, Blumenthal HT: An autopsy study of cerebrovascular accident in diabetes mellitus. Circulation 25:663, 1962

282. Chamorro A, Sacco RL, Mohr JP et al: Clinical-computed tomographic correla-

tions of lacunar infarction in the Stroke Data Bank. Stroke 22:175, 1991

283. Dobkin BH: Orthostatic hypotension as a risk factor for symptomatic occlusive cerebrovascular disease. Neurology 39:30, 1989

284. Biller J, Love BB: Diabetes and stroke. Med Clin N Am 77:95, 1993

285. Asplund K, Hägg E, Helmers C et al: The natural history of stroke in diabetic patients. Acta Med Scand 207:417, 1980

286. McCall AL. The impact of diabetes on the CNS. Diabetes 41:557, 1992

287. Candelise L, Landi G, Orazio EN, Boccardi E: Prognostic significance of hyperglycemia in acute stroke. Arch Neurol 42:661, 1985

288. Berger L, Hakim AM: The association of hyperglycemia with cerebral edema in stroke. Stroke 17:865, 1986

289. Kushner M, Nencini P, Reivich M et al: Relation of hyperglycemia early in ischemic brain infarction to cerebral anatomy, metabolism, and clinical outcome. Ann Neurol 28:129, 1990

290. Sacco RL, Foulkes MA, Mohr JP et al: Determinants of early recurrence of cerebral infarction. The Stroke Data Bank. Stroke 20:983, 1989

291. Hier DB, Foulkes MA, Swiontoniowski M et al: Stroke recurrence within 2 years after ischemic infarction. Stroke 22:155,1991

292. Olsson T, Viitanen M, Asplund K et al: Prognosis after stroke in diabetic patients. A controlled prospective study. Diabetologia 33:244, 1990

293. Foster JW, Hart RG: Hypoglycemic hemiplegia: two cases and a clinical review. Stroke 18:944, 1987

294. Lahat E, Salgado A, Rowan AJ: Transient aphasic episodes due to hypoglycemia. Clin Neurol Neurosurg 90:141, 1988

295. Bell DSH: Stroke in the diabetic patient. Diabetes Care 17:213, 1994

296. Gensler SW, Haimovici H, Hoffert P et al: Study of vascular lesions in diabetic and nondiabetic patients. Arch Surg 91:617, 1965

297. LoGerfo FW, Coffman JD: Vascular and microvascular disease of the foot in diabetes. Implications for foot care. N Engl J Med 311:1615, 1984

298. Orchard TJ, Strandness DE Jr: Assessment of peripheral vascular disease in diabetes. Diabetes Care 16:1199, 1993

299. Young MJ, Veves A, Boulton AJM: The diabetic foot: etiopathogenesis and management. Diabetes Metab Rev 9:109, 1993

300. Vinik AI, Wing RR: The good, the bad, and the ugly in the diabetic diets. Endocrinol Metab Clin North Am 21:237, 1992

301. Williams G: Management of non-insulin-dependent diabetes mellitus. Lancet 343:95, 1994

302. American Diabetes Association: Detection and management of lipid disorders in diabetes. Diabetes Care 16 (suppl 2):106, 1993

303. Horton ES: Exercise and diabetes mellitus. Med Clin North Am 72:1301, 1988

304. Yudkin JS: How can we best prolong life? Benefits of coronary risk factor reduction in non-diabetic and diabetic subjects. BMJ 306:1313, 1993

305. Wang PH, Lau J, Chalmers TC: Meta-analysis of effects of intensive blood-glucose control on late complications of type I diabetes. Lancet 341,1306, 1993

306. Yki-Järvinen H, Kauppila M, Kujansuu E et al: Comparison of insulin regimens in patients with non-insulin-dependent diabetes mellitus. N Engl J Med 327:1426, 1992

307. Groop LC: Sulfonylureas in NIDDM. Diabetes Care 15:737, 1992

308. American Diabetes Association. Policy statement: the UGDP controversy. Diabetes Care 2:1, 1979

309. Bailey CJ: Biguanides and NIDDM. Diabetes Care 15:755, 1992

310. Colwell JA: Is it time to introduce metformin in the U.S.? Diabetes Care 16:653, 1993

311. The Expert Panel: National Cholesterol Education Program Expert Panel on detection, evaluation and treatment of high blood cholesterol in adults. Arch Intern Med 148:36, 1988

312. Frick MH, Elo O, Happa K et al: Hel-

sinki Heart Study: primary-prevention trial with gemfibrozil in middle-aged men with dyslipidemia. Safety of treatment, changes in risk factors, and incidence of coronary heart disease. N Engl J Med 317:1237, 1987

313. Garg A, Grundy SM:. Gemfibrozil alone and in combination with lovastatin for treatment of hypertriglyceridemia in NIDDM. Diabetes 38:364, 1989

314. Pierce LR, Wysowski DK, Gross TP: Myopathy and rhabdomyolysis associated with lovastatin-gemfibrozil combination therapy. JAMA 264:71, 1990

315. Garg A, Grundy SM: Lovastatin for lowering cholesterol levels in non-insulin-dependent diabetes mellitus. N Engl J Med 318:81, 1988

316. Yoshino G, Kazumi T, Iwai M et al: Long-term treatment of hypercholesterolemic non-insulin-dependent diabetics (NIDDM) with pravastatin (CS-514). Atherosclerosis 75:67, 1989

317. Kim DK, Escalante DA, Garber AJ: Prevention of atherosclerosis in diabetes: emphasis on treatment for the abnormal lipoprotein metabolism of diabetes. Clin Ther 15:766, 1993

318. Saad MF, Bergman RN, DeGregorio M et al: Inability of normal beta-cells to compensate completely for experimentally-induced insulin resistance, abstracted. Diabetologia 34:A107, 1991

319. Garg A, Grundy SM: Nicotinic acid as therapy for dyslipidemia in non-insulin-dependent diabetes mellitus. JAMA 264:723, 1990

320. Koev D, Zlateva S, Susic M et al: Improvement of lipoprotein lipid composition in type II diabetic patients with concomitant hyperlipoproteinemia by acipimox treatment. Results of a multicenter trial. Diabetes Care 16:1285, 1993

321. Vaag A, Skott P, Damsbo P et al: Effect of the antilipolytic nicotinic acid analogue acipimox on whole-body and skeletal muscle glucose metabolism in patients with non-insulin-dependent diabetes mellitus. J Clin Invest 88:1282, 1991

322. Pladziewicz DS, Nesto RW: Hypoglyce-

mia-induced silent myocardial ischemia. Am J Cardiol 63:1531, 1989

323. Holmes DR Jr, Vlietstra RE, Smith HC et al: Restenosis after percutaneous transluminal coronary angioplasty (PTCA): a report from the PTCA Registry of the National Heart, Lung, and Blood Institute. Am J Cardiol 53:77C, 1984

324. Weintraub WS, Ghazzal ZM, Douglas JS Jr et al: Long-term clinical follow-up in patients with angiographic restudy after successful angioplasty. Circulation 87:831, 1993

325. Carrozza JP Jr, Kuntz RE, Fishman RF, Baim DS: Restenosis after arterial injury caused by coronary stenting in patients with diabetes mellitus. Ann Intern Med 118:344, 1993

326. Morris JJ, Smith LR, Jones RH et al: Influence of diabetes and mammary artery grafting on survival after coronary bypass. Circulation 84(suppl 5):III,275, 1991

327. Yasuura K, Matsuura A, Sawazaki M et al: Surgical results in diabetics undergoing coronary artery bypass grafting. Nippon Kyobu Geka Gakkai Zasshi 41:363, 1993

328. ISIS-2 (Second International Study of Infarct Survival) Collaborative Group: Randomised trial of intravenous streptokinase, oral aspirin, both or neither among 17,187 cases of suspected acute myocardial infarction: ISIS-2. Lancet 77:349, 1988

329. Barbash GI, White HD, Modan M et al: Significance of diabetes mellitus in patients with acute myocardial infarction receiving thrombolytic therapy. J Am Coll Cardiol 22:707, 1993

330. Granger CB, Califf RM, Young S et al: Outcome of patients with diabetes mellitus and acute myocardial infarction treated with thrombolytic agents. J Am Coll Cardiol 21:920, 1993

331. Lynch M, Gammage MD, Lamb P et al: Acute myocardial infarction in diabetic patients in the thrombolytic era. Diabet Med 11:162, 1994

332. Lew AS, Hod H, Cercek B et al: Mortality and morbidity rates of patients older

and younger than 75 years with acute myocardial infarction treated with intravenous streptokinase. Am J Cardiol 59:1, 1987

333. Gundersen T, Kjekshus J: Timolol treatment after myocardial infarction in diabetic patients. Diabetes Care 6:285, 1983

334. Malmberg K, Herlitz J, Hjalmarson A, Ryden L: Effects of metoprolol on mortality and late infarction in diabetics with suspected acute myocardial infarction. Retrospective data from two large studies. Eur Heart J 10:423, 1989

335. ETDRS Investigators: Aspirin effects on mortality and morbidity in patients with diabetes mellitus. Early Treatment Diabetic Retinopathy Study. Report 14. JAMA 268:1292, 1992

336. The Canadian Cooperative Study Group. A randomized trial of aspirin and sulfinpyrazone in threatened stroke. N Engl J Med 299:53, 1978

337. Fields WS, Lemak NA, Frankowski RF et al: Controlled trial of aspirin in cerebral ischemia. Stroke 8:301, 1977

338. UK-TIA Study Group: The United Kingdom transient ischaemic attack (UK-TIA) aspirin trial: final results. J Neurol Neurosurg Psychiatry 54:1044, 1991

339. Grotta JC, Norris JW, Kamm B: The TASS Baseline and Angiographic Data Subgroup: prevention of stroke with ticlopidine: who benefits most? Neurology 42:111, 1992

340. European Carotid Surgery Trialists' Collaborative Group. MRC European Carotid Surgery Trial: interim results for symptomatic patients with severe (70–99%) or with mild (0–29%) carotid stenosis. Lancet 337:1235, 1991

341. North American Symptomatic Carotid Endarterectomy Trial Collaborators: Beneficial effect of carotid endarterectomy in symptomatic patients with high-grade carotid stenosis. N Engl J Med 325:445, 1991

342. Mayberg MR, Wilson SE, Yatsu F et al: Carotid endarterectomy and prevention of cerebral ischemia in symptomatic carotid stenosis. JAMA 266:3289, 1991

343. Helgason CM: Blood glucose and stroke. Stroke 19:1049, 1988

344. Patrono C, Davi G: Antiplatelet agents in prevention of diabetic vascular complications. Diabetes Metab Rev 9:177, 1993

345. Assal JP, Muhlhauser I, Pernet A et al: Patient education as the basis for diabetes care in clinical practice and research. Diabetologia 28:602, 1985

346. Campbell RK: Clinical update on pentoxifylline therapy for diabetes-induced peripheral vascular disease. Ann Pharmacother 27:1099, 1993

347. Uchikawa T, Murakami T, Furukawa H: Effects of the anti-platelet agent cilostazol on peripheral vascular disease in patients with diabetes mellitus. Arzneimittelforschung 42:322, 1992

348. Stonebridge PA, Murie JA: Infrainguinal revascularization in the diabetic patient. Br J Surg 80:1237, 1993

349. Shah DM, Chang BB, Fitzgerald KM et al: Durability of tibial artery bypass in diabetic patients. Am J Surg 156:133, 1988

350. Johnston KW, Rae M, Hogg-Johnston SA et al: 5-year results of a prospective study of percutaneous transluminal angioplasty. Ann Surg 206:403, 1987

351. Edmonds ME: The diabetic foot: pathophysiology and treatment. Clin Endocrinol Metab 15:889, 1986

352. Rubler S, Dlugash J, Yuceoglu YZ et al: New type of cardiomyopathy associated with diabetic glomerulosclerosis. Am J Cardiol 30:595, 1972

353. Kannel WB, Hjortland M, Castelli WP: Role of diabetes in congestive heart failure: the Framingham study. Am J Cardiol 34:29, 1974

354. Hamby RI, Zoneraich S, Sherman S: Diabetic cardiomyopathy. JAMA 229:1749, 1974

355. Ahmed SS, Jaferi GA, Narang RM, Regan TJ: Preclinical abnormality of left ventricular function in diabetes mellitus. Am Heart J 89:153, 1975

356. Ledet T: Diabetic cardiomyopathy: quantitative histological studies of the heart from young juvenile diabetics.

Acta Pathol Microbiol Scand Sect A Pathol 84:421, 1976

357. Regan TJ, Lyons MM, Ahmed SS et al: Evidence for cardiomyopathy in familial diabetes mellitus. J Clin Invest 60:885, 1977

358. Shirey EK, Proudfit WL, Hawk WA: Primary myocardial disease. Correlation with clinical findings, angiography and biopsy diagnosis. Follow-up of 139 patients. Am Heart J 99:198, 1980

359. Galderisi MI, Anderson K, Wilson P, Levy D: Echocardiographic evidence for the existence of a distinct diabetic cardiomyopathy. Am J Cardiol 68:85, 1991

360. Fein FS, Kornstein LB, Strobeck JE et al: Altered myocardial mechanics in diabetic rats. Circ Res 47:922, 1980

361. Penpargkul S, Fein FS, Sonnenblick EH, Scheuer J: Depressed cardiac sarcoplasmic reticular function from diabetic rats. J Mol Cell Cardiol 13:303, 1981

362. Fein FS: Diabetic cardiomyopathy. Diabetes Care 13:1169, 1990

363. Zarich SW, Nesto RW: Diabetic cardiomyopathy. Am Heart J 118(5 Pt 1):1000, 1989

364. Uusitupa MIJ, Mustonen JN, Airaksinen KEJ: Diabetic heart muscle disease. Ann Med 22:377, 1990

365. Garvey WT, Hardin D, Juhaszova M, Dominguez JH: Effects of diabetes on myocardial glucose transport system in rats: implications for diabetic cardiomyopathy. Am J Physiol 264:H837, 1993

366. Rodrigues B, McNeill JH: The diabetic heart: metabolic causes for the development of a cardiomyopathy. Cardiovas Res 26:913, 1992

367. Dhalla NS, Elimban V, Rupp H: Paradoxical role of lipid metabolism in heart function and dysfunction. Mol Cell Biochem 116:3, 1992

368. Factor SM, Okun EM, Minase T: Capillary microaneurysms in the human diabetic heart. N Engl J Med 302:384, 1980

369. Fischer VW, Barner HB, Leskiw ML: Capillary basal laminar thickness in diabetic human myocardium. Diabetes 28:713, 1979

370. Fisher BM, Gillen G, Lindop GBM et al: Cardiac function and coronary arteriography in asymptomatic Type 1 (insulin-dependent) diabetic patients: evidence for a specific diabetic heart disease. Diabetologia 29:706, 1986

371. Shapiro LM, Leatherdale BA, Mackinnon J, Fletcher RF: Left ventricular function in diabetes mellitus. II: Relation between clinical features and left ventricular function. Br Heart J 45:129, 1981

372. Margonato A, Gerundini P, Vicedomini G et al: Abnormal cardiovascular response to exercise in young asymptomatic diabetic patients with retinopathy. Am Heart J 112:554, 1986

373. Vered Z, Battler A, Segal P et al: Exercise-induced left ventricular dysfunction in young men with asymptomatic diabetes mellitus (diabetic cardiomyopathy). Am J Cardiol 54:633, 1984

374. Mildenberger RR, Bar-Shlomo B, Druck MN et al: Clinically unrecognized ventricular dysfunction in young diabetic patients. J Am Coll Cardiol 4:234, 1984

375. Friedman NE, Levitsky LL, Edidin DV et al: Echocardiographic evidence for impaired myocardial performance in children with Type 1 diabetes Mellitus. Am J Med 73:846, 1982

376. Lababidi ZA, Goldstein DE: High prevalence of echocardiographic abnormalities in diabetic youth. Diabetes Care 6:18, 1982

377. Mustonen J, Uusitupa M, Tahvanainen K et al: Impaired left ventricular systolic function during exercise in middle-aged insulin-dependent and non-insulin-dependent diabetic subjects without clinically evident cardiovascular disease. Am J Cardiol 62:1273, 1988

378. Thuesen L, Christiansen J, Falstie-Jensen N et al: Increased myocardial contractility in short-term type 1 diabetic patients: an echocardiographic study. Diabetologia 28:822, 1985

379. Thuesen L, Christiansen JS, Mogensen CE, Henningsen P: Cardiac hyperfunction in insulin-dependent diabetic patients developing microvascular complications. Diabetes 37:851, 1988

380. Thuesen L: Cardiac function in insulin-dependent diabetic patients without clinical signs of heart disease. Echocardiographic studies with emphasis on the left ventricular systolic function. Dan Med Bull 40:557, 1993

381. Danielsen R, Nordrehaug JE, Lien E, Vik-Mo H: Subclinical left ventricular abnormalities in young subjects with long-term type 1 diabetes mellitus detected by digitized M-mode echocardiography. Am J Cardiol 60:143, 1987

382. Ruddy TD, Shumak SL, Liu PP et al: The relationship of cardiac diastolic dysfunction to concurrent hormonal and metabolic status in type 1 diabetes mellitus. J Clin Endocrinol Metab 66:113, 1988

383. Zarich SW, Arbuckle BE, Cohen LR et al: Diastolic abnormalities in young asymptomatic diabetic patients assessed by pulsed Doppler echocardiography. J Am Coll Cardiol 12:114, 1988

384. Bouchard A, Sanz N, Botvinick EH et al: Noninvasive assessment of cardiomyopathy in normotensive diabetic patients between 20 and 50 years old. Am J Med 87:160, 1989

385. Zoneraich S: Left ventricular diastolic dysfunction evaluated by Doppler echocardiography in patients with diabetes mellitus. Am J Cardiol 64:1037, 1989

386. Paillole C, Dahan M, Paycha F et al: Prevalence and significance of left ventricular filling abnormalities determined by Doppler echocardiography in young type I (insulin-dependent) diabetic patients. Am J Cardiol 64:1010, 1989

387. Borow KM, Jaspan JB, Williams KA et al: Myocardial mechanics in young adult patients with diabetes mellitus: effect of altered load, inotropic state and dynamic exercise. J Am Coll Cardiol 15:1508, 1990

388. Illan F, Valdés-Chávarri M, Tebar J et al: Anatomical and functional cardiac abnormalities in type I diabetes. Clin Invest 70:403, 1992

389. Clarkson P, Wheeldon NM, MacDonald TM: Left ventricular diastolic dysfunction. Q J Med 87:143, 1994

390. Perez JE, McGill JB, Santiago JV et al: Abnormal myocardial acoustic properties in diabetic patients and their correlation with the severity of disease. J Am Coll Cardiol 19:1154, 1992

391. Parving H-H, Rasmussen SM: Transcapillary escape rate of albumin and plasma volume in short- and long-term juvenile diabetics. Scand J Clin Lab Invest 32:81, 1973

392. Fukuhara T, Fujioka H, Kinoshita M: Congestive heart failure associated with diabetes mellitus. Int J Cardiol 23:130, 1989

393. Zoneraich O, Zoneraich S: A vectorcardiographic study of spatial P, QRS and T-loops in diabetic patients without clinically apparent heart disease. J Electrocardiol 10:207, 1977

394. Zoneraich S: Small-vessel disease, coronary artery vasodilator reserve, and diabetic cardiomyopathy. Chest 94:5, 1988

395. Factor SM, Minase T, Sonnenblick EM: Clinical and morphological features of human hypertensive-diabetic cardiomyopathy. Am Heart J 99:446, 1980

396. Van Hoeven KH, Factor SM: A comparison of pathological spectrum of hypertensive, diabetic and hypertensive diabetic heart disease. Circulation 82:848, 1990

397. Sykes CA, Wright AD, Malins JM, Pentecost BL: Changes in systolic time intervals during treatment of diabetes mellitus. Br Heart J 39:255, 1977

398. Shapiro LM, Leatherdale BA, Coyne ME et al: Prospective study of heart disease in untreated maturity onset diabetics. Br Heart J 44:342, 1980

399. Uusitupa M, Siitonen O, Aro A et al: Effect of correction of hyperglycemia on left ventricular function in non-insulin-dependent (type 2) diabetics. Acta Med Scand 213:363, 1983

400. The CONSENSUS Trial Study Group: Effects of enalapril on mortality in severe congestive heart failure: results of the Cooperative North Scandinavian Enalapril Survival Study (CONSENSUS). N Engl J Med 316:1429, 1987

401. Pollare T, Lithell H, Berne C: A comparison of the effects of hydrochlorothizide

and captopril on glucose and lipid metabolism in patients with hypertension. N Engl J Med 321:868, 1989

402. Hitzenberger K: Uber den Blutdruck bei Diabetes mellitus. Wien Arch Inn Med 2:461, 1921

403. Fuller JH, Stevens LK: Epidemiology of hypertension in diabetic patients and implications for treatment. Diabetes Care 14(suppl 4):8, 1991

404. Krolewski AJ, Warram JH: Epidemiology and genetics of hypertension in diabetes mellitus. p. 339. In Draznin B, Eckel RH (eds): Diabetes and Atherosclerosis: Molecular Basis and Clinical Aspects. Elsevier, New York, 1993

405. The Hypertension in Diabetes Study Group: Hypertension in diabetes study: I. Prevalence of hypertension in newly presenting type 2 diabetes patients and the association with risk factors for cardiovascular and diabetic complications. J Hypertens 11:309, 1993

406. Reaven PD, Barrett-Connor EL, Browner DK: Abnormal glucose tolerance and hypertension. Diabetes Care 13:119, 1990

407. Mogensen CE, Christensen CK, Vittinghus E: The stages in diabetic renal disease with emphasis on the stage of incipient diabetic nephropathy. Diabetes 32(suppl 2):64, 1983

408. Seaquist ER, Goetz FC, Rich S, Barbosa J: Familial clustering of diabetic kidney disease. Evidence for genetic susceptibility to diabetic nephropathy. N Engl J Med 320:1161, 1989

409. Borch-Johnson K, Norgaard K, Hommel E et al: Is diabetic nephropathy an inherited complication? Kidney Int 41:719, 1992

410. Pettitt DJ, Saad MF, Bennett PH et al: Familial predisposition to renal disease in two generations of Pima Indians with type 2 (non-insulin-dependent) diabetes mellitus. Diabetologia 33:438, 1990

411. Viberti GC, Keen H, Wiseman MJ: Raised arterial pressure in parents of proteinuric insulin-dependent diabetics. Br Med J 295:515, 1987

412. Krolewski AS, Canessa M, Warram JH,

et al: Predisposition to hypertension and susceptibility to renal disease in insulin-dependent diabetes mellitus. N Engl J Med 318:140, 1988

413. Barzilay J, Warram JH, Bak M, et al: Predisposition to hypertension: a risk factor for nephropathy and hypertension in IDDM. Kidney Int 41:723, 1992

414. Jensen JS, Mathiesen ER, Norgaard K et al: Increased blood pressure and erythrocyte sodium lithium countertransport activity are not inherited in diabetic nephropathy. Diabetologia 33:619, 1990

415. De Chatel R, Weidmann P, Flammer J et al. Sodium, renin aldosterone, catecholamines and blood pressure in diabetes mellitus. Kidney Int 12:412, 1977

416. Feldt-Rasmussen B, Mathiesen ER, Deckert T et al: Central role for sodium in the pathogenesis of blood pressure changes independent of angiotensin, aldosterone and catecholamines in type I (insulin-dependent) diabetes mellitus. Diabetologia 30:610, 1987

417. Hommel E, Mathiesen ER, Giese J et al: On the pathogenesis of arterial blood pressure elevation early in the course of diabetic nephropathy. Scand J Clin Lab Invest 49:537, 1989

418. Trevisan R, Fioretto P, Semplicin A et al: Role of insulin and atrial natriuretic peptide in sodium retention in insulin-treated IDDM patients during isotonic volume expansion. Diabetes 39:289, 1990

419. Blaustein MP, Hamlyn JM: Sodium transport inhibition, cell calcium and hypertension: the natriuretic hormone/Na^+-Ca^{++} exchange/hypertension hypothesis. Am J Med 77(4A):45, 1984

420. Beretta-Piccoli C, Weidmann P: Exaggerated pressor responsiveness to norepinephrine in non-azotemic diabetes mellitus. Am J Med 71:829, 1981

421. Drury PL, Smith GM, Ferriss JB: Increased vasopressor responsiveness to angiotensin II in type I (insulin-dependent) diabetic patients. Diabetologia 27:174, 1984

422. Christensen CK, Krusell LR, Mogensen CE: Increased blood pressure in diabe-

tes: essential hypertension or diabetic nephropathy? Scand J Clin Lab Invest 47:363, 1987

423. Kolterman OG, Insel J, Saekow M, Olefsky JM: Mechanisms of insulin resistance in human obesity: evidence for receptor and postreceptor defects. J Clin Invest 65:1272, 1980

424. DeFronzo RA: The effect of insulin on renal sodium metabolism: a review with clinical implications. Diabetologia 21:165, 1981

425. Rowe JW, Young JB, Minaker KL et al: Effect of insulin and glucose infusions on sympathetic nervous system activity in normal man. Diabetes 30:219, 1981

426. Moore RD: Effects of insulin upon ion transport. Biochim Biophys Acta 737:1, 1983

427. Stout RW, Bierman EL, Ross R: Effects of insulin on the proliferation of cultured primate arterial smooth muscle cells. Circ Res 36:319, 1975

428. Meehan WP, Darwin CH, Maalauf NB et al: Insulin and hypertension: are they related? Steroids 58:621, 1993

429. Creager MA, Liang C-S, Coffman JD: Beta adrenergic-mediated vasodilator response to insulin in the human forearm. J Pharmacol Exp Ther 235:709, 1985

430. Anderson EA, Hoffman RP, Balon TW et al: Hyperinsulinemia produces both sympathetic neural activation and vasodilation in normal humans. J Clin Invest 87:2246, 1991

431. Hall JE, Brands MW, Kivlighn SD et al: Chronic hyperinsulinemia and blood pressure. Interaction with catecholamines? Hypertension 15:519, 1990

432. Brands MW, Hildebrandt DA, Mizelle HL, Hall JE: Sustained hyperinsulinemia increases arterial pressure in conscious rats. Am J Physiol 260:R764, 1991

433. Haffner SM: Insulin and blood pressure: fact or fantasy? J Clin Endocrinol Metab 76:541, 1993

434. Rizza RA, Cryer PE, Haymond MW, Gerich JE: Adrenergic mechanisms of catecholamine action on glucose homeostasis in man. Metabolism 29(suppl 1):1155, 1980

435. Folkow B: Sympathetic nervous control of blood pressure: role in primary hypertension. Am J Hypertens 2:103S, 1989

436. Jéquier E: Energy expenditure in obesity. Clin Endocrinol Metab 13:563, 1984

437. Saad MF, Alger SA, Zurlo F et al: Ethnic differences in sympathetic nervous system-mediated energy expenditure. Am J Physiol 261:E789, 1991

438. Bogardus C, Lillioja S, Mott D et al: Evidence for reduced thermic effect of insulin and glucose infusions in Pima Indians. J Clin Invest 75:1264, 1985

439. Fredrickson M: Racial differences in cardiovascular reactivity to mental stress in essential hypertension. J Hypertens 4:325, 1986

440. Blaustein MP, Hamlyn JM: Role of a natriuretic factor in essential hypertension: an hypothesis. Ann Intern Med 98:785, 1983

441. Mott DM, Clark RL, Andrews WJ, Foley JE: Insulin-resistant Na$^+$ pump activity in adipocytes from obese humans. Am J Physiol 249:E160, 1985

442. DeLuise M, Blackburn GL, Flier JS: Reduced activity of the red-cell sodium-potassium pump in human obesity. N Engl J Med 303:1017, 1980

443. Ferrannini E, Taddei S, Santoro D et al: Independent stimulation of glucose metabolism and Na/K exchange by insulin in the human forearm. Am J Physiol 255:E953, 1988

444. Doria A, Fioretto P, Avogaro A et al: Insulin resistance is associated with high sodium-lithium countertransport in essential hypertension. Am J Physiol 261:E684, 1991

445. Resnick LM, Gupta RK, Gruenspan H et al: Hypertension and peripheral insulin resistance: possible mediating role of intracellular free magnesium. Am J Hypertens 3:373, 1990

446. Aviv A, Gardner J: Racial differences in ion regulation and their possible links to hypertension in Blacks. Hypertension 14:584, 1989

447. Ferrannini E, DeFronzo RA: The association of hypertension, diabetes, and obesity: a review. J Nephrol 1:3, 1989

448. Juhlin-Dannfelt A, Frisk-Holmberg M, Karlsson J, Tesch P: Central and peripheral circulation in relation to muscle-fiber composition in normo- and hypertensive man. Clin Sci 56:335, 1979

449. Lillioja S, Young AA, Culter CL et al: Skeletal muscle capillary density and fiber type are possible determinants of in vivo insulin resistance in man. J Clin Invest 80:415, 1987

450. Annest JL, Sing CF, Biron P, Mongeau J-G: Familial aggregation of blood pressure and weight in adoptive families: II. Estimation of the relative contributions of genetic and common environmental factors to blood pressure correlations between family members. Am J Epidemiol 110:492, 1979

451. Staessen J, Bulpitt CJ, Fagard R et al: Familial aggregation of blood pressure, anthropometric characteristics and urinary excretion of sodium and potassium—a population study in two Belgian towns. J Chronic Dis 38:397, 1985

452. Ferrari P, Weidmann P, Shaw S et al: Altered insulin sensitivity, hyperinsulinemia, and dyslipidemia in individuals with a hypertensive parent. Am J Med 91:589, 1991

453. Berntorp K, Lindgärde F: Familial aggregation of type 2 diabetes mellitus as an etiological factor in hypertension. Diabetes Res Clin Pract 1:307, 1986

454. Haffner SM, Stern MP, Hazuda HP et al: Parental history of diabetes is associated with increased cardiovascular risk factors. Arteriosclerosis 9:928, 1989

455. Ying L-H, Zee RYL, Griffiths LR, Morris BJ: Association of a RFLP for the insulin receptor gene, but not insulin, with essential hypertension. Biochem Biophys Res Comm 181:486, 1991

456. Sawicki PT, Kaiser S, Heinemann L et al: Prevalence of renal artery stenosis in diabetes mellitus—an autopsy study. J Intern Med 229:489, 1991

457. Ritchie CM, McIlrath E, Hadden DR et al: Renal artery stenosis in hypertensive

458. Kincaid-Smith P, Whitworth JA: Hematuria and diabetic nephropathy. p. 81. In Mogensen CE (ed): The Kidney and Hypertension in Diabetes Mellitus. Martinus Nijhof, Boston, 1988

459. Assmann G, Schulte H: The prospective cardiovascular Münster (PROCAM) study: prevalence of hyperlipidemia in persons with hypertension and/or diabetes mellitus and the relationship to coronary heart disease. Am Heart J 116:1713, 1988

460. Hasslacher C, Stech W, Wahl P, Ritz E: Blood pressure and metabolic control as risk factors for nephropathy in type 1 (insulin-dependent) diabetes. Diabetologia 28:6, 1985

461. Baba T, Murabayashi S, Tomiyama T, Takebe K: Uncontrolled hypertension is associated with rapid progression of nephropathy in type 2 diabetic patients with proteinuria and preserved renal function. Tohoku J Exp Med 161:311, 1990

462. Selby JV, FitzSimmons SC, Newman JM et al: The natural history and epidemiology of diabetic nephropathy: implications for prevention and control. JAMA 263:1954, 1990

463. Mauer SM, Steffes MW, Ellis EN et al: Structural-functional relationships in diabetic nephropathy. J Clin Invest 74:1143, 1984

464. Mogensen CE: Progression of nephropathy in long-term diabetics with proteinuria and effect of initial antihypertensive treatment. Scan J Clin Lab Invest 36:383, 1976

465. Berglund J, Lins L-E, Lins P-E: Metabolic and blood pressure monitoring in diabetic renal failure. Acta Med Scand 218:401, 1985

466. Walker WG: Hypertension-related renal injury: a major contributor to end-stage renal disease. Am J Kidney Dis 22:164, 1993

467. Knowler WC, Bennett PH, Ballintine EJ: Increased incidence of retinopathy in diabetics with elevated blood pressure. N Engl J Med 302:645, 1980

diabetic patients. Diabet Med 5:265, 1988

468. Ishihara M, Yukimura Y, Aizawa T et al: High blood pressure as risk factor in diabetic retinopathy development in NIDDM patients. Diabetes Care 10:20, 1987

469. Klein R, Klein BE, Moss SE et al: Is blood pressure a predictor of the incidence or progression of diabetic retinopathy? Arch Intern Med 149:2427, 1989

470. Hypertension Detection and Follow-up Program Cooperative Group. Five-year findings of the Hypertension Detection and Follow-up Program, reduction in mortality of persons with high blood pressure, including mild hypertension. JAMA 242:2562, 1979

471. Systolic Hypertension in the Elderly Program Cooperative Research Group: Implications of the Systolic Hypertension in the Elderly Program. Hypertension 21:335, 1993

472. Mogensen CE: Long-term antihypertensive treatment inhibiting progression of diabetic nephropathy. Br Med J 285:685, 1982

473. Parving H-H: Impact of blood pressure and antihypertensive treatment on incipient and overt nephropathy, retinopathy, and endothelial permeability in diabetes mellitus. Diabetes Care 14:260, 1991

474. Kasiske BL, Kalil RSN, Ma JZ et al: Effect of antihypertensive therapy on the kidney in patients with diabetes: a meta-regression analysis. Ann Intern Med 118:129, 1993

475. The National High Blood Pressure Education Program Working Group: National High Blood Pressure Education Program Working Group report on hypertension in diabetes. Hypertension 23:145, 1994

476. Tuck ML, Sowers JR, Dornfeld L et al: The effect of weight reduction on blood pressure, plasma renin activity, and plasma aldosterone levels in obese patients. N Engl J Med 304:930, 1981

477. Dodson PM, Beevers M, Hallworth R et al: Sodium restriction and blood pressure in hypertensive type II diabetics: randomised blind controlled and crossover studies of moderate sodium restriction and sodium supplementation. BMJ 298:227, 1989

478. Blake GA, Levin SR, Koyal SN: Exercise-induced hypertension in normotensive patients with NIDDM. Diabetes Care 13:799, 1990

479. Uusitupa M: Hypertension in diabetic patients—use of exercise in treatment. Ann Med 23:335, 1991

480. Trost BN: Hypertension in the diabetic patient. Selection and optimum use of antihypertensive drugs. Drugs 38:621, 1989

481. Alkharouf J, Nalinikumari K, Corry D, Tuck M: Long-term effects of the angiotensin converting enzyme inhibitor captopril on metabolic control in non-insulin-dependent diabetes mellitus. Am J Hypertens 6:337, 1993

482. Torlone E, Britta M, Rambotti AM et al: Improved insulin action and glycemic control after long-term angiotensin-converting enzyme inhibition in subjects with arterial hypertension and type II diabetes. Diabetes Care 16:1347, 1993

483. Gans RO, Stehouwer CD, Bilo HJ et al: Effect of cilazapril on glucose tolerance and lipid profile in hypertensive patients with non-insulin-dependent diabetes mellitus. Neth J Med 43:163, 1993

484. Jandrain B, Herbaut C, Depoorter JC, Voorde KV: Long-term (1 year) acceptability of perindopril in type II diabetic patients with hypertension. Am J Med 92(4B):91S, 1992

485. Bakris GL: Angiotensin-converting enzyme inhibitors and progression of diabetic nephropathy. Ann Intern Med 118:643, 1993

486. Remuzzi A, Ruggenenti P, Mosconi L et al: Effect of low-dose enalapril on glomerular size—selectivity in human diabetic nephropathy. J Nephrol 6:36, 1993

487. Parving H-H, Hommel E, Smidt UM: Protection of kidney function and decrease in albuminuria by captopril in insulin-dependent diabetics with nephropathy. BMJ 297:1086, 1988

488. Hermans MP, Brichard SM, Colin I et al: Long-term reduction of microalbuminuria after 3 years of angiotensin-converting enzyme inhibition by

perindopril in hypertensive insulin-treated diabetic patients. Am J Med 92(4 B): 102S, 1992

489. Lewis EJ, Hunsicker LG, Bain RP, Rohde RD: The effect of angiotensin-converting-enzyme inhibition on diabetic nephropathy. The Collaborative Study Group. N Engl J Med 329:1456, 1993

490. Dahloef B, Pennert K, Hansson L: Reversal of left ventricular hypertrophy in hypertensive patients. A metanalysis of 109 treatment studies. Am J Hypertens 5:95, 1992

491. Charpiot P, Rolland PH, Friggi A et al: ACE inhibition with perindopril and atherogenesis-induced structural and functional changes in minipig arteries. Aterioscler Thromb 13:1125, 1993

492. Schuh JR, Blehm DJ, Frierdich GE et al: Differential effects of renin-angiotensin system blockade on atherogenesis in cholesterol-fed rabbits. J Clin Invest 91:1453, 1993

493. Bridoux F, Hazzan M, Pallot JL et al: Acute renal failure after the use of angiotensin-converting-enzyme inhibitors in patients without renal artery stenosis. Nephrol Dial Transplant 7:100, 1992

494. Parving H-H, Rossing P: Calcium antagonists and the diabetic hypertensive patient. Am J Kidney Dis 21(suppl 3):47, 1993

495. Bakris GL, Barnhill BW, Sadler R: Treatment of arterial hypertension in diabetic humans: importance of therapeutic selection. Kidney Int 41:912, 1992

496. Slataper R, Vicknair N, Sadler R, Bakris GL: Comparative effects of different antihypertensive treatments on progression of diabetic renal disease. Arch Intern Med 153:973, 1993

497. Bretzel RG, Bollen CC, Maeser E, Federlin KF: Nephroprotective effects of nitrendipine in hypertensive type I and type II diabetic patients. Am J Kidney Dis 21(Suppl 3):53, 1993

498. Valentino VA, Wilson MD, Weart W, Bakris GL: A perspective on converting enzyme inhibitors and calcium channel antagonists in diabetic renal disease. Arch Intern Med 151:2367, 1991

499. Demarie BK, Bakris GL: Effects of different calcium antagonists on proteinuria associated with diabetes mellitus. Ann Intern Med 113:987, 1990

500. Ferder L, Daccordi H, Martello M et al: Angiotensin converting enzyme inhibitors versus calcium antagonists in the treatment of diabetic hypertensive patients. Hypertension 19 (suppl 2):II237, 1992

501. Melbourne Diabetic Nephropathy Study Group: Comparison between perindopril and nifedipine in hypertensive and normotensive diabetic patients with microalbuminuria. BMJ 302:210, 1991

502. Chan JCN, Cockram CS, Nicholls MG et al: Comparison of enalapril and nifedipine in treating non-insulin dependent diabetes associated with hypertension: one year analysis. BMJ 305:981, 1992

503. Bielen EC, Fagard RH, Lijnen PJ et al: Comparison of the effects of isradipine and lisinopril on left ventricular structure and function in essential hypertension. Am J Cardiol 69:1200, 1992

504. Nayler WG, Panagiotopoulos S: The antiatherosclerotic effect of the calcium antagonists and their implications in hypertension. Am Heart J 125:626, 1993

505. Hedner T, Samuelsson O, Lindholm L: Effects of antihypertensive therapy on glucose tolerance: focus on calcium antagonists. J Intern Med (suppl)735:101, 1991

506. Trost BN, Riesen WF, Mordasini RC, Weidmann P: Antihypertensive long-term monotherapy with the calcium antagonist nitrendipine does not alter serum lipids in type II diabetic patients. Nutr Metab Cardiovasc Dis 1:77, 1991

507. Feher MD: Doxazosin therapy in the treatment of diabetic hypertension. Am Heart J 121:1294, 1991

508. Pollare T, Lithell H, Selinus I, Berne C: Application of prazosin is associated with an increase of insulin sensitivity in obese patients with hypertension. Diabetologia 31:415, 1988

509. Huupponen R, Lehtonen A, Vähätalo M: Effect of doxazosin on insulin sensitivity in hypertensive non-insulin dependent

diabetic patients. Eur J Clin Pharmacol 43:365, 1992

510. Shieh SM, Sheu WH, Shen DC et al: Glucose, insulin, and lipid metabolism in doxazosin-treated patients with hypertension. Am J Hypertension 5:827, 1992

511. Giorda C, Appendino M: Effects of doxazosin, a selective α_1-inhibitor, on plasma insulin and blood glucose response to a glucose tolerance test in essential hypertension. Metabolism 42:1440, 1993

512. Swindell AC, Krupp MN, Twomey TM et al: Effects of doxazosin on atherosclerosis in cholesterol-fed rabbits. Atherosclerosis 99:195, 1993

513. Agabiti-Rosei E, Muiesan ML, Rizzoni D et al: Reduction of left ventricular hypertrophy after longterm antihypertensive treatment with doxazosin. J Hum Hypertens 6:9, 1992

514. Bartels AC, deVries PM, Oe LP et al: Doxazosin in the treatment of patients with mild or moderate hypertension and mild or moderate renal insufficiency. Am Heart J 116:1772, 1988

515. Vardan S, Mehrotra KG, Mookherjee S et al: Efficacy and reduced metabolic side effects of a 15 mg chlorthalidone formulation in the treatment of mild hypertension. A multicenter study. JAMA 258:484, 1987

516. Amery A, Berthaux P, Bulpitt C et al: Glucose intolerance during diuretic therapy. Lancet 1:681, 1978

517. Ames RP: Metabolic disturbances increasing the risk of coronary heart disease during diuretic-based antihypertensive therapy; lipid alterations and glucose intolerance. Am Heart J 106:1207, 1983

518. Warram JH, Laffel LM, Valsania P et al: Excess mortality associated with diuretic therapy in diabetes mellitus. Arch Intern Med 151:1350, 1991

519. Kendall M, Tse WY: Is there a role for beta-blockers in hypertensive diabetic patients? Diabet Med 11:137, 1994

520. Pollare T, Lithell H, Selinus I, Berne C: Sensitivity to insulin during treatment with atenolol and metoprolol: a randomised double blind study of effects on carbohydrate and lipoprotein metabolism in hypertensive patients. BMJ 298:1152, 1989

521. Ostman J: Beta-adrenergic blockade and diabetes mellitus. A review. Acta Med Scand (Suppl)672:69, 1983

522. Deacon SP, Karunanayake A, Barnett D: Acebutolol, atenolol, and propranolol and metabolic responses to acute hypoglycaemia in diabetics. Br Med J 2:1255, 1977

523. Fogari R, Zoppi A, Malamani DG et al: Ambulatory blood pressure monitoring in normotensive and hypertensive type 2 diabetics. Prevalence of impaired diurnal blood pressure patterns. Am J Hypertens 6:1, 1993

524. SHEP Cooperative Research Group: Prevention of stroke by antihypertensive drug treatment in older persons with isolated systolic hypertension: final results of the Systolic Hypertension in the Elderly Program (SHEP). JAMA 265:3255, 1991

525. Ewing DJ, Clarke BF: Diabetic autonomic neuropathy: a clinical viewpoint. p. 66. In Dyck PJ, Thomas PK, Asbury AK et al (eds): Diabetic Neuropathy WB Saunders, Philadelphia, 1987

526. Ewing DJ, Campbell IW, Clarke BF: The natural history of diabetic autonomic neuropathy. Q J Med 49:95, 1980

527. Rathmann W, Ziegler D, Jahnke M et al: Mortality in diabetic patients with cardiovascular autonomic neuropathy. Diab Med 10:820, 1993

528. Ewing DJ, Borsey DQ, Travis P et al: Abnormalities of ambulatory 24 hour heart rate in diabetes mellitus. Diabetes 32:101, 1983

529. Roy TM, Peterson HR, Snider HL et al: Autonomic influence on cardiovascular performance in diabetic subjects. Am J Med 87:382, 1989

530. Thomas JE, Fealey RD, Schirger A: Orthostatic Hypotension p. 201. In Dyck PJ, Thomas PK, Asbury AK et al (eds): Diabetic Neuropathy WB Saunders, Philadelphia, 1987

531. Bellavere F, Ferri M, Guarini L et al: Prolonged QT period in diabetic auto-

nomic neuropathy: a possible role in sudden cardiac death? Br Heart J 59:379, 1988

532. Gonin JM, Kadrofske MM, Schmaltz S et al: Corrected Q-T interval prolongation as diagnostic tool for assessment of cardiac autonomic neuropathy in diabetes mellitus. Diabetes Care 13:68, 1990

533. Ewing DJ, Neilson JMM: QT interval length and diabetic autonomic neuropathy. Diabet Med 7:23, 1990

534. Ong JJC, Sarma JSM, Venkataraman K et al: Circadian rhythmicity of heart rate and QTc interval in diabetic autonomic neuropathy: implications for the mechanism of sudden death. Am Heart J 125:744, 1993

7

End-Stage Renal Disease

Richard A. Preston
Simon Chakko
Barry J. Materson

Cardiovascular complications comprise the major cause of death in the end-stage renal disease (ESRD) population. The effects of chronic renal failure upon the heart are diverse and involve numerous anatomic and functional aspects of the cardiovascular system. We have divided the discussion of cardiac complications of ESRD into the following categories: hypertension, pericarditis, left ventricular dysfunction and congestive heart failure, cardiac arrhythmias, and cardiovascular drug therapy in ESRD.

HYPERTENSION

The association of chronic renal disease and elevated arterial blood pressure has been recognized for over 150 years.[1] Specifically, chronic renal disease and elevation of systemic arterial blood pressure may exist simultaneously in one of two clinically distinct situations. First, the kidney is well known to be a major target organ for the chronic effects of sustained arterial hypertension. Thus, hypertension (in most cases essential hypertension) is an important cause of chronic renal disease. Second, primary disease of the renal parenchyma is a well-established cause of secondary hypertension. In fact, renal parenchymal hypertension is the most common cause of secondary hypertension, accounting for 2.5 to 5.0 percent of all cases.[2] It is more common than renovascular hypertension (renal artery stenosis), pheochromocytoma, or primary hyperaldosteronism. Hypertension is known to occur as a complication of a wide variety of glomerular and interstitial renal diseases and may accelerate the decline in renal function if inadequately controlled.[1-4] Therefore, hypertension is both a cause and a consequence of renal disease, and in some cases it may be difficult to distinguish clinically between these two situations.

The prevalence of hypertension in patients with renal disease depends upon the etiology and the severity of the particular renal disease. Hypertension is often associated with diseases of the small renal vessels such as renal vasculitis, systemic lupus erythematosus, and progressive systemic sclerosis. Hypertension is also often found in several common glomerular diseases such as focal segmental sclerosis, postinfectious glomerulonephritis, and crescentic (rapidly progressive) glomerulonephritis. It is less

175

often found with other glomerular diseases such as minimal change and membranous nephropathy. Interstitial diseases that are frequently associated with hypertension include adult polycystic disease and analgesic abuse nephropathy. Other causes of chronic interstitial kidney disease are less frequently associated with hypertension.[1,2,5]

In many cases, determination of routine blood urea nitrogen and serum creatinine values in addition to careful urinalysis with proper examination of the urinary sediment will exclude the existence of significant underlying renal disease. A few words of caution are in order, however. First, renal function is known to decline progressively with aging, approximately 10 to 15 ml/min/decade after the age of 40 years. In addition, lean body mass (one of the determinants of serum creatinine level) decreases with age. Fat may increase with age, thus maintaining body weight constant. Therefore, even seemingly mild elevations in serum creatinine may reflect significant renal dysfunction in an elderly patient. Second, many interstitial diseases of the kidney may present initially with only mild impairment in urinary concentrating ability or other defects of tubular function in advance of any decline of glomerular filtration rate. Hence, close follow-up and serial screening should be undertaken in any patient suspected of having underlying renal disease.

The precise pathophysiologic mechanisms that produce hypertension in patients with kidney disease remain unclear. Renal parenchymal hypertension most probably represents the combined interactions of multiple mechanisms including impaired sodium handling leading to volume expansion, perturbations of the renin-angiotensin system, altered function of the sympathetic nervous system, and possibly circulating vasoactive substances. It is well known that the dis-

eased kidney has an impaired natriuretic response to salt loading and that many patients will respond favorably to measures that produce salt depletion, but it is probably overly simplistic to ascribe the hypertension associated with many kidney diseases to sodium excess alone.[1,2,5–7] The relationship of volume expansion to pressure elevation is complex and may involve alterations in autonomic baroreflex function and possibly local vascular factors including cytosolic calcium concentration. Several practical considerations may serve as a workable conceptual framework to help guide therapy.

Sodium retention with associated volume expansion plays a central role in the generation of hypertension, and the therapeutic modalities which will reduce total body sodium are frequently very effective in lowering blood pressure. Hence, salt restriction and diuretics will often be effective antihypertensive therapy in patients with renal disease.[4,5,8] It should also be noted that both the prevalence and the severity of hypertension increase as the glomerular filtration rate falls. Thus, it is important to continue close follow-up and frequent reassessment of therapy in patients with renal impairment of any degree.

Despite the importance of sodium homeostasis in the genesis of renal parenchymal hypertension, the most consistently observed hemodynamic alteration is an elevation of peripheral vascular resistance. The mechanism(s) of this increase is not completely explained, but antihypertensive agents that possess vasodilator properties are very effective in controlling blood pressure. As renal insufficiency progresses toward end-stage kidney disease, thiazide diuretics become less effective.

Endogenous renal prostaglandins may play a role in maintaining glomerular filtration rate in the chronically diseased kidney. Agents that inhibit the production of renal prostaglandins, such as the nonsteroidal anti-inflammatory drugs, should be used cautiously, if at all, in patients with chronic renal disease. In addition to potentially deleterious effects on intrarenal hemodynamics and impairment of glomerular filtration rate, the nonsteroidal anti-inflammatory agents may interfere with antihypertensive therapy.

Elevated systemic arterial blood pressure represents a poor prognostic indicator in a number of renal disorders. There is extensive evidence that hypertension accelerates the deterioration of renal function[1,2,4]; this is the major reason for early identification and vigorous treatment of these patients. Regardless of the mechanism(s) involved, treatment of hypertension has been shown to retard the rate of progression of renal impairment in several disease states.

Salt and Water Balance

Restriction of dietary sodium intake will lead to a reduction of blood pressure in a large number of patients with renal parenchymal hypertension.[2,4,8] Sodium restriction should be initiated under close observation since the ability of the failing kidney to adjust to rapid changes in sodium balance is impaired. Thus, caution should be exercised in order to avoid depletion of extracellular fluid volume, prerenal azotemia, and aggravation of existing renal dysfunction. In addition, such care must be used in patients with tubulointerstitial disorders and associated salt wasting. A reasonable guideline to therapy would include:

1. Begin with restriction of dietary sodium to 1 to 2 g/day in the patient without demonstrable peripheral edema. In patients who are nephrotic and actively conserving sodium, more severe (250 to 500 mg NaCl/24 h) sodium restriction will be required.

2. The diseased kidney may adapt poorly to rapid changes in salt intake. It is therefore important to follow a patient carefully for signs of volume depletion (orthostatic blood pressure changes or significant fall in body weight) or worsening azotemia.

3. Caution should be used in patients with suspected salt-wasting syndromes; sodium balance should be monitored closely to prevent hemodynamic compromise or further deterioration of renal function.

4. Many salt substitutes contain potassium and should be avoided in patients with renal impairment.

5. In the patient with end-stage renal failure who is receiving maintenance hemodialysis therapy, close attention should be given to the attainment of "dry weight" through adequate ultrafiltration. In fact, a majority of patients can be rendered normotensive or easily manageable by attainment of ideal weight. The "dry weight" is defined as that weight below which further removal by ultrafiltration will result in hypotension. Hypertension can be controlled in most dialysis patients by rigorous attention to dietary salt, daily weight gain, and adequate ultrafiltration during dialysis therapy.

6. The minority of dialysis patients will fall into a group described as "volume unresponsive."[2,7] This group is characterized by hypertension refractory to sodium restriction and unresponsive to fluid ultrafiltration. In fact, severe hypertension may be seen in the period immediately following dialysis. This group will often require potent antihypertensive agents such as minoxidil or angiotensin converting enzyme inhibitors. Only rarely is bilateral nephrectomy required for the control of blood pressure, except in

the case of uncontrolled hypertension in the pretransplant patient.

Diuretic Therapy

If a trial of sodium restriction does not yield an adequate response of blood pressure, then the initiation of antihypertensive therapy with a diuretic is appropriate.[2,4,5,8]

Thiazide Diuretics

The thiazide diuretics act by inhibiting sodium and chloride reabsorption in the cortical diluting segment of the distal tubule. Early in therapy, the antihypertensive response is dependent upon natriuresis and subsequent reduction in extracellular fluid volume. Later the hypotensive effect may involve vasodilatory mechanisms. The effectiveness of the thiazides is markedly reduced at levels of glomerular filtration rate (GFR) below 30 ml/min, probably as a result of a diminished salt load reaching the distal nephron, as well as an impaired delivery of the drug to its site of action. Therefore, the use of thiazide diuretics is not recommended at low levels of renal function.

The thiazides are known to cause hypokalemia, hyperuricemia (or aggravation of pre-existing hyperuricemia, which is often present in patients with renal insufficiency), impaired glucose tolerance, and renal magnesium wasting.

Loop Diuretics

The loop-acting diuretics become the agents of choice for the management of extracellular fluid volume and hypertension when the GFR falls below 30 ml/min.[2,4,5,8] Unlike the thiazides, the loop agents are effective at GFRs well below 25 ml/min, although very high doses may be required as renal failure progresses. The loop diuretics act by inhibiting active chloride and passive sodium reab-sorption at the medullary thick ascending limb of the loop of Henle, which reabsorbs approximately 25 to 40 percent of the filtered sodium load. Since the natriuretic response depends upon a threshold concentration of drug being delivered to its site of action, a reasonable approach is to increase the dosage of diuretic carefully under close observation until the dosage at which the desired response occurs is established.

Hypokalemia and glucose intolerance accompany therapy with the loop diuretics. The risk of ototoxicity is increased by the presence of renal insufficiency and by the concomitant administration of aminoglycoside antimicrobials. In addition, because of their potency, care must be exercised to avoid intravascular volume depletion and complicating prerenal azotemia.

Nondiuretic Antihypertensive Agents

A few general guidelines should be kept in mind when preparing to add a second agent.

1. The effectiveness of second-line agents may be attenuated if diuretic therapy and attention to salt balance is inadequate.
2. A minority of patients may respond to monotherapy with nondiuretic antihypertensive agents if sodium and water retention are not problems.
3. The presence of concomitant illness must be considered in tailoring therapy to the individual patient.

β-Adrenergic Receptor Blockers

β-Blockers are important agents that have been used successfully to control hypertension in patients with renal impairment.[1,2,4,5,8] A large number of these drugs are marketed and possess a variety of ancillary properties including relative β_1 selectivity (atenolol and metoprolol), intrinsic sympathomimetic activity (pindolol, acebutolol), and combination β-blocking and vasodilator compound (labetalol). In general, β-blockers produce negative chronotropic and inotropic effects and many also inhibit renin release, thus interfering with the renin-angiotensin system. β-Blockers are associated with an initial increase in peripheral vascular resistance that tends to return toward normal with chronic therapy. The effects of β-blockers on renal function are variable and depend upon the individual drug. For example, propranolol has been observed to decrease both renal plasma flow and GFR, while these functions are preserved with nadolol and pindolol.

An important consideration in choosing a β-blocker is its relative lipid solubility. Lipid-insoluble agents such as atenolol, nadolol, and acebutolol are excreted mainly by the kidney, and dosage adjustment is required in the presence of renal insufficiency. It is also important to be aware that the relative β_1 selectivity seen with some agents tends to become less evident at higher doses. Accordingly, all agents should be used with extreme caution, if at all, in patients with congestive heart failure or disease of the cardiac conduction system, diabetes mellitus, bronchospastic airway disease, or peripheral vascular disease. In contrast, these agents are preferred in patients with angina pectoris or in patients with recent myocardial infarction.

Centrally Acting Adrenergic Agonists

Agents including methyldopa, clonidine, guanabenz, and guanfacine act by inhibiting central nervous system adrenergic outflow.[4,5,8] Such drugs, for the most part, do not adversely affect renal blood flow or glomerular filtration rate, but they have adverse effects on the central nervous system that may increase those caused by uremia. Sedation, confusion, and depression may be particularly troublesome, especially in the elderly patient.

When used in high doses and suddenly withdrawn, these drugs may be associated with a discontinuation syndrome characterized by marked "rebound" elevation of blood pressure and evidence of sympathetic nervous system hyperreactivity such as diaphoresis and tachycardia.

Calcium Antagonists

The calcium antagonists, or calcium entry blockers, are effective antihypertensive agents that are generally safe and well tolerated in the setting of chronic renal disease.[4,5,8] Their mechanism involves interference with voltage-dependent calcium channels in vascular smooth muscle and cardiac muscle cells, thereby attenuating the excitation-contraction process. The calcium entry blockers lower peripheral vascular resistance and reduce myocardial contractility. The calcium blockers are not associated with hyperkalemia, magnesium wasting, or hyperuricemia. Also, they do not have significant adverse effects on glucose tolerance or cholesterol metabolism. These are important considerations in assessing the overall cardiovascular risk profile of a patient.

Patients with renal disease may frequently have associated disease states that may make the choice of an antihypertensive agent somewhat difficult. Such disorders as diabetes mellitus, asthma, chronic obstructive pulmonary disease, and peripheral vascular disease are not adversely affected by the calcium channel blockers. In addition, these agents may be preferred in patients with ischemic heart disease and left ventricular hypertrophy. The potential of these agents to delay or attenuate the progression of chronic renal insufficiency and their ability to reverse acute renal ischemia in a number of experimental settings are currently topics of intense interest.

Angiotensin-Converting Enzyme Inhibitors

Angiotensin-converting enzyme (ACE) inhibitors are generally well tolerated agents that have been used successfully in patients with chronic renal disease.[4,5,8] These agents lower blood pressure by causing a decrease in peripheral vascular resistance, probably through a variety of mechanisms. They are known to reduce concentrations of the vasoconstrictor angiotensin II and are thereby especially effective in treating so-called high-renin states such as malignant hypertension and scleroderma renal crisis. In addition, these compounds may exert their antihypertensive effects by enhancing the activities of certain endogenous vasodilator substances such as bradykinin and the vasodilator prostaglandins. The ACE inhibitors may also produce intrarenal vasodilatation by effecting preferential dilatation of the efferent arteriole. In a number of animal models this decrease in efferent arteriolar resistance has resulted in reduction of intraglomerular hypertension and a slowing of the progression of glomerulosclerosis and renal insufficiency.

Most ACE inhibitors are excreted by the kidney, and reduction of dosage is necessary in patients with impaired renal function. Moreover, problems including dysgeusia, leukopenia, and rash are dose related and occur more frequently in patients with renal dysfunction. Hyperkalemia may be encountered in patients with renal insufficiency, especially diabetic patients with hyporeninemic hypoaldosteronism. ACE inhibitors are also known to produce reversible deterioration in GFR in patients with bilateral renal artery stenosis or arterial stenosis in a solitary functioning kidney (for example, a renal allograft). Worsening azotemia may also be seen occasionally in patients with renal disease, possibly as a result of diminished glomerular filtration pressure. Thus, reduction of initial dosage and cautious upward titration should be accompanied by close monitoring of serum electrolytes and creatinine.

The ACE inhibitors lack adverse effects upon lipid or carbohydrate metabolism and are thus suitable agents for patients with diabetes mellitus or hyperlipidemia. In addition, they are of particular value in patients with concomitant bronchospasm, peripheral vascular disease, or congestive heart failure.

α-Adrenergic Blocking Agents

The primary vasodilatory and hypotensive effects of this class of drugs are due to blockade of α_1-adrenoreceptors at postjunctional sites in the precapillary arterioles or peripheral blood vessels.[4,5,8] The α-blockers lower blood pressure without a marked reflex increase in heart rate. The α-blockers generally do not produce a decline in renal blood flow or GFR, but they can be associated with sodium retention. This may produce a blunting of the overall hypertensive effect during chronic therapy. Metabolism is largely hepatic so that little or no adjustment in chronic renal failure is required. An increased sensitivity to the effects of prazosin in patients with renal impairment has been reported, however, so that therapy might better be initiated at a smaller dosage (for example, 3 to 8 mg/day of prazosin).

Current enthusiasm for this group of drugs is based upon their ability to effect favorable changes in blood lipids. α-Blockers lower low-density lipoprotein (LDL) cholesterol by a direct effect upon hepatic metabolism, and thus their use may be particularly appropriate in patients with hypercholesterolemia.

PERICARDITIS

Pericarditis is a common and often severe complication of ESRD. Its presentation may be rapid and may produce profound hemodynamic consequences. Prior to the availability of renal replacement therapy, the appearance of a pericardial friction rub in the patient with ESRD was a harbinger of death within the ensuing 2 weeks. Many authorities prefer to classify pericarditis associated with ESRD into two major categories: early and late.[7,9–11] Early (or uremic) pericarditis occurs in the ESRD patient prior to the initiation of chronic dialysis therapy and is probably secondary to the biochemical perturbations of uremia per se. This form of pericarditis generally responds rapidly to the initiation of dialysis in the large majority of patients. Late (or dialysis-associated) pericarditis occurs in patients who are already receiving renal replacement therapy. In general, this form of pericarditis tends to be more severe, has a higher rate of complications, and responds less readily to dialysis. The pathogenesis of dialysis-associated pericarditis is not clearly understood and, in many cases, may be multifactorial.

Incidence of Uremic Pericarditis

The incidence of uremic (early) pericarditis has fallen in recent years, most likely due to the wider availability and earlier initiation of renal replacement therapy. In 1968, a 41 percent incidence of uremic pericarditis was reported in patients before beginning dialysis.[12] More recent reports indicate a much lower incidence, approximately 15 percent.[13–17] Pericarditis has been found to occur in approximately 10 to 20 percent of patients receiving regular dialysis therapy.[13,14]

Pathology

The basic pathologic process of pericarditis associated with ESRD is an aseptic inflammatory reaction with fibrin formation. Both parietal and visceral pericardia are covered with a fibrinous exudate. Fibrinous bands are usually present and form adhesions and areas of loculation between the two layers. The effusion is usually serosanguinous, but is uniformly hemorrhagic in cases of tamponade. The white blood cell count is variable but usually in the 500 to 700/mm^3 range with a variable proportion of polymorphonuclear and mononuclear leukocytes.

Pathogenesis

Pericarditis in ESRD patients who have not yet begun dialysis is most likely related to the biochemical milieu of untreated uremia. This is evidenced by the rapid response to the initiation of dialysis and the clinical correlation with biochemical control of uremia in most patients.[7,12,13,17] Dialysis-related pericarditis, on the other hand, is less well understood. It is not clear why a substantial percentage of patients receiving regular renal replacement should develop pericarditis. A number of potential pathogenic factors have been proposed including inadequate dialysis therapy, hypercatabolic states, poorly controlled hyperparathyroidism, heparin received during dialysis, and an abnormal immunologic response. Underdialysis has been noted in a significant percent of patients developing dialysis-associated pericarditis, often as a result of vascular access failure or missing dialysis.[12,18] In addition, pericarditis has been observed to occur during periods of hypercatabolism such as following major surgery or during sepsis.

A possible role for severe secondary hyperparathyroidism in the genesis of dialysis-associated pericarditis has been proposed, but the supporting data have been conflicting.[9,15,18,19] Moreover, the occurrence of pericarditis in patients with severe hyperparathyroidism (which reflects poor control of calcium-phosphorous metabolism) may simply indicate poor control of uremia in general, rather than an independent effect of hyperparathyroidism per se.

Heparin most likely does not initiate inflammation of the pericardium, but can contribute to ongoing inflammation by causing bleeding from the friable membranes.[7] Evidence for an infectious etiology has been demonstrated in some patients, but this probably represents a minority of cases.[7] Finally, certain auto-antibodies have been demonstrated in patients with dialysis-associated pericarditis, implying that an immunologic mechanism may be responsible in some cases.[20,21]

Clinical Features

Clinical and laboratory features of the pericarditis of ESRD are shown in Table 7-1. Pericardial friction rub and chest pain are the most important in the diagnosis of pericarditis. In general, dialysis-associated pericarditis is associated with a more severe clinical illness, more systemic manifestations, a higher propensity to tamponade, and a less favorable response to dialysis.[7,9,22]

Chest pain occurs in the majority of patients and may be variable in character and severity. The pain may be located anywhere in the precordium and may precede the development of a friction rub. There is often a pleuritic component

Table 7-1. Clinical Features of Pericarditis Associated With ESRD

Feature	%
Rub	95
Chest pain	60–70
Hypotension	13–56
Fever	63–76
Leukocytosis	35–71
ECG (classical)	2–5
Arrhythmias	20–28
Pericardial effusion (echocardiogram)	89

(Data from Bailey et al.,[12] Silverberg et al.,[14] Comty et al.,[15] Ribot et al.,[16] and Rutsky and Rostand.[24])

to the pain, and the pain may be aggravated by lying supine and partially relieved by sitting forward.

A pericardial friction rub may be detected in more than 90 percent of patients.[7,10,13,14] The rub is typically evanescent in nature and may change in quality from moment to moment. Therefore, the absence of a rub on any given physical examination does not rule out pericarditis.

Hemodynamic compromise, including hypotension during hemodialysis, may occur as a presenting clinical feature.[9,12] Dialysis-associated pericarditis should be suspected and sought in any patient suffering from repeated episodes of hypotension during dialysis or in patients with ESRD presenting with hypotension despite signs of fluid overload.

Fever and leukocytosis may be present more commonly in dialysis-associated pericarditis and, if severe, may predict a less favorable response to dialysis intensification.[23]

The electrocardiogram (ECG) is of limited usefulness in the diagnosis of pericarditis in ESRD. ECG abnormalities are common but lack specificity. The classic ST segment elevations described in several types of acute pericarditis are uncommon in this form of pericarditis[9,11]; the most common findings are non-specific ST- and T-wave abnormalities. Atrial arrhythmias, including atrial flutter and fibrillation, have been observed in a significant number of cases.

Echocardiography is the easiest and most accurate method for diagnosing pericardial effusion. It can be done rapidly and at the bedside, if necessary. The echocardiogram provides useful information regarding the size of a pericardial effusion and can detect early or impending tamponade. This information concerning quantity of effusion and hemodynamic significance is important when reaching a decision regarding early management of uremic pericarditis. A large effusion, or one that causes hemodynamic embarrassment, will generally not respond to conservative management with dialysis alone,[10,23,24] but will often require surgical drainage.

Acute cardiac tamponade is the most serious and potentially lethal complication of pericarditis associated with ESRD and is more common in dialysis-associated pericarditis than in uremic pericarditis. It has been reported that up to 35 percent of patients with dialysis-associated pericarditis will experience tamponade or impending tamponade.[24] Tamponade may occur during or shortly following a dialysis session. It may be difficult to distinguish acute tamponade from hypovolemia-induced hypotension. In cases of unexplained hypotension during or shortly following dialysis, the echocardiogram may be very useful in making this important differential diagnosis.

Management

When uremic pericarditis presents in a patient with renal disease reaching ESRD, then the initiation of renal replacement therapy is indicated. Cardiac tamponade is unusual in this form of pericarditis, and most patients will respond well to dialysis therapy with resolution of the signs and symptoms of pericarditis.

Management of dialysis-associated pericarditis has been less satisfactory. In the patient who does not have evidence of tamponade or impending tamponade, the first line of treatment in the hemodynamically stable patient has been intensification of dialysis, which has yielded a response rate of approximately 60 to 70 percent.[23] In the majority of cases, the response is seen within the first 10 to 14 days of initiating intensive dialysis therapy. In general, tight heparinization or no heparin dialysis protocols are used to avoid the complication of bleeding into the pericardial sac, and the patient is monitored closely for clinical signs of cardiac tamponade. Some authors recommend serial echocardiograms to monitor the size of the effusion during intensification of dialysis therapy. If hemodynamic compromise develops or the effusion fails to reduce in size or becomes larger over a course of 10 to 14 days, then a drainage procedure should be undertaken.

A positive effect from the use of nonsteroidal anti-inflammatory agents in the treatment of pericarditis has been difficult to prove and may be associated with greater gastrointestinal toxicity.[5,7,25,26] Similarly, systemic corticosteroids have been reported to improve the clinical course of pericarditis, but are associated with severe side effects and do not seem to prevent the development of constrictive pericarditis. The use of steroids in pericarditis associated with ESRD is, therefore, controversial.[9,10,15]

Several clinical features predict the failure of intensive dialytic intervention and hence the need for surgical drainage in the treatment of pericarditis. A report by De Pace et al.[23] suggests that the presence of a large pericardial effusion, temperature greater than 102°F, rales, requirement for peritoneal dialysis because the patient is too hemodynamically unstable to permit hemodialysis, systolic blood pressure under 100 mmHg, jugular venous distention, white blood cell count over 15,000/mm³, and white blood cell count left shift all correlated with poor outcome of dialysis treatment alone. The simultaneous presence of several of these features describes a patient at risk of failing to respond favorably to intensive dialysis therapy. Thus, the febrile, toxic patient with a large effusion and evidence of hemodynamic compromise is at high risk of failing to respond to dialysis treatment alone, and the need for a drainage procedure should be anticipated.

Pericardiocentesis, with or without the instillation of local triamcinolone hexacetonide, has been advocated by several authors in the management of pericardial effusion refractory to dialytic management.[27,28] In general, many authors have found pericardiocentesis to be associated with a high rate of severe complications including laceration of atrial or ventricular walls or coronary arteries.[7,9,11,16] Most series report a high morbidity and mortality rate with pericardiocentesis. In addition, pericardiocentesis has a high rate of reaccumulation of pericardial fluid, and thus does not represent a definitive procedure. Therefore, pericardiocentesis is generally recommended only for extreme emergency situations as a lifesaving measure.[7,9]

Subxiphoid pericardiotomy has proved to be a safe, effective, and relatively easy procedure to achieve pericardial drainage.[7,9,24,29,30] It is generally well tolerated in the uremic patient who is ill and who often has hemodynamic compromise, in comparison with the more extensive (albeit more definitive) pericardiectomy. Subxiphoid pericardiotomy is associated with a 6 percent failure rate, but a low rate of complications.

Pericardiectomy is a definitive surgical procedure with an essentially nonexistent rate of fluid reaccumulation; it also prevents the late complication of constrictive pericarditis. It is, however, an extensive major surgical intervention requiring general anesthesia and either a median sternotomy or anterior thoracotomy.[7,9,11] Pericardiectomy remains, nevertheless, the treatment of choice for constrictive pericarditis.

LEFT VENTRICULAR FUNCTION

Among chronic renal failure patients, alterations in cardiac structure and function have been demonstrated using hemodynamic and echocardiographic studies.[31] The etiology of these alterations is multifactorial.[32,33] Knowledge of the pathophysiology of these factors is essential for understanding how renal disease affects cardiac structure and function. They can be divided into four major categories:

1. Loading conditions that affect the myocardial function
2. Conditions that impair systolic function directly by their negative inotropic effect or indirectly by causing myocardial damage
3. Impaired diastolic filling of the heart
4. Alterations in neural control of circulation (Table 7-2)

Loading Conditions

The Frank-Starling mechanism, whereby diastolic cardiac dilatation causes increased force and volume of subsequent systolic contraction, is vital to the mainte-

Table 7-2. Factors Affecting
Myocardial Function in
Chronic Renal Failure

Loading conditions
  Anemia
  Hypertension
  Fluid retention
  AV fistula
  Thiamine deficiency

Systolic dysfunction
  Myocardial ischemia, infarction
  Hyperkalemia
  Hypocalcemia
  Metabolic acidosis
  Uremic toxins (?)
  Myocardial fibrosis
  Valvular disease

Diastolic filling
  Pericardial disease
  Left ventricular hypertrophy
  Myocardial fibrosis

Neural control
  Autonomic neuropathy

nance of cardiac output. As preload (left ventricular end-diastolic volume or pressure) increases, stroke volume increases. However, increase in preload beyond an optimal level does not lead to further increase in stroke volume, but causes pulmonary venous congestion. Usually pulmonary capillary wedge pressure more than 20 mmHg leads to pulmonary congestion, and more than 30 mmHg leads to pulmonary edema. However, if the pulmonary capillary permeability is increased, or plasma oncotic pressure is low, pulmonary congestion and edema may result at lower pressures. Retention of water and sodium may cause pulmonary edema in patients with acute renal failure or chronic renal failure when fluid intake is excessive. In addition, an increase in pulmonary capillary permeability leading to pulmonary edema, even in the absence of elevated pulmonary capillary wedge pressure, has been reported

in end-stage renal failure.[34] The ease with which these patients develop pleural and pericardial effusions supports this possible mechanism. The diluting effect of volume overload on plasma protein concentration, which may already be reduced if significant proteinuria is a feature of the underlying nephropathy, accentuates the tendency for fluid transudation and edema formation.[33]

Afterload refers to the resistance that the ventricle must overcome during systole in order to eject the stroke volume; it includes all factors that oppose ventricular fiber shortening. Arterial pressure is a major determinant of afterload. While increases in afterload have little effect on the stroke volume of the normal ventricle, it can lead to marked decrease in stroke volume when myocardial dysfunction is present. Most patients with chronic renal failure are hypertensive. In end-stage renal failure and in the dialysis population, severe hypertension is usually secondary to sodium and water retention. Such hypertension is present even in anephric patients and is exquisitely dependent on blood volume.[35] In some patients, the hypertension is secondary to elevation of peripheral resistance due to increased plasma renin activity; it is not controlled by lowering the blood volume but responds to bilateral nephrectomy.[36] Thus, retention of water and sodium leads to increases in both preload and afterload in chronic renal failure and may precipitate congestive heart failure. Pressure overload leads to concentric ventricular hypertrophy (symmetric wall thickening with normal cavity size), and volume overload leads to eccentric ventricular hypertrophy (enlarged ventricular cavity with normal or mildly thickened walls).[37] Regression of left ventricular hypertrophy has been demonstrated following renal transplantation.[38]

Heart failure exists when the cardiac output is insufficient to meet the demands of the metabolizing tissue. In anemia and arteriovenous fistula, a high cardiac output state is present; cardiac output and mean arterial pressure are elevated, but the systemic vascular resistance is normal. Using hypertrophy and dilatation as compensatory mechanisms, the normal heart can maintain tissue oxygenation for prolonged periods. But when myocardial function is impaired, these compensatory mechanisms are insufficient, and the high cardiac output state will lead to clinical manifestations of heart failure. Increase in cardiac output occurs when hematocrit falls below 25 percent; lowered blood viscosity is the major cause of increased cardiac output.[39] Increased blood viscosity increases peripheral resistance and arterial blood pressure. Thus, when the anemia is associated with a condition that leads to marked rise in blood viscosity, such as multiple myeloma or macroglobulinemia, cardiac output may fail to rise.[40] Many end-stage renal failure patients treated with erythropoietin experience an increase in arterial pressure due to increase in peripheral vascular resistance.[41] It has also been demonstrated that tissue hypoxia resulting from anemia can lead to an autonomic reflex response resulting in reduced arteriolar resistance.[42] High-output heart failure resulting from the arteriovenous shunts, surgically constructed for vascular access for hemodialysis, is not uncommon.[43] Mean flow rate through these shunts is 1.5 L/min. However, cardiac outputs as high as 11 L/min/m^2, which decrease substantially during the occlusion of the shunt, have been reported.[43] Although anemia may play a role in such high cardiac output states, the added hemodynamic burden of the shunt may explain heart failure. Banding or revising the fistula to an appropriate size may relieve heart failure symptoms.[43] Water-soluble vitamins are dialyzable, and it has been suggested that loss of thiamine may (rarely) lead to high-output heart failure due to beriberi.[44]

Systolic Dysfunction

Although the presence of a cardiomyopathy caused by "uremic toxins" has been suspected for five decades, its existence as a separate entity has not been clearly demonstrated. Since uremic patients often have other conditions that may alter myocardial function (e.g., anemia, arteriovenous fistula, hypertension, and coronary artery disease), it is difficult to establish the independent contribution of uremia to ventricular dysfunction. In an echocardiographic study, uremic patients had left ventricular dilatation, hypertrophy, and a higher ratio of left ventricular radius to wall thickness, indicating inadequate hypertrophy.[45] Myocardial dysfunction associated with uremia is often multifactorial, but is reversible. Left ventricular systolic function has been demonstrated to improve after peritoneal and hemodialysis.[32] However, such improvement may be secondary to reductions in preload and afterload.[46] Following renal transplantation, four patients with dilated cardiomyopathy, normal coronary angiograms, and severe left ventricular dysfunction were reported to have resolution of heart failure symptoms and return of left ventricular ejection fraction to normal.[47] Thus, although the existence of uremic cardiomyopathy is controversial, it is important to remember that the idiopathic cardiomyopathy seen in uremia may be reversible.

Calcium is fundamental to the process of myocardial contraction since its influx through sarcolemmal channels regulates the force of contraction. However, chronic hypocalcemia usually does not cause heart failure. Severe hypocalcemia (<6 mg/dl) in association with congestive heart failure has been described in dialysis patients after parathyroidectomy, with prompt improvement in cardiac function and resolution of heart failure following intravenous calcium replacement.[48] Parathyroid hormone may be a myocardial depressant since cardiac function reportedly improves after parathyroidectomy,[49] but the negative inotropic effect of parathyroid hormone has not been established. Dystrophic calcification of the myocardial fibers occurs in secondary hyperparathyroidism of chronic renal failure.[50] Hyperkalemia has a negative inotropic effect, but its principal detrimental effect is its electrical effect on the heart. Severe metabolic acidosis impairs calcium release from sarcoplasmic reticulum, and myocardial contractility is impaired at a systemic pH below 7.2.[51]

Hypertension, hypertriglyceridemia, and reduced concentrations of high-density lipoprotein cholesterol are common in chronic renal failure and lead to atherosclerotic heart disease. Ectopic calcification in the media of the arteries is a common manifestation of secondary hyperparathyroidism and may lead to luminal narrowing.[50] Myocardial ischemia and infarction may result and cause systolic dysfunction. An increased incidence of calcific aortic stenosis[52] and mitral annular calcification[50] has been reported in chronic renal failure. When valvular lesions are severe, myocardial dysfunction may result.

Diastolic Filling

Recently it has become apparent that diastolic dysfunction may lead to heart failure even in the presence of normal systolic function, especially in patients with left ventricular hypertrophy and in the older population.[53] Doppler echocardiography is now used to evaluate the diastolic function of the ventricles, and numerous studies have shown that diastolic filling is abnormal in the majority of patients with ventricular hypertrophy.[54,55] Echocardiographic left ventricular hypertrophy has been noted in 38 percent of patients with chronic renal failure.[56] Left ventricular hypertrophy develops and progresses with time on dialysis. In a longitudinal study of nondiabetic hemodialysis patients without dilated cardiomyopathy, the prevalence of left ventricular hypertrophy was 71 percent.[57] After a follow-up of 3 to 5 years, the hypertrophy persisted or even increased in the majority of patients. Progression to severe hypertrophy could not be discriminated on the basis of the degree of hypertension, or anemia. Asymmetric septal hypertrophy has also been reported, but this is an unusual manifestation of the hypertrophy resulting from hemodynamic stress, and is not associated with left ventricular outflow obstruction.[58]

A review of the published studies reveals that approximately 15 percent of patients with end-stage renal disease develop pericarditis at some time.[32] Pericarditis may be secondary to inadequate dialysis or an intercurrent illness. Large pericardial effusions, pericardial tamponade, and constriction impair diastolic filling, and an expanded intravascular volume is necessary for adequate filling. Development of hypotension during dialysis that cannot be explained by changes in intravascular volume is a clue to impaired diastolic filling.

Neural Control of Circulation

Although dialysis techniques have improved, autonomic neuropathies are still common, since diabetes mellitus is a common cause of chronic renal failure. Reduced baroreceptor activity in patients with chronic renal failure has been demonstrated by their response to the inhalation of amyl nitrite[59]; amyl nitrite inhalation normally causes vasodilatation and hypotension with reflex vasoconstriction and tachycardia. A blunted heart rate response is evidence for baroreceptor dysfunction. Orthostatic hypotension resulting from autonomic neuropathy may be mistaken for other cardiac disorders.

Factors that affect cardiac function and hemodynamics in chronic renal failure were reviewed. It should be noted that there is continuous interplay of these factors, sometimes with additive and sometimes with opposite effects. An example is increased afterload due to hypertension and decreased afterload due to anemia. Moreover, a cardiac disorder may co-exist as a primary disorder (e.g., rheumatic valvular disease), or as part of a multisystem disorder (e.g., pericarditis and chronic renal failure secondary to a collagen vascular disease).

Hemodynamic and echocardiographic findings in patients with chronic renal failure have been reported. Generally patients with end-stage renal disease have elevated arterial pressure, impaired left ventricular systolic function, increased intravascular volume, and increased peripheral resistance, cardiac index, and cardiac work. The echocardiogram often reveals left ventricular dilatation, hypertrophied septum, free-wall, impaired systolic function, and pericardial effusion.[31,56] Recently, echocardiographic findings of 140 patients on hemodialysis without any cardiovascular disease were compared with those of 120 nonuremic subjects matched for age, sex, and blood pressure.[60] The following echocardiographic abnormalities were observed: increased left atrial and left ventricular dimensions, increased left ventricular wall thickness and mass, normal systolic func-

tion, and altered diastolic filling. It should be noted that these are generalizations and may not apply to individual patients. Since the etiology of cardiac dysfunction in end-stage renal failure is multifactorial, the hemodynamic and echocardiographic manifestations will depend upon the predominant etiology. For example, the findings in a patient with heart failure secondary to anemia, arteriovenous fistula, and volume-dependent hypertension will obviously be different from those of a patient with heart failure due to myocardial infarction, renin-dependent hypertension, and diastolic dysfunction.

CARDIAC ARRHYTHMIAS

End-stage renal failure is associated with a constant disequilibrium of fluid, electrolyte, and acid-base status, left ventricular hypertrophy, congestive heart failure, coronary artery disease, pericardial disease, and altered drug metabolism; all of these conditions may cause arrhythmias.[61–64] It is important to distinguish between primary and secondary arrhythmias.[64] An arrhythmia that results from an electrophysiologic disturbance caused by a disease process, independent of a significant change in hemodynamic or metabolic status, is defined as a primary arrhythmia. An example is ventricular arrhythmia secondary to myocardial infarction in an end-stage renal disease patient with normal hemodynamics and electrolyte levels. In this situation, the aim is to control the arrhythmia and prevent more lethal forms; antiarrhythmic therapy is appropriate. Arrhythmias resulting from hemodynamic or metabolic disturbances are defined as secondary arrhythmias. An example is ventricular arrhythmias secondary to an electrolyte abnormality. In this situation correction of the precipitating factor is the mainstay of therapy, and antiarrhythmic therapy has only a complementary role. In some patients primary arrhythmias may be exacerbated by hemodynamic or metabolic abnormalities. It is often difficult to determine the interrelations among the arrhythmia, arrhythmogenic substrate (underlying heart disease), and factors modifying the arrhythmogenic milieu (electrolyte abnormality, ischemia) in patients with renal failure. It should also be noted that even in the absence of hemodynamic or metabolic fluctuations, the frequency of arrhythmias shows considerable variation on a day-to-day basis. Therefore, it is not surprising that the reported prevalence of arrhythmias in end-stage renal failure varies from normal or low levels, comparable to actively employed middle-aged men, to life-threatening arrhythmias.[61]

Despite these limitations of quantitating arrhythmias in end-stage renal failure, many investigators have reported on the prevalence of arrhythmias. Vizeman and Kramer[61] reviewed 14 studies reporting the prevalence of arrhythmias in end-stage renal disease. Although there was considerable variation in the reported prevalence, atrial and ventricular arrhythmias were common in the majority of studies. The majority of ventricular arrhythmias were unifocal premature ventricular contractions. Among the European patients, it was noted that death was due to cardiac arrest in 9.5 percent of women and 9 percent of men.[61] Ventricular fibrillation is the terminal rhythm noted in 25 percent of deaths occurring in dialysis centers.[65] Although nonsustained ventricular tachycardia is associated with increased mortality, suppression of asymptomatic nonsustained ventricular arrhythmias does not improve survival.[66,67]

Results of the recently reported Cardiac Arrhythmia Suppression Trial and meta-analysis from smaller randomized trials have suggested that there is a net increase in adverse effects of antiarrhythmic drugs used to suppress premature ventricular contractions following myocardial infarction. Thus, antiarrhythmic therapy of asymptomatic nonsustained ventricular arrhythmias is no longer recommended.[68] Patients with sustained ventricular tachycardia and aborted ventricular fibrillation should be treated aggressively. They usually require electrophysiologically guided antiarrhythmic therapy, and, if antiarrhythmic drugs are ineffective, an automatic defibrillator should be implanted. Exceptions to this recommendation are patients in whom ventricular tachycardia or fibrillation is a complication of an acute myocardial infarction or a metabolic abnormality.

Arrhythmias caused by electrolyte abnormalities are common. The effect of hyperkalemia on cardiac rhythm is complex, and virtually any arrhythmia may be seen.[69] A slow elevation of potassium level produces widespread block and depressed automaticity. Sinus bradycardia, sinus arrest, atrioventricular blocks, idioventricular rhythm, and asystole may occur. Rapid rise in potassium level produces ventricular ectopic rhythms and ventricular fibrillation. Ectopic rhythms other than junctional are unusual in clinical hyperkalemia, except as a terminal event. Moderate hyperkalemia has been reported to suppress supraventricular and ventricular ectopic beats.[70] The effects of digitalis are modified by extracellular potassium concentration. This interrelationship is manifested by:

1. Depression of digitalis-induced ectopy by potassium
2. Emergence of digitalis-induced ectopy during hypokalemia
3. Enhancement of digitalis-induced depression of conduction by potassium[69]

It is not clear whether alterations in calcium levels lead to clinical arrhythmia. Hypophosphatemia may depress myocardial performance, but alterations in phosphate levels usually do not cause arrhythmias.[71] Correction of the electrolyte abnormality is obviously the mainstay of therapy.

CARDIOVASCULAR DRUG THERAPY IN ESRD

As the GFR falls toward levels that require hemodialysis (or peritoneal dialysis) in order to sustain life, the dose of drugs that are excreted by the kidneys, or whose metabolites are renally excreted, must be modified. We shall review some important concepts of renal physiology and pharmacology and then review specific drugs likely to be prescribed by cardiologists for patients with renal insufficiency. We shall also review cardiac drug modifications required for patients receiving hemodialysis or peritoneal dialysis.

Renal Physiology

The driving force for renal blood flow and glomerular filtration is the left ventricle. The systolic pressure head generated by left ventricular contraction is reduced in a series of resistance vessels until it traverses the afferent arteriole into the glomerulus. Renal autoregulation preserves glomerular filtration over a wide range of systolic pressure, but pressures less than about 60 mmHg are generally associated with a marked reduction or cessation of glomerular filtration. GFR is regulated in part by the tone of the efferent arteriole. Therefore, drugs such as ACE inhibitors that reduce efferent arteriolar tone may result in decreased GFR.[72,73]

As the left ventricular systolic pressure head decreases due to cardiac failure, the juxtaglomerular apparatus releases renin, which in turn leads to the generation of angiotensin–II and aldosterone. These changes work toward support of systemic blood pressure by generalized vasoconstriction and volume retention by means of avid renal sodium reabsorption. Old-time clinicians recognized that urine that did not glow yellow when flamed (because urine sodium concentration was less than 10 mmol/L) was associated with a poor prognosis.

Acute oliguric or anuric renal failure should be clinically obvious, but acute nonoliguric or chronic renal failure may be subtle. For example, radiocontrast media-associated renal failure may not be noticed unless indicated by a rising serum creatinine concentration.[74]

Serum creatinine concentration alone may be misleading as an index of GFR because it is also a function of lean body mass. Therefore, a serum creatinine concentration of 1.2 mg/dl may be totally normal for a 100-kg 20-year-old athlete but may indicate clinically important renal insufficiency in an 80-year-old woman who weighs 45 kg. The Cockcroft Gault formula permits easy bedside estimation of creatinine clearance as an index of GFR.[75] One needs only a serum creatinine determination, the patient's weight in kg, and the age in years.

estimated GFR =

$$\frac{(\text{weight in kg})(140 - \text{age})}{(72)(\text{serum creatinine in mg/dl})}$$

This number should be multiplied by 0.85 for women.

For example, the athlete discussed above would have an estimated GFR of

$$\frac{(100)(140 - 20)}{(72)(1.2)} = 139 \text{ ml/min}$$

In contrast, the elderly woman with the same serum creatinine level would have an estimated GFR of

$$\frac{(45)(140 - 80)(0.85)}{(72)(1.2)} = 27 \text{ ml/min}$$

Obviously, this very low GFR has significant clinical implications for drug administration and dose of radiocontrast media.

Pharmacology

In simplistic terms, drugs are metabolized by the liver, the kidneys, or both. Drugs that are water soluble or highly lipid insoluble will be renally excreted, while those that are lipid soluble and water insoluble will be excreted by the liver. Some hepatic metabolites may be water soluble and renally excreted, however.

The kidney excretes drugs by glomerular filtration or proximal tubule secretion. In contrast to pressure-driven filtration, tubular secretion is an energy-dependent active transport process. It will not be op-erative in the types of renal failure (such as acute tubular insufficiency) in which tubular energy systems are paralyzed, but is functional to the limit of available intact tubules in most forms of chronic renal failure. Secretion occurs in organic acid and organic base pathways. Renal failure, by definition, will markedly impair or eliminate glomerular filtration as a source of excretion. Drugs that are highly protein bound cannot be effectively filtered. The proximal tubule organic acid secretion pathways must compete with the high levels of retained acids that are typical of uremia. The organic base pathways may be less effected. Tubular secretion does require renal blood flow, but not glomerular filtration. Highly protein-bound drugs can be secreted by the tubules. It is therefore useful to identify the excretion route for drugs used by cardiologists in order to determine whether dose modification is required[76] (Table 7-3).

Drugs vary in their ability to be removed by hemodialysis or peritoneal dialysis. The dose of drug and dosing fre-

Table 7-3. Major Route of Excretion and Dose Modification Required for Selected Drugs

	Major Excretion	Reduction For ESRD	Removed by Dialysis
Antiarrhythmic agents			
Amiodarone	Hepatic	None	No
Bretylium	Renal	Avoid	Yes
Disopyramide	Renal Hepatic	Increase dosing interval	No
Encainide	Hepatic	None	No
Flecainide	Hepatic	50–75%	No
Lidocaine	Hepatic	None	No
Lorcainide	Hepatic	None	?
Mexiletine	Hepatic	50–75%	No
Procainamide	Renal Hepatic	Increase dosing interval	Yes
N-acetylprocainamide	Renal	25% or increase dosing interval	Yes
Quinidine	Hepatic	None	No
Tocainide	Hepatic Renal	50%	Yes

(*Continues*)

Table 7-3. (*continued*)

	Major Excretion	*Reduction For ESRD*	*Removed by Dialysis*
Cardiac glycosides			
Digoxin	Renal	10–25% or increase dosing interval	No
Digitoxin	Hepatic	50–75%	No
Nitrates			
Nitroglycerin	Hepatic	None	?
Isosorbide dinitrate	Hepatic	None	?
Vasodilators			
Diazoxide	Hepatic/Renal	None	Yes
Hydralazine	Hepatic	Increase dosing interval	No
Minoxidil	Hepatic	None	Yes
Sodium nitroprusside	Metabolized to thiocyanate that may be toxic; monitor blood levels	None	Yes
Anticoagulants			
Heparin	Nonrenal	None	No
Streptokinase	—	None	—
Urokinase	—	None	—
Warfarin	Hepatic	None	No
Immunosuppressive Agents			
Azathioprine	Hepatic	75%, dose interval 36 hr	Yes
Cyclophosphamide	Hepatic	50–75%, dose interval 18–24 hr	Yes
Cyclosporine	Hepatic	None	No
Prednisone	Hepatic	None	Yes
Hypolipemic Agents			
Cholestyramine	Not absorbed	None	N/A
Clofibrate	Hepatic	Dose interval 24–84 hr	No
Colestipol	Not absorbed	None	N/A
Gemfibrozil	Renal	25%	?
Nicotinic acid	Hepatic	25%	?
Lovastatin	Hepatic	Do not exceed 20 mg/day	?
Simvastatin	Hepatic	None	?
Pravastatin	Hepatic Renal	Limit dose	?
Probucol	Hepatic	None	No
Inotropic agents			
Dobutamine	Hepatic	None	N/A
Amrinone	Hepatic/Renal	None	N/A
Dopamine	Nonrenal	None	N/A
Milrinone	Renal	Adjust dose by GFR	
Others			
Pentoxifylline	Renal	Avoid	?

[1] *Abbreviation:* GFR, glomerular filtration rate.
(Data from Gambertoglio et al.[77])

quency of drugs normally excreted by the kidney need to be adjusted based on how readily they cross the dialytic membrane. Uremic patients may have nausea and vomiting that prevents them from ingesting or absorbing orally administered medications. Uremia may also decrease the protein binding of drugs and impair hepatic first-pass metabolism of lipid-soluble drugs. Generalized edema may reduce intestinal absorption of drugs and absorption from edematous sites of intramuscular injection. In addition, edema will increase the volume of distribution of water-soluble drugs and thereby prolong their excretion. Table 7-3 provides useful information on the effect of renal failure on the excretion of drugs often prescribed by cardiologists.

REFERENCES

1. Kincaid-Smith P, Whitworth JA: Pathogenesis of hypertension in chronic renal disease. Semin Nephrol 8:155, 1988
2. Smith MC, Dunn MJ: Hypertension in renal parenchymal disease. p. 1583. In Laragh JH, Brenner BM (eds): Hypertension: Pathophysiology, Diagnosis, and Management. Raven Press, New York, 1990
3. Shulman NB, Ford CE, Hall WD et al: Prognostic value of serum creatinine and effect of treatment of hypertension on renal function. Results from the Hypertension Detection and Follow-up Program. Hypertension 13(suppl. I): I-80, 1989
4. Heyka RJ, Vidt DG: Control of hypertension in patients with chronic renal failure. Cleve Clin J Med 56:65, 1989
5. Roy LF, Leenen FHH: Therapy of hypertension in end-stage renal disease. p. 247. In Parfrey PS, Harnett JD (eds): Cardiac Dysfunction in Chronic Uremia. Kluwer Academic Publishers, Boston, 1992
6. Baldwin DS, Neugarten J: Treatment of hypertension in renal disease. p. A57. In:

Hypertension and the Kidney: Proceedings of a Symposium. The National Kidney Foundation, Inc., Philadelphia, 1985
7. Rostand SG, Rutsky EA: Cardiac disease in dialysis patients. p. 408. In Nissenson AR, Fine RN, Gentile DE (eds): Clinical Dialysis, 2nd Ed. Appleton & Lange, Norwalk, 1990
8. Maiorca R, Scolari F, Cancarini G et al: Management of hypertension in chronic renal failure. Contr Nephrol 54:190, 1987
9. Kim KE, Swartz C: Cardiovascular complications of end-stage renal disease. p. 2817. In Schrier RW, Gottschalk CW (eds): Diseases of the Kidney, 5th Ed. Vol. III. Little, Brown, Boston, 1988
10. Suki WN: Pericarditis. Kidney Int 33 (suppl. 24):S10, 1988
11. Pábico RC: Cardiovascular system in uremia. Pericarditis. Part 1. p. 1171. In Massry SG, Glassock RJ (eds): Textbook of Nephrology. 2nd Ed. Vol. 2. Williams & Wilkins, Baltimore, 1989
12. Bailey GL, Hampers CL, Hager EB, Merrill JP: Uremic pericarditis. Clinical features and management. Circulation 38:582, 1968
13. Luft FC, Gilman JK, Weyman AE: Pericarditis in the patient with uremia: clinical and echocardiographic evaluation. Nephron 25:160, 1980
14. Silverberg S, Oreopoulos DG, Wise DJ et al: Pericarditis in patients undergoing long-term hemodialysis and peritoneal dialysis. Incidence, complications and management. Am J Med 63:874, 1977
15. Comty CM, Cohen SL, Shapiro FL: Pericarditis in chronic uremia and its sequels. Ann Intern Med 75:173, 1971
16. Ribot S, Frankel HJ, Gielchinsky I et al: Treatment of uremic pericarditis. Clin Nephrol 2:127, 1974
17. Wray TM, Stone WJ: Uremic pericarditis: a prospective echocardiographic and clinical study. Clin Nephron 6:295, 1976
18. Drüeke T, LePailleur C, Zingraff J et al: Uremic cardiomyopathy and pericarditis. Adv Nephron 9:33, 1980
19. Comty CM, Shapiro FL: Cardiac complications of regular dialysis therapy. p. 595. In Drukker W, Parsons FM, Maher JF (eds): Replacement of Renal Function by

Dialysis, 2nd Ed. Martinus Nijhoff Publishing, Dordrecht, 1983

20. Maisch B, Kochiek K: Humoral immune reaction in uremic pericarditis. Am J Nephrol 3:264, 1983

21. Twardowski ZJ, Alpert MA, Gupta RC et al: Circulating immune complexes: possible toxins responsible for serositis (pericarditis, pleuritis, and peritonitis) in renal failure. Nephron 35:190, 1983

22. Renfrew R, Buselmeier TJ, Kjellstrand CM: Pericarditis and renal failure. Annu Rev Med 31:345, 1980

23. De Pace NL, Nestico PF, Schwartz AB et al: Predicting success of intensive dialysis in the treatment of uremic pericarditis. Am J Med 76:38, 1984

24. Rutsky EA, Rostrand SG: Treatment of uremic pericarditis and pericardial effusion. Am J Kidney Dis 10:2, 1987

25. Minuth ANW, Nottebohm GA, Eknoyan G et al: Indomethacin treatment of pericarditis in chronic hemodialysis patients. Arch Intern Med 135:807, 1975

26. Spector D, Alfred H, Siedlecki M et al: A controlled study of the effect of indomethacin in uremic pericarditis. Kidney Int 24:663, 1983

27. Buselmeier TJ, Simmons RL, Najarian JS et al: Uremic pericardial effusion. Treatment by catheter drainage and local nonabsorbable steroid administration. Nephron 16:371, 1976

28. Fuller TJ, Knochel JP, Brennan JP et al: Reversal of intractable uremic pericarditis by triamcinolone hexacetonide. Arch Intern Med 136:979, 1976

29. Popli S, Ing TS, Daugirdas JT et al: Treatment of uremic pericardial effusion by local steroid instillatior via subxiphoid pericardiotomy. J Dial 4:83, 1980

30. Alcan KE, Zabetakis PM, Marino ND et al: Management of acute cardiac tamponade by subxiphoid pericardiotomy. JAMA 247:1143, 1982

31. Kleiger RE, deMello VR, Malone D et al: Left ventricular function in end-stage renal disease. Echocardiographic classification. South Med J 74:819, 1981

32. Pastan SO, Braunwald E: Renal disorders and heart disease. p. 1856. In Braunwald

E (ed): Heart Disease. WB Saunders, Philadelphia, 1992

33. Delaney VB, Bourke E: The interrelationship of heart disease and kidney disease. p. 1543. In Hurst JW (ed): The Heart. McGraw-Hill, New York, 1990

34. Crosbie WA, Snowden S, Parsons V: Changes in lung capillary permeability in renal failure. Br Med J 4:388, 1972

35. Vertes V, Cangiano JL, Berman LB, Gould A: Hypertension in end-stage renal disease. N Engl J Med 280:978, 1969

36. Kim KE, Onesti G, Schwartz AB et al: Hemodynamics of hypertension in chronic end-stage disease. Circulation 46:456, 1972

37. Hachamovitch R, Strom JA, Sonnenblick EH, Frishman WH: Left ventricular hypertrophy in hypertension and the effects of antihypertensive drug therapy. Curr Probl Cardiol 13:369, 1988

38. Himelman RB, Landzberg JS, Simonson JS et al: Cardiac consequences of renal transplantation: changes in left ventricular morphology and function. J Am Coll Cardiol 12:915, 1988

39. Richardson TQ, Guyton AC: Effects of polycythemia and anemia on cardiac output and other circulatory factors. Am J Physiol 197:1167, 1959

40. Grossman W, Braunwald E: High-cardiac output states. p. 778. In Braunwald E (ed): Heart Disease. WB Saunders, Philadelphia, 1988

41. The US Recombinant Human Erythropoietin Predialysis Study Group: Double-blind, placebo-controlled study of the therapeutic use of recombinant human erythropoietin for anemia associated with chronic renal failure in predialysis patients. Am J Kidney Dis 18:50, 1991

42. Glick G, Plauth WH, Braunwald E: Role of autonomic nervous system in the circulatory response to acutely induced anemia in unanesthetized dogs. J Clin Invest 43:2112, 1964

43. Anderson CB, Codd JR, Graff RA et al: Cardiac failure as a complication of upper extremity arteriovenous dialysis fistulas. Arch Intern Med 136:292, 1976

44. Gotloib L, Servadio C: A possible case of beriberi heart failure in a chronic hemodialysis patient. Nephron 14:293, 1975

45. London GM, Fabiani F, Marchais SJ, et al: Uremic cardiomyopathy: an inadequate left ventricular hypertrophy. Kidney Int 31:973, 1987

46. Blaustein AS, Schmitt G, Foster MC et al: Serial effects on left ventricular load and contractility during hemodialysis in patients with concentric hypertrophy. Am Heart J 111:340, 1986

47. Burt RK, Burt SG, Suki WN et al: Reversal of left ventricular dysfunction after renal transplantation. Ann Intern Med 111:635, 1989

48. Feldman AM, Fivush B, Zakha KG et al: Congestive cardiomyopathy in patients on continuous ambulatory peritoneal dialysis. Am J Kidney Dis 11:76, 1988

49. Drüeke T, Fauchet M, Fleury J et al: Effect of parathyroidectomy on left-ventricular function in haemodialysis patients. Lancet 1:112, 1980

50. Roberts WC, Waller BF: Effect of chronic hypercalcemia on the heart. An analysis of 18 necropsy patients. Am J Med. 71:371, 1981

51. Mitchell JH, Wildenthal K, Johnson RL: The effects of acid-base disturbances on cardiovascular and pulmonary function. Kidney Int 1:375, 1972

52. Maher ER, Pazianas M, Curtis JR: Calcific aortic stenosis: a complication of chronic uremia. Nephron 47:119, 1987

53. Chakko S, Kessler KM: Changes in aging as reflected in noninvasive cardiac studies. p. 235. In Brest AN (ed): Geriatric Cardiology; Cardiovascular Clinics. FA Davis, Philadelphia, 1992

54. Spirito P, Maron BJ: Doppler echocardiography for assessing left ventricular diastolic function. Ann Intern Med 109:122, 1988

55. Chakko S, de Marchena E, Kessler KM et al: Right ventricular diastolic function in systemic hypertension. Am J Cardiol 65:1117, 1990)

56. D'Cruz IA, Bhatt GR, Cohen HC, Glick G: Echocardiographic detection of cardiac involvement in patients with chronic renal failure. Arch Intern Med 138:720, 1978

57. Parfrey PS, Harnett JD, Griffiths SM et al: The clinical course of left ventricular hypertrophy in end-stage renal disease. Nephron 55:114, 1990

58. Abbasi AS, Slaughter JC, Allen MW: Asymptomatic septal hypertrophy in patients on long-term hemodialysis. Chest 74:548, 1978

59. Campese VM, Romoff MS, Levitan D, et al: Mechanisms of autonomic nervous system dysfunction in uremia. Kidney Int 20:246, 1981

60. London GM, Fabiani F. Left ventricular dysfunction in end-stage renal disease: echocardiographic insights. In Parfrey PS, Harnett JD (eds): Cardiac Dysfunction in Chronic Uremia. p. 117. Kluwer Academic Publishers, Boston, 1992

61. Wizemann V, Kramer W: Cardiac arrhythmias in end-stage renal disease: prevalence, risk factors, and management. p. 67. In Parfrey PS, Harnett JD. (eds): Cardiac Dysfunction in Chronic Uremia. Kluwer Academic Publishers, Boston, 1992

62. McLenachan JM, Henderson E, Morris KI, Dargie HJ: Ventricular arrhythmias in patients with hypertensive left ventricular hypertrophy. N Engl J Med 317:787, 1987

63. Chakko S, Gheorghiade M: Ventricular arrhythmias in severe heart failure: incidence, significance and effectiveness of antiarrhythmic therapy. Am Heart J 109:497, 1985

64. Myerburg RJ, Kessler KM: Clinical assessment and management of arrhythmias and conduction disturbances. p. 535. In Hurst JW. (ed.): The Heart. McGraw-Hill, New York, 1990

65. Chazan J: Sudden death in patients with chronic renal failure on hemodialysis. Dial Transplant 16:447, 1987

66. D'elia J, Weinrauch L, Gleason R et al: Application of ambulatory 24-hour electrocardiogram in the prediction of cardiac death in dialysis patients. Arch Intern Med 148:2381, 1988

67. Chakko S, de Marchena E, Myerburg RJ: Sudden death in cardiomyopathy. In Lu-

deritz B, Saksena S. (eds): Interventional Electrophysiology. Futura Publishing, Mount Kisco, NY, 1991

68. Kessler KM, Chakko CS, Myerburg RJ: The management of premature ventricular contractions. Heart Dis Stroke 1:275, 1992

69. Rardon DP, Fisch C: Electrolytes and the heart. p. 1557. Hurst JW (ed): The Heart. McGraw-Hill, New York, 1990

70. Bettinger JC, Surawicz B, Bryfogle JW et al: The effect of intravenous administration of potassium chloride on ectopic rhythms, ectopic beats and disturbances in A-V conduction. Am J Med 21:521, 1966

71. Davis S, Olichwier K, Chakko CS: Reversible depression of myocardial performance in hypophosphatemia. Am J Med Sci 295:183, 1988

72. Hricik DE, Browning PJ, Kopelman R: Captopril-induced functional renal insufficiency in patients with bilateral renal-artery stenosis or renal-artery stenosis in a solitary kidney. N Engl J Med 308:373, 1983

73. Ichikawa I, Brenner BM: Glomerular actions of angiotensin II. Am J Med 76(5B):43, 1984

74. Byrd L, Sherman RL: Radiocontrast-induced acute renal failure: a clinical and pathophysiologic review. Medicine 58:270, 1979

75. Cockcroft DW, Gault MH: Prediction of creatinine clearance from serum creatinine. Nephron 16:31, 1976

76. Materson BJ: Insights into intrarenal sites and mechanisms of action of diuretic agents. Am Heart J 106(1 Part II):188, 1983

77. Gambertoglio JG, Aweeka FT, Blythe WB: Use of drugs in patients with renal failure. p. 3211. In Schrier RW, Gottschalk CW (eds): Diseases of the Kidney. 5th Ed. Little, Brown, Boston, 1993

8

Hematologic and Oncologic Disorders

Laurence A. Harker

Hematologic and oncologic disorders may affect the development, presentation, and management of cardiovascular diseases, and therapies for such disorders may cause or complicate abnormalities of the heart. Conversely, disorders of the heart and their treatment may produce disorders of the blood that complicate the care of patients with cardiac diseases.

DISORDERS OF RED CELLS

Effects of Anemia

In the absence of cardiovascular disease, anemic patients generally have few if any cardiac symptoms. However, resting cardiac output increases when hemoglobin values fall below 7 g/dl. Indeed, anemia is one of the most common causes of increased cardiac output and may give rise to high-output heart failure in association with otherwise asymptomatic heart disease.[1] Symptoms secondary to anemia depend on (1) the rapidity with which the anemia develops, (2) the physical activity of the patient, and (3) the coexistence of underlying cardiac or coronary artery disease.[1–4]

Anemia reduces cardiac reserve and increases fatigue, exertional dyspnea, and edema in proportion to its severity. For example, in association with coronary artery disease, anemia lowers the threshold for developing angina pectoris. If anemia develops gradually, patients with hemoglobin levels below 7 g/dl may compensate sufficiently to carry out all but the most strenuous activities, related perhaps in part to enhanced formation of intercoronary collaterals.

However, congestive heart failure with pulmonary edema may develop solely on the basis of very severe anemia (i.e., hemoglobin < 4 g/dl) in the absence of antecedent heart disease. Tissue hypoxia combined with reduced blood viscosity decreases systemic vascular resistance, leading to increased cardiac output. Left ventricular end-diastolic volume and afterload increases in patients with chronic anemia, resulting in left ventricular end-systolic stress.[5,6] All signs and symptoms of anemia-induced cardiovascular disease disappear when normal hemoglobin levels are restored.

Mechanisms Compensating for Anemia

The extent of circulatory adaptation following chronic anemia depends on (1) hemoglobin concentration, (2) blood flow, (3) tissue oxygen tension, and (4) position of the hemoglobin-oxygen dissociation curve. Normally, for a hemoglobin concentration of 15 g/dl, 100 ml of arterial blood contains 20 ml of oxygen and 100 ml of mixed venous blood having a PO_2 of 40 mmHg and containing 15.5 ml of oxygen. The difference (i.e., 4.5 ml of oxygen/100 ml of arterial blood) is available for delivery to peripheral tissues. However, in patients with anemia, the hemoglobin-oxygen dissociation curve shifts to the right, and more oxygen is released from hemoglobin as the PO_2 declines. Deoxygenated hemoglobin, which is more alkaline than oxyhemoglobin, stimulates the production of 2,3-diphosphoglycerate (2,3-DPG), a byproduct of glycolysis; the intraerythrocytic ratio of deoxy- to oxyhemoglobin regulates the concentration of 2,3-DPG. At a normal arterial PO_2, arterial oxygen saturation remains high despite the reduction in oxygen affinity. However, at the lower PO_2 in the venous blood, elevated 2,3-DPG displaces the hemoglobin-oxygen dissociation curve to the right, facilitating release of oxygen from the cells at any level of PO_2 (Fig. 8-1). Levels of 2,3-DPG are similarly increased in individuals exposed to high altitude and in patients with pulmonary disease.[7,8] Decreased oxygen affinity mediated by increases in red cell 2,3-DPG compensate for up to one-half of the oxygen deficit resulting from anemia.

Oxygen delivery to tissues is directly proportional to blood flow, hemoglobin concentration, and the difference in oxygen saturation between arterial and venous blood, and each of these factors varies independently. Blood flow is a function of total cardiac output and its fractional distribution. Erythropoietin regulates the red cell mass in response to levels of tissue oxygenation. The position of the hemoglobin-oxygen dissociation curve is determined primarily by red cell 2,3-DPG levels and blood pH. Chronic anemia is well tolerated when cardiac output and redistribution of blood flow increases and oxygen affinity decreases.

Clinical Characteristics

Cardiac enlargement develops in response to severe chronic anemia due to dilatation and eccentric hypertrophy with a normal ratio of wall thickness to cavity diameter. On physical examination the precordium is hyperactive, third and fourth heart sounds are often present, and a midsystolic murmur is audible at the left sternal border. The murmur probably arises from the combined effects of increased velocity of blood flow across the pulmonic and aortic valve orifices and reduced blood viscosity. Sometimes a midsystolic rumbling murmur may be heard at the apex, probably related to the increase in blood flow across the mitral or tricuspid valve, and may be difficult to distinguish from the murmurs of mitral or tricuspid stenosis. With hemoglobin levels below 7 g/dl, T-wave depression and T-wave inversion may be found, simulating myocardial disease. Following transfusions, these findings usually return to normal.

The expansion of the blood volume by transfusing whole blood may be poorly tolerated in patients with chronic anemia exhibiting increased cardiac output and decreased oxygen affinity. Consequently, packed red blood cells should be infused slowly in conjunction with diuretics. In addition, intravenous nitroglycerin therapy may improve redistribution of circulating blood volume and blunt the hemodynamic changes caused by transfusion.[9]

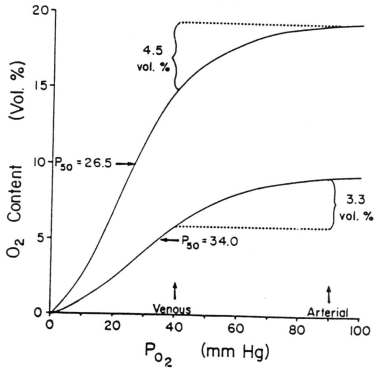

Fig. 8-1. The position of the hemoglobin-oxygen dissociation curve is expressed by the value of P_{50} (i.e., the partial pressure of oxygen at which hemoglobin is 50 percent saturated). A reduction of the oxygen affinity of hemoglobin (i.e., a shift of the dissociation curve to the right) is reflected in an elevation of P_{50}. With a P_{50} of 34 mmHg (as opposed to the normal P_{50} of 26.5 mmHg), 3.3 ml of oxygen is unloaded per 100 ml of blood. As a consequence, an anemic individual with a 50 percent reduction in red cell mass exhibits only a 27 percent reduction in oxygen unloading.

Effects of Hemogloblinopathies

Sickle Cell Disease

Sickle hemoglobin arises from a mutation in the sixth amino acid of the β-globin chain from glutamic acid to valine. Eight to 10 percent of black Americans are heterozygous for this trait. The signs and symptoms in patients homozygous for sickle cell anemia (SS) begin at about 6 months of age, upon completion of the conversion from fetal to adult hemoglo-bin production. When oxygen tension decreases, red cells containing hemoglobin S acquire an elongated crescent (sickle) shape. As red cells remain sickled in vivo, their membranes become damaged and rigid, undergo irreversible sickling, and may block small blood vessels. The continuous formation and destruction of irreversibly sickled cells shortens red cell survival. Factors decreasing oxygen affinity, such as acidosis and increased red cell 2,3-DPG levels, lead to the deoxygenation of hemoglobin, further promoting the production of sickled cells. As anemia worsens, both cardiac output and oxygen extraction by tissues are increased, thereby escalating the sickling process. Importantly, for any given level of hematocrit, the elevation of cardiac output and the auscultatory findings associated with anemia are greater in sickle cell anemia compared with other anemias.[10]

A normal left ventricle tolerates the volume overload of chronic, moderately severe anemia for indefinite periods with no deterioration in functional capacity.[11,12] The increased preload and decreased afterload characteristics of chronic anemia compensate for any left ventricular dysfunction and maintain a normal ejection fraction and high cardiac output in sickle cell anemia.[13] Cardiac decompensation in patients with sickle cell anemia is usually the result of coexisting complications of the SS disease or the presence of underlying cardiovascular abnormalities. Specifically, deaths secondary to congestive heart failure arising in children and young adults with sickle cell anemia are usually precipitated by chronic renal failure, pulmonary thrombosis, or infections.[14]

Pulmonary infarction commonly complicates sickle cell anemia, probably secondary to thrombosis in situ rather than to embolization.[15] Since patients with sickle cell anemia are particularly susceptible to infection, damage to the lung caused by repeated vascular insults creates a suitable milieu for bacterial pneumonias. Mortality and morbidity are high in the setting of pneumonia and hypoxia. Unfortunately, it may be difficult to differentiate pulmonary infection from infarction in patients with sickle cell anemia. Despite the frequency of impaired pulmonary function in sickle cell anemia, pulmonary hypertension and cor pulmonale are uncommon in these patients.

Children with sickle cell disease develop progressive cardiac chamber enlargement with incremental increases in left ventricular mass. At autopsy striking heart weights are noted in a majority of patients despite the absence of other causes of cardiomegaly, such as hypertension, atherosclerosis, or coronary artery disease. The increase in heart weight is secondary to fibrosis, presumably caused by the combination of anemia and papillary muscle infarction.[16] Additionally, patients receiving multiple blood transfusions may show myocardial iron deposition (hemosiderosis) that may contribute to such enlargement and to impairment of cardiac function. However, this complication occurs much less frequently in sickle cell anemia than in patients with thalassemia major.

Acute myocardial infarction is a rare complication of sickle cell disease, although more oxygen is extracted by the myocardium than by any other tissue.[17,18] While transmural infarction due to in situ thrombosis by sickled cells is rare, infarction of the papillary muscles of the heart commonly occurs, presumably explained by the fact that the papillary muscles are at the distal portion of the coronary circulation where collateral vessels are scant and hypoxia is marked.

The majority of patients with sickle cell anemia have an abnormal electrocardiogram, including left ventricular hypertrophy and first-degree atrioventricular (AV) block as well as nonspecific ST-segment and T-wave changes and abnormal septal Q waves.[12] Arrhythmias rarely occur in sickle cell patients between episodes of pain; continuous electrocardiographic monitoring during painful crises reveals both atrial and ventricular arrhythmias in the majority of patients. Echocardiographic measurements in patients with cardiac symptoms are useful in documenting both cardiac hyperactivity and depressed left ventricular performance.[13] With exercise, cardiac dysfunction may exhibit abnormal ejection fraction response.

Thalassemia Syndromes

The thalassemias are a group of inherited disorders caused by an imbalance in the synthesis of hemoglobin chains. α-Thalassemia is the result of absent or reduced synthesis of α-chain (a condition found mainly in Asians), and β-thalassemia represents an absence or reduction in β-chain synthesis. The homozygous form of β-thalassemia is also referred to as Cooley or Mediterranean anemia and is common in individuals of Greek and Italian descent. Heterozygous α- and β-thalassemias are also common in American blacks, particularly in association with sickle cell trait. Since the result in either type of thalassemia is decreased production of hemoglobin A (Hb A), the resultant hemoglobin-deficient red cells are both microcytic and hypochromic. In addition, the red cells are target-shaped and demonstrate basophilic stippling. A diagnosis of β-thalassemia is established by quantitative hemoglobin electrophoresis showing decreased levels of Hb A and elevated levels of Hb A_2 and fetal hemoglobin (Hb F). The anemia in homozygous β-thalassemia represents a combination of hemolysis and ineffective erythropoiesis.

The cardiac complications of heart failure and arrhythmias are the major cause of death in patients with thalassemia; they arise from a combination of chronic anemia and cardiac siderosis.[19] Iron overload arises from a combination of extravascular hemolysis, frequent transfusions, and inappropriately increased intestinal iron absorption. Although anemia undoubtedly contributes to cardiomegaly, iron overload of the heart is undoubtedly the principal cause of myocardial damage.[20,21] Patients with transfusion-dependent, chronic severe refractory thalassemia typically manifest serious cardiac involvement, usually by the second decade of life, with death occurring after a few months following the development of congestive heart failure; occasionally patients die suddenly, presumably secondary to arrhythmic events. At postmortem examination, iron is characteristically deposited in all viscera, including the hypertrophied heart, similar to hemochromatosis. Cardiac dysfunction depends on the quantity of iron deposited in the ventricles and is attributed to myocardial damage resulting from iron-induced release of acid hydrolases from lysosomes.

Pericarditis occurs in about one-half of all patients with thalassemia and often presents as recurrent fever, precordial pain, and electrocardiographic changes characteristic of acute pericarditis. The creation of a pericardial window may be required to relieve tamponade.

The chest x-ray may show cardiac enlargement, and echocardiographic assessment may disclose increased left ventricular end-diastolic, left atrial, and aortic root dimensions as well as a thickened left ventricular wall.[19] The electrocardiogram frequently shows left ventricular hypertrophy, nonspecific ST-segment and T-wave abnormalities, supraventricular or ventricular premature contractions, and first- or second-degree AV block. At cardiac catheterization, the usual findings comprise a normal or elevated cardiac index with moderate elevations in left ventricular end-diastolic pressure and volume and end-systolic volume with a reduced ejection fraction.[22]

Supportive therapy consists primarily of an adequate transfusion program (often hypertransfusion), splenectomy, and early treatment of infections. In children, cardiomegaly regresses when hemoglobin is maintained above 10 g/dl. In addition, chelating agents for both treatment and prevention of iron overload helps prolong life for many years (see below).

Effects of Polycythemia

Polycythemia, or erythrocytosis, includes a variety of conditions characterized by an increase in the concentration of blood red cells, as determined by hematocrit, hemoglobin, or red blood cell count.[23] Absolute polycythemias refer to conditions in which there is an absolute increase in red cell mass. They are subclassified as primary or secondary, depending on whether the elevation in red cell mass is autonomous (primary) or under hormonal (erythropoietin) control. Primary polycythemia (polycythemia vera) is a clonal myeloproliferative disorder.[24] Secondary polycythemia includes disorders arising from pathophysiologic hypoxia-induced erythropoietin secretion (i.e., cyanotic forms of congenital heart disease or pulmonary disease) and autonomous inappropriate increase in erythropoietin production (i.e., tumors and various renal diseases). Relative polycythemia refers to elevations in hematocrit, hemoglobin, or red cell counts, with normal red cell mass but reduced plasma volume.

Although the symptoms of secondary polycythemia depend on the underlying disease, they are also usually the result of increased blood volume and viscosity.[25] Viscosity increases exponentially with increased hematocrit. When flow rate through a capillary tube is determined at various levels of hematocrit, flow decreases essentially as a linear function of hematocrit (Fig. 8-2). The product of flow rate and arterial oxygen content provides a relative measure of the rate of oxygen transport through a single blood vessel. Optimal hematocrit is just below 40 percent. Delivery of oxygen to the body depends on the product of total blood flow and the oxygen content of arterial blood, which tends to be high in polycythemia vera, in which blood volume, cardiac output, and arterial blood oxygen content are all elevated, despite the increase in viscosity. Whereas the increases in oxygen content, blood volume, and cardiac output in polycythemia vera are not required for adequate tissue oxygenation, the increases in blood oxygen content and cardiac output in polycythemia secondary to hypoxemia improve oxygen delivery.

Polycythemia Vera

Polycythemia vera is classified as a myeloproliferative disorder because of the clonal nature of the disease process.[24] Since erythropoietin is not the stimulus for increased red cell production, erythropoietin production is suppressed in this condition.

The diagnosis of polycythemia vera is confirmed when erythrocytosis is accompanied by an increased red cell mass, arterial oxygen saturation greater than 92 percent, and splenomegaly.[26-28] In the absence of splenomegaly, any two of the following laboratory findings satisfy the diagnostic criteria: thrombocytosis, leukocytosis (absent infection); elevated leukocyte alkaline phosphatase activity, or a combination of elevated serum vitamin B_{12} concentration and unsaturated B_{12} binding capacity. Clinical manifestations may be divided into symptoms secondary to the increased red cell mass and increased blood volume, including headache, plethora, pruritus, dyspnea, and bleeding; those due to increased blood viscosity, including paresthesias and thrombosis; and those due to hypermetabolism, including weight loss (despite a good appetite) and night sweats. There

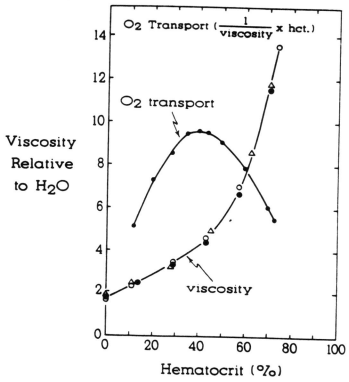

Fig. 8-2. Viscosity of heparinized normal blood related to hematocrit. Viscosity was measured with an Ostwald viscosimeter at 37°C and expressed in relation to viscosity of water. Oxygen transport was calculated from the product of hematocrit and 1/viscosity and is recorded in arbitrary units.

are also frequent occurrences of angina pectoris, intermittent claudication, and arterial hypertension.

Paradoxically, both bleeding and thrombosis complicate this disease and occur in about one-half of patients.[22,29] They are the major causes of morbidity and mortality. Bleeding is caused by the distention of veins and capillaries due to the increased blood volume, defective platelet function, or both. Thrombosis is attributed to increased blood viscosity, thrombocytosis, and abnormally increased aggregation of platelets. Thrombus formation develops in coronary and cerebral arteries as well as those in the

extremities. Less frequently, thrombosis may involve the mesenteric and portal veins. Surgical morbidity is high in patients with polycythemia vera who are inadequately treated, and anesthesia and the stress of operation amplify the risk of hemorrhagic and thrombotic events during the immediate postoperative period.

The overall clinical severity of polycythemia is usually related to the degree of hypervolemia and hyperviscosity.[30] In older patients with underlying atherosclerotic vascular disease, the incidence of ischemic episodes may be higher, although cardiac output is usually not elevated. Since in vitro studies show that white blood cells also contribute to blood viscosity and because leukocytosis is characteristic of polycythemia vera, the elevated viscosity seen in this disease may be attributable to these cells.[30]

In approximately one-half of the patients with hematocrits averaging 54 percent, cerebral blood flow is significantly reduced and is associated with cerebral symptoms, reflecting the reciprocal relationship between cerebrovascular insufficiency and blood viscosity.[27] When hematocrit is reduced to approximately 45 percent, viscosity declines by nearly one-third, and cerebral blood flow increases substantially. Indeed, with hematocrit values ranging from 46 to 52 percent, cerebral blood flow is less than normal. These results imply that patients with polycythemia vera should undergo phlebotomy until hematocrit levels reach the low 40s, rather than the previously recommended level of about 45 percent.

Therapy is directed toward decreasing the potential for both hemorrhage and thrombosis and often consists of phlebotomy alone. However, in order to control thrombocytosis, hydroxyurea is generally used, although anagrelide will probably become the drug of choice because of its specificity for platelet effects.[31]

Secondary Polycythemia

The secondary polycythemias are divided into two subgroups: (1) those in which the increased red cell mass compensates for a reduction in oxygen transport with appropriate stimulation by erythropoietin, and (2) those in which erythrocytosis is associated with an inappropriate increase in erythropoietin production. Hypoxia stimulates the production of erythrogenin by the kidney, which gives rise to erythropoietin via enzymatic conversion of a putative plasma protein substrate, possibly of hepatic origin. If an individual living at sea level is transported to a high altitude, plasma erythropoietin increases and hemoglobin concentrations will rise, with secondary elevated levels of urinary erythropoietin.[32] Similarly, severe chronic hypoxemia in chronic obstructive pulmonary disease, with arterial PO_2 less than 60 mmHg, stimulates erythropoietin production, producing an increase in red cell mass. However, in most patients with chronic pulmonary disease, hemoglobin values do not exceed 17 g/dl, and hematocrit does not rise above 57 percent, although values as high as 24 g/dl and 75 percent, respectively, have been reported.[33] In cyanotic congenital heart disease, red cell mass increases reciprocally as resting arterial oxygen saturation falls. Hematocrits as high as 86 percent, almost three times normal,[34] may be seen with red blood cell masses. Although plasma volume may be diminished, total blood volume remains significantly elevated because of the striking increase in red cell mass. Tetralogy of Fallot, transposition of the great arteries, and persistent truncus arteriosus are typical congenital defects resulting in these striking changes.

Signs and symptoms of hyperviscosity accompany elevations in hematocrit above 60 percent. Unfortunately, cardiac function may be compromised by the combination of hypervolemia and the constant volume load and augmented vascular resistance consequent to the increased viscosity of the blood. Ruddy cyanosis, headache, dizziness, roaring in the ears, thrombotic episodes, and bleeding are the major clinical findings; these symptoms are successfully treated by phlebotomy. Careful monitoring during phlebotomy is necessary, and the effects of acute reduction in blood volume are minimized by the simultaneous administration of plasma expanders.[35] After isovolemic phlebotomy to reduce the hematocrit from the 70s to the 60s, cardiac output increases, and despite the fall in arterial oxygen content, systemic oxygen transport usually improves. These favorable changes are attributable to decreases in blood viscosity and vascular resistance. Thus, while erythrocytosis reflects a homeostatic mechanism compensating for chronic arterial hypoxemia, marked increases in hematocrit may actually impair overall oxygen transport.[36] Secondary polycythemia due to cyanotic congenital heart disease has been reported to cause myocardial infarction in the absence of coronary atherosclerosis.[37]

Phlebotomy, or preferably erythropheresis, in secondary polycythemia reduces blood viscosity, increases systemic oxygen transport without lowering compromising peripheral oxygen consumption, and simultaneously increases effective renal plasma flow.[38,39] The optimal hematocrit for patients with cyanotic congenital heart disease and other chronically hypoxemic states is poorly defined and presents an interesting and perplexing dilemma, requiring careful evaluation of the presenting symptoms. Cerebral blood flow is reduced in secondary erythrocytosis as well as in polycythemia vera and improves with phlebotomy.[40] If phlebotomy is deemed necessary, close monitoring of the patient's blood pressure, heart rate, arterial oxygen saturation, and general condition is necessary. As might be expected from the decreased oxygen transport associated with right-to-left shunts, P_{50} and red cell 2,3-DPG are increased, but the relationship between decreased arterial PO_2 and the rise in P_{50} and red cell 2,3-DPG varies greatly. Successful surgical correction of the underlying cardiac defect obviates the need for compensatory erythrocytosis, and hematocrit and blood volume are returned to normal.

Hemoglobin variants with increased oxygen affinity give rise to erythrocytosis.[41,42] These variants generally have amino acid substitutions at structural sites crucial to hemoglobin function, and are transmitted in an autosomal dominant fashion. These mutants cause a shift in the oxygen dissociation curve to the left with reduced levels of P_{50}. The shift to the left of the hemoglobin-oxygen dissociation curve reduces oxygen extraction by the tissues. Oxygen delivery is maintained by increasing hemoglobin concentration and blood flow. However, the primary compensating response appears to be secondary erythrocytosis.[43] Cardiac output is usually normal. Polycythemia compensates effectively in patients with hemoglobin variants to ensure adequate oxygen delivery in the absence of myocardial ischemia or other forms of organ hypoxia.

True erythrocytosis without demonstrable cause, other than excessive cigarette smoking, occurs in a significant number of individuals exhibiting increased levels of carboxyhemoglobin and shifts of the hemoglobin-oxygen dissociation curve to the left.[44] In most cases of polycythemia secondary to inappropriate erythropoietin production (e.g., tumors, renal cysts, and hydronephrosis), the red cell mass does not generally cause symptoms of hyperviscosity despite measurable increases.

Relative Polycythemia

Relative polycythemia is a distinct and commonly encountered entity alternatively referred to as spurious polycythemia or stress erythrocytosis. It is not a primary disease process but a physiologic state characterized by slightly reduced plasma volume and slightly increased red cell mass.[42] Hematocrit rarely exceeds 60 percent, and other cellular blood elements are normal. This disorder is differentiated from polycythemia vera by measuring the red cell mass, which is normal in relative polycythemia and elevated in polycythemia vera. Patients are often hypertensive, likely to have thromboembolic complications, and obese.[26,27,45] Since these complications do not appear to reflect the hematologic changes, it is not appropriate to reduce the red cell mass by phlebotomy or chemotherapy. When present, hypertension and thromboembolic complications should be treated independently of the stress erythrocytosis.

Mechanical Fragmentation Hemolysis

Direct mechanical destruction of red cells leading to chronic anemia may arise from (1) diseased heart valves,[46,47] (2) mechanical heart valves,[48,49] (3) other intracardiac or intravascular prostheses,[50,51] (4) hypertrophic obstructive cardiomyopathy,[52] coarctation of the aorta, (6) ruptured aneurysms of sinus of Valsalva, or (7) postoperative complication of mitral valvulotomy or repairs of tetralogy of Fallot. Characteristically, microangiopathic red cell changes are present in the peripheral blood films, consisting of fragmented red cells, burr cells, and schistocytes.[50] Red cell survival studies confirm that the half-life of both donor and autologous red cells are shortened, indicating an extrinsic red cell defect. Intravascular hemolysis may be evidenced by the presence of free hemoglobin in plasma and urine if destruction is severe. The amount of iron excreted in the urine (hemosiderinuria) is the most reliable measure of the rate at which red cells are being destroyed. Intravascular red cell destruction induces compensatory increases in red cell production, as shown by elevations in the reticulocyte count and marrow erythroid hyperplasia.

Turbulence is the most common feature of fragmentation hemolytic anemias secondary to valvular disease and cardiac surgery. For example, after insertion of a prosthetic valve, perivalvular regurgitation will increase the stroke volume and therefore the turbulence of flow through the narrowed orifice. Experiments in vitro demonstrate that shearing stresses in excess of 3,000 dyne/cm^2 disrupt red cells, causing hemolysis. Such degrees of stress may readily develop with perivalvular leaks, regurgitant jets from the aorta to the left ventricle, and situations involving the relatively small flow channel of aortic valve prosthesis compared with the stroke volume or a relatively large ball value compared with the diameter of the aorta.[53] Similar phenomena occur after implanting prosthetic mitral valves. Chronic intravascular hemolytic anemia in the presence of hypertrophic cardiomyopathy is probably secondary to abnormal turbulence associated with the underlying cardiac disease. Definitive treatment of the hemolytic process consists of surgical repair of the cardiac abnormality (i.e., either replacement or correction of the prosthesis or correction of the perivalvular leak). If a patient is not readily operable, rest improves the condition by decreasing the rate of red cell fragmentation, and iron and folate replacement will help sustain the increased red cell production.

DISORDERS OF IRON METABOLISM

Effects of Iron Deficiency on Cellular Performance

In addition to anemia, iron deficiency produces disturbances in cellular metabolism and function in many tissues, including the heart.[54–56] Iron deficiency is defined as a decrease in the content of iron in the body. The earliest stage of iron deficiency is iron depletion, in which storage iron is decreased or absent, but serum iron concentration and blood hemoglobin levels are normal. Iron deficiency without anemia is a more advanced stage of iron deficiency, characterized by decreased or absent storage iron, low serum iron concentration, and transferrin saturation, without frank anemia. More advanced iron deficiency causes iron deficiency anemia, which is characterized by decreased or absent iron stores, low serum iron concentration, low transferrin saturation, and low hemoglobin concentration or hematocrit value. Iron deficiency may be caused by inadequate dietary iron intake, malabsorption of iron, chronic blood loss, diversion of iron to fetal and infant erythropoiesis during pregnancy and lactation, intravascular hemolysis with hemoglobinuria, or a combination of these causes.

Additional changes arise as other tissues in the body become depleted of iron. The activity of many other important iron proteins (cytochrome c, cytochrome oxidase, succinic dehydrogenase, aconitase, xanthine oxidase, and myoglobin is decreased.[57,58] Reduced activity has also been reported for some enzymes that do not contain or require iron. Many affected enzymes are required for oxidative glycolysis (Krebs cycle) in the mitochondria.[59] Accordingly, the activities of several mitochondrial matrix enzymes may be increased in skeletal muscle of iron-deficient animals, presumably as an adaptive response. For example, dysfunction in the nervous system occurs with iron deficiency, as suggested by the fact that some iron-deficient patients complain of paresthesias, and other neurologic manifestations.[54] Other neurophysiologic aberrations have been ascribed to iron deficiency in adults. These include asymmetries in electroencephalographic recording and ST-T segment changes in electrocardiograms obtained during treadmill tests.

There is no doubt that iron deficiency anemia results in deceased muscular work capacity.[55,56,58,60] Numerous metabolic processes require iron-containing enzymes such as cytochrome c, α-glycerophosphate oxidase, NADH cytochrome c reductase, succinic cytochrome c reductase, succinic dehydrogenase, and NADH ferricyanide oxidoreductase. There is evidence that these enzymes may be depleted to levels that prevent adequate oxidative metabolism before iron deficiency anemia occurs and impairs oxygen delivery. Finch et al.[55,56] showed, and others have since confirmed,[58] that profound tissue iron deficiency greatly compromises exercise performance despite transfusion-restored peripheral red cell concentration. Energy transport pathways of submitochondrial particles of liver and skeletal muscle show the skeletal muscle to be less sensitive to iron depletion than the liver.[59] In addition to these metabolic aberrations of muscle cells in iron deficiency, ultrastructural studies show swollen mitochondria with distorted cristae.[60] Subsequently, "nonanemic" hypoferritinemic athletes with normal hemoglobin concentrations have been administered therapeutic iron while measuring athletic performance.[60] The supplemental iron increases the ferritin levels and improves athletic performance. Although controlled clinical trials have yet to be carried out, these data support the practice of including supplemental iron in the management of iron-deficient patients with cardiac failure, in addition to restoring red cell mass by transfusions and administering diuretics.

Effects of Iron Overload

Bodily iron stores characteristically increase in a number of disease states. When significant amounts of iron accumulate in different organs, including the myocardium, liver, pancreas, and gonads, they become dysfunctional.[61] Insofar as the heart is concerned, myocardial deposits of iron may lead to congestive heart failure, conduction disturbances, and arrhythmias. Significant siderosis is most often encountered in patients with idiopathic hemochromatosis or in anemic patients with large and long-standing transfusion requirements.

In idiopathic hemochromatosis, excessively large quantities of iron are absorbed from the gastrointestinal tract. This inherited disorder, which develops slowly and has a variable clinical expression, depends partially upon environmental factors, such as the magnitude of dietary iron intake, alcohol intake, and the severity of any underlying liver disease. HLA subtyping suggests a recessive mode of transmission linked to chromosome 6, and has been helpful in distinguishing idiopathic hemochromatosis from iron overload secondary to liver disease.[62,63]

Clinical manifestations of hemochromatosis occur more frequently in men than in women. The disease rarely manifests before individuals are 20 years old and reaches its peak when they are in their forties. Diabetes is the most common initial manifestation, occurring in one-half the patients. The classic clinical presentation includes increased pigmentation of the skin, hepatomegaly, and cardiac dysfunction. Loss of libido and other endocrinopathies, such as hypopituitarism, may also develop. Cellular damage has been attributed to iron-induced release of lysosomal acid hydrolases.

The frequency of cardiac symptoms increases with time.[62,63] Dyspnea, edema, and ascites are noted early in the course in 15 to 20 percent of the patients, but about one-third eventually develop symptoms referable to the heart, and approximately the same proportion of patients eventually die of cardiac failure. Arrhythmias are common and include paroxysmal atrial tachycardia and flutter, chronic atrial fibrillation, and frequent premature ventricular contractions. Varying degrees of AV block have also been noted. Heart block and arrhythmias are often associated with iron deposits in the AV node and supraventricular arrhythmias with deposits in the atria. Low-voltage and nonspecific T-wave changes are also frequently present.

Radiographic studies in symptomatic patients usually reveal a globular heart with biventricular enlargement and weak pulsations. Some patients may have elevated right ventricular and right atrial pressures, consequent to the restrictive cardiomyopathy and secondary to iron deposition in the myocardium, as well as involvement of the pericardium itself.[64]

Transfusional hemosiderosis may become a clinical problem in patients with severe chronic anemia who survive long enough to accumulate toxic quantities of iron from transfused blood; each milliliter of transfused red cells contains 1 mg of iron. Thus, patients with thalassemia, other serious chronic refractory anemias, myeloid metaplasia, pure red cell aplasia, and aplasia anemia readily accumulate 50 g of iron from transfusions, which results in clinical problems similar to those encountered in idiopathic hemochromatosis.[61] For example, children with β-thalassemia major maintained by hypertransfusion are generally spared the cardiac consequences of severe anemia, but ultimately die of heart failure as a consequence of myocardial siderosis. In adults with chronic anemias, cardiac iron deposition secondary to transfusional hemosiderosis may contribute to cardiovascular disability, which is often incorrectly attributed to high-output heart failure. The combination of impaired cardiac function secondary to iron deposition and the increased cardiac demands of persistent, incompletely treated anemia imposes a double burden on the heart.[65,66]

In a review of hearts studied at autopsy, grossly visible iron deposits in the heart are accompanied by a prior history of cardiac dysfunction, including chronic heart failure.[67] Deposits are extensive in patients with idiopathic hemochromatosis and in patients who receive more than 100 units of blood without evidence of equivalent blood loss.[68] In patients with cardiac hemosiderosis, histologic examination reveals that the ventricular free wall and septum contain heavier deposits than the atrial wall. The quantity of iron in the different areas of the ventricular myocardium is variable, with the epicardium and papillary muscles containing the most iron, the subendocardium containing intermediate amounts, and the midmyocardium and conduction tissue containing the least.

It is often difficult to determine whether myocardial dysfunction results from chronic anemia or hemosiderosis. With the use of atomic absorption spectrophotometry, the exact concentrations of iron may be measured in various body organs or tissues. Rarely is iron deposition limited to the heart. Since the liver is easily accessible by biopsy and its iron concentration is closely related to that in the myocardium, liver biopsy is a useful procedure to establish the diagnosis of myocardial siderosis. In some patients, echocardiography may detect early left ventricular dysfunction prior to the development of symptoms. In a group of patients with severe β-thalassemia or transfusion-dependent anemias without clinical cardiac symptoms, left ventricular dysfunction may be measured by radionuclide angiography during exercise but not at rest.[66,67] Noninvasive assessment of the left ventricular end-systolic pressure-dimension relation (using a methoxamine challenge) detects preclinical left ventricular dysfunction not evident on resting or dynamic exercise studies and not due to chronic anemia per se.

This technique may be a sensitive means of monitoring therapeutic response to iron overload.

Reversal of the iron overload is indicated because the majority of patients with myocardial siderosis will ultimately die of irreversible cardiac failure and arrhythmias without therapy. In patients with idiopathic hemochromatosis, it is possible to mobilize iron stores by repeated phlebotomies, which is the preferred mode of therapy.[69,70] Decreases in hepatic iron stores and fibrosis, improvement of liver function, amelioration of diabetes, and reversal of cardiomyopathy will follow such treatment if initiated before irreversible changes develop. Since the average patient with idiopathic hemochromatosis has 20 to 40 g of stored iron, weekly to bimonthly phlebotomies must be continued for several years. Although the hematocrit will initially drop, it will return toward normal as weekly phlebotomies are continued. Removal of excess body iron by phlebotomy has been possible in patients with hematocrits as low as 30 percent.

The distribution of iron in the tissues differs somewhat between individuals with idiopathic hemochromatosis and those with transfusion siderosis, since transfused patients have relatively more iron stored in the reticuloendothelial cells. However, repeated transfusion in such patients produces organ dysfunction similar to that found in idiopathic hemochromatosis.[66,68] Obviously, phlebotomy is not a therapeutic alternative in managing iron overload caused by chronic blood transfusions for anemia. Chelation therapy is the only approach available for removing iron in anemic patients. Desferrioxamine is the most widely used iron chelator.[71–73] This hydroxamic acid compound has a very high affinity for trivalent iron. It must be administered parenterally, and most of the chelated iron will be excreted in the

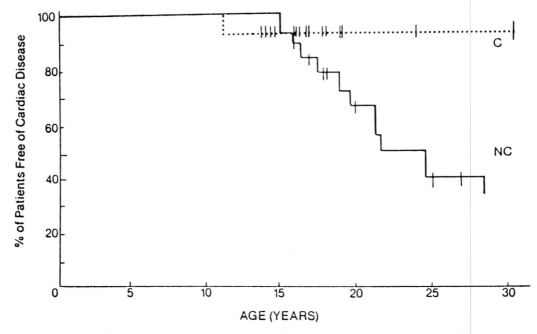

Fig. 8-3. Life-table depiction of survival free of cardiac disease in patients with thalassemia major treated with desferrioxamine. Dotted line represents the compliant group (C) and solid line represents the noncompliant group (NC). The vertical slashes represent the current ages of patients still free of cardiac disease. (From Wolfe et al.,[71] with permission.)

urine within 4 hours of the injection. Intramuscular desferrioxamine does not sustain negative iron balance without the addition of oral ascorbic acid, which doubles iron excretion. Ascorbic acid loading in combination with continuous subcutaneous administration of desferrioxamine, achieves a negative iron balance in children with thalassemia. Unfortunately, ascorbate supplementation in patients with iron overload may be hazardous. For example, clinical cardiotoxicity manifested as fatal congestive heart failure and arrhythmias occurs in patients treated simultaneously with ascorbic acid and desferrioxamine. Not only does ascorbate make more cellular iron available for chelation, but it also liberates free intracellular iron, generating membrane-damaging free oxygen. The adverse effects of ascorbate may be prevented by adding this agent after the

patient has been started on chelation therapy.

Long-term desferrioxamine iron chelation therapy is effective not only in delaying organ damage caused by transfusional iron overload, but also in reversing it (Fig. 8-3). In children with thalassemia major, regular treatment with iron chelation appears to protect from the development of cardiac disease induced by iron overload.

DISORDERS PREDISPOSING TO THROMBOSIS

Patients predisposed to thrombosis are grouped into inherited and acquired categories (Table 8-1).[74,75] The group of inherited thrombotic disorders comprises

Table 8-1.   Disorders Predisposing
to Thrombosis

Inherited
  Antithrombin III deficiency
  Protein C deficiency
  Protein S deficiency
  Dysfibrinogenemias
  Inherited abnormalities of fibrinolysis
  Heparin cofactor II deficiency
  Homocystinemia

Acquired
  Cardiac abnormalities
  Lupus anticoagulant
  Thrombocytosis
  Activated constituents of blood
  Risk factors for thrombosis

specific defects in one of the major natural anticoagulant mechanisms, including vascular heparin sulfate-antithrombin III, protein C-thrombomodulin-protein S, and plasminogen-plasminogen activator mechanisms. The second category consists of heterogeneous clinical conditions exhibiting increased risk for the development of thrombotic complications as compared with the general population. These prothrombotic conditions include lupus anticoagulant syndrome, atherosclerosis, malignancy, postpartum state, nephrotic syndrome, myeloproliferative disorders, paroxysmal nocturnal hemoglobinuria, immobilization, postoperative state, obesity, advancing age, prosthetic valves, artificial surfaces, hyperviscosity, thrombotic thrombocytopenic purpura, oral contraceptive or estrogen therapy, and heparin-induced platelet activation/destruction.

Kinetic studies using labeled platelets and fibrinogen demonstrate significant distinctions between arterial and venous thrombogenesis.[76] The important role of platelets in the thrombotic process in patients with ongoing arterial thromboembolism is shown as selective platelet consumption (i.e., shortened platelet survival and increased platelet turnover

without increased turnover of circulating fibrinogen). Ongoing venous thrombosis, however, manifests kinetically as increased turnover of both platelets and fibrinogen at equal rates, since venous thrombogenesis reflects thrombus formation under static or low shear flow conditions. The nature of the thrombus, therefore, has therapeutic implications [i.e., fibrin formation in venous thrombosis is effectively inhibited by anticoagulants (heparin or warfarin)], but arterial thrombi may be prevented by agents that block platelet activation.

Thrombogenesis

Vascular endothelium generates an array of molecules that regulate interactions of circulating blood cells and plasma factors with constituents of the vessel wall (Fig. 8-4). Maladaptive modulation of these endothelial-dependent regulatory pathways may lead to vascular thrombus formation, vascular inflammatory processes, and vascular lesion formation.

Following denuding, arterial injury platelets and plasma coagulation factors rapidly interact with exposed subendothelial connective tissue structures under high-flow conditions, leading to the formation of localized mechanical thrombotic masses in flow-dependent patterns variably composed of deposited platelets, insoluble fibrin, leukocytes, and entrapped erythrocytes. Thrombus formation remains localized to the site of vascular injury because of (1) multiple protease inhibitor systems in plasma, including antithrombin III and (2) modulating inhibitory pathways involving elements in blood and the vessel wall, including thrombomodulin.

Platelets initially attach to subendothelial connective tissue structures and subsequently spread, expressing functional receptors for adhesive molecules (pri-

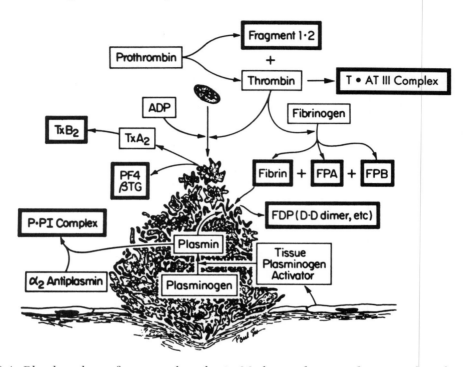

Fig. 8-4. Blood markers of ongoing thrombosis. Markers indicative of ongoing thrombosis are shown in the bold boxes. These include the amino-terminal half of prothrombin (fragment 1 · 2) from thrombin generation, thrombin/antithrombin III complex, or the effects of thrombin on platelet release stimulation of β-thromboglobulin (βTG) or platelet factor 4 (PF4). Platelet reactivity can be further documented by measuring plasma levels of the more stable metabolite, thromboxane B_2. Blood levels of fibrinopeptides A and B reflect the proteolysis of fibrinogen by thrombin, and soluble fibrin monomers can also be detected. As the result of fibrinolysis, circulating levels of plasmin-α_2-antiplasmin complex (P-PI) as well as specific fibrin degradation products (FDP) can be shown. With the exception of the Bβ form of fibrinopeptide B, which is found after plasmin degradation of the amino-terminal portion of the Bβ-chain of fibrinogen (following thrombin cleavage of the Aα-chain), other tests cannot distinguish between thrombin formation in disseminated intravascular coagulation and ongoing thrombotic disorders. ADP, adenosine diphosphate; FPA, fibrinopeptide A; FPB, fibrinopeptide B; T·AT III, thrombin/antithrombin III; TF, tissue factor; TxA_2, thromboxane A_2; TxB_2, thromboxane B_2.

marily fibrinogen), resulting in cohesion with ambient platelets. This self-amplifying process of platelet recruitment is mediated by three independent, yet interrelated agonists: (1) thrombin, generated on phospholipid platelet surfaces, activates platelet thrombin receptors by a novel catalytic mechanism; (2) adenosine diphosphate (ADP), secreted from storage granules of activated platelets, initi-ates receptor signaling of ambient platelets; and (3) thromboxane A_2, arising via platelet arachidonic acid metabolic pathways, induces receptor activation. At sites of vascular injury, thrombin is the principal mediator of platelet recruitment. The membranes of adherent activated platelets provide efficient and localizing phospholipid surfaces for the amplified generation of thrombin via the assembly of interactive enzyme-cofactor complexes.

Thrombin also initiates endothelial-dependent protective mechanisms that prevent the unrestricted extension of thrombus formation beyond the site of vascular injury. These antithrombotic mechanisms include (1) the inactivation of coagulation cofactors Va and VIIIa by activated protein C (APC) and its cofactor protein S, which prevents further thrombin generation; (2) the release of endothelial antiaggregatory products, prostacyclin and nitric oxide; and (3) the release of endothelial tissue plasminogen activator, which enhances local thrombolysis. Finally, excess thrombin escaping into the circulation is inactivated by inhibitor-enzyme complex formation (thrombin: antithrombin III) catalyzed by endothelial heparin-like glycosaminoglycans and thrombomodulin.

Thus, the site, size, and composition of forming thrombi are determined by (1) mechanical hemodynamic blood flow effects, (2) extent and type of exposed intimal thrombogenic elements, (3) concentrations and reactivity of responding plasma and cellular blood constituents, and (4) effectiveness of the physiologic protective mechanisms. Subsequent removal of the thrombus proceeds by gradual fibrinolysis and healing responses.

Molecules synthesized by vascular endothelial cells that exhibit known antithrombotic effects include (1) prostacyclin, (2) nitric oxide, (3) thrombomodulin, (4) heparin-like glycosaminoglycans, (5) tissue plasminogen activator, and (6) ectoenzymes. Since the generation of these protective molecules is impaired when endothelium becomes dysfunctional as a consequence of disease or the administration of various pharmacologic agents, the risk of thrombotic or thromboembolic complications may increase. The most important mechanisms for limiting thrombus formation are related to the in-

activation of thrombin activity, the reduction in thrombin production, and the thrombin-stimulated production of antithrombotic and vasodilating factors of intact endothelium.

Molecules synthesized by vascular endothelial cells that exhibit known prothrombotic effects include (1) tissue factor (TF), (2) plasminogen activator inhibitor-1 and -2 (PAI-I and PAI-2), and (3) von Willebrand factor (vWF). Inflammation is characterized by the sequential attachment of blood neutrophils, monocytes, and lymphocytes to, and transmigration through, endothelium subserving inflammatory sites with the subsequent infiltration and localization of inflammatory cells.[77–80] The stimulated endothelium expresses specific adhesive molecules that bind with counterreceptors expressed on stimulated blood leukocytes. Monocytes and lymphocytes may produce TF and cytokines that may participate in thrombotic responses associated with inflammatory processes. The molecules generated by endothelium that mediate inflammatory responses that may contribute to thrombotic outcomes include (1) E-selectin and P-selectin, (2) intercellular adhesion molecules 1 and 2 (ICAM-1 and ICAM-2), (3) vascular cell adhesion molecule (VCAM), and (4) leukocyte-activating cytokines, including interleukin-1 (IL-1), tumor necrosis factor (TNF), IL-8, and platelet activating factor (PAF).

Blood tests of ongoing thrombosis in vivo that detect fibrin formation, fibrinolysis, and platelet release have been developed (Fig. 8-4). Two platelet-specific proteins have been studied as markers of platelet activation: β-thromboglobulin and platelet factor 4.[7] These proteins are localized in the α-granules of resting platelets, and approximately 70 percent are released during platelet activation. Although sensitive radioimmunoassays for these platelet-specific proteins are commercially available, care must be taken in drawing blood and in preparing the blood samples for assay to prevent artifactual release of these proteins during blood collection and processing. Failure to comply with these rigorous conditions produces artifactually elevated and variable plasma levels.

Fibrinopeptide A (FPA) is increased in patients with venous thrombosis and pulmonary embolism. This test is sensitive to intravascular thrombin but is not entirely specific for intravascular thrombosis, since positive results are also found in patients with cellulitis and with generalized infections, indicating that FPA is derived from extravascular microvascular thrombosis located at sites of infection and inflammation.

Prothrombin activation fragment F1.2 circulates in humans under normal conditions and is detectably elevated in various thrombotic syndromes. Similarly, levels of thrombin-antithrombin complex, fibrinopeptide A, and protein C activation peptide are also increased in patients with disseminated intravascular coagulation, deep-vein thrombosis, and pulmonary emboli.

Assays for the detection of plasmin-antiplasmin complex and D-dimer in plasma have been developed. The D-dimer assay may be particularly useful in monitoring the effects of thrombolytic agents in patients with thromboembolic disease.

At present, these blood tests of ongoing thrombus formation are useful primarily for monitoring the effects of therapy, with less certain interpretation in identifying individual patients at risk.

Effects of Inherited Prothrombotic Disorders

The frequency of an inherited basis for a thrombotic disorder has been evaluated in several cross-sectional investigations of thrombotic patients with a positive family history or a personal history of spontaneous venous thrombosis. In such unrelated patients under age 45, deficiencies of protein C and protein S comprise 4 and 5 percent, respectively. Deficiencies of antithrombin III, identifiable plasminogen, and fibrinogen abnormalities constitute 3, 2, and 1 percent, respectively. Thus, with currently available tests, a diagnosis of a specific hereditary disorder can be identified in 10 to 20 percent of young patients presenting with a documented prior episode of venous thromboembolism (Fig. 8-5). Those clinical features suggesting the presence of one of these disorders and prompting laboratory evaluation, include thrombosis occurring at an early age, a family history of thrombotic disease, thrombosis occurring at unusual sites (for example, mesenteric venous thrombosis, cerebral venous thrombosis), or recurrent thrombosis without apparent precipitating factors. Most individuals with thrombophilia in association with congenital deficiencies of the proteins of the natural anticoagulant mechanisms (e.g., antithrombin III, protein C, protein S) primarily develop venous thromboembolic disease (Fig. 8-5). The relative absence of arterial thromboses in these disorders is attributed to the dependence of venous thrombosis on stasis and changes in blood constituents and association of arterial thrombosis with platelets and local vascular injury.

When a patient with an inherited thrombotic disorder is discovered, family studies should be conducted because almost one-half of the members of a given kindred may be affected, and these individuals should receive counseling regarding the implications of the diagnosis, as well as advice regarding the types of symptoms that require immediate medical attention. In view of the increased thrombotic risk associated with the use of oral contraceptives or estrogen, these medications are contraindicated in

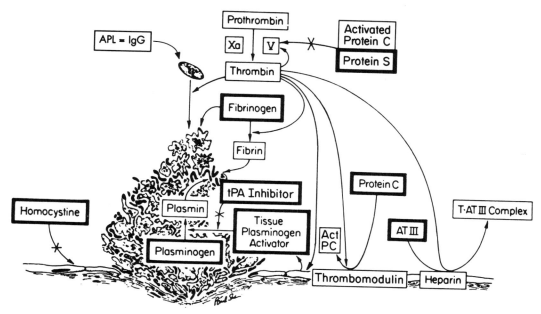

Fig. 8-5. Prothrombotic mechanisms of inherited deficiencies. Kindreds with various abnormalities affecting thrombus formation and its regulation have a predisposition to thrombosis. Established inherited disorders are identified by the bold boxes. tPA, tissue plasminogen activator; APL·IgG, antiphospholipid antibodies, T·AT III complex, thrombin/antithrombin III complex.

women. All biochemically affected persons should be carefully evaluated before undergoing surgical, medical, or obstetric procedures that carry an increased thrombotic risk, and they should be placed on appropriate prophylactic anticoagulation regimens. If specific concentrates are available for patients with particular deficiency states, they can be given to raise the plasma levels of the protein to the normal range during the perioperative period. All women with previous thrombotic episodes should receive prophylactic anticoagulation throughout pregnancy; asymptomatic women should generally receive such treatment as well.

In patients with an inherited thrombotic disorder who have experienced two or more spontaneously occurring thromboembolic episodes, treatment with oral anticoagulants should continue for life.

Chronic warfarin therapy is generally not recommended until a patient has had at least one documented thrombotic episode.

Inherited deficiencies of antithrombin III, protein C, and protein S may be responsible for thrombophilia, but the rates of thrombosis probably represent overestimates due to diagnostic biases and reporting biases for subjects from families with the most severe thrombotic diatheses. Furthermore, some of the reported episodes of venous thrombosis have not been confirmed by objective tests. Because future events in an asymptomatic patient or in a patient with only one prior thrombotic episode cannot currently be predicted with certainty, and because there is a risk of bleeding associated with warfarin therapy, recommendations relating to long-term anticoagulation must be individualized. The clinical features to be considered in making such decisions include (1) number, sites, and severity of the thromboses; (2) spontaneous or precipitated presentation; (3) sex and life-style of the patient; and (4) the history of thromboembolism in other biochemically affected members of the family.

Antithrombin III Deficiency

Antithrombin III deficiency is inherited in an autosomal dominant pattern and affects both sexes equally.[81-89] The true prevalence of antithrombin III deficiency in the general population ranges from approximately 1 in 2,000 to 1 in 5,000.[88,89] Approximately one-half of the biochemically affected patients experience at least one thrombotic event, but rarely before puberty, and the number of patients reporting such events increases as they reach the age of 50.[84-86] Usually, the initial clinical manifestation is spontaneous deep vein thrombosis of the leg, the iliofemoral veins, or the mesenteric veins. About two-thirds of patients develop recurrent thrombotic episodes, and clinical signs of pulmonary embolism are evident in approximately one-third.

Two major types of inherited antithrombin III deficiency have been delineated.[86-88] The classic deficiency state (type I) is a result of the reduced synthesis of biologically normal protease inhibitor molecules. In these instances, the immunologic and biologic activity of antithrombin III is equivalently reduced, and the molecular basis of this disorder is attributable to either a complete deletion of the entire gene, nonsense mutations, or base substitutions at splice sites. The second type of antithrombin III deficiency represents a defective protease inhibitor (type II). Under these circumstances, the plasma levels of antithrombin III are reduced, as judged by biologic activity measurements, whereas the immunologic determinations of this inhibitor are normal.

The mean concentration of antithrombin III in normal pooled plasma is approximately 140 μg/ml. In the plasma from normal patients, the range of antithrombin III concentrations as determined by immunologic or functional tests is quite narrow, 80 to 120 percent for cofactor activity and a slightly wider range for immunoassay results. Because of the various subtypes of the familial deficiency state that might be encountered, the best single screening test for the disorder is the antithrombin III-heparin cofactor assay. Healthy newborns have about one-half the normal adult concentration and gradually attain the adult level by 6 months of age. The levels may be considerably lower in premature infants.

A variety of pathophysiologic conditions reduce the concentration of antithrombin III within the blood. Although acute thrombosis does not characteristically decrease antithrombin III levels, reductions in antithrombin III levels are commonly found in patients with disseminated intravascular coagulation (DIC), liver disease (due to decreased protein synthesis), the nephrotic syndrome (because of urinary excretion), and estrogen therapy, including women receiving oral contraceptives. Infusions of L-asparaginase, a chemotherapeutic agent employed in the treatment of acute lymphocytic leukemia, substantially reduces the plasma concentration of this inhibitor.[90] In addition, the administration of heparin significantly decreases plasma antithrombin III levels, presumably on the basis of accelerated clearance of the inhibitor in vivo.[91] Accordingly, evaluation of plasma samples from patients suspected of having congenital antithrombin III deficiency during a period of heparinization may lead to an erroneous diagnosis of the disorder.

Because of the number of clinical conditions associated with acquired reductions in the plasma concentration of antithrombin III, definitive diagnosis of the hereditary deficiency state is often difficult in the setting of the acute thrombosis. While an antithrombin III level within the normal range obtained upon clinical presentation is usually sufficient to exclude the presence of the disorder, low levels should be confirmed by a second determination. This determination is ideally performed when the patient is no longer receiving oral anticoagulants, as these medications have been reported to raise plasma antithrombin III concentrations into the normal range in patients with the hereditary deficiency state;[92] clinical assessment as to the patient's risk of recurrent thrombosis will determine whether this approach is feasible. In most antithrombin III-deficient subjects, however, oral anticoagulants do not obscure the diagnosis. Confirmation of the hereditary nature of the disorder requires investigation of other family members. Diagnosis of other biochemically affected family members also allows for appropriate counseling regarding the need for prophylaxis against venous thrombosis.

These patients are treated successfully for venous thrombotic events with intravenous heparin. High doses of heparin may be required to achieve adequate anticoagulation, and the diagnosis of antithrombin deficiency is in the differential diagnosis of heparin resistance. In antithrombin III-deficient patients receiving heparin for the treatment of acute thrombosis, the adjunctive role of antithrombin III concentrate is not established since controlled trials have not been performed. The indications for thrombolytic therapy in heterozygous antithrombin III-deficient patients are similar to those in other populations with acute venous thromboembolic episodes.

Antithrombin III-deficient subjects may be treated with human antithrombin III concentrates before major surgery or in obstetric cases in which the risk of bleeding in the presence of full anticoagulation is deemed unacceptable.[93–95] Antithrombin III concentrate is more than 95 percent pure, and the viruses responsible for the hepatitis B and acquired immunodeficiency syndrome (AIDS) are inactivated by commercial manufacturing processes. It is therefore better to administer antithrombin III concentrate rather than fresh-frozen plasma in these clinical settings. The biologic half-life of antithrombin III is approximately 48 hours. Infusion of antithrombin III concentrate in a bolus of 50 units/kg body weight (1 unit is defined as the amount of antithrombin in 1 ml of pooled normal human plasma) will usually raise the plasma antithrombin III level to approximately 120 percent in a congenitally deficient patient with a baseline level of 50 percent. Plasma levels should be monitored to ensure that plasma levels remain above 80 percent. The administration of 60 percent of the initial dose at 24-hour intervals is recommended to maintain inhibitor levels in the normal range.

Oral anticoagulants are highly effective in the management of patients with antithrombin III deficiency. Warfarin should be continued indefinitely in patients with recurrent venous thrombosis. Asymptomatic antithrombin III-deficient persons from thrombophilic kindreds are not generally anticoagulated prophylactically unless they are exposed to situations predisposing them to developing thrombosis such as prolonged immobilization, surgery, and pregnancy.

The management of pregnancies in women with congenital antithrombin III deficiency poses special problems.[96] Affected persons who have not experienced thrombotic events should probably be given antithrombotic prophylaxis with heparin throughout pregnancy. Patients with a history of previous thrombotic episodes should definitely receive treatment. In women treated with oral anticoagulants chronically, several approaches can be taken while planning pregnancy to minimize the risk of thrombotic complications as well as warfarin embryopathy. One way is to stop warfarin and commence subcutaneous heparin therapy. This potentially exposes the patient to many months of heparin therapy while she is trying to conceive. Another approach is to use replacement therapy with antithrombin III concentrates until conception, although concentrates must be administered intravenously at frequent intervals. Finally, warfarin therapy could be continued with the performance of pregnancy tests on a frequent basis. As soon as pregnancy is diagnosed and prior to the sixth week of gestation, oral anticoagulants must be discontinued and heparin therapy initiated. Although the risk of warfarin embryopathy appears to be quite small during the first 6 weeks of pregnancy, even the small risk of this complication makes this the least preferable of the three approaches.

Protein C Deficiency

This biochemical deficiency state is inherited as an autosomal dominant gene and has clinical features quite similar to those of hereditary antithrombin III deficiency.[97–101] Approximately 75 percent of these persons experience one or more thrombotic events. The initial episode occurs spontaneously in the majority of patients, while about one-fourth have the usual associated risk factors at the time they develop acute thrombotic events (for example, pregnancy, delivery, oral contraceptive ingestion, surgery, or trauma). These patients are not, however, usually symptomatic until the age of 20, with increasing numbers of individuals experiencing thrombotic events as they reach the age of 50. The most common sites of disease are the deep veins of the legs, the iliofemoral veins, and the mesenteric veins. Approximately two-thirds

of affected patients develop recurrent venous thrombosis, with about 40 percent exhibiting signs of pulmonary embolism. Some kindred have a high frequency of superficial thrombophlebitis of the leg veins, while other families show predisposition to cerebral venous thrombosis.[98]

Kindred with heterozygous protein C deficiency have minimal symptoms. By contrast, a number of case reports have described a homozygous or double-heterozygous state in which newborns develop purpura fulminans and laboratory evidence of DIC in association with protein C antigen levels less than 1 percent of normal.[102,103] The frequency of heterozygous protein C deficiency is as high as 1 in 200 in a healthy adult population, but biochemically affected persons may not exhibit thrombotic manifestations.[101] These data suggest that other, undefined, factors are likely to modulate the phenotype expression of heterozygous protein C deficiency. Two major subtypes of heterozygous protein C deficiency have been delineated by means of immunologic and functional assays.[104,105] The classic, or type I, deficiency state has equivalent reduction in the immunologic and biologic activity of the zymogen in the blood (while type II reflects the presence of a dysfunctional protein).

Protein C circulates in human plasma at a concentration of 4 μg/ml. The levels of protein C antigen in healthy adults are normally distributed. Ninety-five percent of the values range from 70 to 140 percent. There is no significant gender dependence, but mean protein C antigen concentrations increase by approximately 4 percent each decade. This is largely a reflection of the tendency for some older subjects to have higher values rather than individual change at the lower end of the normal range. The relatively wide normal range of protein C measurements in the general population will frequently make it more difficult to identify a given patient definitively as having heterozygous protein C deficiency. If medical and pharmacologic causes of low levels are excluded, protein C values of less than 55 percent lead to a high likelihood that the person has the genetic abnormality. Levels from 55 to 65 percent are consistent with either a deficiency state or the lower end of the normal distribution. To document this disorder, it is useful to perform repeat determinations on the patient suspected of being protein C deficient, as well as to perform family studies to document the presence of an autosomal dominant inheritance pattern for the abnormality. Protein C levels in newborns are 20 to 40 percent of normal adult levels. Preterm infants have even lower levels. Newborns may develop purpura fulminans in association with protein C antigen levels less than 1 percent of normal.[102,103]

Acquired protein C deficiency occurs in a number of clinical disorders, including liver disease, DIC, adult respiratory distress syndrome (ARDS), and the postoperative state, and in association with L-asparaginase therapy.[106,107] In contradistinction to antithrombin III, the antigen concentrations of vitamin K-dependent plasma proteins including protein C are often elevated in patients with the nephrotic syndrome.

Warfarin therapy reduces functional and immunologic measurements of protein C, which makes it quite difficult to diagnose heterozygous protein C deficiency in patients who are being treated with oral anticoagulants.[108] A reduced ratio of protein C antigen to prothrombin antigen may be used to identify patients with a type I deficiency state. This approach requires a stable phase of oral anticoagulation. In addition, the diagnostic criteria for the disorder vary with the intensity of warfarin therapy. Actually, it is preferable to investigate patients suspected of having the deficiency after oral anticoagulation has been discontinued for at least a 1-week period and to perform family studies. If it is not possible to discontinue warfarin due to the severity of the thrombotic tendency, such patients should be studied while receiving heparin therapy, since heparin has not been shown to alter plasma protein C levels.

Thromboembolic events in heterozygous protein C-deficient patients are managed like venous thrombosis in subjects without this disorder. It is advisable to keep the subject fully anticoagulated with heparin during the initiation of oral anticoagulation. Large loading doses of warfarin must be avoided.[108,109] Oral anticoagulants are effective in managing the patient with protein C deficiency, similar to their use in patients with congenital antithrombin III deficiency. Many of the general guidelines for the management of pregnancies in women with this latter disorder are also relevant to this situation in protein C deficient women.

Coumarin-induced skin necrosis may be associated with the presence of heterozygous protein C deficiency.[110,111] During the first several days of warfarin therapy, often with large loading doses, the skin lesions occur on the extremities, breasts, and trunk, as well as the penis, and may develop within hours of the initial central erythematous macule. The explanation of warfarin-induced skin necrosis is related to the emergence of a transient decrease in protein C anticoagulant activity levels at a greater rate than its action on factor VII. These effects are likely to be augmented when loading dose schedules are used or the patient has an underlying hereditary deficiency of protein C. However, only approximately one-third of patients with warfarin-induced skin necrosis have an inherited deficiency of protein C, and this complication is infrequent among patients with the heterozygous deficiency state. When starting oral anticoagulants in a patient who is already known or likely to be protein C deficient, it is prudent to start the drug under the cover of full heparinization, and also to increase the dose of warfarin gradually, starting from a relatively low level (for example, 2 mg for the first 3 days, and then increasing in increments of 2 to 3 mg until therapeutic anticoagulation is achieved).

Neonatal purpura fulminans in association with severe protein C deficiency is more complicated to manage since neither heparin therapy nor antiplatelet agents has proven effective. Protein C administration is critical in the initial treatment of these patients, by administering either fresh-frozen plasma or concentrates of protein C. However, the half-life is relatively short (approximately 6 to 16 hours). Warfarin has been administered to these infants without the redevelopment of skin necrosis during the phased withdrawal of fresh-frozen plasma infusions.

Protein S Deficiency
Patients with heterozygous protein S deficiency present similarly to that of antithrombin III deficiency or protein C deficiency.[112–116] The first thrombotic event occurs between 15 to 68 years; one-half of the episodes are spontaneous, and the remainder have an identifiable predisposing factor. Thrombosis occurs in the axillary, mesenteric, and cerebral veins.

Approximately one-half of the total protein S antigen is normally complexed to a plasma complement component, C4b-binding protein.[117] Only free protein S is functionally active as a cofactor in mediating the anticoagulant effects of activated protein C.[114,117] The classic deficiency state is associated with approximately 50 percent of the normal total S antigen level and free protein S antigen and protein S functional activity to about 40 percent or less of normal values. The molecular basis for these disorders is usually a point mutation.[118] Another type

of hereditary deficiency state has been described in which total protein S antigen measurements are within the normal range but in which the levels of free protein S and protein S functional activity are disproportionately reduced.[119]

The concentration of total protein S antigen in normal adults is approximately 23 μg/ml. Plasma levels increase significantly with advancing age and are significantly lower and more variable in females than in males. These factors may confound the reliable estimation of the prevalence of heterozygous protein S deficiency in the normal population and complicate the diagnosis of heterozygous protein S deficiency when performing assays on a given patient at a single point in time. The re-examination of patients and family studies are required to establish a firm diagnosis.

Acquired protein S deficiency occurs during pregnancy and in association with the use of oral contraceptives.[120] Reduced protein S levels have been noted in association with L-asparaginase therapy, in patients with DIC, and in acute thromboembolic disease.[121] C4b-binding protein is an acute-phase protein, and the decline in protein S activity in inflammatory disorders is attributable to a shift of the protein to the complexed, inactive form.[121] Levels of total protein S antigen are generally increased in patients with the nephrotic syndrome, although functional assays give reduced values, partly explained by the loss of free protein S in the urine and elevations in C4b-binding protein levels.[122] Total and free protein S antigen concentrations are moderately decreased in liver disease.[121] Because total protein S antigen values in healthy newborns at term are 15 to 30 percent of normal, and C4b-binding protein is markedly reduced to less than 20 percent, the free form of the protein predominates in this setting. Reductions in the ratio of total protein S antigen to prothrombin antigen may be used to infer a diagnosis of the classic type of protein S-deficient state, as for protein C-deficient subjects.

The treatment of protein S-deficient patients with anticoagulants and thrombolytic agents is similar to those for patients without this deficiency. Heparin therapy is effective for the acute treatment of thrombotic episodes, and standard warfarin schedules are effective in preventing recurrent venous thromboembolism.

Dysfibrinogenemias

Generally, qualitative abnormalities of fibrinogen are usually inherited in an autosomal dominant manner. The dysfibrinogenemias are a heterogeneous group of clinical disorders that rarely present with a history of recurrent venous or arterial thromboembolic episodes.[123–125] These defects are discovered by screening patients with thrombin and reptilase times and by fibrinogen assays. Those abnormal fibrinogens associated with thromboembolic disease exhibit defects in the release of activation peptides or in thrombin binding. Other mutants produce abnormal fibrin polymerization. Some of the abnormal fibrinogens resist or promote fibrinolysis upon incorporation into a fibrin clot. These types of abnormalities have the potential to decrease fibrinolytic activity in vivo, which could result in a familial thrombotic tendency in biochemically affected persons.

Inherited Abnormalities of Fibrinolysis

Dysfunction of the fibrinolytic system predisposes to thrombus formation.[126–131] Although individuals with inherited abnormalities of the fibrinolytic mechanism have recurrent venous thromboembolism, the clinical association between these two conditions is considerably less striking than that observed in many kindreds with deficiencies of antithrombin III, protein C, or protein S. Dysplasminogenemia or hypoplasminogenemia has

been reported in patients with thromboembolic disease.[127–129] Immunochemical methods measuring tissue-type plasminogen activator and functional assays for the inhibitor suggest that defective synthesis or release of tissue-type plasminogen activator as well as an increased concentration of the inhibitor of this serine protease may be important pathogenetic factors. Reduced fibrinolytic activity due to increased plasma levels of a rapid inhibitor of tissue-type plasminogen activator has been found in young survivors of myocardial infarction, but the measurements of this inhibitor correlated strongly with serum concentrations of triglycerides.[132]

Heparin Cofactor II Deficiency

Heparin cofactor II is an anticoagulant protein that inactivates thrombin without affecting other serine proteases.[133] Heparin cofactor II is of lesser importance in this regard than antithrombin III. The rate of thrombin inactivation by heparin cofactor II is greatly potentiated by heparin, as also occurs with antithrombin III. Venous or arterial thrombotic symptoms may be associated with half-normal levels of heparin cofactor II, inherited as a dominant disorder.[134,135]

Homocystinemia

The rare genetic recessive disorder of homocystinemia leads to focal endothelial denudation involving both the arterial and the venous endothelial surfaces so that thrombotic events in either or both systems may be observed.[136]

Effects of Acquired Prothrombotic Disorders

Cardiac Abnormalities

Cardiogenic cerebral embolism is the mechanism responsible for nearly 100,000 strokes each year among North Americans, and perhaps a million or more worldwide.[137–143] These thrombotic episodes derive from a diversity of cardiac disorders. There is a history of atrial fibrillation in just under one-half of patients, valvular heart disease in one-fourth, and left ventricular mural thrombi in almost one-third.

Epidemiologic studies have estimated the risk of stroke and systemic embolism associated with atrial fibrillation as five to six events per 100 patient-years, at least five times the rate among comparable patients without this cardiac rhythm disturbance, and accumulating to a 35 percent lifetime risk of stroke for patients with atrial fibrillation. The risk appears related to age, so that among stroke victims over 85 years of age, a history of atrial fibrillation can be found in nearly one-half.

Sixty percent of the emboli of left ventricular origin are associated with acute myocardial infarction. The remainder occur in patients with chronic ventricular dysfunction resulting from coronary disease, hypertension, or other forms of dilated cardiomyopathy. Each year, over a million survivors of myocardial infarction with large anterior infarcts face a risk of stroke that is over 5 percent within the first few weeks. Within the even larger population of patients with chronic left ventricular dysfunction, the potential for cerebral emboli persists.

Cardioembolic stroke is usually associated with substantial functional disability, and yet the warning signs of transient cerebral ischemia are absent. This makes a preventive strategy for defined high-risk groups the only sensible clinical approach. The additional incidence of subclinical silent strokes is unknown, and this mechanism may take an uncounted toll on cognitive function, perhaps contributing to the problem of multi-infarct dementia among the elderly.

The pathogenesis of intracavitary mural thrombosis arises from endocardial damage, circulatory stasis, and genera-tion of prothrombotic factors in blood.[144] In addition, the clinical significance derives from the potential for systemic embolism, which also depends upon dynamic forces of the circulation. In the first few days following acute myocardial infarction, leukocytic infiltration produces endothelial denudation, which serves as the nidus for thrombus development. Specific endocardial abnormalities have also been identified histologically in surgical and postmortem specimens from patients with left ventricular aneurysms, and at necropsy in patients with idiopathic dilated cardiomyopathy.[145,146] Wall motion abnormalities are of primary importance in the development of left ventricular mural thrombi; stasis of blood in regions of akinesia or dyskinesia is the essential factor. Similarly, stasis is important in the development of atrial thrombi when effective mechanical atrial activity is impaired, as occurs in atrial fibrillation, atrial enlargement, mitral stenosis, and cardiac failure.[147-149] Stasis with low shear rate and activation of the coagulation system play the predominant pathogenetic role in the development of intracavitary thrombi. Platelet activation and activation of the coagulation cascade leading to fibrin deposition have been implicated in the process of intravascular thrombus formation. During the process of mural thrombosis in the cardiac chambers, fibrin and thrombin accumulate to a greater degree. Thrombin is even more powerful than collagen as an activator of platelet aggregation. Since platelets and the coagulation system are closely interrelated in the genesis of left ventricular mural thrombosis, a potential role exists for both platelet inhibitor and anticoagulant medication for the prevention of these thrombi and the embolic phenomena they can produce. Factors leading to thrombus formation are not the same, however, as those that produce systemic embolism, and this contradictory result must not be neglected in the selection of therapeutic options.

Patients with atrial fibrillation (e.g., with rheumatic valvular heart disease or with prosthetic heart valves) are at risk of stroke and systemic embolism.[139–141,149] These patients have at least an 8 to 10 percent annual risk of ischemic thromboembolic events, which is at least ten times that of patients in normal sinus rhythm, according to the Framingham Heart Study. Furthermore, these patients are considered at risk with maintenance anticoagulant therapy using drugs such as warfarin.

Among those with nonvalvular atrial fibrillation, the risk is highest when stroke or systemic embolism has occurred within the previous 2 years. These patients face a risk of more than 10 percent per year.[149–152] The mechanism responsible for this incremental risk is unknown, but may be related to the potential for the surface of freshly formed thrombus to stimulate additional coagulation, or it may be related to the association of other clinical factors (e.g., hypertension or atherosclerotic vascular disease), which may contribute to ischemic events in these patients.

In patients with very localized forms of chronic left ventricular dysfunction following ventricular aneurysm formation beyond 3 months after myocardial infarction, thrombi can be identified in approximately 50 percent of the cases by echocardiography or other imaging techniques, but the incidence of systemic embolism is no more than 1 event in 100 patient-years. Alternatively, when left ventricular systolic function is more diffusely reduced, as occurs in dilated cardiomyopathy, the risk of cerebral embolism is 3 to 4 percent a year. These results demonstrate the difference between the effect of regional circulatory stasis, which favors thrombus formation within the aneurysmal cavity, and the isolation from the dynamic forces of the circulation, which protects against embolic migration. In contrast, protrusion and mobility of the thrombotic mass within the ventricular chamber are associated with much greater embolic potential.

Transesophageal echocardiography is more effective in identifying potential sources of cerebral embolism in patients with acute brain infarction than is transthoracic echocardiography.[153] This is especially true for detection of thrombi in the left atrial appendage. Two-dimensional echocardiography is the best means of detecting left ventricular thrombi, but its sensitivity and specificity are not clearly established.

Within the cardiac chambers, stasis of blood flow causes coagulation to predominate over platelet activation as the principal mechanism of thrombus formation, and anticoagulant therapy alone seems most appropriate for managing these patients. The patients at highest risk are those with atrial fibrillation and prior embolism. Patients with mitral stenosis or prosthetic heart valves are considered to be at substantial risk, whereas immediately following large anterior myocardial infarction and uncompensated dilated cardiomyopathy patients are at medium risk. For all of these patients, there is sufficient evidence to indicate chronic anticoagulation.[154,155] Some patients with nonvalvulopathic atrial fibrillation also benefit from warfarin therapy, but subgroups within this population have not been clearly defined. Patients under 60 years old who have only experienced atrial fibrillation without overt heart disease and those with chronic left ventricular aneurysm who do not require anticoagulants are considered to be at lowest risk.

Atrial fibrillation is now recognized as a major risk factor for the development of ischemic stroke, particularly among elderly patients.[156] Rhythm disturbance is indicative of associated cardiovascular pathology, which may be the cause of more cases of stroke than atrioembolic mechanisms alone. The effectiveness and relative safety of chronic anticoagulant therapy with warfarin has now been validated in four separate clinical trials (Table 8-2).[157–160] The results of these trials suggest a thrombotic mechanism for most of the strokes that occur in patients with nonvalvular atrial fibrillation. The success of therapy with aspirin in younger individuals in one of the studies suggests that administration of this platelet inhibitor may be sufficient for some patients with nonvalvular atrial fibrillation.

Lupus Anticoagulant

Lupus anticoagulants are antibodies that interfere with coagulation tests in vitro by prolonging phospholipid-dependent clotting assays.[161,162] The presence of lupus anticoagulants has been associated with an apparent increased risk of both arterial and venous thromboembolism and habitual abortions in some women.[163] Approximately one-third of patients with these inhibitors have a history of thrombotic events. Thrombophilic patients with this abnormality, however, are more likely to be diagnosed than are asymptomatic subjects. Cutaneous lesions associated with lupus anticoagulants, including livedo reticularis and skin necrosis, may be manifestations of thrombosis in underlying vessels. Lupus anticoagulants frequently occur in patients without systemic lupus erythematosus (SLE), including other autoimmune diseases, following drug exposure or various infectious agents, in malignancy, and in patients without apparent underlying disease.[161–164] The presence of lupus anticoagulants has also been associated with biologic false-positive tests for syphilis because the veneral disease research laboratory (VDRL) assay is dependent on the presence of cardiolipin. Some of

Table 8-2.   Randomized Trials of Antithrombotic Therapy in Nonvalvular Atrial Fibrillation: Outcome[a]

	AFASAK[157]	SPAF[158]	BAATAF[159]	CAFA[160]
Control				
Event rate	6.0	6.3	3.0[b]	4.6
Warfarin				
Event rate	2.6	2.3	0.4	3.0
Percent reduction	57	67	86	35
Aspirin				
Event rate	5.0	3.6	—	—
Percent reduction	17	42		
Control mortality				
(Percent per year)	6.1	6.5	6.0[b]	3.3
Warfarin bleeding				
Risk[c]		0.8		1.2

Abbreviations: AFASAK, Atrial Fibrillation, Aspirin, Anticoagulant Study, Copenhagen Denmark; BAATAF, Boston Area Anticoagulation Trial for Atrial Fibrillation; CAFA, Canadian Atrial Fibrillation Anticoagulation; SPAF, Stroke Prevention in Atrial Fibrillation.

  [a] Intention-to-treat analysis.

  [b] Not placebo-controlled; values refer to control group, nearly one-half of which used aspirin for unspecified periods.

  [c] Major hemorrhage, variably defined, but generally implying central nervous system involvement, hospitalization, transfusion, surgery, or death.

these antibodies react with anionic phospholipids. Sensitive radioimmunoassays (RIAs) or enzyme-linked immunosorbent assays (ELISAs) detect antiphospholipid antibodies with more sensitivity than does the VDRL test.[165] There are complex relationships among lupus anticoagulants, antiphospholipid antibodies, and a thrombotic predisposition. The presence of such immunoglobulins does not necessarily confer an increased thrombotic risk on these persons.

Patients with lupus anticoagulants constitute a heterogeneous population, and several mechanisms have been implicated in the pathogenesis of their thrombotic complications. Most studies have attempted to demonstrate alterations in the function of one of the natural anticoagulant mechanisms of the endothelium, as phospholipids are essential components of vascular cell membranes.[166]

The presence of lupus anticoagulants or anticardiolipin antibodies has also been associated with obstetric complications, such as habitual abortions, intrauterine death, and intrauterine growth retardation. Occasionally, pathologic examination has demonstrated placental infarction due to decidual vessel thrombosis. The administration of prednisone (40 to 60 mg/day) and low-dose aspirin (75 to 81 mg/day) or full-dose heparin may improve the outcome of pregnancies in women with lupus anticoagulants and poor obstetric histories.

The management of acute venous thromboembolism in patients with lupus anticoagulants is similar to that of other patients without this abnormality. The initial treatment of such subjects is, however, complicated by the practitioner's inability to use activated partial thromboplastin time reliably to monitor heparin dosage. The best approach to monitoring anticoagulant therapy in such patients is to perform plasma heparin measurements using either factor Xa or thrombin with an appropriate chromogenic substrate. The range for therapeutic anticoagulation is 0.2 to 0.5 units of heparin/ml, which usually corresponds to an activated partial thromboplastin time of 1.5 to 2.5 times the pretreatment value in patients without circulating inhibitors. The presence of lupus anticoagulants may also interfere with heparin monitoring during cardiac surgery.

The clinical heterogeneity of patient populations that develop lupus anticoagulants makes it difficult to formulate general long-term antithrombotic management strategies for them. Patients who develop transient lupus anticoagulants in association with infections do not appear to develop thromboembolic episodes, whereas drug-associated lupus anticoagulants appear to be associated with such complications. The presence of a persistent lupus anticoagulant or a high titer of antiphospholipid antibody in an asymptomatic subject with no prior thrombotic history is therefore not currently an indication for anticoagulant or antiplatelet medications. While it is not yet possible to determine the risk of thrombosis in an asymptomatic patient manifesting laboratory abnormalities, all such patients should be administered antithrombotic prophylaxis in conjunction with major surgical procedures or a prolonged period of immobilization unless there is a strong contraindication to such treatment. Corticosteroids may lead to a normalization of clotting assay times or to a reduction in antiphospholipid antibody titers in patients with lupus anticoagulants. These and other immunosuppressive medications have not been reported to be effective in preventing recurrent thrombosis in such subjects.

Thrombocytosis

Primary thrombocythemia is a chronic myeloproliferative disorder characterized by a sustained proliferation of megakaryocytes, leading to increased numbers of circulating platelets, with profound marrow megakaryocyte hyperplasia, splenomegaly, and a clinical course punctuated by hemorrhagic and/or thrombotic episodes.[167] Ten new patients with primary thrombocythemia per million population are diagnosed each year. Primary thrombocythemia and polycythemia vera appear to have approximately a 1:4 relative incidence.

The disorder appears to affect primarily middle-aged persons, the average age at diagnosis being between 50 and 60 years.[168,169] One-fourth of patients present with symptoms related to hemorrhagic events, while three-fourths of patients report thromboembolic complications. The thrombotic events primarily involve the microvasculature, with thrombosis of large vessels occurring far less frequently. Neurologic complications are common, consisting of paresthesias of the extremities and high incidence of transient ischemic attacks involving both the anterior and posterior cerebral circulations.

Microvascular occlusions involving the toes and fingers are frequent.[170–173] Such events may lead to digital pain that is aggravated by warmth, leading to distal extremity gangrene. The term *erythromelalgia* refers to a syndrome of redness and burning pain in the extremities. The relief of such pain for several days after a single dose of aspirin is diagnostic of erythromelalgia.

Thrombosis of large veins and arteries in patients with primary thrombocythemia occurs frequently, involving coronary, renal, carotid, and mesenteric arteries. Venous thrombosis involving either the splenic vein, hepatic veins, or veins of the legs and pelvis may also occur. Unexplained thrombosis of the hepatic veins leads to the Budd-Chiari syndrome, while thrombosis of the renal vein can result in development of the nephrotic

syndrome. Priapism is a rare complication of primary thrombocythemia and is presumably caused by platelet aggregate formation obstructing flow from the corpus cavernosum. In addition, myocardial ischemia and/or infarction associated with normal coronary angiograms has been reported in patients with primary thrombocythemia, as has a high incidence of anginal symptoms. Acute renal failure was observed after thrombosis of renal arteries and veins in one patient with primary thrombocythemia.

Primary thrombocythemia must be distinguished from reactive or secondary forms of thrombocytosis and from other myeloproliferative disorders such as polycythemia vera, agnogenic myeloid metaplasia, and chronic granulocytic leukemia, which are also characterized by thrombocytosis. The causes of secondary or reactive forms of thrombocytosis are numerous and include acute or chronic infections, rheumatoid arthritis, ankylosing spondylitis, chronic inflammatory bowel disease, iron deficiency anemia, nonhematologic malignancies, and sickle cell anemia. Thrombocytosis also occurs frequently postoperatively especially following splenectomy.

Since chemotherapeutic agents generally require 18 to 20 days before platelet counts can be reduced to normal levels, many hematologists recommend reducing the platelet count to 500,000/mm^3 by each platelet pheresis by exchanging two blood volumes over a 3- to 4-hour period. Such a therapeutic approach has been employed to treat acutely ill patients with problems such as cerebrovascular accidents, myocardial infarction, transient ischemic attacks, or life-threatening gastrointestinal hemorrhage.[174,175]

Transient ischemic attacks and erythromelalgia associated with primary thrombocythemia have been reported to respond rapidly to aspirin alone, aspirin and dipyridamole in combination, or indomethacin alone.[170–173] Symptoms disappear for 2 to 4 days after administration of a single 500-mg dose of aspirin. Although these agents surely have a role in the treatment of these specific complications, their use should be pursued with extreme caution because of the increased risk of hemorrhage.

At present, hydroxyurea (15 mg/kg for the first week, followed by a maintenance dose adjusted to maintain an acceptable platelet count but avoiding leukopenia) would seem to be the drug of choice.[176] Hydroxyurea is quite efficient in lowering the platelet count, and its leukemogenic effect has been said to be less than that associated with other chemotherapeutic alkylating agents. Intermittent use of busulfan (4 mg/day until the platelet count falls to 400,000/mm^3) has proved to be a relatively nontoxic but effective regimen.[177] Of great interest has been the development of a new drug, anagrelide, which is currently under investigation for the treatment of primary thrombocythemia.[31] The drug acts primarily by inhibiting megakaryocyte maturation and platelet release from the marrow; it does not appear to affect DNA metabolism. This new agent is very promising for the treatment of primary thrombocythemia.

Activated Constituents of Blood

Platelets and coagulation factors may become activated by local exposure to thrombogenic endovascular or nonvascular tissue or to prosthetic surfaces, or by the entry of activators into the bloodstream.[75,76] The activated species may circulate temporarily in a partially or fully activated state, and the activated constituents may contribute directly to the enhanced development of thrombosis, especially in association with stasis (Fig. 8-4). Under some conditions, rate of activation and removal are sufficiently abnormal that the clinical presentation is that of consumptive coagulopathy with or without symptomatic thrombosis.

Clinical thrombosis may follow the entry of some activators of coagulation into the bloodstream [e.g., acute severe brain trauma (brain tissue factor), infusion of concentrates of vitamin K-dependent factors (activated serine proteases), neoplasms (release of breakdown or secretory product), viremia or bacteremia (monocyte and neutrophil-derived tissue factor), and some animal venoms].[76]

Clinical Risk Factors for Thrombosis

Table 8-3 lists the clinical states that have been statistically associated with increased risk of arterial and venous thrombotic disease.[75,76]

In venous thrombosis, increased stasis is produced by immobilization, obesity, congestive heart failure, pregnancy, or varicosities. Other important risk factors include recent trauma or surgery, neoplastic disease, myeloproliferative disorders, or the nephrotic syndrome.

One clinical controversy relates to the risk imposed by the estrogens in oral contraceptive agents in women predisposed to arterial or venous thromboembolic disease. Two epidemiologic studies have concluded that the use of oral contraceptives is a definite risk factor contributing to thrombosis. It appears that decreasing the content of estrogens decreases the risk of venous, but not arterial, complications. The risk of arterial thrombosis in women appears to be increased if they are smokers.

Risk factors for arterial disease include hypertension, cigarette smoking, hyperlipidemia, diabetes, and, infrequently, essential thrombocytosis. High blood pressure causes a greater risk to cerebral arteries, whereas smoking and diabetes causes a greater risk to peripheral arteries. An increase in platelet count occurs

Table 8-3. Clinical Risk Factors
Predisposing to Thrombosis

Venous thrombosis
  Increased venous stasis
    Immobilization
    Pregnancy
    Congestive heart failure
    Varicosities
    Previous thrombotic history
    Obesity
    Age

  Coagulation activation
    Trauma
    Surgery
    Malignancies
    Factor IX concentrates
    Lupus inhibitor
    Myocardial infarction
    ?Myeloproliferative disorders
    ?Pregnancy

  Inadequate regulation
    Genetic disorder
    ?Nephrotic syndrome
    ?Oral contraceptives

Arterial thrombosis
  Abnormal vascular surface
    Atherosclerosis
    Hyperlipidemia
    Diabetes
    Homocystinemia
    Hypertension
    Cigarette smoking
    Estrogen therapy
    Prosthetic cardiovascular device

  Vascular occlusive
    Hyperviscosity
    Sickle cell disease
    Polycythemia
    Plasma cell dyscrasias (especially
      macroglobulinemia)

  Increased platelet reactivity
    Thrombocytosis
    ?Nephrotic syndrome

  Others
    ?Personality
    ?Lack of physical exercise

---

after splenectomy and other operative procedures. Although there is a consistent relationship between the circulating platelet count and the amount of throm-bus formed in laboratory experiments, the clinical association is not at all as well established. Lack of physical exercise has also been implicated in the increased risk of coronary artery disease. The frequency of arterial thrombosis in nephrotic syndrome is also increased; it has been attributed to hyper-responsive platelets.

DISORDERS OF MALIGNANT DISEASE

Primary tumors of the heart occur in less than 0.1 percent of autopsies, whereas tumors metastatic to the pericardium or heart are more common, occurring in 1.5 to 20.6 percent of autopsies on patients with malignant disease. The metastases usually involve the pericardium and myocardium.[178] The right side of the heart is affected more frequently than the left, but the valves or endocardium are rarely affected. Solitary metastases to the heart are rare. Although metastatic nodules in the heart are generally multiple, they may become diffuse and lead to manifestations of restrictive cardiomyopathy. Malignant extension occurs by direct spread (e.g., lung cancer), by the hematogenous route (e.g., malignant melanoma), or via lymphatic channels (e.g., lymphoma).

Carcinoma of the bronchus is the most common primary tumor producing cardiac metastases. The next most frequently occurring malignancies are carcinoma of the breast, malignant melanoma, lymphomas, and leukemias, respectively.[179] At autopsy, about one-third of patients dying with primary lung cancer show cardiac involvement, while over 60 percent of patients with melanoma have cardiac metastases. Hematologic malignancies, especially lymphomas, account for 15 percent of all cardiac and pericardial metastases, and approximately 15 percent of patients dying of malignant lymphomas demonstrate metastases to the heart.

Many metastatic cardiac lesions are found only at necropsy. There may be little evidence of cardiac dysfunction, despite massive heart involvement. Clinical manifestations of cancer involvement of the heart reflect (1) involvement of the pericardium, myocardium, or endocardium; (2) consequences of circulating mediators arising from the tumor; (3) embolization in patients in a hypercoagulable state; or (4) the effects of specific tumor therapy (e.g., chemotherapy and radiation therapy).

The most common clinical manifestations result from pericardial effusion with tamponade, tachyarrhythmias, AV block, or congestive heart failure.[180] Metastatic cardiac disease is seldom the presenting symptom of a tumor. Routine chest radiographs, computed chest tomography, magnetic resonance imaging, echocardiography, and/or radionuclide imaging with gallium or thallium are useful in establishing cancer involving the heart. Osteogenic sarcoma, which may metastasize to the heart, is unique because the metastases contain bone and may be radiographically visible.

In a necropsy study of patients with solid tumors, 4 percent died of myocardial infarction. Patients with carcinoma of the lung, malignant lymphoma, and leukemia are most commonly afflicted; whereas patients with breast cancer and cancer of the gastrointestinal tract and malignant melanoma are less affected. The etiology of coronary artery disease (CAD) in cancer patients is usually coincidental spontaneous atherosclerosis. The most common cause of tumor-related myocardial infarction is extrinsic compression of a coronary artery, occurring in two-thirds of the patients; tumor emboli are responsible for approximately one-third of events. Widespread thromboses, such as coronary artery thromboses due to disseminated intravascular coagulation, infrequently occur in patients with metastatic tumors (usually mucin-secreting adenocarcinomas).[181] One-half of all patients with acute myocardial infarction secondary to malignant disease have a history of typical chest pain prior to death, but an acute event in a patient with advanced malignant disease is a particularly poor prognostic sign because more than two-thirds die within 3 weeks of the event.

Arrhythmias and many electrocardiographic changes are common in patients with metastatic disease. Such conditions are often the result of altered electrolyte concentrations, anemia, hypoxia, and so on, although they may be caused directly by tumor involvement of the heart. It may be clinically difficult to determine whether abnormalities, such as nonspecific ST-segment and T-wave changes, low voltage, and sinus tachycardia are attributable to cardiac metastases or the result of an associated cardiac problem, irradiation, or the cardiotoxic effects of drugs.[182] Atrial arrhythmias, such as fibrillation and flutter, may occur secondary to either neoplastic involvement of autonomic fibers supplying the atria or tumor invasion of the coronary arteries perfusing the atria, giving rise to atrial infarction or to neoplastic infiltration of the atrial myocardium or sinus node. Similarly, the electrocardiographic changes of acute myocardial infarction can be produced by tumor infiltration of hemorrhage into the ventricle or occlusion of one of the coronary arteries. Occasionally, the exact area of tumor involvement may be pinpointed by acute electrocardiographic changes. Involvement of the AV node is a rare cause of complete heart block, but may be the presenting symptom of the tumor. In addition, tumor involvement of cervical lymph nodes without mediastinal involvement has been associated with carotid sinus syncope.

Roentgenographic evidence of cardiac enlargement and the development of congestive heart failure may be the only clinical signs of malignant involvement of the heart. Unexplained pansystolic or late systolic murmurs may occur with intraluminal invasion or external compression of the carotid or pulmonary arteries by the tumor. In addition to coincidental atherosclerosis, CAD in cancer patients may be caused by tumor emboli, extrinsic compression of the coronary arteries or ostia, or thromboemboli secondary to tumor-associated coagulation disorders.

Pericardial Involvement

Symptoms of pericarditis with pericardial effusion and cardiac tamponade are typical in patients with carcinoma of the lung and breast, in Hodgkin's disease, in non-Hodgkin's lymphoma, and in leukemia, particularly acute myelogenous, lymphoblastic leukemia and the blast crisis of chronic myelogenous leukemia.[183] Pericardial involvement is usually diagnosed ante mortem because of the resultant symptomatology (cardiac tamponade or adhesive pericarditis, associated with extensive nodular tumor infiltration of the pericardium) and radiographic/echocardiographic evidence. Lymphomatous involvement usually manifests as chylous pericardial effusion. With increased use of serial M-mode echocardiography in patients with advanced malignant disease, the incidence of pericardial effusions seems to be higher than was previously thought. Pericardiocentesis may be necessary to differentiate tumor from radiation effects, because pericardial tumor or fibrosis secondary to radiation therapy may mimic chronic constrictive pericarditis or chronic effusive pericardial disease. Radiation-induced pericarditis is common in patients with carcinoma of the lung, Hodgkin's disease, and non-Hodgkin's lymphoma, as a consequence of irradiation to the thorax. In addition, radiation-induced pericarditis may occur as late as 8 years after therapy. In patients with leukemia, massive involvement of the pericardium and epicardium is a common finding at autopsy, with the extent of infiltration usually related to the degree of leukocytosis. Leukemic infiltration of the heart is more common in the acute leukemias and in the blast crisis phase of chronic myelogenous leukemia.

Myocardial Involvement

Direct myocardial involvement or endocardial involvement by tumor may result in arrhythmias, congestive heart failure, ventricular outflow tract obstruction, and peripheral emboli. Cardiac metastases found on two-dimensional echocardiography have been described. For example, melanoma favors the endocardium and may often appear as an intracavitary mass.[184]

Valvular and Endocardial Involvement

Metastatic tumors may affect cardiac valves in a number of different ways: (1) direct invasion of valves; (2) interference with valvular function by compression; (3) valvular dysfunction secondary to carcinoid tumors; and (4) noninfective (marantic) endocarditis, occurring with several types of malignant disease (e.g., adenocarcinoma, leukemia, and lymphoma). Such tumors may be diagnosed only at autopsy.[185,186] The pathogenesis is unclear. Nonbacterial thrombotic endocarditis is most frequently associated with Hodgkin's disease; carcinoma of the pancreas, stomach, colon, and lung; and the unusual condition of acute eosinophilic leukemia. It is possible that immune complexes, elicited by the underlying malignant process, play an important role in the pathogenesis of thrombus formation in noninfective thrombotic endocarditis. Although the exact connection between this condition and endomyocardial fibrosis is unclear, there is a high correlation between eosinophilia in the bone marrow and peripheral blood and the occurrence of endomyocardial fibrosis, which may cause restrictive cardiomyopathy. In some patients, the cardiac manifestations predominate (most often cardiomegaly, congestive heart failure, arrhythmias, and heart murmurs), whereas in others, all or most of the clinical manifestations are secondary to the eosinophilic leukemia. Pathologically, these syndromes are characterized by local or widespread eosinophilic infiltrates with fibrous scarring and thickening of the endocardium, including the atrioventricular valves. In many patients, the course is chronic and insidious, but death is usually the direct result of cardiac involvement.

Vena Cava Involvement

Another reported complication in patients with carcinoma of the lung and malignant lymphoma is the superior vena cava syndrome, which results from obstruction of the vessel by tumor.[187] Enlarged mediastinal nodes or the primary tumor may encroach upon or occlude the superior vena cava, causing dyspnea, distention of the neck veins, edema of the face and arms, proptosis, headache, and syncope. Because of the potential life-threatening nature of these problems, local irradiation may be required before any diagnostic procedure. Similar enlargement of nodes or tumor may cause obstruction of the inferior vena cava, with massive leg edema, congestive hepatomegaly, and hypotension.

Amyloidosis

Most patients with primary amyloidosis evidence cardiac involvement. Moreover, the majority of patients with amyloidosis secondary to multiple myeloma exhibit amyloidosis of the heart.[188,189] Symptoms include congestive heart failure, hypotension, cardiac arrhythmias, and conduction disturbances. The diagnosis may be established using (1) echocardiography, (2) contrast tomography, and (3) endomyocardial biopsy. Cardiac amyloidosis may result in reduced myocardial density on contrast-aided tomography, diffuse myocardial thickening, and diffuse hypokinetic wall motion. Hypertrophic cardiomyopathy may also develop. Endomyocardial biopsy may be necessary to confirm the diagnosis.

DISORDERS OF DRUG THERAPIES

Hematologic Effects of Cardiac Drugs

Drugs used to treat cardiac disorders frequently cause complicating blood dyscrasias, including unexplained anemia, neutropenia, or thrombocytopenia. Generally, diuretics, antihypertensive drugs, or antiarrhythmic agents are implicated. The mechanisms underlying the hematologic abnormalities include suppression of one or more of the cellular elements in the bone marrow as well as a variety of immune phenomena with increased peripheral destruction of the formed elements. The drug effect may be dose related or idiosyncratic.

Anemia

Anemia may be the consequence of aplastic, hemolytic, megaloblastic, or sideroblastic processes.[190]

Many therapeutic agents are capable of suppressing marrow function and producing hypoplasia or aplasia.[191] Chloramphenicol, benzene, cytostatic agents, or phenylbutazone are most commonly involved. Antibiotics, such as sulfonamides, hypoglycemic agents, and insecticides are less frequently associated and less well documented in the production of hypoplasia or aplasia. Among drugs used to treat cardiovascular disease, phenytoid (an antiarrhythmic agent), acetazolamide (a diuretic agent), and captopril (the angiotensin-converting enzyme inhibitor), have infrequently been reported to lead to hypoproliferative responses.[192,193] The onset of aplastic anemia is usually insidious, and the symptoms are directly related to the degree of pancytopenia. If the causative agent is discontinued upon detection of the blood dyscrasia, marrow function is generally restored.

Megaloblastic anemia may be caused by drugs impairing the absorption of folic acid or acting as folate antagonists. Pancytopenia with macrocytosis may also be caused by vitamin B_{12} or folate deficiency or by purine and pyrimidine inhibitors due to impairment of DNA synthesis. Phenytoin, oral contraceptives, and a variety of other drugs inhibit folate absorption by interfering with the liver conjugases needed to break down the polyglutamate structure of naturally occurring folates to the monoglutamate form appropriate for absorption by the gastrointestinal tract. Triamterene, a potassium-sparing diuretic, is a pteridine analog that exhibits antifolate activity, similar to aminopterin, in vitro. Its propensity for producing megaloblastic anemia is dose related.

Hemolytic anemia may develop by several different mechanisms, all of which produce a positive direct Coombs or antiglobulin test. The first involves binding of the drug to plasma protein. The resulting complex acts as the antigenic stimulus. These drugs include quinidine and the sulfonamides. The resultant antibody forms a complex with the drug that deposits on the red cell surface and causes agglutination by anticomplement sera. Hemolysis may be severe. Fortunately, improvement quickly follows withdrawal of the drug.

The second type of reaction resulting in a positive Coombs test involves the antihypertensive drug α-methyldopa. The mechanism of antibody formation is unknown; presumably, antibody induced by α-methyldopa has an affinity for the Rh locus of the red cell, similar to that of IgG antibodies in idiopathic immunohemolytic anemia. The frequency of Coombs test positivity varies from 11 percent in patients who are receiving 0.75 g/day for over 3 months to 40 percent in those receiving 2 g/day for the same period of time. The affinity of the α-methyldopa antibody for red cells is low, and fewer than 1 percent of patients whose antiglobulin test is positive will manifest significant hemolytic anemia. Nonetheless, α-methyldopa surpasses all other drugs in causing immunohemolytic anemia. On withdrawal of the drug, hemolysis improves within 1 or 2 weeks, with full recovery within 1 month, although the positive Coombs test may persist for 6 to 24 months. A positive Coombs test without hemolysis is not an indication to discontinue α-methyldopa, if its administration is otherwise indicated in the treatment of hypertension.

The other two mechanisms of drug-related positive antiglobulin reactions do not involve cardiovascular drugs. The third occurs, for example, with penicillin; the drug binds to the red cell membranes, creating a cell-drug complex and antigenic stimulation of an IgG antibody. The fourth mechanism involves cephalothin, which is bound to the red cell membrane; normal serum proteins adhere nonspecifically to red cell membranes.

Neutropenia

A reduction in circulating neutrophils is the most threatening hematologic complication produced by drugs. It may be secondary to depression of the marrow, or it may be an immune mechanism causing peripheral destruction. In immune neutropenia, examination of the marrow reveals active myeloid precursors. On the other hand, the absence of myeloid elements suggests marrow suppression. Generally, the marrow-depressive effect is dose related. Anticoagulants (e.g., phenindione), antiarrhythmics (e.g., procainamide and tocainide), antihypertensives (e.g., captopril), and diuretics (e.g., the thiazides) have all been reported to produce neutropenia.[194,195] The cardiac drug most frequently causing granulocytopenia is procainamide. Patients may present with a sore throat, ulcerations of mucus membranes, fever, malaise, fatigue, and weakness. Discontinuation of the drug may be followed by a rebound in the white blood cell count and, occasionally, a leukemoid picture. Because laboratory tests are not conclusive for white cell antibodies, an accurate definition of the immune mechanism responsible for white cell destruction remains to be established.

Thrombocytopenia

Many of the drugs used to treat cardiovascular disorders cause thrombocytopenia, either by a direct effect on the bone marrow or by inducing formation of drug-specific antibody.[196] The thiazide diuretics, for example, directly suppress megakaryocyte production. Thiazide-induced thrombocytopenia is usually mild, with the platelet count rarely falling below $50,000/\mu l$. It is unique in that it persists for 6 to 8 weeks after withdrawal of the drug. Thrombocytopenia caused by amrinone, a positive inotropic agent with vasodilator properties, is less well studied, but is obviously related to the total dose of drug administered and to peripheral destruction of platelets. Other common agents, such as alcohol, may cause thrombocytopenia by a direct depressant effect on the bone marrow.

Shortened platelet survival secondary to antibody or complement binding to platelets can cause severe thrombocytopenia and life-threatening hemorrhage. The onset is abrupt and is not related to the dose of medication or the duration of its use. In most cases of immunologic thrombocytopenia, the offending agent induces a specific antibody. The resulting drug-antibody complex then binds to the platelet and shortens its survival. Quinidine, one of the first cardiac drugs identified as producing this response, has been well studied as a cause of immune thrombocytopenia. The defect may be transferred to a normal individual by administering serum from a patient with quinidine-induced thrombocytopenia, followed by a quinidine challenge to the normal subject. A similar defect is caused by antibodies to quinine, including the small quantities present in tonic drinks.

Acetaminophen (a common analgesic given to cardiac patients), acetazolamide, digitoxin, phenytoin, ethacrynic acid, α-methyldopa, and spironolactone have all been implicated in various cases of suspected drug-induced thrombocytopenia, although the mechanism has not always been well defined.

The results of laboratory tests for drug-dependent platelet antibodies are not always helpful in explaining clinical events. The best evidence of drug-induced thrombocytopenia is early recovery of the platelet count after drug withdrawal (or a second episode of thrombocytopenia upon readministration of the suspected drug, although such a challenge is not recommended). If serious hemorrhage persists after the drug is withdrawn, treatment with 1 mg/kg prednisone or its equivalent may be necessary. Corticosteroids may hasten the return of a normal platelet count and may also protect capillaries and small vessels without effecting an elevation in the platelet count. Platelet transfusions are not usually helpful but may be indicated when the hemorrhage is acutely life-threatening. Such transfusions are most useful if thrombocytopenia persists long after the drug-antibody complex has been cleared.

Heparin is one of the most significant causes of thrombocytopenia. In cardiac patients the frequency averages about 5 percent.[197–200] There is no persuasive evidence that heparin derived from beef lung is more commonly associated with thrombocytopenia than other types of heparin. Some preparations of heparin may contain fractions that exhibit direct platelet-aggregating effects; these may contribute nonspecifically to thrombocytopenia. This effect may be most marked in those fractions with the highest molecular weight and the lowest affinity for antithrombin. By contrast, an immune etiology is established in many patients in vitro by demonstrating IgG-dependent aggregation or serotonin release of normal platelets, upon the addition of heparin in the presence of patient's test plasma obtained during periods of thrombocytopenia. The nature of the offending antigen in heparin, or complexes formed by heparin with blood elements, and its relationship to the biologically active heparin fractions, however, remain to be defined. In addition, some patients with heparin-induced thrombocytopenia develop paradoxical thrombosis and DIC.

The development of thromboembolism in association with thrombocytopenia is unique to heparin and is presumably related to the capacity of the heparin : antibody complex to activate platelets.

Other Hematologic Abnormalities Caused by Cardiac Drugs

Amyl nitrite, sodium nitrite, and nitroglycerin oxidize hemoglobin to methemoglobin, a molecule note capable of carrying oxygen. The patient with methemoglobinemia appears cyanotic but has a normal arterial PO_2, and oxygen therapy will not improve the pallor. Although symptomatic methemoglobinemia may occur in adults, most cases are seen in children who accidentally ingest medications prescribed for adults. Occasionally, adults with mild congenital methemoglobinemia will become markedly symptomatic when exposed to small doses of these same medications.[201] This complication may become more frequent with the increasing use of intravenous nitroglycerin. If venous blood is chocolate brown, and if this color persists after the blood is shaken in air, the diagnosis of methemoglobinemia is almost certain. The diagnosis is confirmed when the addition of a few drops of 10 percent potassium cyanide leads to the rapid production of the bright red cyanmethemoglobin. Symptoms are nonspecific and consist of dyspnea, headache, fatigue, and dizziness. Since normal red cells enzymatically reduce the methemoglobin, these events are usually self-limited if the responsible drug is discontinued. In severe cases or in patients with enzyme defects, methylene blue may be administered to stimulate reduction of the methemoglobin.

Other medications may interfere with oxygen delivery to tissues. For example, sodium nitroprusside (used in the treatment of hypertensive emergencies and to reduce afterload in heart failure) may cause fatigue, nausea, abnormal behavior, and muscle spasm when the medication reacts with oxyhemoglobin to produce cyanmethemoglobin and free cyanide ions.[202,203]

Hydralazine, procainamide, and occasionally phenytoin may cause a lupus erythematosus-like syndrome, with urticaria, erythema multiforme, photosensitivity, delirium, and immune-mediated blood cell destruction.[204,205] Although patients with drug-induced lupus have positive antinuclear antibody tests and many of the clinical manifestations of the systemic form, renal function is not usually impaired, and all these manifestations usually remit within several months when the offending drug is discontinued. The syndrome is of particular importance in cardiac patients, since the onset of chest pain, pleurisy, or pericardial effusion in the patient with heart disease could lead to an erroneous diagnosis unless drug-induced lupus is suspected.

Cardiac Effects of Anticancer Therapies

With the advent of intensive radiation therapy and aggressive chemotherapy, cardiac toxicity of antitumor therapies has increased greatly (Table 8-4). Formerly, the heart was considered to be relatively radioresistant and seemed to be spared most of the side effects of chemotherapy. The frequency of cardiovascular complications, however, has risen sharply with the use of curative forms of radiation therapy for Hodgkin's disease and non-Hodgkin's lymphoma and the addition of the anthracyclines, a potent class of chemotherapeutic agents.

Radiation Therapy

Therapeutic radiation causes heart damage by either acute or chronic injury to various structures.[206,207] The pericardium is most commonly affected, with less damage to the myocardium, endocardium, and papillary muscles; the heart valves and coronary arteries are least

Table 8-4. Cardiovascular Complications of Chemotherapeutic Drugs

Agent	Cardiac Toxicity
Amsacrine	Arrhythmia, cardiomyopathy
Busulfan	Pulmonary fibrosis
	Pulmonary hypertension
Cisplatin	Endocardial fibrosis
Cyclophosphamide	ECG changes
Cytosine arabinoside	Cardiac necrosis
	Congestive heart failure
Diethylstilbestrol	Pericarditis
Doxorubicin	Cardiovascular deaths
Etoposide	ECG changes, cardiomyopathy
5-Fluorouracil	? Sudden death, myocardial infarction
Methotrexate	? Myocardial infarction
Mitomycin	ECG changes
Mitoxantrone	Myocardial damage
Taxol	Cardiomyopathy
Vincristine	Sudden death, myocardial dysfunction
	Hypotension, myocardial infarction

damaged. Severe pericardial damage with pericarditis, acute myocardial infarction, valvular disease, cardiomyopathy, and arrhythmias are recognized complications.

Pericardial abnormalities have been divided into early, intermediate, and late changes.[206] Pericarditis, the most common acute cardiovascular complication of radiation therapy, occurs in 10 to 15 percent of patients with Hodgkin's disease who receive over 4,000 rads to the mediastinum. These episodes are characterized by fever, pleuritic pain, pericardial friction rub, and the echocardiographic changes to be expected with this condition. The time from completion of chemotherapy to the clinical onset of pericarditis ranges from 0 to 85 months, with the peak frequency occurring between 5 and 9 months. Echocardiography demonstrates a pericardial effusion in almost all patients. Long-term follow-up of patients cured of underlying neoplastic disease shows that symptoms of pericarditis may not develop for 8 to 10 years. The frequency of pericarditis appears to be a function of the fractional and total dose of radiation to the pericardium and the proportion of the heart irradiated. When the entire dose of radiation is delivered through an anterior port, the incidence of pericarditis is increased.[208] However, when chest irradiation is delivered in divided doses to anterior and posterior ports and with a subcarinal shield, the incidence of pericarditis decreases to 2.5 percent, without increasing the risk of relapse of Hodgkin's disease. If the entire heart receives therapeutic doses of radiation, up to 50 percent of patients may develop pericardial complications. To ensure adequate therapy of large mediastinal masses, total heart irradiation has been replaced with curative forms of chemotherapy.

Echocardiographic studies carried out before and within 6 months after conventional irradiation therapy in women with breast cancer demonstrate decreases in the fractional systolic shortening of the left ventricular minor-axis diameter and in the systolic blood pressure/end-systolic diameter ratio. This transient depression of left ventricular function, occurring within the first 6 months after postoperative radiation, disappears over the subsequent 6 months. Accordingly, it is recommended that routine follow-up during the first year after radiation therapy should consist of frequent echocardiograms and chest roentgenograms. If cardiac diameter is increased, or if clinical manifestations suggest pericarditis or pericardial effusion (and there is no reason to suspect another cause of pericarditis), patients may be treated symptomatically. They may occasionally require pericardiocentesis and/or pericardiectomy.

Radiation-induced endocardial fibrosis may lead to restrictive cardiomyopathy, detected by a variety of nonspecific electrocardiographic changes and varying degrees of AV block.[209] Additionally, regurgitation may develop secondary to radiation-induced papillary muscle dysfunction; aortic regurgitation may occur as a consequence of endocardial valvular thickening.[210] The onset of new murmurs after radiation therapy should alert the physician to these possibilities. Three-fourths of the patients exposed to more than 3,500 rads, particularly with more exposure of the anterior thorax, develop myocardial fibrosis with more involvement of the right than of the left ventricle. Functional abnormalities on echocardiography and radionuclide angiocardiography may occur 5 to 15 years after radiation, although newer radiotherapy techniques should permit earlier detection.[207]

Since myocardial infarction may develop many months after receiving, 4,000 rads to the heart, it has been proposed that radiation induces CAD.[211] This hypothesis is supported by (1) the occurrence of CAD in very young subjects with no predisposing factors and with disease limited to coronary vessels within the path of the radiation beam; (2) absence of atherosclerosis in arteries not exposed to irradiation; (3) reports of occlusive lesions in other arteries (e.g., the carotid artery after irradiation); (4) the presence of distinctive pathologic changes; and (5) the production of similar lesions in experimental models. Coronary artery lesions induced by radiotherapy appear to be pathologically distinct and to contain severe medial and adventitial fibrosis in continuity with overlying epicardial fibrous tissue and a near absence of lipid in the intimal lesions. Affected younger patients examined at autopsy demonstrate that the proximal portions of the arteries are significantly narrower than the distal portions with significant loss of smooth muscle cells from the media.[212]

Radiation-induced coronary artery or carotid artery obstruction or occlusion may require surgical treatment. Since this complication is infrequent and because lowering the dose of radiation might prejudice therapeutic efficacy for the neoplastic process, no systematic attempts have been made to prevent this complication other than considering chemotherapeutic alternatives when total heart irradiation is otherwise deemed necessary.

Chemotherapeutic Drugs

There have been major advances over the last 25 years in the management of many neoplastic disorders by combination chemotherapy. Therapies have become more aggressive, and new agents have been introduced that produce significant patient responses and longer survival. Unfortunately, increased toxicity often accompanies these improved responses. Although most of the complications caused by anticancer drugs primarily affect those tissues exhibiting active proliferation, such as the bone marrow and gastrointestinal tract, both early and late cardiotoxicity occurs with increasing frequency (Table 8-4).[213–216]

The incidence of cardiac toxicity resulting from chemotherapy for neoplastic disease has increased dramatically following the advent of the anthracycline drugs (e.g., doxorubicin, daunorubicin). Prior to the appearance of the anthracyclines, the only notable cardiopulmonary complications of chemotherapy for neoplastic diseases were orthostatic hypotension and the rare myocardial infarctions that occurred in the course of therapy with vincristine, a periwinkle alkaloid, and the interstitial lung disease and mild pulmonary hypertension secondary to pulmonary fibrosis created by bleomycin or busulfan.

Doxorubicin, an anthracycline with potent antitumor effects, binds to both strands of the DNA helix, inhibiting nucleic acid synthesis and intercalating between base pairs, and thereby inhibiting the normal function of DNA and RNA polymerases. Its inhibitory ability results in a potent antitumor activity. Doxorubicin has received more attention than the related compound, daunorubicin, because of its wider spectrum of antitumor activity in solid tumors and hematologic malignancies. Complete remissions in 30 to 40 percent of patients with Hodgkin's disease and non-Hodgkin's lymphoma, as well as all the acute leukemias, are produced by doxorubicin. Its effectiveness is enhanced when it is combined with other chemotherapeutic agents. Remission rates of 60 to 80 percent are attained in adults with acute leukemia when doxorubicin is used in combination with cytosine arabinoside, bleomycin, cyclophosphamide, vincristine, and corticosteroids in patients with lymphomas. Although the majority of toxic manifestations produced by these drugs, including alopecia, gastrointestinal distress, myelosuppression, and mucositis, were predictable from animal studies, the occurrence of cardiac toxicity and the interactions with radiation therapy were unexpected.[217,218]

Cardiotoxicity may be early or late. Early cardiotoxicity includes arrhythmias, electrocardiographic abnormalities, left ventricular dysfunction, a pericarditis-myocarditis syndrome, and (rarely) sudden death with myocardial infarction.[217,218] Arrhythmias, (including supraventricular tachyarrhythmias and premature atrial and ventricular contractions) and abnormalities of conduction (e.g., left axis deviation, decreased QRS voltage, and other nonspecific ST-segment and T-wave abnormalities) occur in approximately 10 percent of patients. These electrocardiographic changes are usually transient, may occur even at low doses of the anthracycline, and are usually seen within several days after administration of the drug.

The pericarditis-myocarditis syndrome and acute left ventricular dysfunction (LVD) are rare events. Acute LVD may occur in patients with marginal cardiac reserve, whereas acute pericarditis-myocarditis syndrome has been seen in patients with no previous cardiac history. Sudden death may occur as a result of an arrhythmia, myocardial infarction, or acute LVD.

Late or chronic cardiotoxicity usually results from dose-dependent degenerative cardiomyopathy, which manifests as sinus tachycardia, tachypnea, cardiomegaly, peripheral and pulmonary edema, hepatomegaly, venous congestion, and pleural effusion.[219] Cardiomyopathy develops as a cumulative consequence of the drug, occurring with increasing frequency at higher doses (Fig. 8-6). Congestive heart failure occurs within days to months after the administration of the last dose.[220] It is usually refractory to therapy. When it is severe, as in patients who present with marked dyspnea and with evidence of heart failure within 4 weeks of the last dose of doxorubicin, survival is short (i.e., usually less than 2 weeks). The majority of patients with less severe symptoms may be treatable with digitalis and diuretics, but the frequency of cardiac death is high.

In chronic anthracycline toxicity, pathologic examination discloses enlarged, pale, flabby hearts with dilated ventricles. Mural thrombi are occasionally found, but the coronary arteries and cardiac valves appear normal. Light microscopy reveals a severe cardiomyopathy with fewer myocardial cells showing degenerative changes. Electron microscopy shows extensive depletion of myofibrillar bundles, myofibrillar lysis, and distortion and disruption of the Z-lines. The mitochondria are swollen, with disrupted cristae and inclusion bodies. Routine autopsy studies on patients who received anthracycline chemotherapy may reveal little pathologic change despite clinical evidence of toxicity.[221,222] On the other hand, histologic signs of drug toxicity may be seen without clinical signs or symptoms.

The incidence of cardiomyopathy with doxorubicin is 1.7 percent, and with daunorubicin it is 4.4 percent. It is fatal in over one-half the affected patients.[217] With anthracycline, there is a clear dose-related incidence of cardiomyopathy (Fig. 8-6). In a study of this response involving 764 patients, none who received cumulative doses of less than 500 mg/m^2 showed cardiomyopathy, whereas a progressive increase in the frequency of this complication was noted with higher doses (Fig. 8-6).[222] Cumulative doses of doxorubicin should accordingly be held to less than 450 to 500 mg/m^2 (500 to 600 mg/m^2 for daunorubicin). However, car-

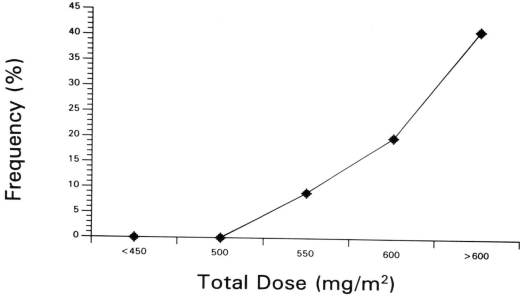

Fig. 8-6. Correlation of cardiomyopathy and the total dose of doxorubicin in adults. Whereas a cumulative dose of less than 500 mg/m² generally fails to produce cardiomyopathy in previously asymptomatic adults, the frequency of cardiomyopathy is directly related to increasing cumulative doses greater than this level.[222]

diomyopathy is increasingly being reported when doxorubicin doses are below 450 mg/m². Use of these agents in combination with other types of therapy (such as radiation or cyclophosphamide) may be synergistic in the pathogenesis of cardiomyopathy, since both radiation and cyclophosphamide alone have been described as potentially cardiotoxic.

No mechanism for doxorubicin cardiotoxicity has been established. Lipid peroxidation may be caused by DNA binding, specifically to spectrin, actin, or cardiolipin. Doxorubicin inhibits adenosine triphosphate (ATP) production, interferes with the sarcolemmal sodium-potassium pump, inhibits oxidative phosphorylation, may provoke an autoimmune response, binds to DNA precursors, interferes with mitochondrial respiration by inhibiting coenzyme Q, and causes myocardial necrosis by allowing the build-up of myocardial calcium.[223]

Because of the importance of these drugs in cancer chemotherapy and the high incidence of serious cardiac toxicity, several approaches have been suggested for early detection of this complication and for predicting suceptibility.[224] Radionuclide angiography appears to provide a sensitive and reproducible measurement of left ventricular dysfunction due to doxorubicin cardiotoxicity.[225] Sequential studies demonstrate the frequent presence of subclinical left ventricular abnormalities but may not be clinically significant if the studies are performed after exercise.

Endomyocardial biopsy is the definitive diagnostic procedure. When administration of doxorubicin is associated with a dose-related increase in the degree of myocyte damage, drug-associated degenerative changes are identified in patients receiving doses of 240 mg/m² or more.[226] Simultaneous studies using endomyocardial biopsy and radionuclide angiography demonstrate good correlation. While other noninvasive studies reveal an accelerating decrease in myocardial function with drug levels exceeding 400 mg/m^2, biopsy studies show a fairly constant progression of myocardial damage as a function of cumulative dose.[227] These findings suggest that compensatory mechanisms are available to maintain myocardial function despite pathologic damage.

Cardiac monitoring has demonstrated a reduction in the severity and mortality of doxorubicin-associated cardiac failure. Unfortunately, endomyocardial biopsy is invasive and moderately expensive. It has therefore been suggested that different strategies be devised for patients at high risk for cardiotoxicity. Patients at low risk for cardiac toxicity would undergo noninvasive cardiac monitoring, with measurements of ejection fraction at rest and during exercise at a dose of 400 mg/m^2 of doxorubicin. In patients at high risk, baseline ejection fraction would be measured at rest and with exercise at 100 mg/m^2 with repeat studies for each dose increment of 100 mg/m^2. If the results of any of the screening tests are abnormal, cardiac catheterization and endomyocardial biopsy may be advised. The histopathologic features found on endomyocardial biopsy can provide an estimate, for purposes of continuing therapy, of the risk of congestive heart failure if higher doses are administered.

There are several possibilities for preventing doxorubicin-induced cardiotoxicity.[228] Lowering the peak blood levels of the drug seems to be the best means for reducing cardiac toxicity. In a controlled study monitoring cardiac toxicity by both noninvasive techniques and endomyocardial biopsy, drug-related damage was significantly reduced but not eliminated when the drug was administered by prolonged continuous intravenous infusion rather than by bolus injection. The reduction in toxicity appears to be related to reduced peak plasma levels. Similarly, lower dosages given more frequently reduce peak plasma levels and seem to decrease the incidence of cardiac toxicity. Such changes in the drug regimen do not appear to compromise antitumor activity.[229]

Cardiomyopathies have also been reported secondary to high doses of intravenous cyclophosphamide.[230,231] In contrast to doxorubicin, the cardiotoxicity of cyclophosphamide is acute and not due to cumulative doses. It causes reductions in ECG voltage and systolic function. Although mortality is appreciable, survivors exhibit no residual cardiac abnormalities. In addition, the antineoplastic amsacrine (AMSA) has been associated with acute cardiac arrhythmias and cardiomyopathy.[232] Although AMSA-related cardiac events occur, they are less common than those due to doxorubicin. Manifestations of toxicity include ECG abnormalities, sudden death, and congestive heart failure. Hypokalemia appears to be a risk factor for the development of severe arrhythmias with this agent. The antraquinones (mitoxantrone and nonvantrone) are a new group of antineoplastic agents with significant clinical activity; they have been shown to produce favorable results in leukemias as well as in advanced breast cancer.[233,234] Deterioration in ejection fraction and congestive heart failure have also been reported.

Bone marrow transplantation, either allogenic or autologous, involves the combination of large doses of whole-body irradiation therapy and high-dose chemotherapy. Cardiac complications are frequent during transplant procedures of this type, including fatal cardiomyopathies, pericarditis, and significant arrhythmias.[235] High-dose cyclophosphamide and cytosine arabinoside are commonly associated with cardiotoxicity.

Also, the effect of whole-heart irradiation in conjunction with anthracycline drugs and cyclophosphamide appears to be additive.

REFERENCES

1. Duke M, Abelmann WH: The hemodynamic response to chronic anemia. Circulation 39:503, 1969
2. Varat MA, Adolph RJ, Fowler NO: Cardiovascular effects of anemia. Am Heart J 83:415, 1972
3. Torrance JD, Jacobs P, Restrepo A et al: Intraerythrocyte adaptation to anemia. N Engl J Med 283:165, 1970
4. Oski FA, Marshall BD, Cohen PJ et al: Exercise with anemia. The role of the left or right shifted oxygen-hemoglobin equilibrium curve. Ann Intern Med 74:44, 1971
5. Quinones MA, Gaasch WH, Alexander JK: Influence of acute changes in preload, afterload, contractile state and heart rate on ejection and isovolumic indices of myocardial contractility in man. Circulation 53:293, 1976
6. Reichek N, Wilson J, Sutton MS et al: Noninvasive determination of left ventricular end systolic stress: validation of the method and initial application. Circulation 65:99, 1982
7. Lenfant C, Torrance J, English E et al: Effect of altitude on the oxygen binding by hemoglobin and on organic phosphate levels. J Clin Invest 47:2652, 1968
8. Oski FA, Gottlieb AJ, Delivoria-Papadopoulos M, Miller WW: Red-cell 2,3-diphosphoglycerate levels in subjects with chronic hypoxemia. N Engl J Med 280:1165, 1969
9. Varriale P, Kwa RP, Vyas P: Intravenous nitroglycerin in transfusion therapy for severe anemia. Association with congestive heart failure. Arch Intern Med 144:401, 1984
10. Shubin H, Kaufmann R, Shapiro M, Levinson DC: Cardiovascular findings in children with sickle cell anemia. Am J Cardiol 6:875, 1960
11. Denenberg BS, Criner G, Jones R, Spann JF: Cardiac function in sickle cell anemia. Am J Cardiol 51:1674, 1983
12. Falk RH, Hood WB: The heart in sickle cell anemia. Arch Intern Med 142:1680, 1982
13. Rees AH, Stefadouras MA, Strong WB et al: Left ventricular performance in children with homozygous sickle cell anemias. Br Heart J 40:690, 1978
14. Gerry JL, Bulkley BH, Hutchins GM: Clinicopathologic analysis of cardiac dysfunction in 52 patients with sickle cell anemia. Am J Cardiol 42:211, 1978
15. Rubler S, Fleischer RA: Sickle cell states and cardiomyopathy. Sudden death due to pulmonary thrombosis and infarction. Am J Cardiol 19:867, 1967
16. Lippman SM, Ginzton LE, Thigpen T et al: Mitral valve prolapse in sickle cell disease: presumptive evidence for a linked connective tissue disorder. Arch Intern Med 145:435, 1985
17. Barrett O, Saunders DE, McFarlend DE, Humphries JO: Myocardial infarction in sickle cell anemia. Am J Hematol 16:139, 1984
18. Martin CR, Cobb C, Tatter D et al: Acute myocardial infarction in sickle cell anemia. Arch Intern Med 143:830, 1983
19. Ehlers LH, Levin AR, Klein AA et al: The cardiac manifestations of thalassemia major: natural history, noninvasive cardiac diagnostic studies, and results of cardiac catheterization. p. 171. In Engle MA (ed): Pediatric Cardiovascular Disease. Cardiovascular Clinics II. FA Davis, Philadelphia, 1981
20. Sapoznikov D, Lewis N, Rachmilewitz EA et al: Left ventricular filling and emptying patterns in anemia due to beta thalassemia. A computer-assisted echocardiographic study. Cardiology 69:276, 1982
21. Lewis BS, Lewis N, Degan I et al: Studies of left-ventricular function in anemia due to beta-thalassemia. Isr J Med Sci 18:928, 1982
22. Berk PD, Goldberg JD, Donovan PB: Therapeutic recommendations in polycythemia vera based on Polycythemia

Vera Study Group protocols. Semin Hematol 23:132, 1986

23. Braunwald E: Hypoxia, polycythemia, and cyanosis. p. 224. In Wilson JD, Braunwald E, Isselbacher KJ et al (eds): Harrison's Principles of Internal Medicine. McGraw-Hill, New York, 1991

24. Adamson JW, Fialkow PJ: Polycythemia vera: stem cell and probable clinical origin of the disease. N Engl J Med 245:913, 1976

25. Castle WB, Jandl JH: Blood viscosity and blood volume: opposing influences upon oxygen transport in polycythemia. Semin Hematol 3:193, 1966

26. Golde DW, Hocking WG, Koeffler HP, Adamson JW: Polycythemia: mechanism and management. Ann Intern Med 95:71, 1981

27. Berlin NI: Polycythemia vera: an update. Semin Hematol 23:131, 1986

28. Murphy S: Polycythemia vera. p. 193. In Williams WJ, Beutler E, Erslev AJ, Lichtman MA (eds): Hematology. 4th Ed. McGraw-Hill, New York, 1990

29. Schafer AL: Bleeding and thrombosis in the myeloproliferative disorders. Blood 64:1, 1984

30. Dintenfass L: Viscosity of the packed red and white blood cells. Exp Mol Pathol 4:597, 1965

31. Silverstein MN, Petitt RM, Solberg LA, Jr: Anagrelide: a new drug for treating thrombocytosis. N Engl J Med 318:1292, 1988

32. Torrance JD, Lenfant C, Cruz J: Oxygen transport mechanisms in residents at high altitude. Respir Physiol 11:1, 1970

33. Balcerzak SP, Bromberg PA: Secondary polycythemia. Semin Hematol 12:353, 1976

34. Rosenthal A, Button LN, Nathan DG: Blood volume changes in cyanotic congenital heart disease. Am J Cardiol 29:162, 1971

35. Rosenthal A, Nathan DG, Marty AT et al: Acute hemodynamic effects of red cell production in polycythemia of cyanotic congenital heart disease. Circulation 42:197, 1970

36. Erslev AJ, Caro J: Secondary polycythemia: a boon or a burden? Blood Cells 10:177, 1984

37. Yeager SB, Freed MD: Myocardial infarction as a manifestation of polycythemia in cyanotic heart disease. Am J Cardiol 53:952, 1984

38. Wallis PJ, Skehan JD, Newland AC et al: Effects of erythropheresis on pulmonary hemodynamics and oxygen transport in patients with secondary polycythemia and cor pulmonale. Clin Sci 70:91, 1986

39. Wallis PJ, Cunningham J, Few JD et al: Effects of packed cell volume reduction on renal hemodynamics and the renin angiotensin aldosterone system in patients with secondary polycythemia and hypoxic cor pulmonale. Clin Sci 70:81, 1986

40. York EL, Junes RL, Menon D, Sproule BJ: Effects of secondary polycythemia on cerebral blood flow in chronic obstructive pulmonary disease. Am Rev Respir Dis 121:813, 1980

41. Charache S, Weatherall DJ, Clegg JB: Polycythemia associated with hemoglobinopathy. J Clin Invest 45:813, 1966

42. Adamson JW, Finch CA: Erythropoietin and the polycythemias. Ann NY Acad Sci 149:560, 1968

43. Charache S, Achuff S, Winslow R et al: Variability of the homeostatic response to P50. Blood 52:1156, 1978

44. Smith J, Landow SA: Smoker's polycythemia. N Engl J Med 298:6, 1978

45. Weinreb NJ, Shih CF: Spurious polycythemia. Semin Hematol 12:397, 1975

46. Westring DW: Aortic valve disease and hemolytic anemia. Ann Intern Med 65:203, 1966

47. Miller DS, Mengel CE, Kremer WB et al: Intravascular hemolysis in a patient with valvular heart disease. Ann Intern Med 65:210, 1966

48. Rose JC, Hufnagel CA, Freis CD et al: The hemodynamic alterations produced by a plastic valvular prosthesis for severe aortic insufficiency in man. J Lab Clin Med 33:891, 1954

49. Sayed HM, Dacie JV, Handley DA et al: Hemolytic anemia of mechanical origin after open-heart surgery. Thorax 16:356, 1961

50. Dacie JV: The Hemolytic Anemias, Part III. Grune & Stratton, New York, 1967

51. Sears AD, Crosby WH: Intravascular hemolysis due to intracardiac prosthetic devices. Diurnal variations related to activity. Am J Med 39:341, 1965

52. Zezulka A, Schapiro L, Sind S: Chronic haemolytic anemia in hypertrophic cardiomyopathy. Br Heart J 52:474, 1984

53. Nevaril CG, Lynch EC, Alfrey CP Jr, Hellums J: Erythrocyte damage and destruction induced by shearing stress. J Lab Clin Med 71:784, 1968

54. Fairbanks VF, Beutler E: Iron deficiency. p. 482. In Williams WJ, Beutler E, Erslev AJ, Lichtman MA (eds): Hematology. McGraw-Hill, New York, 1990

55. Finch CA, Miller LR, Inamdar AR et al: Iron deficiency in the rat. Physiological and biochemical studies of muscle dysfunction. J Clin Invest 58:447, 1976

56. Finch CA, Gollnick PD, Hlastala MP: Lactic acid acidosis as a result of iron deficiency. J Clin Invest 64:129, 1979

57. MacDonald VW, Charache S, Hathaway PJ: Iron deficiency anemia: mitochondrial α-glycerophosphate dehydrogenase in guinea pig skeletal muscle. J Lab Clin Med 105:11, 1985

58. Mackler B, Person R, Grace R: Iron deficiency in the rat: effects on energy metabolism in brown adipose tissue. Pediatr Res 19:989, 1985

59. Evans TC, Mackler B: Effects of iron deficiency on energy conservation in rat liver and skeletal muscle submitochondrial particles. Biochem Med 34:93, 1985

60. Galan P, Hercberg S, Touitou Y: The activity of tissue enzymes in iron-deficient rat and man: an overview. Comp Biochem Physiol 77B:647, 1984

61. Brittenham GM: Disorders of iron metabolism: iron deficiency and overload. p. 327. In Hoffman R, Benz EJ Jr, Shattil SJ et al (eds): Hematology: Basic Principles and Practice. Churchill Livingstone, New York, 1991

62. Swan WGA, Dewar HA: The heart in hemochromatosis. Br Heart J 14:117, 1952

63. Finch SC, Finch CA: Idiopathic hemochromatosis, an iron storage disease. Medicine 34: 381, 1955

64. Wasserman AJ, Richardson DW, Baird CL, Wyso EM: Cardiac hemochromatosis simulating constrictive pericarditis. Am J Med 32:316, 1962

65. Fairbanks VF, Baldus WP: Iron overload. p. 752. In Williams WJ, Beutler E, Erslev AJ, Lichtman MA (eds): Hematology. McGraw-Hill, New York, 1990

66. Leon MD, Borer JS, Bacharach SL et al: Detection of early cardiac dysfunction in patients with severe beta-thalassemia and chronic iron overload. N Engl J Med 301:1143, 1979

67. Buja LM, Roberts WC: Iron in the heart. Etiology and clinical significance. Am J Med 51:209, 1971

68. Schafer AI, Cheron RG, Dluhy R et al: Clinical consequences of acquired transfusional iron overload in adults. N Engl J Med 304:319, 1981

69. Easley RM, Schreiner BF, Yu PN: Reversible cardiomyopathy associated with hemochromatosis. N Engl J Med 287:866, 1972

70. Skinner C, Kenmore CF: Haemochromatosis presenting as congestive cardiomyopathy and responding to venesection. Br Heart J 35:466, 1973

71. Wolfe L, Olivieri N, Sallan D et al: Prevention of cardiac disease by subcutaneous deferoxamine in patients with thalassemia major. N Engl J Med 312:1600, 1985

72. Schafer AI, Rabinowe S, LeBoff MS, et al: Long term efficacy of deferoxamine iron chelation therapy in adults with acquired transfusional overload. Arch Intern Med 145:1217, 1985

73. Cohen A, Schwartz E: Iron chelation therapy with deferoxamine in Cooley anemia. J Pediatr 92:643, 1978

74. Harker LA: Pathogenesis of thrombosis. p. 1559. In Williams WJ, Beutler E, Erslev AJ, Lichtman MA (eds): Hematology. McGraw-Hill, New York, 1990

75. Bauer KA: Pathobiology of the hypercoagulable state: clinical features, laboratory evaluation, and management. p. 1415. In Hoffman R, Benz EJ Jr, Shattil SJ et al (eds): Hematology: Basic

Principles and Practice. Churchill Livingstone, New York, 1991

76. Harker LA, Slichter SJ: Platelet and fibrinogen consumption in man. N Engl J Med 287:999, 1972

77. Pober JS, Cotran RS: Cytokines and endothelial cell biology. Physiol Rev 70:427, 1990

78. Harlan JM, Lie DY: Adhesion: Its Role in Inflammatory Disease. WH Freeman, New York, 1991

79. Huber AR, Kunkel S, Todd RF III, Weiss SJ: Regulation of transendothelial neutrophil migration by endogenous interleukin-8. Science 254:99, 1991

80. Gimbrone MA Jr: Vascular Endothelium in Hemostasis and Thrombosis. Churchill Livingston, Edinburgh, 1986

81. Egeberg O: Inherited antithrombin deficiency causing thrombophilia. Thromb Diath Haemorrh 13:516, 1965

82. Gruenberg JC, Smallridge RC, Rosenberg RD: Inherited antithrombin-III deficiency causing mesenteric venous infarction: a new clinical entity. Ann Surg 1975:791, 1981

83. Mackie M, Bennett B, Ogston D, Douglas AS: Familial thrombosis: inherited deficiency of antithrombin III. Br Med J 1:136, 1978

84. Vikydal R, Korninger C, Kyrle PA: The prevalence of hereditary antithrombin-III deficiency in patients with a history of venous thromboembolism. Thromb Haemost 54:744, 1985

85. Winter JH, Fenech A, Ridley W: Familial antithrombin III deficiency. Q J Med 204:373, 1982

86. Cosgriff TM, Bishop DT, Hershgold EJ: Familial antithrombin III deficiency: its natural history, genetics, diagnosis and treatment. Medicine 62:209, 1983

87. Bock SC, Prochownik EV: Molecular genetic survey of 16 kindreds with hereditary antithrombin III deficiency. Blood 70:1273, 1987

88. Prochownik EV, Antonarkis S, Bauer KA: Molecular heterogeneity of inherited antithrombin III deficiency. N Engl J Med 308:149, 1983

89. Finazzi G, Caccia R, Barbui T: Different prevalence of thromboembolism in the subtypes of congenital antithrombin deficiency: review of 404 cases. Thromb Haemost 58:1094, 1987

90. Buchanan GR, Holtkamp CA: Reduced antithrombin III levels during L-asparaginase therapy. Med Pediatr Oncol 8:7, 1980

91. Marciniak E, Gockemen JP: Heparin-induced decrease in circulating antithrombin III. Lancet II:581, 1978

92. Kitchens CS: Amelioration of antithrombin III deficiency by coumarin administration. Am J Med Sci 293:403, 1987

93. Hoffman DL: Purification and large-scale preparation of antithrombin III. Am J Med 87, suppl. 3B:23S, 1989

94. Mannucci PM, Boyer C, Wolf M: Treatment of congenital antithrombin III deficiency with concentrates. Br. J Haematol 50:531, 1982

95. Schwartz RS, Bauer KA, Rosenberg RD: Clinical experience with antithrombin III concentrate in treatment of congenital and acquired deficiency of antithrombin. Am J Med 87, suppl. 3B:53S, 1989

96. Hirsh J, Piovella F, Pini M: Congenital antithrombin III deficiency. Incidence and clinical features. Am J Med 87, suppl. 3B:34S, 1989

97. Griffin JH, Evatt B, Zimmerman TS et al: Deficiency of protein C in congenital thrombotic disease. J Clin Invest 68:1370, 1981

98. Broekmans AW, Veltkamp JJ, Bertina RM: Congenital protein C deficiency and venous thromboembolism: a study of three Dutch families. N Engl J Med 309:340, 1983

99. Horellou MH, Conard J, Bertina RM, Samama M: Congenital protein C deficiency and thrombotic disease in nine French families. Br Med J 289:1285, 1984

100. Bovill EG, Bauer KA, Dickerman JD: The clinical spectrum of heterozygous protein C deficiency in a large New England kindred. Blood 73:712, 1989

101. Miletich J, Sherman L, Broze G Jr: Absence of thrombosis in subjects with heterozygous protein C deficiency. N Engl J Med 317:991, 1987

102. Branson HE, Katz J, Marble R, Griffin

JH: Inherited protein C deficiency and coumarin-responsive chronic relapsing purpura fulminans in a newborn infant. Lancet 2:1165, 1983

103. Seligsohn U, Berger A, Abend M et al: Homozygous protein C deficiency manifested by massive venous thrombosis in the newborn. N Engl J Med 310:559, 1984

104. Bertina RM, Broekmans AW, Krommenhoek-van EsC, van Wijngaarden A: The use of a functional and immunologic assay for plasma protein C in the study of the heterogeneity of congenital protein C deficiency. Thromb Haemost 51:1, 1984

105. Comp PC, Nixon RR, Esmon CT: Determination of functional levels of protein C, an antithrombotic protein, using thrombin-thrombomodulin complex. Blood 63:15, 1984

106. Griffin JH, Mosher DF, Zimmerman TS, Kleiss AJ: Protein C, an antithrombotic protein, is reduced in hospitalized patients with intravascular coagulation. Blood 60:261, 1982

107. Rodeghiero F, Mannucci PM, Vigano S: Liver dysfunction rather than intravascular coagulation as the main cause of low protein C and antithrombin III in acute leukemia. Blood 63:965, 1984

108. D'Angelo SV, Comp PC, Esmon CT, D'Angelo A: Relationship between protein C antigen and anticoagulant activity during oral anticoagulation and in selected disease states. J Clin Invest 77:416, 1986

109. Peters C, Casella JF, Marlar RA: Homozygous protein C deficiency: observations on the nature of the molecular abnormality and the effectiveness of warfarin therapy. Pediatrics 81:272, 1988

110. Zauber NP, Stark MW: Successful warfarin anticoagulation despite protein C deficiency and a history of warfarin necrosis. Ann Intern Med 104:659, 1986

111. McGehee WG, Klotz TA, Epstein DJ, Rapaport SI: Coumarin necrosis associated with hereditary protein C deficiency. Ann Intern Med 100:59, 1984

112. Comp PC, Esmon CT: Recurrent venous thromboembolism in patients with a partial deficiency of protein S. N Engl J Med 311:1525, 1984

113. Schwarz HP, Fischer M, Hopmeier P: Plasma protein S deficiency in familial thrombotic disease. Blood 64:1297, 1984

114. Comp PC, Nixon RR, Cooper MR, Esmon CT: Familial protein S deficiency is associated with recurrent thrombosis. J Clin Invest 74:2082, 1984

115. Broekmans AW, Bertina RM, Reinalda-Proot J: Hereditary protein S deficiency and venous thrombo-embolism. A study in three Dutch families. Thromb Haemost 53:273, 1985

116. Engesser L, Broekmans AW, Briet E: Hereditary protein S deficiency: clinical manifestations. Ann Intern Med 106:677, 1987

117. Comp PC, Doray D, Patton D, Esmon CT: An abnormal plasma distribution of protein S occurs in functional protein S deficiency. Blood 67:504, 1986

118. Ploos van Amstel HK, Huisman MV, Reitsma PH: Partial protein S gene deletion in a family with hereditary thrombophilia. Blood 73:479, 1989

119. Bertina RM, van Wijngaarden A, Reinalda-Poot J: Determination of plasma protein S-the protein cofactor of activated protein C. Thromb Haemost 53:268, 1985

120. Comp PC, Thurnau GR, Welsh J, Esmon CT: Functional and immunologic protein S levels are decreased during pregnancy. Blood 68:881, 1986

121. D'Angelo A, Vigano-D'Angelo S, Esmon CT, Comp PC: Acquired deficiencies of protein S. Protein S activity during oral anticoagulation, in liver disease, and in disseminated intravascular coagulation. J Clin Invest 81:1445, 1988

122. Gouault-Heilmann M, Gadelha-Parente T, Levent M: Total and free protein S in nephrotic syndrome. Thromb Res 49:37, 1988

123. Egeberg O: Inherited fibrinogen abnormality causing thrombophilia. Thromb Diath Haemorrh 17:175, 1967

124. Henschen A, Kehl M, Southan C: Genetically abnormal fibrinogens—some current characterization strategies. p. 125.

In Haverkate F, Henschen A, Nieuwenhuizen W, Straub PW (eds): Fibrinogen-Structure Functional Aspects of Metabolism. Vol. 2. Walter de Gruyter, Berlin, 1983

125. Carrell N, McDonagh J: Functional defects in abnormal fibrinogens. p. 155. In Henschen A, Hessel B, McDonagh J, Saldeen T (eds): Fibrinogen: Structural Variants and Interactions. Vol. 3. Walter de Gruyter, Berlin, 1985

126. Johansson L, Hedner U, Nilsson IM: A family with thromboembolic disease associated with deficient fibrinolytic activity in vessel wall. Acta Med Scand 203:477, 1978

127. Aoki N, Moroi M, Sakata Y: Abnormal plasminogen. A hereditary abnormality found in a patient with recurrent thrombosis. J Clin Invest 61:1186, 1978

128. Wohl RC, Summaria L, Robbins KC: Physiological activation of the human fibrinolytic system. Isolation and characterization of human plasminogen variants, Chicago I and Chicago II. J Biol Chem 254:9063, 1979

129. Jorgensen M, Mortensen JZ, Madsen AG et al: A family with reduced plasminogen activator activity in blood associated with recurrent venous thrombosis. Scand J Haematol 29:217, 1982

130. Nilsson IM, Ljungner H, Tengborn L: Two different mechanisms in patients with venous thrombosis and defective fibrinolysis: low concentration of plasminogen activator or increased concentration of plasminogen activator inhibitor. Br Med J 290:1453, 1985

131. Wiman B, Ljungberg B, Chmielewska J: The role of the fibrinolytic system in deep venous thrombosis. J Lab Clin Med 105:265, 1985

132. Hamsten A, Wiman B, de Faire U, Blomback M: Increased plasma levels of a rapid inhibitor of tissue plasminogen activator in young survivors of myocardial infarction. N Engl J Med 313:1557, 1985

133. Tollefsen DM, Majerus DW, Blank MK: Heparin cofactor II. Purification and properties of a heparin-dependent inhibitor of thrombin in human plasma. J Biol Chem 257:2162, 1982

134. Sie P, Dupouy D, Pichon J, Boneu B: Constitutional heparin cofactor II deficiency associated with recurrent thrombosis. Lancet 2:414, 1985

135. Bertina RM, van der Linden IK, Engesser L: Hereditary heparin cofactor II deficiency and the risk of development of thrombosis. Thromb Haemost 57:196, 1987

136. Harker LA, Ross R, Slichter S, Scott C: Homocystine-induced arteriosclerosis: the role of endothelial cell injury and platelet response in its genesis. J Clin Invest 58:731, 1976

137. Cerebral Embolism Task Force: Cardiogenic brain embolism. Arch Neurol 43:71, 1986

138. Cerebral Embolism Task Force: Cardiogenic brain embolism: the second report of the Cerebral Embolism Task Force. Arch Neurol 46:727, 1989

139. Kannel WB, Abbott RD, Savage DD, McNamara PM: Epidemiologic features of chronic atrial fibrillation: the Framingham Study. N Engl J Med 306:1018, 1982

140. Wolf PA, Abbott RD, Kannel WB: Atrial fibrillation: a major contributor to stroke in the elderly: the Framingham Study. Arch Intern Med 147:1561, 1987

141. Halperin JL, Hart RG: Atrial fibrillation and stroke: new ideas, persisting dilemmas. Stroke 19:937, 1988

142. Sherman DG, Dyken ML, Fisher M et al: Cerebral embolism. Chest 89 (suppl):82S, 1986

143. Fuster V, Halperin JL: Left ventricular thrombi and cerebral embolism: an emerging approach. N Engl J Med 320:392, 1989

144. Hochman JS, Platia EB, Bulkley BH: Endocardial abnormalities in left ventricular aneurysms: a clinicopathologic study. Ann Intern Med 100:29, 1984

145. Roberts WC, Siegel RJ, McManus BM: Idiopathic dilated cardiomyopathy: analysis of 152 necropsy patients. Am J Cardiol 60:1340, 1987

146. Mikell FL, Asinger RW, Elsperger KJ, Anderson WR, Hodges M: Regional stasis of blood in the dysfunctional left ventricle: echocardiographic detection and

differentiation from early thrombosis. Circulation 66:755, 1982

147. Cabin HS, Roberts WC: Left ventricular aneurysm, intra-aneurysmal thrombus and systemic embolus in coronary heart disease. Chest 77:586, 1980

148. Fuster V, Gersh BJ, Giuliani ER et al: The natural history of idiopathic dilated cardiomyopathy. Am J Cardiol 47:525, 1981

149. Wolf PA, Dawber TR, Thomas HE, Kannel WB: Epidemiologic assessment of chronic atrial fibrillation and risk of stroke: the Framingham Study. Neurology 28:973, 1978

150. Sage JI, Van Uitert RL: Risk of recurrent stroke in patients with atrial fibrillation and nonvalvular heart disease. Stroke 14:537, 1983

151. Hart RG, Coull BM, Hart PD: Early recurrent embolism associated with nonvalvular atrial fibrillation. Stroke 14:688, 1983

152. Chesebro JH, Fuster V, Halperin JL: Atrial fibrillation—risk marker for stroke. N Engl J Med 323:1556, 1990

153. Aschenberg W, Schluter M, Kremer P et al: Transesophageal two-dimensional echocardiography for the detection of left atrial appendage thrombus. J Am Coll Cardiol 7:163, 1986

154. Dunn M, Alexander J, de Silva R: Antithrombotic therapy in atrial fibrillation. Chest 95(suppl):118S, 1989

155. Sherman DG, Dyken ML, Fisher M: Antithrombotic therapy for cerebrovascular disorders. Chest 96(suppl):140S, 1989

156. Halperin JL, Petersen P: Thrombosis in the cardiac chambers: ventricular dysfunction and atrial fibrillation. p. 215. In Fuster V, Verstraete M (eds): Thrombosis in Cardiovascular Disorders. WB Saunders, Philadelphia, 1992

157. Petersen P, Boysen G, Godtfredsen J et al: Placebo controlled, randomised trial of warfarin and aspirin for prevention of thromboembolic complications in atrial fibrillation: the Copenhagen AFASAK study. Lancet 1:175, 1989

158. Stroke Prevention in Atrial Fibrillation Study Group Investigators: Preliminary report of the Stroke Prevention in Atrial Fibrillation Study. N Engl J Med 322:863, 1990

159. The Boston Area Anticoagulation Trial for Atrial Fibrillation Investigators: The effect of low-dose warfarin on the risk of stroke in patients with nonrheumatic atrial fibrillation. N Engl J Med 323:1505, 1990

160. Connolly SJ, Laupacis A, Gent M et al: Canadian Atrial Fibrillation Anticoagulation (CAFA) study. J Am Coll Cardiol 18:349, 1991

161. Mueh JR, Herbst KD, Rapaport SI: Thrombosis in patients with the lupus anticoagulant. Ann Intern Med 92:156, 1980

162. Thiagarajan P, Shapiro S, DeMarco L: Monoclonal immunoglobulin M coagulation inhibitor with phospholipid specificity. Mechanism of a lupus anticoagulant. J Clin Invest 66:397, 1980

163. Carreras LO, Defreyn G, Machin SJ: Arterial thrombosis, intrauterine death and "lupus" anticoagulant: detection of immunoglobulin interfering with prostacyclin production. Lancet 1:244, 1981

164. Schleider MA, Nachman RL, Jaffe EA, Coleman M: A clinical study of the lupus anticoagulant. Blood 48:499, 1976

165. Brandt JT, Triplett DA, Musgrave K, Orr C: The sensitivity of different coagulation reagents to the presence of lupus anticoagulants. Arch Pathol Lab Med 11:120, 1987

166. Harris EN, Gharavi AE, Boey ML et al: Anticardiolipin antibodies: detection by radioimmunoassay and association with thrombosis in systemic lupus erythematosus. Lancet 2:1211, 1983

167. Hoffman R, Silverstein MN: Primary thrombocythemia. p. 881. In Hoffman R, Benz EJ, Jr, Shattil SJ et al (eds): Hematology: Basic Principles and Practice. Churchill Livingstone, New York, 1991

168. Murphy S, Iland H, Rosenthal D, Laszlo J: Essential thrombocythemia: an interim report from the Polycythemia Vera Study Group. Semin Hematol 23:177, 1986

169. Hehlmann R, Jahn M, Baumann B, Kopcke W: Essential thrombocythemia:

clinical characteristics and course of 61 cases. Cancer 61:2487, 1988

170. Jabaily J, Iland HJ, Laszlo J: Neurologic manifestations of essential thrombocythemia. Ann Intern Med 99:513, 1983

171. Michiels JJ, Abels J, Stekette J: Erythromelalgia caused by platelet-mediated arteriolar inflammation and thrombosis in thrombocythemia. Ann Intern Med 102:466, 1985

172. Preston FE, Martin JF, Stewart RM, Davies-Jones GAB: Thrombocytosis, circulating platelet aggregates and neurological dysfunction. Br Med J 2:1561, 1979

173. Preston FE, Emmanuel IG, Winfield DA, Malia RG: Essential thrombocythaemia and peripheral gangrene. Br Med J 3:548, 1974

174. Panlilio AL, Reiss RF: Therapeutic plateletpheresis in thrombocythemia. Transfusion 19:147, 1979

175. Taft EG, Babcock RB, Scharfman WB, Tartaglia AP: Plateletpheresis in the management of thrombocytosis. Blood 50:927, 1977

176. Lofunberg E, Wahlin A: Management of polycythaemia vera, essential thrombocythaemia and myelofibrosis with hydroxyurea. Eur J Haematol 41:375, 1988

177. Bensinger TA, Logue GL, Rendler RW: Hemorrhagic thrombocythemia: control of postsplenectomy thrombocytosis with melphalan. Blood 36:61, 1970

178. Kapoor AS: Clinical manifestations of neoplasia of the heart. p. 21. In Kapoor AS (ed): Cancer and the Heart. Springer-Verlag, New York, 1986

179. Schoen FJ, Berger BM, Guerina NC: Cardiac effects of noncardiac neoplasms. Cardiol Clin 657:1984

180. Waller BF, Gottdiener JS, Virmni R, Roberts WC: Structure-function correlations in cardiovascular and pulmonary diseases. The charcoal heart. Chest 77:671, 1980

181. Stewart JR, Fajardo LF: Cancer and coronary artery disease. Int J Radiat Oncol Biol Phys 11:915, 1978

182. Koiwaya Y, Nakamura M, Yamamoto K: Progressive ECG alterations in metastatic cardiac mural tumor. Am Heart J 105:339, 1983

183. Haedersdal C, Hasselbach H, Devantier A, Saunamak K: Pericardial hematopoiesis with tamponade in myelofibrosis. Scand J Haematol 34:270, 1985

184. Kutalek SP, Panidis IP, Kotler M et al: Metastatic tumors of the heart detected by two-dimensional echocardiography. Am Heart J 109:343, 1985

185. Parker BM: Valvular involvement in cancer. p. 64. In Kapoor AS (ed): Cancer and the Heart. Springer-Verlag, New York, 1986

186. Deppisch LM, Fayemi AO: Nonbacterial thrombotic endocarditis. Am Heart J 92:723, 1976

187. Perez CA, Presant CA, Amburg AL: Management of superior vena caval syndrome. Semin Oncol 5:123, 1978

188. Wahlin A, Olofsson B, Eriksson A, Backman C: Myeloma-associated cardiac amyloidosis. Acta Med Scand 215:189, 1984

189. Alpert MA: Cardiac amyloidosis. p. 162. In Kapoor AS (ed): Cancer and the Heart. Springer-Verlag, New York, 1986

190. Rosenthal DS, Braunwald E: Hematological-oncological disorders and heart disease. p. 1734. In Heart Disease. A Textbook of Cardiovascular Medicine. WB Saunders, Philadelphia, 1988

191. Adamson JW, Erslev AJ: Aplastic anemia. p. 158. In Williams WJ, Beutler E, Erslev AJ, Lichtman MA (eds): Hematology. McGraw-Hill, New York, 1990

192. Gavras F, Graff LG, Rose BD et al: Fatal pancytopenia associated with the use of captopril. Ann Intern Med 94:58, 1981

193. Lundh B, Hasselgren KH: Hematological side effects from antihypertensive drugs. Acta Med Scand (Suppl)628:73, 1979

194. Volosin K, Greenberg RM, Grenspon AJ: Tocainide-associated agranulocytosis. Am Heart J 109:1392, 1985

195. Dale DC: Neutropenia. p. 807. In Williams WJ, Beutler E, Erslev AJ, Lichtman MA (eds): Hematology. McGraw-Hill, New York, 1990

196. Hackett T, Kelton JG, Powers P: Drug-induced platelet destruction. Semin Thromb Hemost 8:116, 1982

197. Salzman EW, Rosenberg RD, Smith MH et al: Effect of heparin and heparin frac-

tins of platelet aggregation. J Clin Invest 65:64, 1980

198. Kelton JG, Sheridan D, Santos A, et al: Heparin-induced thrombocytopenia: Laboratory studies. Blood 72:925, 1988

199. Atkinson JL, Sundt TM, Kazmier FJ et al: Heparin-induced thrombocytopenia and thrombosis in ischemic stroke. Mayo Clin Proc 63:353, 1988

200. Chong BH: Heparin-induced thrombocytopenia. Blood Rev 2:108, 1988

201. Gibson GR, Hunter JB, Raabe DS et al: Methemoalbuminemia produced by high-dose intravenous nitroglycerin. Ann Intern Med 96:615, 1982

202. Shoemaker C, Meyers M: Sodium nitroprusside for control of severe disease of pregnancy: a case report and discussion of potential toxicity. Am J Obstet Gynecol 149:171, 1984

203. Vesey CJ, Cole PV: Blood cyanide and thiocyanate concentrations produced by long-term therapy with sodium nitroprusside. Br J Anaesth 57:148, 1985

204. Cush JJ, Goldings EA: Drug-induced lupus: clinical spectrum and pathogenesis. Am J Med 290:36, 1985

205. Weisbart RH, Yee WS, Colburn KK et al: Antiguanosine antibodies: a new marker for procainamide-induced systemic lupus erythematosus. Ann Intern Med 104:310, 1986

206. Niemtzow RC, Reynolds RD: Radiation therapy and the heart. p. 232. In Kapoor AS (ed): Cancer and the Heart. Springer-Verlag, New York, 1986

207. Gottdeiner JS, Katin MJ, Borer JS et al: Late cardiac effects of therapeutic mediastinal irradiation: assessment by echocardiography and radionuclide angiography. N Engl J Med 308:569, 1983

208. Taymor-Luria H, Kohn K, Pasternak RC: Radiation heart disease. J Cardiovasc Med 8:113, 1983

209. Gomez GA, Park JJ, Panahoh AM et al: Heart size and function after radiation therapy to the mediastinum in patients with Hodgkin's disease. Cancer Treat Rep 67:1099, 1983

210. Shashaty GG: Aortic insufficiency following mediastinal radiation for Hodgkin's disease. Am J Med Sci 287:46, 1984

211. Simon EB, Ling J, Mendizabal RC, Midawell J: Radiation-induced coronary artery disease. Am Heart J 108:1031, 1984

212. Brosius FC, Waller BF, Roberts WC: Radiation heart disease: analysis of 16 young (aged 15 to 33 years) necropsy patients who received over 3500 rads to the heart. Am J Med 7:519, 1981

213. Kantrowitz NE, Bristow MR: Cardiotoxicity of antitumor agents. Prog Cardiovasc Dis 27:195, 1984

214. Sunnenberg D, Kramer B: Long-term effects of cancer chemotherapy. Compr Ther 11:58, 1985

215. Perry MC: Effects of chemotherapy on the heart. p. 223. In Kapoor AS (ed): Cancer and the Heart. Springer-Verlag, New York, 1986

216. Lancaster LD, Ewy GA: Cardiac consequences of malignancy and their treatment. Adv Intern Med 30: 275, 1984

217. Lena L, Page JA: Cardiotoxicity of Adriamycin and related anthracyclines. Cancer Treat Rev 3:111, 1976

218. Ali MK, Soto PA, Maroongroge D et al: Electrocardiographic changes after Adriamycin chemotherapy. Cancer 43:465, 1979

219. Bristow MR, Billingham ME, Mason JW, Daniels JR: Clinical spectrum of anthracycline antibiotic cardiotoxicity. Cancer Treat Rep 62:873, 1978

220. Wortman JE, Lucas VS Jr, Schuster E et al: Sudden death during doxorubicin administration. Cancer 44:1588, 1979

221. Haq MM, Legha SS, Choksi J et al: Doxorubicin-induced congestive heart failure in adults. Cancer 56:1361, 1985

222. Greene HL, Reich SD, Dalen JE: How to minimize doxorubicin toxicity. J Cardiovasc Med 7:306, 1982

223. Milei J, Bovevis A, Llesoy S et al: Amelioration of Adriamycin-induced cardiotoxicity in rabbits by prenylamine and vitamin A + E. Am Heart J 111:95, 1986

224. Lee BH, Goodenday LS, Muswick GJ et al: Alterations in left ventricular diastolic function with doxorubicin therapy. J Am Coll Cardiol 9:184, 1987

225. Alexander J, Dainiak T, Berger HJ et al: Serial assessment of doxorubicin car-

diotoxicity with quantitative radionu-clide angiocardiography. N Engl J Med 300:278, 1979

226. Bristow MR, Mason JW, Billingham ME, Daniels JR: Doxorubicin cardio-myopathy. Evaluation by phonocardiog-raphy, endomyocardial biopsy, and cardiac catheterization. Ann Intern Med 88:168, 1978

227. Bristow MR, Mason JW, Billingham ME, Daniels JR: Dose effect and struc-ture-function relationships in doxorubi-cin cardiomyopathy. Am Heart J 102: 709, 1981

228. Doroshow HJ, Locker GY, Ifrim I, Myers CE: Prevention of doxorubicin cardiac toxicity in the mouse by N-acetylcysteine. J Clin Invest 68:1053, 1981

229. Legla SS, Benjamin RS, MacKay B et al: Reduction of doxorubicin cardiotoxicity by prolonged continuous intravenous infusion. Ann Intern Med 96:133, 1982

230. Baello EB, Ensberg ME, Ferguson DW et al: Effect of high-dose cyclophos-phamide and total-body irradiation on left ventricular function in adult patients with leukemia undergoing allogeneic bone marrow transplantation. Cancer Treat Rep 70:1187, 1986

231. Goldberg MA, Antin JH, Guinan EC, Rappeport JM: Cyclophosphamide car-diotoxicity: an analysis of dosing as a risk factor. Blood 68:1114, 1986

232. Lindpainter K, Lindpainter LS, Went-worth M, Burns CP: Acute myocardial necrosis during administration of am-sacrine. Cancer 57:1284, 1986

233. Pratt CG, Vietti TJ, Etcubanas E et al: Nonvantrone for childhood malignant solid tumors. A pediatric oncology group phase II study. Invest New Drugs 4:43, 1986

234. Landys K, Bergstom S, Andersson T, Noppa H: Mitoxantrone as a first line treatment of advanced breast cancer. In-vest New Drugs 3:133, 1985

235. Cazin V, Gorin C, Laport JP et al: Car-diac complications after bone marrow transplantation. A report on a series of 63 consecutive transplantations. Cancer 57: 2061, 1986

9

Tumors of the Heart and Pericardium

Hugh A. McAllister, Jr.
Robert J. Hall
Denton A. Cooley

Primary tumors of the heart and pericardium are rare, and reports have estimated that metastatic tumors are 16 to 40 times more common.[1,2] Nevertheless, attention should be focused on the detection of primary tumors since many tumors or cysts that would have been fatal in the past are now amenable to surgical removal. These tumors can often be life-threatening and are complicated by symptoms that may mimic other types of heart conditions. It is therefore important for cardiologists to enhance their knowledge of the distribution, histologic identification, and biologic behavior of primary cardiac tumors to achieve the most timely and successful clinical outcome.

Metastatic Neoplasms

The heart is involved in approximately 10 percent of patients with malignant neoplasms; of these, 85 percent have tumor

in the pericardium.[3] Approximately 10 percent of patients with secondary neoplasms of the heart have clinical evidence of cardiac disease; in 90 percent of these, the clinical dysfunction is the result of pericardial involvement, usually a pericardial effusion or neoplastic thickening of the pericardium, or both.[3] Although hemorrhagic pericardial effusion is frequent in patients with cardiac metastases, serous pericardial effusion is also common in patients who have malignant neoplasms without cardiac metastases. These "nonmetastatic" serous pericardial effusions are most commonly secondary to hypoalbuminemia. Pericardial injury secondary to chemotherapy or radiation therapy, as well as infective pericarditis in an immunologically compromised host, must also be considered.[4]

Nearly every type of malignant tumor from any organ and tissue has been reported to metastasize to the heart, with the exception of tumors primary to the central nervous system. In absolute numbers, the most common neoplasms with cardiac metastases are those of the lung in males and breast in females, followed

(Portions of this text adapted from McAllister,[144] with permission, and McAllister and Fenoglio.[5])

by leukemia and lymphoma, especially reticulum cell sarcoma. Approximately 10 percent of patients with carcinoma of the lung or breast will have cardiac metastases.[3] Among specific malignant neoplasms, those with the highest percentage of metastases to the heart are melanoma (70 percent), leukemia, and lymphoma.[3]

Forms of metastatic growth in the heart depend somewhat on the mode of spread and origin of the tumor. Some malignant neoplasms, especially carcinoma of the lung, breast, and esophagus, frequently involve the heart and pericardium by direct extension from contiguous structures. However, the primary tumor is far removed from the heart in approximately 50 percent of patients with carcinoma of the lung and breast with cardiac metastasis. In this case, there is no evidence of direct extension of the primary tumor to the heart; frequently, however, there is evidence of retrograde lymphatic spread of the tumor. Indeed, most carcinomas appear to reach the heart by retrograde lymphatic spread; if so, multiple small nodules, many of microscopic size, are found throughout the myocardium and epicardium.

Besides direct extension from contiguous structures and lymphatic spread, carcinoma may occasionally reach the heart by direct venous extension. This is especially true for renal cell carcinoma and hepatoma, which may extend along the inferior vena cava into the right atrium. Hematogenous spread, although unusual for carcinoma, is the main route of metastasis for sarcoma, lymphoma, and leukemia, as well as melanoma involving the heart.

Carcinomatous metastases are usually grossly visible, multiple, discrete, small, firm nodules; microscopically, they resemble the primary tumor and metastases in other organs (Fig. 9-1). Diffuse infiltration is characteristic of sarcomatous me-

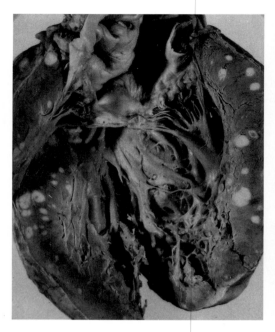

Fig. 9-1. Multiple nodules of malignant cells throughout the pericardium and myocardium are often found when the heart is involved by metastatic carcinoma. Nodules of metastatic papillary carcinoma of the thyroid were apparent microscopically in this heart. Cardiac metastases from carcinoma are usually well circumscribed, both macroscopically and microscopically. (From McAllister and Fenoglio.[5])

tastases. In either case, tumor necrosis is uncommon.

PRIMARY TUMORS OF THE HEART AND PERICARDIUM

Primary tumors of the heart and pericardium are rare, with an incidence of 0.001 to 0.28 percent in reported or collected autopsy series. At the Armed Forces Institute of Pathology (AFIP), we reviewed 533 primary tumors and cysts of the heart and pericardium; their relative incidence is summarized in Table 9-1.[5] Considering all age groups, the most common cardiac tumor is the myxoma. Forty percent of all benign cardiac tumors are myxomas, and 25 percent of all tumors and cysts of the heart and pericardium are myxomas.[6] In adults, almost one-half of the benign tumors are cardiac myxomas[5] (Table 9-2). Approximately one-fourth of all tumors and cysts of the heart and pericardium are malignant. Of these, 33 percent are angiosarcomas, 20 percent are rhabdomyosarcomas, 15 percent are mesotheliomas, and 10 percent are fibrosarcomas.

In infants and children, the most common cardiac tumor is the rhabdomyoma[7] (Tables 9-3 and 9-4). In infants (under 1 year of age) more than 75 percent of these tumors and cysts are rhabdomyomas or teratomas. Rhabdomyomas, fibromas, and myxomas are the most common cardiac tumors in children aged 1 to 15 years, accounting for 80 percent of benign tumors and 60 percent of all tumors and cysts in this age group. Malignant tumors are rare in the pediatric age group and comprise less than 10 percent of all tumors and cysts of the heart and pericardium.

Table 9-1.   Tumors and Cysts of the Heart and Pericardium in all Ages

Type	No.	%
Benign		
Myxoma	130	24.4
Lipoma	45	8.4
Papillary fibroelastoma	42	7.9
Rhabdomyoma	36	6.8
Fibroma	17	3.2
Hemangioma	15	2.8
Teratoma	14	2.6
Mesothelioma of the AV node	12	2.3
Granular cell tumor	3	—
Neurofibroma	3	—
Lymphangioma	2	—
Subtotal	319	59.8
Pericardial cyst	82	15.4
Bronchogenic cyst	7	1.3
Subtotal	89	16.7
Malignant		
Angiosarcoma	39	7.3
Rhabdomyosarcoma	26	4.9
Mesothelioma	19	3.6
Fibrosarcoma	14	2.6
Malignant lymphoma	7	1.3
Extraskeletal osteosarcoma	5	—
Neurogenic sarcoma	4	—
Malignant teratoma	4	—
Thymoma	4	—
Leiomyosarcoma	1	—
Liposarcoma	1	—
Synovial sarcoma	1	—
Subtotal	125	23.5
Total	533	100.0

(From McAllister and Fenoglio.[5])

Table 9-2. Tumors and Cysts of the Heart and Pericardium in Adults

Type	No.	%
Benign		
Myxoma	118	26.6
Lipoma	45	10.1
Papillary fibroelastoma	42	9.5
Hemangioma	11	2.5
Mesothelioma of the AV node	9	1.1
Fibroma	5	—
Teratoma	3	—
Granular cell tumor	3	—
Neurofibroma	2	—
Lymphangioma	2	—
Rhabdomyoma	1	—
Subtotal	241	54.3
Pericardial cyst	80	18.0
Bronchogenic cyst	6	1.4
Subtotal	86	19.4
Malignant		
Angiosarcoma	39	8.8
Rhabdomyosarcoma	24	5.4
Mesothelioma	19	4.3
Fibrosarcoma	13	2.9
Malignant lymphoma	7	1.6
Extraskeletal osteosarcoma	5	1.1
Thymoma	4	—
Neurogenic sarcoma	3	—
Leiomyosarcoma	1	—
Liposarcoma	1	—
Synovial sarcoma	1	—
Subtotal	117	26.3
Total	444	100.0

(From McAllister and Fenoglio.[5])

Diagnostic Studies

Although angiography characterizes the size, location, and mobility of the tumor, echocardiography and other imaging techniques have largely supplanted contrast angiography and usually permit immediate operative intervention without additional invasive studies. Echocardiography, transthoracic and transesophageal echocardiography, and computed tomography (CT) facilitate identification of pericardial effusion and intracavitary and pericardial masses. Magnetic resonance imaging (MRI) provides a global view of cardiac anatomy and plays an important role in the diagnosis and evaluation of both primary and secondary tumors of the heart, providing information about the location, extent, and attachment of the tumor. Pericardiocentesis may afford prompt symptomatic relief from pericardial tamponade and often provides a definitive cytologic diagnosis. The results of endomyocardial biopsy may contribute to the diagnosis in some cases. Calcification in myoxomas and other tumors as well as bone formation in metastatic

Table 9-3. Tumors and Cysts of the Heart and Pericardium in Infants

Type	No.	%
Benign		
Rhabdomyoma	28[a]	58.3
Teratoma	9	18.8
Fibroma	6	12.5
Hemangioma	1	2.1
Mesothelioma of the AV node	1	2.1
Subtotal	45	93.7
Bronchogenic cyst	1	2.1
Subtotal	1	2.1
Malignant		
Fibrosarcoma	1	2.1
Rhabdomyosarcoma	1	2.1
Subtotal	2	4.2
Total	48	100.0

[a] Includes three stillborn infants.
(From McAllister and Fenoglio.[5])

total excision would compromise any of these structures.[10] The technique for tumor excision varies because of the diversity of tumor presentations. Valve replacement may be necessary when the tumor encroaches on the valve. Tumors of the myocardium may be removed by ventriculotomy and enucleation.

Fragmentation and embolization are ever present threats in patients with cardiac tumors, and often the initial diagnosis is made after microscopic examination of a removed peripheral embolus. Thus, one should avoid vigorous palpation or other manipulations of the heart during cannulation and until cardiopulmonary bypass is started. Cardioplegia is important to prevent embolization into the lungs. The aortic cross-clamp prevents systemic embolization.

osteogenic sarcoma may occasionally be visible radiographically.

Operative Management

Operative management of cardiac tumors varies, depending upon the site and extent of the tumor. Alternate routes of cannulation are sometimes necessary. Surgical treatment of pericardial tumors includes drainage, biopsy, pericardial window, or resection.[8] Intrapericardial tumors may be excised without cardiopulmonary bypass, since they are sometimes only superficially attached. Most cardiac tumors, however, require cardiopulmonary bypass.

Total excision is the goal for benign or recurring tumors.[8,9] However, it is always necessary to consider the extent of involvement of the valves, coronary arteries, septum, and conduction system, and partial excision may be necessary when

Table 9-4. Tumors and Cysts of the Heart and Pericardium in Children

Type	No.	%
Benign		
Rhabdomyoma	35	39.3
Fibroma	12	13.5
Myxoma	12	13.5
Teratoma	11	12.4
Hemangioma	4	4.5
Mesothelioma of the AV node	3	3.4
Neurofibroma	1	1.1
Subtotal	78	87.6
Pericardial cyst	2	2.2
Bronchogenic cyst	1	1.1
Subtotal	3	3.4
Malignant		
Malignant teratoma	4	4.5
Rhabdomyosarcoma	2	2.2
Neurogenic sarcoma	1	1.1
Fibrosarcoma	1	1.1
Subtotal	8	9.0
Total	89	100.0

(From McAllister and Fenoglio.[5])

PRIMARY CARDIAC TUMORS

Myxoma

Before 1960, cardiac myxomas were generally misdiagnosed as chronic rheumatic heart disease. Since that time, clinicians have become increasingly aware of the ability of cardiac myxomas to imitate mitral valve disease. As newer diagnostic methods of cardiology have become available, these tumors have been correctly diagnosed and surgically excised in most cases. The clinical presentation of a cardiac myxoma mostly depends on the cardiac chamber involved by the tumor. The presentations of 130 patients in the AFIP series are summarized in Table 9-5.[5] Of the 57 patients with clinical signs and symptoms of mitral valve disease in this series, 56 had a myxoma in the left atrium; the other had a myxoma in the right atrium. Signs and symptoms included dyspnea, progressive or refractory congestive heart failure, systolic and

Table 9-5.   Cardiac Myxoma: Clinical Presentation in 130 Patients

Clinical Presentation[a]	No.
Signs and symptoms of mitral valve disease	57
Embolic phenomena	36
No cardiac symptoms—incidental finding	16
Signs and symptoms of tricuspid valve disease	6
Sudden unexpected death	5
Pericarditis	4
Myocardial infarction	3
Signs and symptoms of pulmonary valve disease	2
Fever of undetermined origin	2

[a] One patient with multiple myxomas had signs and symptoms of mitral and tricuspid valve disease.
(From McAllister and Fenoglio.[5])

diastolic murmurs, and atrial arrhythmias. Although the distinction between those patients with cardiac myxoma and those with intrinsic mitral valve disease may be difficult by physical examination, diagnosis may be aided by murmurs of changing intensity and laboratory findings such as an elevated erythrocyte sedimentation rate or increased gamma globulin levels. Either anemia or polycythemia may be present in these patients. Evidence has been presented that myxomas may produce erythropoietin.

The second most common clinical presentation of patients with cardiac myxoma is that of embolic phenomena. In 36 patients in the AFIP series, the initial event was embolic and occurred in patients with myxomas arising in either the left or right side of the heart. Diagnosis was difficult in the six patients with pulmonary emboli from right atrial myxoma. Each had persistent fever, changing murmurs, and progressive congestive heart failure. Slightly more than one-third of patients with a myxoma located in the left ventricle or the left atrium died of a cerebrovascular accident, and an embolic myxoma was found at autopsy. Symptoms or signs in the remaining 18 patients were sudden hemiparesis, sudden diplopia, or sudden loss of blood supply to an extremity. The common denominator in these patients was sudden onset of symptoms or signs suggesting arterial occlusion. Many of these tumors were diagnosed following arterial embolectomy. Occasionally, the myxoma was not identified microscopically, and some patients had repeated episodes of peripheral embolization before a cardiac myxoma was suspected. All but one of the patients with a myxoma in the left ventricle presented with signs or symptoms of emboli. An additional 18 had episodes of arterial embolic occlusion during the course of their disease, or evidence of myxoma emboli at autopsy. Three patients who presented with signs or symptoms of myocardial infarction had a myxoma embolus in at least one coronary artery at autopsy. Thus, patients with a myxoma in the left side of the heart most frequently have symptoms of mitral valve disease or of embolic phenomena. These were the presenting symptoms of 86 of 108 patients with myxomas of the left atrium or left ventricle in the AFIP series.

By contrast, myxomas arising in the right side of the heart may mimic any number of clinical entities. In addition to pulmonary emboli, patients with myxomas in the right atrium or ventricle may have signs or symptoms of tricuspid valve disease or pulmonary stenosis. Occasionally, patients with a myxoma in the right atrium or ventricle may present with pericarditis or with fever of undetermined origin. Rhythm disturbances are frequently present, especially right bundle branch block and atrial flutter or fibrillation. As with myxomas on the left side of the heart, advances in diagnostic cardiology have greatly aided the diagnosis of right atrial and ventricular myxomas.

More than 50 percent of patients with cardiac myxoma are in their fourth, fifth, and sixth decades; however, myxomas occur in all age groups. Twelve percent of patients in the AFIP series were older than 70 years, and 9 percent were in the pediatric age group (15 years or under). Most published series have indicated a nearly equal sex distribution. It appears, however, that nonfamilial cardiac myxoma is mainly a disorder of middle-aged women (mean age, 51 years), usually occurs in the left atrium, presents as a single tumor, and is not associated with any particular lesions elsewhere.

By contrast, familial cardiac myxoma is mainly a disorder of young men (mean age, 24 years), and is less commonly found in the left atrium. This type of disease is often multicentric and is occasionally associated with unusual or rare conditions, including skin pigmentation, such as lentigo and several types of nevi, which commonly affect the lips and oral cavity; cutaneous myxomas; pigmented nodular adrenocortical disease (with or without Cushing syndrome); myxoid mammary fibroadenomas; pituitary adenomas; and testicular tumors.[11] This familial myxoma syndrome appears to follow a pattern of mendelian dominant inheritance.[12]

The locations of the myxomas in this series are summarized in Table 9-6.[5] The myxomas were multiple in 5 percent of the patients, and in one patient a myxoma was present in each of the four cardiac chambers. The majority of myxomas arising in the atria, either left or right, are attached to the atrial septum, usually in the region of the limbus of the fossa ovalis; however, 10 percent originate in sites in the atria other than the septum. After the atrial septum, the most common site is the posterior atrial wall, followed by the anterior wall and the atrial appendage. By contrast, only 1 of the 10 ventricular myxomas originated from the ventricular septum. Although myxoma imitators such as papillary fibroelastomas, sarcomas, and (rarely) metastatic carcinomas have been localized to valves, we are not aware of a documented example of a true myxoma arising from a cardiac valve.

Table 9-6. Cardiac Myxoma: Location of 138 Myxomas in 130 Patients

Site[a]	No.	%
Left atrium	103	74.5
Right atrium	25	18.1
Right ventricle	5	3.7
Left ventricle	5	3.7

[a] Multiple myxomas were present in six patients.

(From McAllister and Fenoglio.[5])

Although cardiac myxomas differ in clinical presentation, depending on the chamber in which they are located, they are similar in gross and microscopic appearance, irrespective of their location. Grossly, most have a short, broad-based attachment and are pedunculated, gelatinous, and polypoid (Fig. 9-2), although some tumors have a rounded smooth surface. True sessile myxomas are distinctly rare (Fig. 9-3). The majority of so-called sessile myxomas have previously embolized, leaving only the broad base of the polypoid tumor attached to the endocardium. Characteristically, myxomas are

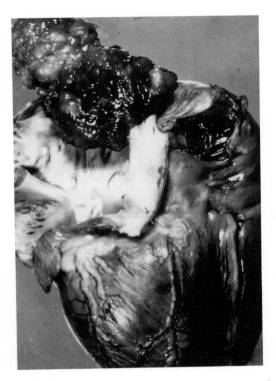

Fig. 9-2. Most cardiac myxomas consist of multiple, friable, polypoid fronds and have a distinctive mucoid or gelatinous appearance. Approximately 75 percent of cardiac myxomas arise in the left atrium, as shown here, and 18 percent arise in the right atrium. (From McAllister and Fenoglio.[5])

soft and gelatinous and frequently contain areas of hemorrhage. Their size varies from 1 to 15 cm in diameter, although most myxomas are 5 to 6 cm in diameter.

Microscopically, myxomas have a myxoid matrix composed of acid mucopolysaccharide within which are polygonal cells with scant eosinophilic cytoplasm (Fig. 9-4). These cells are arranged singly, often assuming a stellate shape, and in small nests; they are occasionally multinuclear.[13] The surface of the myxoma is covered by the polygonal cells, usually in a monolayer with focal clustering in crevasses. These cells also form vascular-like channels throughout the myxoid stroma, simulating primitive capillaries. Ultrastructurally, the polygonal cells closely resemble multipotential mesenchymal cells.[14-16] Occasionally, glandular elements are present within myxomas. These usually stain positively with both mucicarmine and periodic acid-Schiff (PAS) reagent with diastase pretreatment. Immunoperoxidase studies demonstrate positivity of the glandular cells for carcinoembryonic antigen (CEA), epithelial membrane antigen (EMA), and keratin.[17,18] Factor VIII-related antigen (FVIIIAg) is identified only in cells lining vascular spaces. An electron microscopy study of one tumor revealed well-formed glands having basement membranes, junctional complexes, and apical secretory granules.[18] The stroma contains variable amounts of reticular fibers, collagen, elastic fibers, and smooth muscle cells. Large arteries and veins are commonly present at the base of the tumor and communicate with the subendocardium. Lymphocytes and plasma cells are not infrequent, especially at the site of attachment to the subendocardium, and foci of extramedullary hematopoiesis are commonly found throughout the tumor. Foci of microscopic calcification are present in approximately 10 percent of myxomas, and areas of metaplastic bone

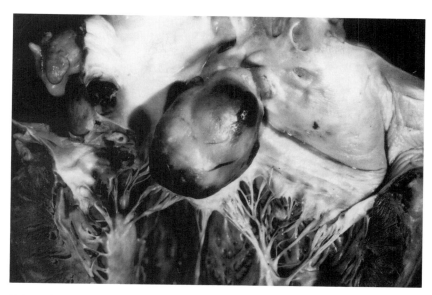

Fig. 9-3. Although most cardiac myxomas are polypoid and friable, a significant percentage are rounded and solid. Their surface is smooth, glistening and gelatinous, and foci of hemorrhage and thrombus are frequently present. (From McAllister and Fenoglio.[5])

occasionally occur. Rarely, a cardiac myxoma infarcts or undergoes degenerative changes to produce the so-called Gamna body of the heart.[19,20]

Although arguments supporting a thrombotic origin of cardiac myxomas have appeared in the literature,[21] they do not account for the following points:

1. True thrombi, even in the atria, organize into fibrous tissue; myxomas do not.

2. Fluid influx into the lesion in the low-pressure system of the atria cannot explain the myxomatous appearance of myxomas arising in the ventricles.

3. True thrombi are most frequent in patients with underlying cardiac disease and occur most frequently in the right atrium and right atrial appendage, whereas underlying cardiac disease is infrequent in patients with myxomas, and most myxomas arise in the left atrium, usually from the atrial septum. Myxomas

arising from the atrial appendage of either atrium are a distinct rarity, whereas this is the most common location for atrial thrombi. The most compelling argument against the thrombotic origin of the cardiac myxoma is based on tissue-culture work.[22] When thrombi are placed in tissue culture, fibroblasts overgrow the culture, as is true of cultured granulation tissue, whereas the cells obtained from cardiac myxomas grown in tissue culture are mononuclear and polygonal or multinuclear, and collagen formation does not occur. These tissue-cultured cells closely resemble the primitive multipotential mesenchymal cells characteristic of the cardiac myxoma.

Embryonal rests have been reported in the heart in the region of the limbus of the fossa ovalis, and many investigators have speculated that these tissue rests contain the cells of origin of the cardiac myxoma.[23] Although embryonal rests

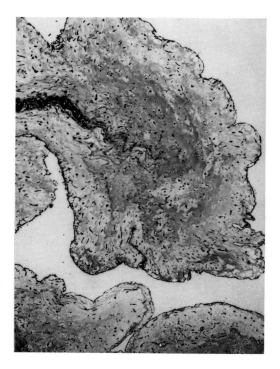

Fig. 9-4. Histologically, the cardiac myxoma consists of an acid mucopolysaccharide matrix within which are embedded polygonal cells and occasional blood vessels. The surface of the fronds of the myxoma is covered by cells similar to those embedded in the matrix. (H&E, × 305.) (From McAllister and Fenoglio.[5])

may occur in this region, more frequently clusters of "cardiac reserve" cells (multipotential mesenchymal cells) are found. In either case, the cardiac myxoma is most likely derived from these multipotential mesenchymal cells of the subendocardium. Although an occasional report has suggested that myxoma originates from endothelial or endocardial cells,[24] the overwhelming evidence gathered from immunoperoxidase,[25–28] ultrastructural,[15,16] and cytogenetic[29] studies supports the theory (originally proposed in the AFIP fascicle) that cardiac myxomas arise from subendocardial mesenchymal cells.

Complete surgical excision of a myxoma and its base along with a small rim of unaffected endocardium and myocardium is the treatment of choice. Surgical excision should not be unduly delayed because of the high incidence of embolization. It is not well recognized that special care must be taken during the operation to avoid embolization, and all cardiac chambers should be explored for the occasional multicentric tumor. If not completely excised, the cardiac myxoma can recur, although in many cases recurrence is probably caused by multiple foci of tumor growth.[30] Despite this tendency for recurrence, the existence of a true malignant cardiac myxoma remains in doubt. The malignant cardiac myxomas reported in the literature that we reviewed have either been malignant tumors of other types that had extensive areas of myxoid degeneration, or multiple myxomas that were benign.[5]

Papillary Fibroelastoma

Forty-two patients with fibroelastomas were identified in the AFIP series. They ranged in age from 25 to 86 years, although 55 percent were older than 60 years. Fibroelastomas are usually found incidentally at autopsy, or on surgically excised valves, and are not associated with cardiac dysfunction in most patients. However, in at least three reported cases, these tumors were associated with paroxysmal angina pectoris or sudden unexpected death.[5] In those three patients, the papillary tumor was located on the aortic side of the aortic valve and partially obstructed the ostium of a coronary artery.

Although they most frequently arise from the valvular endocardium, papillary fibroelastomas may arise anywhere in the heart, and occasionally are multiple. When these tumors occur on the atrioventricular (AV) valves they usually project into the atria. Although they may arise from the free edge of the valve, more commonly they arise from its mid portion (Fig. 9-5). On the semilunar valves, these tumors arise with nearly equal frequency on the ventricular and arterial side and may be situated anywhere on the valve.[5]

Grossly, papillary fibroelastomas resemble a sea anemone, with multiple papillary fronds attached to the endocardium by a short pedicle. Histologically and ultrastructurally, the papillary fronds consist of a central core of dense connective tissue surrounded by a layer of loose connective tissue and covered by endothelial cells, which are frequently hyperplastic. The mantle of loose connective tissue consists of an acid mucopolysaccharide matrix, within which are embedded collagen fibrils, elastic fibers, scattered smooth muscle cells, and occasional mononuclear cells. Usually, a fine meshwork of elastic fibers surrounds a central collagen core. Occasionally, however, the entire central core appears to consist of elastic fibers. The central core of the papillary fibroelastoma is continuous with the connective tissue of the endocardium and merges imperceptibly with it. Similarly, the endothelial cells covering the papillary fronds are contiguous with the normal endothelial cells covering the endocardium or the cardiac valve.

The papillary fronds of these tumors are microscopically similar in structure to normal chordae tendineae, and the tumors replicate all components of normal endocardium. These observations suggest that the papillary fibroelastoma is a hamartoma; however, the fact that the tumors are rarely found in children and are

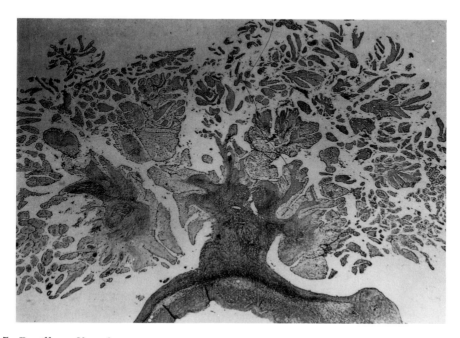

Fig. 9-5. Papillary fibroelastomas are most frequently located on the cardiac valves. These tumors consist of multiple papillary fronds arranged on a stalk that merges imperceptibly with the valve substance. (H&E, × 12.) (From McAllister and Fenoglio.[5])

more frequent in older patients, many of whom have had long-standing cardiac disease, has suggested to some authors that the tumors are secondary to mechanical damage and represent a degenerative process.[31]

The frequent occurrence of papillary fibroelastomas on the atrial surface of the AV valves and on the ventricular surface of the semilunar valves parallels the location of Lambl's excrescences; however, Lambl's excrescences do not usually occur on the arterial side of the semilunar valves or on the mural endocardium, whereas the papillary fibroelastomas do. Lambl's excrescences are most frequently located along the line of closure of the valves, whereas papillary fibroelastomas are located more frequently on the midportion or body of the valve, away from the contact surface. Lambl's excrescences have been reported in 70 to 80 percent of adult heart valves, whereas papillary fibroelastomas are rare. Lambl's excrescences are multiple in more than 90 percent of affected hearts, whereas papillary fibroelastomas are rarely multiple. Finally, Lambl's excrescences, unlike papillary fibroelastomas, contain deposits of fibrin, lack an abundant acid mucopolysaccharide matrix, and do not contain smooth muscle cells as a significant component.[32,33]

Papillary fibroelastomas are not to be confused with polypoid myxomatous valvular lesions of childhood (incompletely differentiated or dysplastic valves),[5] nor should the papillary fibroelastoma of the endocardial surface be confused with papillary projections from the epicardium. The fronds of the serosal papilloma are composed of loose connective tissue, covered by mesothelial cells, often with a central blood vessel. Unlike the papillary fibroelastoma, they lack a collagen core surrounded by an elastic tissue mantle. The epicardial papillomas are occasionally complex structures with multiple papillary fronds; however, they more frequently consist of only one or two fibrous tissue stalks. Histologically, the epicardial papilloma resembles a fibrous pericardial adhesion. Surgical excision would appear to be indicated in those patients with symptoms of angina pectoris secondary to obstruction of a coronary ostium by the fronds of a papillary fibroelastoma.

Rhabdomyoma

The most common primary cardiac tumor in infancy and childhood is the rhabdomyoma. In the AFIP series of 36 patients with rhabdomyoma, 78 percent were under 1 year of age, and only one patient was over age 15 years. Ninety percent of rhabdomyomas were multiple and occurred with nearly equal frequency in the right or left ventricles, including the ventricular septum. Although reportedly infrequent in the atria, rhabdomyomas involved either one or both atria in 30 percent of these patients. In no case did a rhabdomyoma originate in a cardiac valve. In 50 percent of patients, at least one of the tumor masses was intracavitary and obstructed 50 percent or more of one of the cardiac chambers or valve orifices (Fig. 9-6). Symptoms referable to obstruction of intracardiac blood flow were present in nine patients, none of whom had tuberous sclerosis and all of whom would appear to have been good surgical candidates. The incidence of tuberous sclerosis associated with rhabdomyomas in the 30 patients in whom the brain was examined was 37 percent.

Grossly, these tumors are white to yellow-tan and vary in diameter from millimeters to centimeters. Microscopically, they are circumscribed but not encapsulated and are easily distinguished from the surrounding myocardium. The rhabdomyoma cells are large—up to 80 μm in

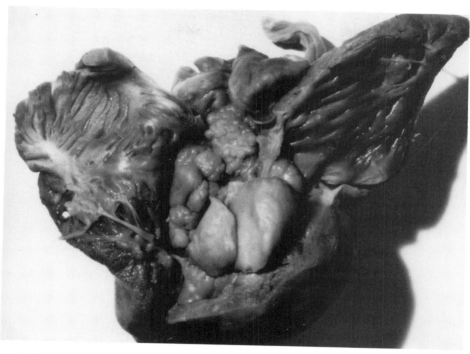

Fig. 9-6. This rhabdomyoma fills the right ventricle of a newborn infant and clearly obstructs the tricuspid valve. In approximately 50 percent of children with rhabdomyomas, at least one of the tumors is intracavitary and partially obstructs at least one valve orifice. (From McAllister and Fenoglio.[5])

diameter—and contain abundant glycogen. Classic "spider cells," with centrally placed cytoplasmic masses containing the nucleus and elongated projections of slender myofibrils extending to the periphery of these cells, are present in each tumor (Figs. 9-7 and 9-8). Rarely, microscopic calcification is found within rhabdomyoma cells.

Ultrastructurally, cellular junctions resembling intercalated discs are located around the total periphery of the rhabdomyoma cells interconnecting them. This ultrastructural feature is unlike that seen in normal myocardial cells or Purkinje cells (in which intercalated discs are located at the poles of the cell), but is suggestive of embryonic cardiac myoblasts.[34] Thus, rhabdomyomas are probably not

abnormal proliferations of specialized Purkinje cells or of nonspecialized myocardium, nor is the rhabdomyoma a localized form of glycogen storage disease. In glycogen storage disease (types II, III, and IV), the contractile elements are compressed around the periphery of the cardiac muscle cells by the accumulated glycogen. The cell, however, maintains its cylindrical shape, and intercalated discs are located at the two poles of the cell. The preservation of a relatively normal cell shape distinguishes glycogen-laden cardiac muscle cells in glycogen storage disease from rhabdomyoma cells. The preponderance of multiple, as opposed to solitary, cardiac rhabdomyomas and their most frequent occurrence in infants suggest that the cardiac

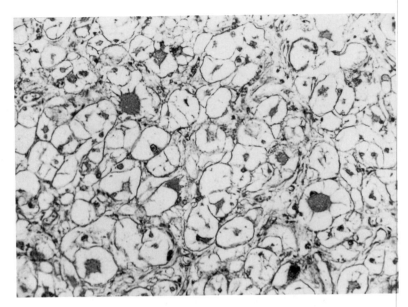

Fig. 9-7. Rhabdomyomas are composed of vacuolated, large, ovoid cells. Islands and strands of cytoplasm are present against the cell membrane and occasionally in the center of the cell. If the tissue is fixed in methyl alcohol, the vacuolated areas seen in the formaldehyde-fixed tissue are easily demonstrated to contain abundant glycogen. (H&E, × 125.) (From McAllister and Fenoglio.[5])

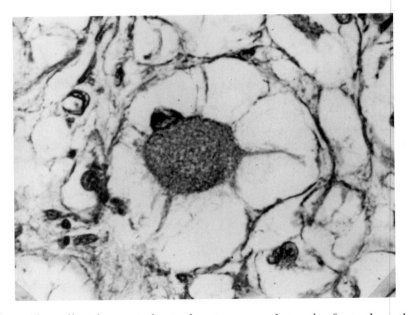

Fig. 9-8. The spider cell with a central cytoplasmic mass and strands of cytoplasm that extend to the cell membrane is pathognomonic of the cardiac rhabdomyoma. The nucleus is usually centrally located, but may be eccentrically placed, as in this cell. (H&E, × 525.) (From McAllister and Fenoglio.[5])

rhabdomyoma is a hamartoma or malformation rather than a true neoplasm. The clinical behavior and microscopic appearance of these tumors suggest that rhabdomyoma cells eventually lose their ability to divide. A similar loss of mitotic activity occurs in normally differentiated human cardiac muscle cells soon after birth. The rhabdomyoma cells appear to undergo arrest of development and to lose the ability to differentiate fully. The ovoid shape and the peripheral location of cellular junctions of intercalated disc type in rhabdomyoma cells are reminiscent of cardiac myoblasts and suggest that the tumor is a fetal hamartoma derived from embryonic cardiac myoblasts.

Although the cardiac rhabdomyoma has been described repeatedly in the literature as a nonsurgical lesion because of its tendency to multiplicity, cardiac rhabdomyomas have been excised successfully.[5] Surgical management is only necessary in patients presenting with symptoms related to obstruction of intracardiac blood flow or with arrhythmias that are resistant to conventional medical treatment.[35] Since there is no evidence to suggest that rhabdomyoma cells are capable of mitotic division after birth,[36] and, indeed, regression of the tumor has been demonstrated in infancy by two-dimensional echocardiography,[37] these patients should be considered for surgical treatment.

Fibroma

Cardiac fibromas are almost always solitary, and they are located in the ventricular myocardium—frequently in the ventricular septum. The clinical findings in 17 patients with cardiac fibromas in the AFIP series depended on the location of the tumor. Ten fibromas of the ventricular septum were inoperable, and the patients either died suddenly or developed intractable congestive heart failure. Most of these tumors encroached on, or invaded, the conduction system, usually the left and right bundle branches, and the patients either developed ventricular fibrillation or died suddenly and unexpectedly. Seven patients with fibromas located in the left ventricular free wall or atrium presented with cardiomegaly, often as an incidental finding on a chest x-ray. In five patients, the mass lesion was identified by cardiac catheterization, and surgical excision was attempted. One of these patients died postoperatively, but four were alive and well, without evidence of recurrence, at least 2 years after surgery.

Cardiac fibromas occur at all ages and in both sexes; however, they are more frequent in children and, as such, are the second most common primary cardiac tumor in the pediatric age group.[5] These firm gray-white tumors are often large and sometimes exceed 10 cm in diameter.[38] Grossly, they appear sharply demarcated, but microscopically they interdigitate with the adjacent myocardium (Fig. 9-9). There may be an impression of satellite nodules, but when traced, these nodules connect to the main tumor mass in a different plane. The central portion of the tumor is composed of hyalinized fibrous tissue, often with multiple foci of calcification and cystic degeneration, probably secondary to a poor blood supply. This central calcification may often be seen on chest x-rays. Elastic tissue may also be prominent, as in many of the fibromatoses of the superficial soft tissues.[5] Indeed, fibromas of the heart are connective tissue tumors derived from fibroblasts, and they have the same spectrum of appearance and behavior as the soft tissue fibromatoses in other areas of the body. These definable masses of proliferating connective tissue should not be confused with reactive fibrous tissue proliferation in the endocardial or epicardial

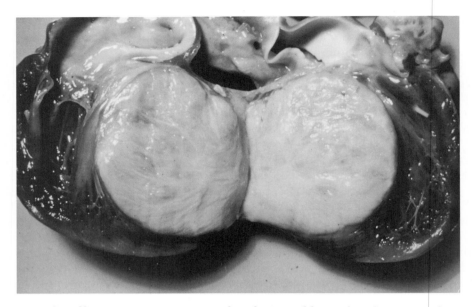

Fig. 9-9. Cardiac fibromas are most commonly solitary and located in the ventricular septum. This fibroma virtually replaces the ventricular septum and encroaches on the left ventricular chamber. (From McAllister and Fenoglio.[5])

layers of the heart. Areas of cellular fibrous tissue are present in each tumor, usually at the periphery. Mitotic figures are rare in the areas of cellular fibrous tissue, and, as in the extracardiac fibromatoses, cellularity is not an indication of malignancy. Because of the invasive growth of these tumors, normal cardiac muscle cells are frequently entrapped in the growing fibrous tissue and are left intact deep within the tumor, occasionally in central locations. The myocardial cells eventually degenerate and become vacuolated as they are separated from the syncytium of the contracting myocardium; this observation led pathologists to speculate that the fibroma is a "healing rhabdomyoma" or a "mesoblastic tumor."[5] However, both light and electron microscopy has shown that they are degenerating cardiac muscle cells, not embryonic (rhabdomyoma) muscle cells, and they are not an intrinsic, developing part of the fibroma. True "spider cells," diagnostic of the rhabdomyoma, are not found in the cardiac fibroma.

Cardiac fibromas located outside the ventricular septum are amenable to surgical excision, and patients usually do well after surgery. Surgical resection of ventricular septal fibromas may not be possible, especially if the tumor is close to the conduction system; such patients often succumb to ventricular arrhythmias.[39] Cardiac transplantation should be a consideration in these patients. The efficacy of permanent cardiac pacing in patients with large ventricular septal fibromas has not been adequately evaluated.

Lipomatous Hypertrophy of the Atrial Septum and Lipoma

Lipomatous hypertrophy (interatrial lipoma) is a nonencapsulated mass of adipose tissue in the atrial septum that is in continuity with the epicardial fat. Most probably, it represents atypical hyperplasia of primordial fat rather than a true neoplasm. The clinical significance of the lesion has been debated in the literature;[40] however, we believe that it may be associated with cardiac symptoms, especially cardiac arrhythmias.

The clinical and pathologic findings in 45 patients with abnormal accumulations of adipose tissue in the heart and pericardium were reviewed at the AFIP.[5] Thirty-two of the 45 patients had lipomatous hypertrophy of the atrial septum. In 28 percent of these 32 patients, the cause of death appeared to be directly related to the atrial tumor. The patients died either suddenly or after prolonged episodes of arrhythmia (atrial or ventricular), or of intractable congestive heart failure. The etiology of the cardiac symptomatology was clinically uncertain in each case, and at autopsy no abnormality or cardiac disease other than lipomatous hypertrophy of the atrial septum was found. Of the remaining patients, approximately 50 percent had either conduction disturbances or evidence of congestive heart failure; however, in each case the relationship of these findings to coexistent cardiopulmonary disease was unclear. In only 10 of the 32 patients was lipomatous hypertrophy an incidental finding at autopsy.

Ten patients in this series had chronic or debilitating diseases; however, this did not correlate with the size of the interatrial lipoma or with the presence of rhythm disturbance. Similarly, the body habitus of the patient and the amount of epicardial fat did not correlate with the interatrial lipoma or with the rhythm disturbances.

Although most patients with lipomatous hypertrophy of the atrial septum are over 60 years of age, approximately 25 percent of the patients in this series were younger, with one dying at age 22 years.

In lipomatous hypertrophy of the atrial septum, the mass of accumulated fat frequently causes the atrial septal endocardium to bulge, most frequently into the right atrium (Fig. 9-10). This may be detected by either two-dimensional echocardiography[41] or MRI.[42] Rarely, an interatrial lipoma protrudes so far into the atrium that this entity must be considered in the angiographic differential diagnosis of intracavitary masses. Interatrial lipomas vary in size from 1 or 2 cm up to 7 or 8 cm in maximum diameter. They may extend into the region of the AV node, but most often they are located anterior to the foramen ovale. The interatrial lipoma is situated in the area of at least two proposed interatrial conduction pathways. The interruption of these pathways could be the major reason for rhythm disturbances in these patients.

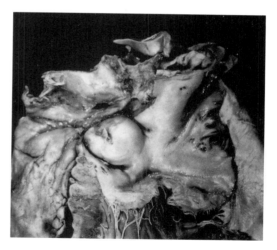

Fig. 9-10. Occasionally, a portion of the tumor in lipomatous hypertrophy of the atrial septum projects into the atrial cavity, usually the right atrium. The intracavitary portion of the tumor may be large enough to be detected by angiography and mistakenly interpreted as a myxoma. The intracavitary portion of this tumor is situated just proximal to the region of the AV node. (From McAllister and Fenoglio.[5])

Microscopically, there are varying proportions of mature adipose tissue and granular or vacuolated cells.[40] By both light and electron microscopy, the granular cells are identical to fetal fat cells.[43] The presence of fetal fat is a hallmark of lipomatous hypertrophy of the atrial septum; occasionally, these interatrial masses consist almost entirely of fetal fat. Myocardial cells are invariably entrapped in the mass, especially at the periphery (Fig. 9-11). Varying amounts of fibrosis and foci of chronic inflammatory cells, predominantly lymphocytes and plasma cells, are frequently present.

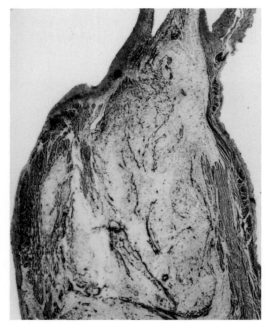

Fig. 9-11. In lipomatous hypertrophy, the atrial septum is thickened by adipose tissue, and the myofibers are compressed against the endocardium. Islands of atrial myofibers are trapped in the lipoma and often do not appear to be in contact with the myofibers compressed against the endocardium. Blood vessels and fibrous tissue septae are·abundant. (H&E, × 8.) (From McAllister and Fenoglio.[5])

When located within the myocardium, lipomas are usually small and irregular in contour and have a barely definable, but definite capsule; varying numbers of myocardial cells are entrapped in the tumor. An association of cardiac lipoma and tuberous sclerosis has been reported, however, and lipomas may be present in the heart and other viscera of patients with tuberous sclerosis in the absence of cardiac rhabdomyoma.

Hemangioma

Hemangiomas are composed of benign proliferations of endothelial cells, usually forming channels containing blood. They may occur at any site in the heart or pericardium and may be mainly intramural or mainly intracavitary. The clinical and pathologic findings in 15 patients with cardiac hemangioma have been reviewed at the AFIP.[5] In greater than 50 percent of these patients, who ranged in age from 7 months to 80 years, the tumors were incidental findings at autopsy. Signs and symptoms in the remaining patients depended on the location of the tumor. In three patients, the tumors were intracavitary and mimicked the symptoms of patients with myxomas. In two patients, a mass was discovered on routine chest x-ray. Both underwent surgery with the probable diagnosis of pericardial cyst. A hemangioma was present in both patients. The final two patients presented with cardiomegaly and recurrent pericardial effusion. In both, the cardiac enlargement suggested a mass lesion and, in both, an intramyocardial hemangioma was discovered at surgery.

Grossly, hemangiomas are red and hemorrhagic. Microscopically, they are classified according to the morphologic pattern and interrelationship of the vascular channels, endothelial cells, and supporting stroma. This microscopic classification (capillary, cavernous, intramuscular, hemangioendothelioma) is descriptive of varying growth patterns and does not necessarily imply differences in prognosis.[44]

When the tumors produce symptoms, the treatment of choice is surgical excision. The varied presentation of hemangiomas underscores the importance of a complete clinical evaluation in all patients with cardiac symptoms.

Varix

Varices are dilated blood vessels in the subendocardium that are frequently mistaken for hemangiomas. They may occur at any site in the heart but are most common in the subendocardium of either the atrial or ventricular septum. Varices are microscopically different from hemangiomas and consist of normally formed vascular channels, usually veins, found either singly or in a cluster; they are dilated and frequently thrombosed, resembling hemorrhoids. The exact frequency of varices is unknown; however, they are usually incidental findings.[45]

Blood Cysts

Blood cysts are found on the endocardium, particularly the valvular endocardium, in newborns and infants. These cysts are usually lined by normal-appearing endothelial cells that are not delimited by a basement membrane. Occasionally, the lining cells are absent in the intravalvular portion of the blood cyst, in which case the cyst wall consists of endocardial stroma.[46] They contain blood, probably derived from the cavitary blood of the heart. These cysts are not true blood vessels or hemangiomas; they have no clinical significance.

Mesothelioma of the Atrioventricular Node

Mesotheliomas are always located in the region of the AV node. They most likely originate in mesothelial rests, like adenomatoid tumors of the ovary and testis, and are always benign.[47] Most patients with mesotheliomas have partial or complete heart block, usually of long duration, and often die of either complete heart block or ventricular fibrillation. This tumor has appropriately been designated as the smallest tumor capable of causing sudden death. The 12 patients studied at the AFIP ranged in age from 11 months to 71 years, a distribution similar to that reported in the literature.

Grossly, the tumors are usually poorly circumscribed, slightly elevated nodules, located in the atrial septum immediately cephalad to the junction of the septal and anterior leaflets of the tricuspid valve in the region of the AV node (Fig. 9-12). On cross section, they are usually multicystic. Microscopically, the cysts are lined by uniform polygonal cells, frequently multilayered, with a suggestion of a "brush border." Interspersed with these cysts are multiple nests of cells of markedly varying size. The small nests appear solid, whereas the large nests frequently have a central lumen. The cellular nests and cystic structures are set in a dense connective tissue stroma. Within this stroma, collagen and elastic fibers are abundant and mast cells are frequent. The tumor usually replaces part or all of the AV node, and may extend proximally into the atrial septum and distally into the AV bundle.

Ultrastructurally, these tumors are strikingly similar to adenomatoid tumors of the ovary and testis. The luminal surfaces of the polygonal cells lining the cysts have numerous, widely spaced microvilli. These cells are multilayered, and there are numerous intercellular

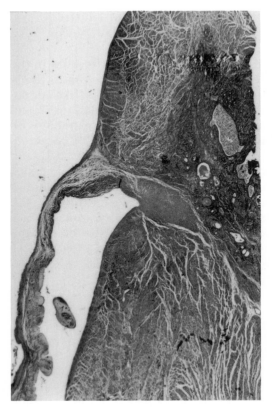

Fig. 9-12. Mesotheliomas of the AV node are located in the atrial septum at or close to the region of the AV node and are delineated from the ventricular myocardium by the fibrous annulus. The tumor is primarily subendocardial and only rarely replaces the full thickness of the atrial septum. This tumor completely replaced the AV node. (H&E, × 6.) (From McAllister and Fenoglio.[5])

spaces bound on all sides by tight junctions and desmosomes. These are features of mesothelial cells and present further evidence that the tumors are of mesothelial origin with focal metaplasia.[48] Although some immunohistochemical studies have been interpreted to indicate that the tumors have an endodermal origin,[49,50] these findings have not been correlated with ultrastructural observations, so such a conclusion seems premature.

Since AV block, both complete and partial, is the major clinical manifestations of this tumor, the use of a pacemaker to maintain normal ventricular function appears indicated. However, even with cardiac pacing, two patients in our series developed ventricular fibrillation. Cardiac pacing, coupled with drug therapy to suppress residual AV nodal activity and possible accessory AV pathways, is probably indicated.

Teratoma

Most true teratomas of the heart and pericardium are extracardiac, but intrapericardial, and arise from the base of the heart. They are usually attached to the root of the pulmonary artery and aorta and receive their blood supply from the vasa vasora of these vessels (Fig. 9-13). Although intracardiac teratomas have been reported, most of the reports describe cysts that do not include all three germ layers. Teratomas may occur in adults, but the majority present in the pediatric age group. Females are affected much more commonly than males.[5]

The clinical and pathologic findings in 14 patients with intrapericardial teratomas were available for study at the AFIP. The patients ranged in age from less than 1 day to 42 years; however, 11 were in the pediatric age group. All were female, with the exception of one 10-week-old boy. Two patients in this series died suddenly and unexpectedly; the remaining 12 all presented with signs and symptoms relating to the heart. Dyspnea and cardiomegaly were among the presenting symptoms and signs in each patient. The infants were usually cyanotic and occasionally had cardiac murmurs. With the aid of newer diagnostic techniques in cardiology, a diagnosis of an extracardiac mass was established in each case occurring after 1960. The teratoma was excised

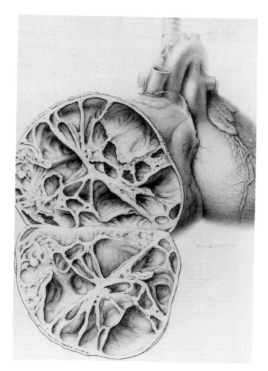

Fig. 9-13. Cardiac teratomas are usually intrapericardial and attached to the root of a pulmonary artery and aorta. These tumors may reach massive proportions. On section, the teratoma contains numerous multiloculated cysts and intervening solid areas similar to teratomas occurring elsewhere in the body. (From McAllister and Fenoglio.[5])

in eight patients; six were alive and well without evidence of recurrence at least 2 years after surgery, and two died during the postoperative period.

Intrapericardial teratomas may assume massive proportions, measuring up to 15 cm in diameter. They are pear-shaped, usually smooth surfaced, and lobulated. On section, the teratoma contains numerous multiloculated cysts and intervening solid areas. Microscopically, intrapericardial teratomas resemble teratomas elsewhere in the body, and derivatives of all three germ layers are present. Like all teratomas, intrapericardial teratomas

have a malignant potential, although this is decidedly unusual. Nevertheless, all teratomas should be adequately sampled in order to avoid overlooking the rare malignant example.

Surgical excision following diagnosis is the only effective therapy. Since these tumors usually receive their blood supply from the vasa vasora of the aorta and pulmonary artery, effective removal must include a careful dissection of the root of these great arteries.

Bronchogenic Cysts

Bronchogenic cysts are usually contained within the myocardium, especially the ventricular myocardium, although occasionally they may project into a cardiac chamber or into the pericardial space. They rarely exceed 1 to 2 cm in diameter. Bronchogenic cysts are misplaced elements of the respiratory tract, and, unlike teratomas, contain only elements derived from mesoderm and ectoderm, arranged in an orderly manner resembling a bronchus.

Of the seven patients with cardiac bronchogenic cysts in the AFIP collection, five were male and two were female, a sex distribution similar to that of bronchogenic cysts in the skin and subcutaneous tissues. In six of the seven patients, the cyst was an incidental finding at autopsy. These six patients ranged in age from 36 to 75 years. The other patient, a 6-month-old infant, presented with cardiomegaly and a loud systolic murmur. At autopsy, a large cyst protruded from the ventricular septum into the right ventricle displacing the tricuspid valve into the right atrium.

Intracardiac bronchogenic cysts are, with rare exceptions, incidental findings of no clinical significance. In the unusual exception, surgical excision would be indicated for relief of symptoms.[51]

Granular Cell Tumor

The granular cell tumor is a rare and apparently incidental finding in the heart that occurred in only three patients in the AFIP series.[52] All were adults, and none had cardiac symptoms. The tumors are frequently multiple.[52] Histologically, they are identical to granular cell tumors elsewhere in the body.

Lymphangiomas and Hamartomas

Lymphangiomas are proliferations of lymphatic channels without proliferations of blood-carrying channels. They are uncommon in the heart but, as elsewhere in the body, are frequently diffuse proliferations rather than distinct tumors. Therefore, total excision is often not practical.[53,54] Cardiac transplantation may be considered an alternative treatment in these cases.[9] There were two cardiac lymphangiomas in the AFIP collection; one was found in the parietal pericardium and the other in the left ventricular myocardium. Lymphatic ectasia, which may occur in the heart, must be distinguished from lymphangioma.

Approximately 12 primary cardiac tumors composed of more than one type of mesenchymal tissue have been reported. Anbe and Fine[55] reviewed these tumors and concluded that all but two were, in fact, lymphangiomas of the heart. The two exceptions were considered best classified as arterial or venous malformations (vascular hamartomas).

Intrapericardial Paraganglioma

Paragangliomas, such as pheochromocytomas and chemodectomas, may rarely be localized within the pericardium. Al-though these tumors may be found overlying or within any cardiac chamber, they most commonly occur over the base of the heart in the major region of vagus nerve distribution.[56] Detection and localization have been provided by iodine-131 metaiodobenzylguanidine (^{131}I-MBIG) nuclear scanning. MRI can further localize cardiac paragangliomas without the need for contrast material and may provide detailed information for better guidance of surgical excision. Although definitive diagnosis can only be made histologically, benign pathologic characteristics do not necessarily predict a favorable outcome, as these tumors are highly vascular, adherent, and difficult to resect. Human cardiac explantation and autotransplantation have been applied in a case involving a large cardiac paraganglioma.[57]

Neurofibroma

Although exceedingly rare, neurofibromas have been reported in the heart, especially as a complication of von Recklinghausen's disease. In the AFIP collection, three neurofibromas involved the heart. One was present in the parietal pericardium, and two in the left ventricular myocardium. Two of the patients had von Recklinghausen's disease, and the third had a neuroblastoma that had been treated with radiation in childhood. Neurofibromas occurring in the heart are identical grossly and microscopically to those occurring elsewhere in the body.

Angiosarcoma

Angiosarcoma is the most frequently occurring primary cardiac sarcoma and is two to three times more common in men than in women. The site of origin is most frequently the right side of the heart, especially the right atrium, followed by the pericardium. Eighty percent of the primary cardiac angiosarcomas in the 39 patients in the AFIP series originated in the right atrium or pericardium.[5] In approximately 25 percent of these patients, a portion of the angiosarcoma was intracavitary and obstructed a valve orifice. The tricuspid valve was most frequently obstructed by a right atrial tumor mass (seven patients), although the pulmonary valve was obstructed in two patients and the mitral valve in one. All 39 patients ranged in age from 15 to 76 years, although 70 percent were between 20 and 50 years. Seventy-seven percent of patients had clinical findings of right-sided heart failure or of pericardial disease. These findings included congestive heart failure, pericardial effusion, dyspnea, and pleuritic chest pain. However, a significant number of patients (10 percent) had symptoms suggestive of malignancy (fever, weight loss, and malaise) without cardiac findings or before cardiac findings were noted. Systolic murmurs and atrial arrhythmias were present in six patients, each of whom also had evidence of right-sided heart failure. All patients presented with cardiomegaly by chest x ray and with electrocardiogram (ECG) abnormalities, such as nonspecific ST-segment and T-wave changes and/or low voltage. Only 11 patients had distant metastases; in 3 they were confined to the nervous system. Five additional patients had local spread of the tumor either to the adjacent pleura or mediastinum, or both.

These tumors are often subclassified on the basis of their microscopic appearance; however, since their clinical course and prognosis appear to be identical, irrespective of the subclassification, the all-inclusive term *angiosarcoma* is preferable. Without treatment, prognosis is poor; most patients die within a year of the onset of the symptoms. In the future, newer pathologic techniques for identification of sarcomas, aggressive surgical resection, and advanced chemotherapy and radiotherapy may contribute to better survival for patients with these tumors.

Kaposi's Sarcoma

Metastatic Kaposi's sarcoma to the epicardium and myocardium has been described in autopsy studies of patients with acquired immune deficiency syndrome (AIDS),[58] and primary Kaposi's sarcoma has also been reported in this group of patients.[59]

Rhabdomyosarcoma

Rhabdomyosarcoma, the second most common primary sarcoma of the heart, is a neoplasm composed of malignant cells with features of striated muscle. Rhabdomyosarcomas have been reported in patients ranging in age from 3 months to 80 years, but, like other primary sarcomas, they are rare in the pediatric age group. In the AFIP collection of 26 rhabdomyosarcomas primary in the heart, the ages range from 1 to 66 years, with only two patients in the pediatric age group. The incidence of cardiac rhabdomyosarcoma in the adult population is nearly equal in all decades. A slightly increased incidence in men over women has been reported.[5]

The majority of patients in the AFIP collection had nonspecific symptoms characterized by fever, anorexia, malaise, and weight loss—symptoms more indicative of malignancy than of cardiac disease. However, findings of pericardial disease, pleuritic chest pain, pleural effusion, dyspnea, and embolic phenomena, both pulmonary and cerebral, were common in patients with rhabdomyosarcoma. A common denominator in all patients was cardiomegaly by chest radiograph and nonspecific electrocardiographic changes, such as ST-segment and T-wave changes, low voltage, and/or varying degrees of bundle branch block. Most frequently the heart borders were irregular and the contour of the heart was distorted. In addition, 50 percent of patients had unexplained murmurs, usually systolic and of recent onset and/or intractable atrial or ventricular arrhythmias. Findings of obstruction to blood flow, such as congestive heart failure, were common. In each patient in which a cardiac murmur was noted, a large portion of the rhabdomyosarcoma was intracavitary, and there was significant obstruction of at least one valve orifice. Approximately 50 percent of the patients in this series had partial obstruction of at least one valve orifice, the mitral and pulmonic orifices being the most frequently obstructed. Unlike benign intracavitary tumors, the cardiac valves are often invaded, occasionally with extensive valve replacement by adjacent intracavitary rhabdomyosarcoma.[5]

Unlike angiosarcoma, rhabdomyosarcoma does not have a propensity for arising in a particular cardiac chamber. These tumors originate with equal frequency in the left and right heart; in approximately 60 percent of patients, the tumor involves multiple sites within the heart at autopsy. The pericardium is involved in 50 percent of these patients, usually by direct extension of the tumor from the myocardium. However, diffuse pericardial involvement characteristic of mesothelioma or angiosarcoma is not a feature of rhabdomyosarcoma. Occasionally, the tumor extends beyond the parietal pericardium to the contiguous mediastinum or pleural cavity.

Excision of the main tumor mass, followed by combined radiation therapy and chemotherapy, is recommended. In spite of therapy, prognosis is generally poor, although 3-year survivals following treatment have been reported. Most patients, however, die within 1 year of diagnosis.

Fibrosarcoma and Malignant Fibrous Histiocytoma

Fibrosarcoma and malignant fibrous histiocytoma are malignant mesenchymal tumors that are primarily fibroblastic in their differentiation. The clinical and pathologic findings of 14 patients with malignant cardiac fibroblastic tumors were available at the AFIP.[5] The clinical findings associated with these tumors are often multiple and confusing. The most common findings in patients with fibrosarcoma of the heart include systolic murmurs, often of changing intensity and recent onset; nonspecific ECG changes including ST-segment and T-wave changes, low voltage, and bundle branch block; arrhythmias, especially atrial arrhythmias; and findings of pericardial disease including chest pain, fever, and dyspnea. Eight percent of the patients in this series had one or more of these signs or symptoms. In addition, two patients had symptoms usually suggestive of malignancy, including weight loss, fever, and malaise.

Five of the 14 patients had distant metastases involving other viscera, and in 2 additional patients there was a direct spread of the tumor to involve adjacent structures. The patients in this series ranged in age from less than 1 year to 87 years.

These tumors arise with equal frequency on the left and right sides of the heart, with no predilection for any single site. They may be nodular or infiltrative, and are firm and gray-white. In slightly more than one-half of the patients, they involve multiple sites within the heart at autopsy. The pericardium is invaded in approximately one-third, and a portion of the tumor protrudes into a cardiac chamber causing significant obstruction of a valve orifice, or invasion of a valve leaflet, in 50 percent of patients. The mitral valve was involved in four patients, the pulmonary valve in two, and the tricuspid valve in one.

Malignant fibrous histiocytoma has fibrosarcomatous areas, but it is differentiated from fibrosarcoma in that the former has a whorled pattern of the spindle cells, and giant cells, often with multiple nuclei, are present. Immunohistochemical studies may aid in establishing the fibroblastic origin of these sarcomas.

Although radiation and chemotherapy have been tried with minimal success, no therapy has been especially effective for treating malignant fibroblastic tumors of the heart; however, in the future, aggressive surgical resection with advanced chemotherapy and radiotherapy may contribute to better survival.

Cardiac transplantation may also have a therapeutic role for patients with localized disease.[60]

Lymphoma

By definition, a primary lymphoma of the heart must involve only the heart and pericardium. Lymphomas primary in the heart have been found in patients from 14 months to 84 years of age.

The AFIP series included seven examples. The patients ranged in age from 18 to 77 years, with a nearly equal incidence among men and women. In three of these patients, lymphoma was an incidental finding at autopsy. In the remaining four, the most common findings were congestive heart failure, cardiomegaly, and pericardial effusion. All four patients died of intractable congestive heart failure without clinical suspicion of malignant disease.[5] An increased incidence of lym-

phoma, including cardiac lymphoma, has been noted in patients with AIDS[61,62] and in transplant patients receiving immunosuppressive therapy.[63] Most of these cardiac lymphomas have been of B-cell lineage.

In the AFIP series, all sites in the heart were involved without apparent predilection for any specific site. In two patients, the lymphoma diffusely involved the pericardium (both visceral and parietal) and the myocardium. Both patients had cardiomegaly by chest radiograph and died of intractable congestive heart failure. In the remaining five patients, the lymphoma was localized, although there were multiple sites of involvement in three patients. A portion of the lymphoma was intracavitary in two patients and partially obstructed the pulmonary valve in another.

Surgical excision followed by radiation therapy or chemotherapy is the treatment of choice. Endomyocardial biopsy may be helpful in establishing the diagnosis without resorting to thoracotomy.

Extraskeletal Osteosarcoma

When extraskeletal osteosarcoma is primary in the heart, it most commonly arises in the left atrium, usually from the posterior wall, near the entrance of the pulmonary veins. Of the five tumors in the AFIP series, three were primary in the left atrium, one was in the right atrium, and one in the right ventricle. The five patients in this series—four men and one woman—ranged in age from 16 to 58 years.[5] Their clinical findings were similar to those associated with other sarcomas of the heart: progressive congestive heart failure, dyspnea, and cardiac murmurs of recent onset. Systolic murmurs were present in three of the patients; in all three, an intracavitary tumor was diagnosed with the aid of angiography, and the intracavitary portion of the tumor was excised surgically.

A portion of the tumor was intracavitary in four of the five patients; the mitral valve was obstructed in two, the tricuspid valve in one, and the pulmonary in another. In the fifth patient, both the mitral and aortic valves were invaded by the tumor, although neither valve orifice was obstructed.

Four patients in the series died within 2 years in spite of surgery, radiation therapy, and/or chemotherapy. The remaining patient, who lived 4 years after onset of symptoms, was treated with radiation therapy and chemotherapy following excision of the intracavitary portion of the tumor.

Malignant Nerve Sheath Tumors

All four patients with malignant nerve sheath tumors in the AFIP series were male and ranged in age from 9 to 52 years. All presented with pleuritic chest pain, dyspnea, and pericardial effusion. Two patients had nonspecific ECG findings of low voltage and left ventricular strain. A systolic murmur was present in one patient. In three of these patients, a diagnosis of pericardial tumor was made ante mortem with the aid of echocardiography and angiocardiography. Surgical excision was attempted in each patient.[5]

All four tumors involved the visceral pericardium over the base of the heart. In three patients, primary involvement was over the outflow tract of the right ventricle and pulmonary artery. In the fourth, the bulk of the tumor was situated over the right atrium. In each patient, the underlying myocardium was invaded; in two, the parietal pericardium was involved. The main mass of the tumor was intrapericardial in all four patients. In one, the adjacent mediastinum was involved and there were metastases to the lungs in two patients.

These tumors are presumably derived from the cells of nerve sheaths. In all probability, when they primarily involve the heart, they originate in the cardiac plexus or the vagus nerve innervation of the heart.

All reported malignant nerve sheath tumors, as well as the four tumors in this series, were located on the visceral pericardium at the base of the heart on the right side—the precise location of the vagus nerve innervation of the heart.

Three of the patients in this series were diagnosed ante mortem. Of these, two died within a year despite radiation and chemotherapy following surgical excision of the main intrapericardial mass. The third patient had evidence of recurrent disease 1 year after surgery.

Leiomyosarcoma

Malignant tumors derived from smooth muscle are extremely rare in the heart and pericardium. Approximately eight leiomyosarcomas of the heart have been reported; however, in at least one-half of the cases the heart was not unequivocally the primary site of the tumor.[5]

PERICARDIAL TUMORS

Pericardial Cysts

Most patients with pericardial cysts are asymptomatic; the cysts are first noted either on a chest radiograph or as an incidental finding at autopsy. However, slightly more than one-third of the 82 patients with pericardial cysts in the AFIP series were symptomatic.[5] Chest pain, usually precordial or substernal, was the most frequent symptom. These patients ranged from 4 to 82 years of age, although 62 percent were in their twenties or thirties at the time the cyst was discovered. Most series in the literature indicate a nearly equal incidence in males and females.

Sites of pericardial cysts in this series are summarized in Table 9-7. Pericardial cysts are most commonly located at the right heart border, and a small but significant number (8 percent) project into either the anterosuperior or posterior mediastinum.[64] They range in size from 1 to 15 cm or more in diameter. Commonly they appear multilobulated externally; however, although the cyst lining is frequently trabeculated, most are unilocular. They contain clear yellow fluid and occasionally communicate with the pericardial sac. The wall of the cyst is composed mainly of collagen with scattered elastic fibers and is lined by mesothelial cells. Although these mesothelial cells usually form a single layer, foci of hyperplastic mesothelial cells are occasionally encountered. Rarely, foci of calcification and accumulations of lymphocytes and plasma cells are present.

Malignant Teratoma

Malignant teratomas, unlike most primary cardiac sarcomas, occur most commonly in children. Like their benign counterparts, they are primarily intra-

Table 9-7. Pericardial Cyst: Location in 82 Patients

Site	No.	%
Right costophrenic angle	57	70
Left costophrenic angle	18	22
Anterior or superior mediastinum	4	4
Posterior mediastinum	3	4
Total	82	100

(From McAllister and Fenoglio.[5])

pericardial, attached to the base of the heart, and more common in females. A malignant teratoma is a teratoma in which one of the elements has undergone a malignant change, either metastasizing to or invading adjacent structures. The malignant portion may be a carcinoma or a sarcoma. When the malignant portion of the tumor is embryonal carcinoma, the tumor is termed *teratocarcinoma*. The most common malignancy is embryonal carcinoma, but examples of choriocarcinoma and squamous cell carcinoma have also been recognized.[65]

All four malignant teratomas in the AFIP collection occurred in children—three girls and one boy—ranging in age from 1 to 4 years. Each child in this series had congestive heart failure, usually associated with anorexia and vomiting. All four had cardiomegaly by chest x-ray; two had arrhythmias and nonspecific electrocardiographic findings, and one had a systolic murmur. Three of the tumors were primarily intrapericardial, attached to the root of the aorta and pulmonary artery. In each, elements derived from all three germ layers were identified. Two patients had metastases to the lungs and mediastinum, and another patient had extensive invasion of the myocardium of the left and right ventricles. In the fourth patient, the tumor was situated over the anterior surface of the heart and had invaded the ventricular septum and right ventricle. A large portion of the tumor was intracavitary within the right ventricle, but it did not appear to obstruct either the tricuspid or pulmonary valve. The main masses of this tumor and the pulmonary metastases were both embryonal carcinoma and choriocarcinoma.

Surgical excision of the pericardial mass was attempted in one patient; however, the tumor had invaded the heart so extensively that excision was impossible. All four children died within 3 months of the onset of symptoms.

The pericardial cyst and the pericardial diverticulum are microscopically identical, and both probably originate as persistent blind-ending parietal pericardial recesses.[66]

The pericardial cysts were successfully excised from 78 patients in this series, and the 30 symptomatic patients experienced prompt relief of all symptoms. All 78 patients were alive and well without evidence of recurrence or symptoms at least 2 years following surgery. The four remaining pericardial cysts were incidental findings at autopsy.

Some tumors of the pericardium may simulate the clinical and radiologic picture of a pericardial cyst.[67] Ultrasound diagnosis, CT scanning, and MRI may help differentiate pericardial cysts from these solid pericardial tumors.[68–70]

Solid tumors of the pericardium include lipoma, hemangioma, lymphangioma, leiomyoma, neurofibroma, heterotopic tissue, benign and malignant teratomas, mesothelioma, thymoma, liposarcoma, angiosarcoma, and synovial sarcoma.

Lipoma

Lipomas, exclusive of lipomatous hypertrophy of the atrial septum, occur throughout the heart, including the pericardium. They are less frequent than interatrial lipomas and are usually not associated with symptoms unless they are situated in the visceral or parietal pericardium and protrude into the pericardial sac. Parietal pericardial lipomas are often mistaken clinically for pericardial cysts, and visceral pericardial lipomas are frequently associated with a pericardial effusion. Relief of symptoms follows surgical excision of visceral or parietal pericardial lipomas. In contrast to interatrial lipomas, these tumors are encapsulated masses of adult adipose tissue. The pericardial lipomas are frequently bosselated and may be 10 cm or more in diameter. Grossly, these lipomas are identical to adult fat or lipomas elsewhere in the body. Microscopically, they consist of mature fat cells with varying amounts of fibrous tissue, myxoid matrix, and blood vessels. Rarely, fetal fat cells are present.

Leiomyoma

In the AFIP series, there are no examples of a leiomyoma arising in the heart, and a search of the literature has not yielded any report of one. There is, however, one report of a leiomyoma arising in the parietal pericardium.[71]

Heterotopic Tissue

Heterotopic islands of thymic tissue and thyroid have been described in the parietal pericardium.[70] Thyroid rests in the heart have also been reported.[72]

Mesothelioma

Mesotheliomas are malignant tumors of either visceral or parietal pericardium and are derived from mesothelial cells. They represent the third most common primary malignant neoplasm of the heart and pericardium. The clinical and pathologic findings of 19 patients dying of mesothelioma of the pericardium were available in the AFIP series. Dyspnea, usually with cough and signs of pericardial effusion, is the most common clinical finding. Frequently, pericardial effusion is recurrent, and cytologic examination of the aspirated fluid may be of diagnostic value. Many patients have symptoms of pericarditis and nonspecific ST-segment and T-wave changes on the ECG. Clinical findings of pericarditis and pericardial effusion are frequently present without a history or accompanying signs of an inflammatory disease. Other patients have signs and symptoms of constrictive pericarditis, often with severe right-sided congestive heart failure.[73] Occasionally, the only clinical findings are fever, malaise, and weight loss. Cardiomegaly may be present on chest radiograph.

The patients in the AFIP series ranged in age from 17 to 83 years. Although there were no children in this series, mesotheliomas have been reported in the pediatric age group. Most series indicate a male-to-female ratio of nearly 2 : 1 in frequency.

The majority of pericardial mesotheliomas diffusely cover the parietal and visceral pericardium, encasing the heart. Solitary or localized pericardial mesotheliomas exist but are distinctly rare. Histologically, a localized mesothelioma is identical to a diffuse mesothelioma and may be an epithelioid or fibrous type.

The mesothelioma, whether nodular or sheetlike, invades contiguous structures, including the heart, only superficially (Fig. 9-14). This is an important differential diagnostic point in that other primary sarcomas, most notably angiosarcoma, can diffusely involve the pericardium but, unlike mesotheliomas, almost invariably have a significant intramyocardial or intracavitary component.

Pericardial mesotheliomas frequently spread to the adjacent pleura and mediastinum and may involve mediastinal lymph nodes. Occasionally, pericardial mesotheliomas spread through the diaphragm and involve the peritoneum. Distant metastases are extremely unusual. Cytologic examination of the pericardial fluid may aid diagnosis. The distinction between hyperplastic and malignant mesothelial cells is, however, extremely difficult. Indeed, differentiation of mesothelial hyperplasia and mesothelioma on a pericardial biopsy poses a major diagnostic problem to the pathologist. Exfoliative cytology is usually helpful in establishing the diagnosis of metastatic carcinoma of the pericardium. Most metastatic carcinomas that are likely to be confused with mesothelial hyperplasia can be identified by differential histochemical staining of a pericardial biopsy. However, mesothelial hyperplasia may be a complication of treatment by radiotherapy, or be second-

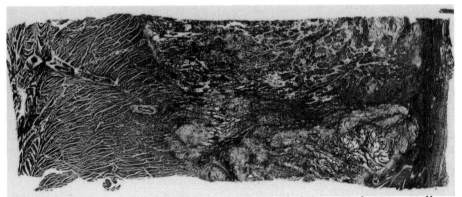

Fig. 9-14. Mesothelioma tends to obliterate the pericardial space and may actually constrict the heart, causing symptoms of constrictive pericarditis. Occasionally, the parietal pericardium is not invaded. The tumor may extend along blood vessels from the epicardium into the heart, although the myocardium is usually not directly invaded. (H&E, × 5.)

ary to pericarditis following the spread of carcinoma to the pericardium. Finding only mesothelial hyperplasia in a patient suspected of having metastatic pericardial carcinoma, therefore, does not exclude the diagnosis of metastatic carcinoma involving the pericardium.

There is no specific treatment for pericardial mesothelioma. Surgical excision is usually not possible. Although chemotherapy and radiotherapy may produce temporary improvement, there is no well-established correlation between this treatment and the course of the disease. Prognosis is generally poor, with as many as 60 percent of patients dying within 6 months of diagnosis; survivals of 5 and 6 years were reported in an AFIP series.[5]

Thymoma

Thymomas are primarily tumors of the anterior mediastinum; however, they are occasionally primary within the pericardium. Presumably, they are derived from thymic rests, which, incidentally, are not infrequently encountered in the parietal pericardium. The pericardium can be accepted as the primary sight of origin only in those tumors in which there is no evidence of anterior mediastinal involvement.

Four thymomas originating in the parietal pericardium were in the AFIP series. Three of the four patients were women. In one, thymoma was an unexpected finding at autopsy. The remaining three patients had clinical findings of intractable congestive heart failure, pericardial effusion, and a mediastinal or pericardial mass by chest x-ray. At operation, each patient had an intrapericardial thymoma attached to the pericardium, either at the base of the heart or over its anterior aspect. No patient had myasthenia gravis.

Liposarcoma

Although lipomas of the heart are relatively frequent, liposarcomas of the heart and pericardium are distinctly rare. Only six primary liposarcomas in the heart or pericardium have been reported in the literature.[5]

Synovial Sarcoma

The only reported case of primary synovial sarcoma in the heart was that of a 30-year-old man who had progressive dyspnea, syncopal episodes, and a systolic ejection murmur that was believed to represent pulmonic stenosis.[5] At autopsy, a 15 × 10-cm tumor was found at the base of the heart involving the pericardium and invading the outflow tract of the right ventricle and pulmonary artery. It extended into the right ventricle, obstructing the pulmonary valve. No metastases were found. Microscopically, the tumor had the classic biphasic pattern and staining properties characteristic of synovial sarcoma.

Other Tumors

Benign and malignant teratomas are most commonly extracardiac, but intrapericardial examples occur. Because these tumors are usually attached to the base of the heart and derive their blood supply from the vasa vasorum of the aorta and pulmonary artery, they are discussed under the section on primary tumors of the heart. Hemangiomas, lymphangiomas, and angiosarcomas may primarily involve the pericardium, myocardium, or both. They are discussed under primary tumors of the heart. Serosal papillomas are discussed as part of the differential diagnosis of papillary fibroelastomas of the endocardium or cardiac valves.

THE CARCINOID SYNDROME

Carcinoid tumors arise from enterochromaffin cells (Kulchitsky cells), which are found throughout the gastrointestinal tract, bronchi, bile duct, and pancreatic ducts.[74] Carcinoid tumors in ovarian or testicular teratomas have also been reported.[75,76] Most commonly, primary carcinoid tumors arise in the small intestine (chiefly in the terminal ileum) or in the appendix. Usually, appendiceal carcinoids are localized and seldom metastasize to produce the carcinoid syndrome.[77] The functional carcinoid syndrome most frequently occurs with carcinoid tumors of the small intestine after metastases to regional lymph nodes and liver have occurred. Carcinoid tumors of the stomach and bronchi produce syndromes that may differ from the classic syndrome associated with ileal carcinoids.[78,79] The tumor produces several biologically active substances, including serotonin (5-hydroxytryptamine), histamine, and kinin peptides (bradykinin). Dermal flushing and diarrhea occur in almost all patients with the syndrome; wheezing occurs in approximately one-third; and thickening of valvular and mural endocardium of the heart is present in more than one-half of affected patients.[80] Telangiectasia may develop in the skin over the nasal bridge, malar area, and upper chest. Rarely, a permanent cyanotic hue may result in the flush area.[74]

In carcinoid heart disease, there is either focal or diffuse plaquelike thickening of valvular and mural endocardium, and occasionally of the intima of the great veins, coronary sinus, pulmonary trunk, and main pulmonary arteries.[75,76] These plaques usually appear only in patients with hepatic metastases or when the venous blood from the tumor bypasses the liver, as with bronchial or ovarian carcinoids. The fibrous tissue is atypical and is limited in most instances to the right side of the heart. When the pulmonary valve is involved, deposition is almost exclusively on the arterial aspect of the valve cusps. The fibrous tissue is located predominantly on the ventricular aspect of the posterior and septal leaflets of the tricuspid valve, and about equally on the ventricular and atrial aspect of the anterior leaflet when the latter is affected.[74,75,81] Involvement of the tricuspid valve often causes the leaflets to adhere to the adjacent ventricular wall, producing regurgitation as the principal functional defect. The pulmonic valve becomes predominantly stenotic, although some regurgitation may occur.[82] These carcinoid fibrous plaques are also deposited on the endocardial surface of the right atrium, especially on the atrial septum immediately proximal to the junction of the septal and anterior tricuspid leaflets. When there is diffuse deposition of fibrous tissue on the endocardium of the right atrium, its walls become relatively noncompliant.[81] Fibrous plaques are less extensive in the right ventricle than in the atrium, and usually consist of capping of the papillary muscles, most commonly resulting in no functional significance.[74]

Similar lesions may be observed in the mitral and aortic valves in patients with predominantly right-sided carcinoid heart disease and a patent foramen ovale, or in those with a functioning bronchial carcinoid tumor, or with pulmonary metastases.[83,84] In some patients with predominant right-sided carcinoid heart disease, the mitral and aortic valves also may be involved to a lesser degree.[81] Involvement of the left side of the heart appears to be a late development of the disease, except in the presence of a right-to-left shunt or a bronchial carcinoid.[74] When the mitral valve is extensively involved, the posterior mitral leaflet may adhere to the underlying mural endocardium, resulting in mitral regurgitation. When the aortic valve is extensively involved, the fibrous plaquing is usually on the arterial surface within the sinuses of Valsalva, predisposing of the valve to stenosis or insufficiency.[75]

Microscopically, these lesions contain fibroblasts, myofibroblasts, and smooth muscle cells embedded in a distinctive stroma rich in collagen and proteoglycans but lacking in elastic fibers.[75] The valvular cusps and the mural endocardium, per se, are morphologically normal and clearly separated from the atypical fibrous tissue by intact elastic lamellae.[75]

The pathogenesis of the carcinoid plaque is uncertain. It has not been possible to produce the valvular and endocardial lesions in animals by giving serotonin; and urinary levels of the breakdown product of serotonin, 5-hydroxyindoleacetic acid (5-HIAA), and blood serotonin levels have been similar in patients with the carcinoid syndrome with and without cardiac involvement.[85,86] However, serotonin does stimulate fibroblast growth in tissue culture.[87] Initially, serotonin was also believed to be responsible for the dermal flush in this syndrome, but this hypothesis has been challenged.[88] A kinin peptide such as bradykinin appears the more likely cause of the flush, and may also contribute to the development of the carcinoid endocardial lesions, although this has not been demonstrated.[89]

Although the valvular and endocardial lesions were once believed pathognomonic of this condition, identical lesions lacking in elastic fibers have been described in patients being treated with methysergide and, less commonly, with ergotamine tartrate.[90–92] The similarity of the chemical structure of methysergide to that of serotonin to which it is an antagonist is striking.[93] The major difference between the cardiac lesions in carcinoid syndrome and those associated with methysergide is the predominant right-sided cardiac involvement in the carcinoid syndrome, compared with the preponderance of left-sided disease associated with methysergide.[92]

CARDIOVASCULAR EFFECTS OF CORTICOSTEROIDS AND OTHER ANTINEOPLASTIC DRUGS

Long-term treatment with corticosteroids may be accomplished by arteritis involving small and medium arteries. In most cases, it is not clear whether the arteritis is caused by the underlying disease or causally related to the treatment with steroids. Most of the available evidence points to the first possibility.[94] Corticosteroids alter carbohydrate metabolism, inducing abnormal glucose tolerance, especially in patients with a family history that predisposes them to diabetes mellitus.[95] Treatment with steroids also predisposes to an increased incidence of thromboembolic complications in both adults and children.[94] Although the evidence is not conclusive, it has been suggested that corticosteroids may induce intimal proliferation in arteries and veins of susceptible individuals similar to that seen in patients receiving oral contraceptives. The combination of damage to the arterial wall with arteritis, an increased tendency to thrombosis, alteration of carbohydrate metabolism, and possible intimal proliferation suggests that the long-term administration of corticosteroids may accelerate atherosclerosis. Steroid-induced hypertension must also be considered an additional risk factor in accelerating atherogenesis.

Although focal myocardial necrosis has been induced in experimental animals receiving large doses of corticosteroids, the induction of these lesions in human subjects has not been documented.[96] Some patients who die while receiving large doses of corticosteroids will have cytoplasmic vacuoles in myocytes, similar to those seen in patients with Cushing syndrome or hypokalemia. Patients with cardiac sarcoidosis treated with steroids have an increased incidence of ventricular aneurysm.[97] The immunosuppressive effect of corticosteroids predisposes the patient to infection of the heart and blood vessels by opportunistic organisms.

The antineoplastic drugs most commonly associated with cardiotoxicity are the anthracycline antibiotics (daunomycin and its analogs, especially doxorubicin hydrochloride [Adriamycin]) and cyclophosphamide. Although the anthracycline antibiotics can produce acute and subacute cardiac toxicity, these agents are more notoriously known for the chronic congestive cardiomyopathy that they produce in human subjects and experimental animals. The cardiotoxic effects of doxorubicin hydrochloride are dose-related, and the critical dose is 500 mg per square meter. An accumulative dose below 500 mg per square meter yields a low incidence of cardiomyopathy, whereas approximately 30 percent of the patients receiving a larger dose will develop cardiomyopathy.[98]

The pathogenesis of this complication remains uncertain; however, a number of possible mechanisms have been proposed, including damage to DNA in cardiac muscle cells and peroxidative damage to cell membranes, mitochondrial membranes, and membranes of sarcoplasmic reticulum.[99] Mural thrombi are frequently present in both ventricles. Microscopically, the lesions are both focal and disseminated. The earliest lesions are most common in the subendocardium. In these early lesions, single isolated myocytes with degenerative changes are often dispersed in an otherwise morphologically intact myocardium.[100]

The degeneration induced by anthracyclines is manifested microscopically by myofibrillar loss and cytoplasmic vacuolization.[101–103] The latter is a prominent but focal finding that involves individual cells rather than large, confluent areas of myocardium, and it is caused by massive dilatation of tubules of sarcoplasmic reticulum; some dilatation of T tubules also occurs. This vacuolar degeneration can occur with apparent preservation of the nucleus and mitochondria. The two types of degeneration may occur concomitantly in the same cell or in separate cells. There does not appear to be a relation between the two types of injury and the severity of the course of the cardiotoxicity.[100]

These lesions eventually progress to the death of the myocytes, at which time the nuclei become pyknotic and disintegrate, and the mitochondria swell and develop myelin figures. When the myocardial cells die, they are replaced by fibrous tissue, resulting in patchy stellate scars throughout the myocardium. Although the microscopic and ultrastructural changes of anthracycline cardiotoxicity are characteristic, these changes are not specific and can be seen in cardiomyopathy due to other conditions. The severity of the cardiac morphologic changes induced by anthracyclines has been evaluated by myocardial biopsies, and these have been useful in determining whether patients suspected of developing anthracycline cardiomyopathy can receive additional amounts of the drug.[100] In addition to the myocardial degenerative lesions just described herein, which characteristically are not accompanied by an inflammatory cell infiltrate, patients receiving anthracycline antibiotics may develop acute myopericarditis, which is thought to be reversible.

Cyclophosphamide, an alkylating

agent used in the treatment of cancer, also is associated with a high incidence of cardiac toxicity, especially when administered in high-dose combination chemotherapy.[104,105] Cyclophosphamide-induced cardiotoxicity usually has an acute onset within hours or days after the beginning of treatment. Morphologically, there may be numerous large foci of hemorrhagic necrosis in the myocardium associated with extensive capillary microthrombosis, erythrocytes, and fibrin in the interstitium and necrotic myocytes.[106] Subpericardial and subendocardial ecchymosis with an acute inflammatory infiltrate may also be present. Treatment with cyclophosphamide may result in acute myopericarditis with or without hemorrhagic necrosis of the myocardium.[100] Electron microscopic examination of the myocardial lesions reveals capillary endothelial damage and unraveling of nuclear chromatin in both myocytes and endothelial cell nuclei, producing prominent thick, thin, and intermediate filaments.[106]

Antineoplastic drugs may indirectly cause damage to the cardiovascular system by their immunosuppressive effect, resulting in infective vasculitis, endocarditis, myocarditis, or pericarditis by opportunistic organisms.

RADIATION INJURY TO THE HEART

First reported by Seguy and Quenisset in 1897, radiation-induced heart disease is not widely understood. The consequences of mediastinal radiation have been characterized by many investigators and involve the pericardium,[107–115] coronary arteries,[116–119] myocardium,[120–124] endocardium and cardiac valves,[125] and the conduction tissues.[126–128]

Of the cardiac tissues, the pericardium is most commonly affected by radiation. Doses of radiation usually in excess of 40 Gy produce acute pericarditis, usually after 1 to 6 or more months, in more than 30 percent of individuals so exposed. Pericarditis may occur acutely during the course of radiation, or in some patients it may be considerably delayed. Chronic pericarditis may be manifested by pericardial effusion or chronic constriction, or both.[129]

Pericardial effusion is the most common manifestation of radiation injury,[130] and this may progress to tamponade[111] or chronic constrictive pericarditis.[109] Clinical features include pericarditic pain; elevated jugular venous pressure; an early diastolic filling sound (pericardial "knock"); and to varying degrees, features of systemic venous hypertension, such as hepatic enlargement, ascites, and edema. There is enlargement of the cardiac silhouette on chest x-ray, and the ECG reveals evidence of changes compatible with pericarditis. Two-dimensional echocardiography is excellent for documenting pericardial effusion. CT aids in identifying both pericardial thickening and fluid, as well as malignant tumor involvement, which may coexist or mimic radiation involvement of the heart. Pericardiocentesis may be required to differentiate malignant from radiation pericarditis.[131] The differential diagnosis must also include myxedematous pericardial effusion because hypofunction of the thyroid may follow mediastinal irradiation.[132] Treatment consists of salicylates and indomethacin.[130] The successful use of corticosteroid therapy also has been reported.[133] Pericardiocentesis may be required and aggressive surgical pericardiectomy has been recommended, even early in the course of effusive disease.[113] Constrictive pericarditis may occur many years after therapy,[134,135] and the patient may require surgical decortication, although differentiation from a restrictive myopathy may be difficult. In this regard, CT is particularly helpful in confirming major thickening of the pericardium.[136]

The genesis of postirradiation pericarditis has been the subject of some debate. A direct radiation effect is considered the most likely cause, but hypersensitivity reaction, radiation-induced vasculitis, and reaction to tumor-cell necrosis are possible factors.[130,135] Others have also considered radiation-induced obstruction of lymphatic vessels within the pericardium to be important in this process.[137]

Myocardial necrosis and hyalinization secondary to radiation were first described by Davis[138] in 1924; Fajardo and Stewart[139] noted pericarditis with neutrophilic infiltration within days of exposure of hearts in rabbits to 20 Gy of radiation. A long period of time followed during which no changes were evident on light microscopy; however, during this period, electron microscopy disclosed abnormalities within the capillaries. After 8 to 10 weeks, a fibrotic reaction was visible on light-microscopic examination. These investigators postulate that the early capillary damage was responsible for the ultimate myocardial fibrosis, probably mediated by acute capillary endothelial injury and subsequent loss of capillaries, resulting in a chronic state of ischemia, late death of myocytes, and interstitial fibrosis.[121,122,139,140] These changes can ultimately result in clinical features of restrictive or congestive cardiomyopathy.[130] In some patients, the right ventricle was involved more severely than the left, probably because of its anterior location. The consequent selective clinical features of right-sided heart failure may make the differential diagnosis of radiation-induced cardiomyopathy and constrictive pericarditis even more difficult.

Clinical abnormalities in the period following radiation may be of either myocardial or pericardial origin. Electrocardiographic changes usually consist of transitory ST-T-wave abnormalities. Cardiac enzymes may occasionally be elevated. Technetium-pyrophosphate uptake by the heart may also be noted after chest radiation,[119,141] and radiation-induced cardiomyopathy has been documented by gated radionuclide ventriculography.[142]

Additionally, the cancer chemotherapeutic agents may act synergistically with radiation in the genesis of a cardiomyopathic picture.

Coronary occlusion following mediastinal radiation therapy was first reported by Pearson[143] in 1957. Irradiation can cause coronary artery occlusive disease, either by coronary artery fibrosis or by accelerated atherosclerosis. Chest irradiation of experimental animals has produced coronary fibrosis and myocardial infarction.[119] These lesions were related to doses and demonstrated angiographically. Experimental animals, fed an atherogenic diet and exposed to cardiac irradiation, developed severe atherosclerotic coronary occlusive disease related in magnitude to the severity of the atherogenic diet and to the radiation dose.[119] The occurrence of coronary disease in patients older than 40 years of age who have received radiation therapy may be coincidental. Such does not appear to be the case, however, in younger subjects, many of whom lacked any other risk factors, who have developed postradiation angina, infarction, or sudden coronary death together with angiographically or anatomically demonstrable coronary occlusive disease.[119] These patients have anatomically demonstrated either fibrous changes or accelerated atherosclerosis in the coronary arteries.[116–118] An occasional patient with postradiation coronary artery occlusive disease has required aortocoronary saphenous vein bypass grafting as treatment for angina at a young age.[124]

Fajardo et al.[121] in 1968 were the first to describe focal fibrosis endocardial changes. If severe, these changes may resemble congenital fibroelastosis. Valvular lesions, usually incompetence of the aortic or mitral valve, have been reported, and deformity and thickening of the valves have been described in postmortem findings.[113,135] Stenosis of cardiac valves is frequent,[125] but may lead to hemodynamic and clinical sequelae.

There have been several reported examples of complete heart block following radiation therapy.[126–128] Bundle branch block has also been reported.

Radiation effects on the heart to varying degrees involve all of the cardiac tissues. Involvement is a function of the dose and the type of radiation exposure and, in lesser degrees, may be clinically inapparent yet evident on postmortem examination. Furthermore, the length of time the patient is alive after exposure to radiation may be an important factor in the character and degree of the clinical expression of radiation injury.

REFERENCES

1. Bearman RM: Primary leiomyosarcoma of the heart: report of a case and review of the literature. Arch Pathol 98:62, 1974
2. Griffiths GC: A review of primary tumors of the heart. Prog Cardiovasc Dis 7:465, 1965
3. Roberts WC, Spray TL: Pericardial heart disease. Curr Probl Cardiol 2:1, 1977
4. McAllister HA, Jr, Hall RJ: Iatrogenic heart disease. p. 871. In Cheng TO (ed): The International Textbook of Cardiology. Pergamon Press, New York, 1986
5. McAllister HA, Jr, Fenoglio JJ, Jr: Tumors of the Cardiovascular System. Fascicle 15, Second Series. Atlas of Tumor Pathology. Armed Forces Institute of Pathology, Washington, DC, 1978
6. McAllister HA, Jr: Primary tumors of the heart and pericardium. p. 325. In Sommers SC, Rosen PP (eds): Pathology Annual. Appleton-Century-Crofts, East Norwalk, CT, 1979
7. McAllister HA, Jr: Primary tumors of the heart and pericardium. p. 1. In Harvey WP (ed): Current Problems in Cardiology. Year Book Medical Publishers, Chicago, 1979
8. Cooley DA: Surgical management of cardiac tumors. p. 126. In Kapoor AS (ed): Cancer and the Heart. Springer-Verlag, New York, 1986
9. Hall RJ, Cooley DA, McAllister HA, Jr et al: Neoplastic heart disease. p. 1382. In Hurst JW, Logue RB, Rackley CE et al (eds): The Heart. 7th Ed. McGraw-Hill, New York, 1989
10. McAllister HA, Jr, Cooley DA: Cardiac tumors. p. 437. In Cooley DA (ed): How To Do It—Cardiac Surgery: State of the Art Reviews. Hanley and Belfus, Philadelphia, 1990
11. Carney JA: Differences between non-familial and familial cardiac myxoma. Am J Surg Pathol 9:53, 1985
12. Carney JA, Hruska LS, Beauchamp GD, Gordon H: Dominant inheritance of the complex of myxomas, spotty pigmentation, and endocrine overactivity. Mayo Clin Proc 61:165, 1986
13. Fine G, Morales A, Horn RC: Cardiac myxoma: a morphologic and histogenetic appraisal. Cancer 22:1156, 1968
14. Ferrans VJ, Roberts WC: Structural features of cardiac myxomas. Hum Pathol 4:111, 1973
15. Tanimara A, Kitazono M, Nagayama K et al: Cardiac myxoma: morphologic, histochemical, and tissue culture studies. Hum Pathol 19:316, 1988
16. Valente M: Structural profile of cardiac myxoma. Appl Pathol 1:251, 1983
17. Abenoza P, Sibley RK: Cardiac myxoma with glandlike structures: an immunohistochemical study. Arch Pathol Lab Med 110:736, 1986
18. Goldman BI, Frydman C, Harpaz N et al: Glandular cardiac myxomas: histo-

logic, immunohistochemical and ultra-structural evidence of epithelial differentiation. Cancer 59:1767, 1987

19. Coard KC, Silver MD: Gamna body of the heart. Pathology 16:459, 1984
20. Wang S-C, Dirkman SH, Goldberg SL, Deppisch LM: Gamna-Gandy body in a cardiac myxoma. Mt Sinai J Med 41:524, 1974
21. Salyer WR, Page DL, Hutchins GM: The development of cardiac myxomas and papillary endocardial lesions from mural thrombus. Am Heart J 89:4, 1975
22. Glasser SP, Bedynek JL, Hall RJ et al: Left atrial myxoma. Report of a case including hemodynamic, surgical, histologic and histochemical characteristics. Am J Med 50:113, 1971
23. Mahaim I: Les tumeurs et les polypes du coeur. Masson, Paris, 1945
24. Morales AR, Fine G, Casto A, Nadji M: Cardiac myxoma (endocardioma): an immunocytochemical assessment of histogenesis. Hum Pathol 12:896, 1981
25. Boxer ME: Cardiac myxoma: an immunoperoxidase study of histogenesis. Histopathology 8:861, 1984
26. Govani E, Severi B, Cenacchi G et al: Ultrastructural and immunohistochemical contribution to the histogenesis of human cardiac myxoma. Ultrastruct Pathol 12:221, 233, 1988
27. McComb RD: Heterogenous expression of factor VIII/von Willebrand factor by cardiac myxoma cells. Am J Surg Pathol 8:539, 1984
28. Schuger L, Ron N, Rosenmann E: Cardiac myxoma: a retrospective immunohistochemical study. Pathol Res Pract 182:63, 1987
29. Dewald GW, Dahl RJ, Sparbeck JL et al: Chromosomally abnormal clones and nonrandom telomeric translocations in cardiac myxomas. Mayo Clin Proc 62:558, 1987
30. Gray IR, Williams WG: Recurring cardiac myxoma. Br Heart J 53:645, 1985
31. Heath D, Best PV, Davis BT: Papilliferous tumors of the heart valves. Br Heart J 23:20, 1961
32. Magarey FR: On the mode of formation of Lambl's excrescences and their rela-

tion to chronic thickening of the mitral valve. J Pathol 61:203, 1949
33. Pomerance A: Papillary "tumours" of the heart valves. J Pathol 81:135, 1961
34. Fenoglio JJ, Diana DJ, Bowen TE et al: Ultrastructure of a cardiac rhabdomyoma. Hum Pathol 8:700, 1977
35. Ott DA, Garson A, Cooley DA, McNamara DG: Definitive operation for refractory cardiac tachyarrhythmias in children. J Thorac Cardiovasc Surg 90:681, 1985
36. Fenoglio JJ, McAllister HA, Jr, Ferrans VJ: Cardiac rhabdomyoma: a clinicopathologic and electron microscopic study. Am J Cardiol 38:241, 1976
37. Allenlay AL, Ferry DA, Lin B et al: Spontaneous regression of cardiac rhabdomyoma in tuberous sclerosis. Clin Pediatr 26:532, 1987
38. Heath D: Cardiac fibroma. Br Heart J 31:656, 1969
39. James TN, Carson DJ, Marshall TK: De subitaneis morbitus. 1. Fibroma compressing His bundle. Circulation 48:428, 1973
40. Page DL: Lipomatous hypertrophy of the cardiac interatrial septum: its development and probable clinical significance. Hum Pathol 1:151, 1970
41. Fyke FE, Tajik AJ, Edwards WD, Seward JB: Diagnosis of lipomatous hypertrophy of the atrial septum by two-dimensional echocardiography. J Am Coll Cardiol 1:1352, 1983
42. Levine RA, Weyman AE, Dinsmore RE et al: Noninvasive tissue characterization: diagnosis of lipomatous hypertrophy at the atrial septum by nuclear magnetic resonance imaging. J Am Coll Cardiol 7:688, 1986
43. Heggtveit HA, Fenoglio JJ, McAllister HA, Jr: Lipomatous hypertrophy of the interatrial septum: an assessment of 41 cases. Lab Invest 34:318, 1976
44. Baroldi G, Colombo F, Manion WC: Benign primary hemangioma of the right atrium of the heart: report of a case. Med Ann DC 36:287, 1967
45. Heggtveit HA: Thrombosed varices of the heart. Am J Pathol 48:50a, 1966
46. Begg JG: Blood-filled cysts in the car-

diac valve cusps in foetal life and infancy. J Pathol 87:177, 1964

47. Fine G, Morales AR: Mesothelioma of the atrioventricular node. Arch Pathol 92:402, 1971

48. Fenoglio JJ, Jacobs DW, McAllister HA, Jr: Ultrastructure of the mesothelioma of the atrioventricular node. Cancer 40:721, 1977

49. Fine G, Raju U: Congenital polycystic tumor of the atrioventricular node: a histogenetic appraisal with evidence for its endodermal origin. Hum Pathol 18:791, 1987

50. Linder J, Shelburne JD, Surge JP et al: Congenital endodermal heterotopia of the atrioventricular node: evidence for the endodermal origin of so-called mesotheliomas at the atrioventricular node. Hum Pathol 15:1093, 1984

51. Fine G: Neoplasms of the pericardium and heart. p. 868. In Gould SE (ed): Pathology of the Heart and Blood Vessels. Charles C Thomas, Springfield, IL, 1968

52. McAllister HA, Jr, Fenoglio JJ: Granular cell tumor of the heart: a report of three cases. Arch Pathol 100:276, 1976

53. Trout HH, McAllister HA, Jr: Treatment of vascular anomalies in infancy and childhood. p. 380. In Ernst CB, Stanley JC (eds): Current Therapy in Vascular Surgery. BC Decker, Philadelphia, 1987

54. Trout HH, McAllister HA, Jr, Giordano JM, Rich NM: Vascular malformations. Surgery 97:36, 1985

55. Anbe DT, Fine G: Cardiac lymphangioma and lipoma. Report of a case of simultaneous occurrence in association with lipomatous infiltration of the myocardium and cardiac arrhythmia. Am Heart J 86:227, 1973

56. Hui G, McAllister HA, Jr, Angelini P: Left atrial paraganglioma: report of a case and review of the literature. Am Heart J 113:1230, 1987

57. Cooley DA, Reardon MJ, Frazier OH: Human cardiac explantation and autotransplantation: application in a patient with a large cardiac pheochromocytoma. Tex Heart Inst J 12:171, 1985

58. Cammarosano C, Lewis W: Cardiac le-sions in acquired immune deficiency syndrome (AIDS). J Am Coll Cardiol 5:703, 1985

59. Autran B, Gorin I, Leibowitch M: Aids in a Haitian woman with cardiac Kaposi sarcoma and Whipple disease. Lance 1:767, 1983

60. McAllister HA, Jr: Cardiac fibrous histiocytoma—is heart transplantation a therapeutic option? Tex Heart Inst J 16:303, 1989

61. Constantino A, West TE, Gupta M, Loghmanee F: Primary cardiac lymphoma in a patient with acquired immune deficiency syndrome. Cancer 60:2801, 1987

62. Guarner J, Brynes RK, Chan WC et al: Primary non-Hodgkin's lymphoma of the heart in two patients with the acquired immunodeficiency syndrome. Arch Pathol Lab Med 111:254, 1987

63. Rodenburg CJ, Kluin P, Maes A, Paul LC: Malignant lymphoma confined to the heart, 13 years after cadaver kidney transplant. N Engl J Med 313:122, 1985

64. Feigin DS, Fenoglio JJ, McAllister HA, Jr, Madewell JE: Pericardial cysts: a radiologic-pathologic correlation and review. Radiology 125:15, 1977

65. Berry CL, Keeling J, Hilton C: Teratoma in infancy and childhood: a review of 91 cases. J Pathol 98:241, 1969

66. McAllister HA, Jr, Hall RJ, Cooley DA: Surgical pathology of tumors and cysts of the heart and pericardium. p. 343. In Waller BF (ed): Contemporary Issues in Surgical Pathology. Churchill Livingstone, New York, 1988

67. Wychulis AR, Connolly DC, McGoon DC: Pericardial cysts, tumors, and fat necrosis. J Thorac Cardiovasc Surg 62:294, 1971

68. Vasile N, Nicoleau F, Mathieu D: CT features of cardio-pericardial masses. Eur J Radiol 1:21, 1986

69. Williamson BR, Sturtevant NV, Black WC et al: Epicardial lipoma: a CT diagnosis. Comput Radiol 9:169, 1985

70. Zanca P, Chuang TH, DeAvila R: True congenital mediastinal thymic cyst. Pediatrics 36:615, 1965

71. Brandes WW, Gray JAC, MacLeod NW: Leiomyoma of the pericardium: report of a case. Am Heart J 23:426, 1942

72. Rogers AM, Kesten HD: A thyroid mass in the ventricular septum obstructing the right ventricular outflow tract and producing a murmur. J Cardiovasc Surg 4:175, 1963

73. Sytman AL, MacAlpin RN: Primary pericardial mesothelioma: report of two cases and review of the literature. Am Heart J 81:760, 1971

74. Ludwig GD: Carcinoid heart disease. Part 4. p. 1309. In Conn HL Jr, Horwitz O (eds): Cardiac and Vascular Disease. Vol II. Lea & Febiger, Philadelphia, 1971.

75. Bancroft JHJ, O'Brien DJ, Tickner A: Carcinoid syndrome due to carcinoid tumour of the ovary. Br Med J 2:1440, 1964

76. Hall RJ, McAllister HA Jr, Cooley DA, Frazier OH: Neoplastic heart disease. p. 2021. In Schlant RD, Alexander RW (eds): Hurst's The Heart. 8th Ed. McGraw-Hill, New York, 1993

77. Kieraldo J, Eversole S, Allen R: Carcinoid tumor of vermiform appendix with distant metastasis: review of the literature and report of two cases, one in a 14-year-old girl. Calif Med 99:161, 1963

78. Melmon KL, Sjoerdsma A, Mason DT: Distinctive clinical therapeutic aspects of the syndrome associated with bronchial carcinoid tumors. Am J Med 39:568, 1965

79. Oates JA, Sjoerdsma A: A unique syndrome associated with secretion of 5-hydroxytryptophan by metastatic gastric carcinoids. Am J Med 32:333, 1962

80. Grahame-Smith DG: The carcinoid syndrome. p. 1703. In Bondy PK, Rosenberg LE (eds): Metabolic Control and Disease. 9th Ed. WB Saunders, Philadelphia, 1980

81. McAllister HA Jr, Ferrans VJ: The cardiovascular system. p. 787. In Silverberg SG (ed): Principles and Practice of Surgical Pathology. 2nd Ed. Churchill Livingstone, New York, 1990

82. Carpena C, Kay JH, Mendez AM et al: Carcinoid heart disease. Surgery for tricuspid and pulmonary valve lesions. Am J Cardiol 32:229, 1973

83. Azzopardi JG, Bellau AR: Carcinoid syndrome and oat-cell carcinoma of the bronchus. Thorax 20:393, 1965

84. Roberts WC, Sjoerdsma A: The cardiac disease associated with the carcinoid syndrome (carcinoid heart disease). Am J Med 36:5, 1969

85. Sjoerdsma A, Weissbach H, Terry LL, Undenfriend S: Further observations on patients with malignant carcinoid. Am J Med 23:5, 1957

86. Tammes AR: Exogenous serotonin administered to rats with liver damage. Arch Pathol 79:626, 1965

87. Bowcek RJ, Alvarez TR: 5-hydroxytryptamine: a cytospecific growth stimulator of cultured fibroblasts. Science 167:898, 1970

88. Oates JA, Melmon K, Sjoerdsma A et al: Release of a kinin peptide in the carcinoid syndrome. Lancet 1:514, 1964

89. Oates JA, Pettinger WA, Doctor RR: Evidence for the release of bradykinin in carcinoid syndrome. J Clin Invest 45:173, 1966

90. Bana DS, McNeal PS, LeCompte PM et al: Cardiac murmurs and endocardial fibrosis associated with methysergide therapy. Am Heart J 88:640, 1975

91. McAllister HA Jr, Hall RJ: Iatrogenic heart disease. p. 871. In Cheng TO (ed): The International Textbook of Cardiology. Pergamon Press, New York, 1986

92. McAllister HA Jr, Mullick FG: Pathology of drug-induced and toxic diseases in the cardiovascular system. In Riddell R (ed): Pathology of Drug-Induced and Toxic Diseases. Churchill Livingstone, New York, 1982

93. Grahan JR: Cardiac and pulmonary fibrosis during methysergide therapy for headache. Am J Med Sci 254:1, 1967

94. von Eickstedt KW: Corticotrophins and corticosteroids. pp. 727–743. In Dukes MNG (ed): Meyler's Side Effects of Drugs. Vol. 10. Elsevier, New York, 1984

95. McKiddie MT, Jasani MK, Buchanan KD et al: The relationship between glu-

cose tolerance, plasma insulin and corticosteroid therapy in patients with rheumatoid arthritis. Metabolism 17:730, 1968

96. Karstad L, Tabel H, Gordon D: Myocardial necrosis and mineralization in normal and Aleutian disease in mink fed dexamethasone. Can J Comp Med 33:253, 1969

97. Roberts WC, McAllister HA Jr, Ferrans VJ: Sarcoidosis of the heart: a clinicopathologic study of 35 necropsy patients (group I) and review of 78 previously described necropsy patients (group II). Am J Med 63:86, 1977

98. Lefrak EA, Pitha J, Rosenheim S, Gottlieb JA: A clinicopathologic anatomy of Adriamycin cardiotoxicity. Cancer 32:302, 1973

99. Ferrans, VJ: Overview of morphologic reactions of the heart to toxic injury. p. 83. In Balazs T (ed): Cardiac Toxicology. CRC Press, Boca Raton, Fl, 1981

100. Billingham ME: Some recent advances in cardiac pathology. Hum Pathol 10:367, 1979

101. Jaenke RS, Fajardo LF: Adriamycin-induced myocardial lesions: report of a workshop. Am J Surg Pathol 1:55, 1977

102. Buja LM, Ferrans VJ, Mayr RJ, Roberts WC et al: Cardiac ultrastructural changes induced by daunorubicin therapy. Cancer 32:771, 1973

103. Billingham ME, Mason JW, Bistow MR, Daniels JR: Anthracycline cardiomyopathy monitored by morphologic changes. Cancer Treat Rep 62:865, 1978

104. Buckner CD, Rudolf RH, Fefer A et al: High dose cyclophosphamide therapy for malignant disease. Cancer 29:357, 1972

105. Applebaum FR, Strauchen JA, Graw R et al: Acute lethal carditis caused by high dose combination chemotherapy. Lancet 1:58, 1976

106. Buja LM, Ferrans VJ: Myocardial injury produced by antineoplastic drugs. p. 487. In Fleckenstein A, Rona G (eds): Recent Advances in Studies on Cardiac Structure and Metabolism. Vol. 6. University Park Press, Baltimore, 1975

107. Seguy G, Quenisset F: Action des rayons X sur le coeur, abstracted. Comput Rendu Acad Sci 124:790, 1897

108. Maslund DS, Rotz CT, Harris JH: Postradiation pericarditis with chronic pericardial effusion. Ann Intern Med 69:97, 1968

109. Muggia FM, Cassileth PA: Constrictive pericarditis following radiation therapy. Am J Med 44:116, 1968

110. Blumenfeld H, Thomas SF: Chronic massive pericardial effusion following roentgen therapy for carcinoma of the breast. Radiology 44:335, 1945

111. Hurst DW: Radiation fibrosis of pericardium with cardiac tamponade. Can Med Assoc J 81:377, 1959

112. Teng CY, Nemickas R, Robin JR Jr, Szanto PB: Pericardial effusion following radiation to the chest. Report of a case. Dis Chest 52:549, 1967

113. Morton DL, Glancy DL, Joseph WL, Adkins PC: Management of patients with radiation induced pericarditis with effusion: a note in the development of aortic regurgitation in two of them. Chest 64:291, 1973

114. Stewart JR, Fajardo LF: Dose response in human and experimental radiation-induced heart disease. Radiology 99:403, 1971

115. Byhardt R, Brace K, Ruckdeschel J, Chang P et al: Dose and treatment factors in radiation related pericardial effusion associated with the mantle technique for Hodgkin's disease. Cancer 35:795, 1975

116. Dollinger MR, Lavine DM, Foye LV Jr: Myocardial infarction due to postirradiation fibrosis of the coronary arteries. JAMA 195:316, 1966

117. Huff H, Saunders EM: Coronary artery occlusion after radiation. N Engl J Med 286:780, 1972

118. McReynolds RA, Gold GL, Roberts WC: Coronary heart disease after mediastinal irradiation for Hodgkin's disease. Am J Med 60:39, 1976

119. Kopelson G, Herwig KJ: The etiologies of coronary artery disease in cancer patients. Int J Radiat Oncol Biol Phys 4:895, 1978

120. Bolti RE, Driscol TE, Pearson OH,

Smith JC: Radiation myocardial fibrosis simulating constrictive pericarditis. Cancer 22:1254, 1968

121. Fajardo LF, Stewart JR, Cohn KE: Morphology of radiation-induced heart disease. Arch Pathol 86:512, 1968
122. Fajardo LF, Stewart JR: Experimental radiation induced heart disease. Am J Pathol 59:299, 1970
123. Rubin E, Camara J, Grayzel DM, Zak FG: Radiation-induced cardiac fibrosis. Am J Med 34:71, 1963
124. Ali MK, Khalil KG, Fuller LM, et al: Radiation-related myocardial injury: management of two cases. Cancer 38:1941, 1976
125. Warda M, Khan A, Massumi A et al: Radiation-induced valvular dysfunction. J Am Coll Cardiol 2:180, 1983
126. Cohn SI, Saroja B, Glass J, Lev M: Radiotherapy as a cause of complete atrioventricular block in Hodgkin's disease. Arch Intern Med 141:676, 1981
127. Tzivoni D, Ratzkowski E, Biran S et al: Complete heart block following therapeutic irradiation of the left side of the chest. Chest 71:231, 1977
128. Kremer DN, Laplace LB: Heart block following x-ray treatment for thyrotoxicosis. Am Heart J 11:227, 1936
129. Wolf GL, Kumar PP: Radiation-induced pericarditis. Pract Cardiol 6:41, 1980
130. Cohn KE, Stewart JR, Fajardo LF, Hancock EW: Heart disease following irradiation. Medicine 46:281, 1967
131. Posner MR, Cohn GI, Skarin AT: Pericardial disease in patients with cancer. The differentiation of malignant from idiopathic and radiation-induced pericarditis. Am J Med 71:407, 1981
132. Schimpff SC, Diggs CH, Salvatore PC, Wiernik PH: Radiation-related thyroid dysfunction: implications for treatment of Hodgkin's disease. Ann Intern Med 92:91, 1980
133. Keelan MH Jr, Rudders RA: Successful treatment of radiation pericarditis with corticosteroids. Arch Int Med 134:145, 1974
134. MacLeod CA, Schwartz H, Linton OB: Constrictive pericarditis following irradiation therapy. JAMA 207:2281, 1969
135. Haas, JM: Symptomatic constrictive pericarditis developing 45 years after radiation therapy to the mediastinum: a review of radiation pericarditis. Am Heart J 77:89, 1969
136. Moncada R, Baker M, Salinas M et al: Diagnostic role of computed tomography in pericardial heart disease: congenital defects, thickening, neoplasms, and effusions. Am Heart J 103:263, 1982
137. Miller AJ, Jain S, Levin B: Radiographic visualization of lymphatic drainage of heart muscle and pericardial sac in the dog. Chest 59:271, 1971
138. Davis KS: Intrathoracic changes following x-ray treatment: clinical and experimental study. Radiology 3:301, 1924
139. Fajardo LF, Stewart JR: Pathogenesis of radiation-induced myocardial fibrosis. Lab Invest 29:244, 1973
140. Totterman KJ, Pesonen E, Siltanen P: Radiation-related chronic heart disease. Chest 88:875, 1983
141. Soin JS, Cox JD, Youker JE, Swartz HM: Cardiac localization of ^{99m}Tc-(Sn)-pyrophosphate following irradiation of the chest. Radiology 124:165, 1977
142. Burns RJ, Bar-Schlomo B-Z, Druck MN et al: Detection of radiation cardiomyopathy by gated radionuclide angiography. Am J Med 74:297, 1983
143. Pearson HES: Coronary occlusion following thoracic radiotherapy, two cases. Proc R Soc Med 50:516, 1957
144. McAllister HA Jr: Tumors of the heart and pericardium. p. 1297. In Silver MD (ed): Cardiovascular Pathology. Churchill Livingstone, NY, 1991

10

Autonomic Dysfunction and the Heart

H. Cecil Coghlan

Leonardo da Vinci postulated that the heart's action depended on both its morphology and its nerves.[1] Claude Bernard defined the vasoconstrictor function of the sympathetic nerves supplying the peripheral blood vessels between 1851 and 1853, and DeCyon and Ludwig[1a] found in 1866 that "the stimulation of the central end of a nerve emerging from the cardiovascular system itself, lying parallel to but separate from the cervical vagus and sympathetic trunks, caused marked bradycardia and hypotension." These landmark discoveries set the stage for the remarkable evolution of our understanding of the fascinating servocontrol of the circulatory system by the autonomic nervous system (ANS).

The autonomic nervous system affects functions of all other systems and influences behavior. It is the orchestrator for adaptive responses to stress, be it emotional, environmental or sociologic. It is not surprising, therefore, that clinical manifestations of any illness are influenced by the autonomic nervous system which also affects interactions of individuals with their surroundings. Because published work in this field is so extensive and the issues are so big, most physicians do not get beyond nebulous concepts of autonomic dysfunction.

> O. Appenzeller[2]

As practicing physicians, however, we need to keep Professor Plum's admonition clearly in mind:

> Autonomic control extends to almost every organ of the body and perturbations in these regulatory systems probably take more American patients to doctors than all other conditions combined.

> F. Plum[3]

Despite the fact that studies of many pathologic conditions that we will discuss later have highlighted the causative role of autonomic dysfunction, no systematic analysis of the interrelationship between dysfunction in the nervous and cardiovascular systems was published until Johnson, Lambie, and Spalding[4] released their landmark monograph of 1984 in which they coined the term "neurocardiology." In 1985, Natelson re-emphasized the importance of this approach[5] and inspired a meeting in 1987 of anatomists, pathologists, physiologists, neurophysiologists, neurologists, psychiatrists, and cardiologists, whose contributions are contained in a monograph published in 1988.[6]

Progress in this field has continued to produce increasingly sophisticated methods for evaluation of baroreceptors and sympathetic neural traffic in humans,[7-9] enzymatic and membrane receptor studies,[10-14] radioisotope imaging of the cardiac adrenergic system in patients,[15-16] and cardiac electrophysiologic and neuroanatomic studies.[17-21] It is therefore timely to try to put the interrrelationship of the autonomic and cardiovascular systems in perspective for the practicing physician.

PHYSIOLOGY OF THE AUTONOMIC NERVOUS SYSTEM (CARDIOVASCULAR REGULATION)

The precise and immediate adjustment of the heart and blood vessels to meet highly variable organ and tissue requirements, maintain homeostasis, and counteract gravitational shifts of blood volume is essential for our normal, enjoyable performance and health. Neural regulation, essential because it provides both stability, rapid adaptive change, and even anticipatory adjustments, is based on closed loop feedback systems that depend on multiple reflex arcs; such arcs permit processing of afferent information at various levels within the nervous system, and they also allow for the control and influence exerted by higher brain centers. Autonomic control of various functions is accomplished through the extensive innervation of multiple organs by the sympathetic and parasympathetic divisions of the autonomic nervous system.

Physicians are most familiar with the sympathetic and parasympathetic divisions of the peripheral ANS. The third (or enteric) division is being increasingly recognized (as suggested by Langley in 1898), but is out of the scope of the present chapter. The ANS is integrally connected to neocortical regions, the limbic system, the hypothalamus, and somatosensory pathways, and is also subject to neurohumoral influences. The definition of the central component has come later than that of the peripheral, but has advanced significantly in recent years.[22] The ANS determines immediate cardiovascular homeostatic adjustments, whereas long-term changes are mediated by the endocrine system, in particular the renin-angiotensin-aldosterone system. The heart itself acts as a "sensory organ,"[23] providing important input to the medullary integrating centers from receptors in the venoatrial junctions and the ventricular myocardium.

A detailed description of the autonomic regulation of the circulatory system is beyond the scope of this chapter. Several excellent reviews have recently been published describing the authors' valuable and extensive research in depth; these studies represent an important contribution to our knowledge of this field and offer a solid information base for the interested reader.[24-39] Specific examples of autonomic dysfunction-related cardiovascular problems have been selected as likely to be important in the daily practice of medicine; additional information on the specific pathophysiologic situations will be provided, with the pertinent references.

The diagram of the central and peripheral cardiovascular control (Fig. 10-1), inspired particularly by Shepherd and Mancia[29] and by Abboud and Thames's comprehensive review,[25] should help to visualize how the neural control of the heart and blood vessels operates as a highly integrated multiaccess, smoothly functioning controller capable of producing large or small variations in sympathetic and parasympathetic outflow. The medullary cardiovascular "control centers" (functionally committed pools of neurons rather than anatomically defined structures) respond to multiple afferent signals integrated fundamentally in the nucleus tractus solitarius of the medulla oblongata, under the instant-to-instant modulation from "higher centers" that exert inhibitory or facilitory influence on the complex multisynaptic neural pathways that control cardiovascular reflex responses.[36–40] This very simplified diagram does not acknowledge documented autonomic-hormonal interactions, such as modulation of vasopressin release by cardiac sensory afferents,[31] the central and peripheral autonomic effects of angiotensin II,[31,38,41,42] the reduction of the release of norepinephrine by prostaglandins during sympathetic stimulation,[43,44] the growing importance of opioids and peptides[38] including atrial natriuretic peptide,[33,45,46] and the modulation of norepinephrine release at the sympathetic neuroeffector junction by the action on prejunctional receptors (positive by epinephrine and angiotensin II and negative by histamine, serotonin, norepinephrine, adenosine, and acetylcholine).[33]

Figure 10-1 shows the highly important central antagonism of excitatory-inhibitory effects that are expressed as a change of the "balance" between sympathetic and parasympathetic efferent traffic, but does not stress that this balance is fine-tuned by interactions at the level of the intermediolateral column synapses, the ganglia, and the sympathetic nerve endings themselves, where vagal stimulation decreases norepinephrine release by acting on prejunctional receptors and

by inhibition of adenylate cyclase via muscarinic postjunctional receptors (what M.N. Levy has termed "accentuated antagonism").[47–50]

Figure 10-1 also fails to emphasize that traffic in efferent autonomic nerves is controlled selectively from the central nervous system and targeted to specific vascular beds and even to particular segments of a vascular bed,[9,51] and that autonomic tone has a circadian variation. Thus, sympathetic vasoconstrictor activity determines higher forearm vascular resistance in the morning than the evening.[52] Likewise there is higher systemic blood pressure[53–55] and increased frequency of episodes of myocardial ischemia in the early morning hours.[56–57] This circadian variation is important in view of the well-documented morning increase in the risk of acute cardiovascular disorders (transient myocardial ischemia, myocardial infarction, sudden cardiac death, and stroke).[58] Heart rate variability, considered a measure of cardiac autonomic function of great clinical utility, also varies throughout the day[54,59] and decreases with age.[60] Other age-induced autonomic changes (decreased baroreflex sensitivity, increased plasma catecholamine concentrations, and impulse traffic in recordings from cutaneous and muscle sympathetic nerves without a change in adrenoceptor number or affinity) are nicely detailed by Davies and Sever[12] and others.[61] The effects of age-induced changes on the clinical evaluation of autonomic function are well established.[60,62–66]

There is also a centrally mediated oscillation of vasomotor tone that results in a mild low-frequency variation in digital blood flow measured by infrared flow probe, which is markedly increased in frequency and amplitude in patients with mitral valve prolapse and dysautonomia, with no neurologic disease on prolonged

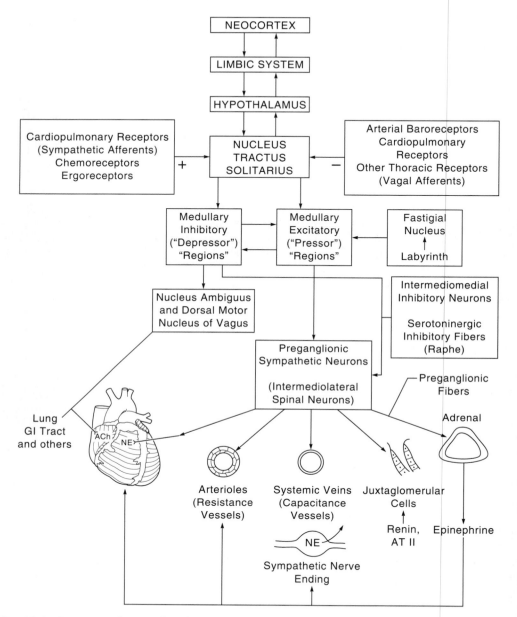

Fig. 10-1. Diagram of central and peripheral cardiovascular control. (From Coghlan,[67] with permission.)

follow-up.[67] (Fig. 10-2). The frequency of oscillation of subcutaneous microvascular flow measured by laser-Doppler flowmetry is greater in patients who develop syncope during tilt testing than in controls under baseline conditions. It decreases in patients (but not in control subjects) in the first quartile of the tilt test, and increases markedly just prior to the onset of syncope. This autonomic in-

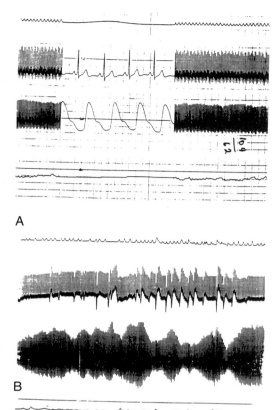

Fig. 10-2. Comparison of the mild oscillation of peripheral vasomotor tone of the subject with normal autonomic control (**A**) and the marked oscillation in a subject with autonomic dysregulation (**B**). The tracings in each panel represent, from top to bottom: respiratory motion from a chest bellows, electrocardiographic tracing from chest electrodes simulating standard lead one, finger plethysmography from infrared flow probe, and tachograph depiction of heart rate. Note that changes in digital flow signal are not synchronous with the changes of respiratory signal. (From Coghlan,[67] with permission.)

stability that precedes syncope (and is thus similar to that of our patients who are symptomatic because of autonomic dysregulation) is very striking and deserves further study.[68]

There is an extensive interaction between reflexes in the moment-by-moment regulation of the cardiovascular and respiratory systems.[22] Both baroreceptors and lung stretch afferents terminate within the nucleus tractus solitarius, which also contains a major population of inspiratory neurons.[69] It appears that any action of lung stretch inputs must be mediated at sites between the nucleus tractus solitarius and the nucleus ambiguus of the vagus.[22] This interaction is the basis for the use of heart rate variation induced by breathing in autonomic assessment of vagal activity and has been postulated to have a possible role in sudden infant death syndrome. A number of vagal reflexes referred from the upper aerodigestive tract may be responsible for abnormal cardiovascular regulation resulting from pathology of or diagnostic manipulations of the pharynx, larynx, and esophagus.[70]

Anticipatory changes are essential for adequate circulatory adjustment to daily activity. The autonomic responses that accompany "familiar" activities are a form of learned behavior[71] and form the basis of the fundamental training effect. Studies of athletes and instrumented animals have shown that the higher control centers resort to the "memory bank" and provide a pattern of integration utilized previously by the circulatory system. This allows a "trained" person to perform with particular efficiency. "Faulty or disturbed central planning," which may lead to inappropriate processing of afferent inputs centrally or even initiate abnormal cardiovascular responses in the absence of afferent "requirement signals," may play a crucial role in cardiovascular autonomic dysfunction or dysautonomia. In addition, afferent signals may interfere in central modulation, causing important changes in the expected pattern of a circulatory response. We demonstrated that atrial mechanoreceptor afferent stimuli caused by distention of atrial appendages significantly changed the normally highly stereotyped response of the serotonin cardiogenic hypertensive chemoreflex.[72] Profound changes of autonomic regulation by "conflicting signals" from dyskinetic areas in experimental myocardial infarction have been correlated with human observations.[23,73–77] The possibility has been raised that "conflicting signals" originating from the valve cusp distended during systole in mitral valve prolapse (at a time when ventricular receptors are "reporting" declining stress) may play a role in the dysautonomia present in a subset of patients with symptomatic mitral valve prolapse by disturbing central modulation of cardiovascular reflexes.[67]

Centrally triggered integrated cardiovascular responses, representing "playing dead" (depression) or "fight or flight" (anxiety) reactions, are important in human physiology as well as in the experimental animal. Plum has reminded us that:

> Most psychosomatic disorders produce their symptoms at least partly and often predominantly through the limbic-autonomic system. Autonomic influences act in subtle ways, and abnormal responses to life stress are often highly individual matters, not easy to separate from the nervous system's routine adjustments to living. Clinical sensitivity to the possibility that the brain rather than the target organ sometimes causes the symptoms represents perhaps the most important first step in detecting pathologic autonomic adjustments to life stress.
>
> F. Plum[3]

The physiology and pathophysiology of exercise has been comprehensively analyzed by Blomqvist.[78] The physiologic response to exercise, so vital in daily activity, requires a complex set of adjustments of central and peripheral components of the cardiovascular system, in order to meet the increased demand for oxygen transport. The neurogenic mechanisms have recently been reviewed by Shepherd and co-workers[79] and by Mitchell.[80] The cardiovascular control centers receive signals from the motor areas of the brain where the voluntary contraction of the skeletal muscles is initiated and from ergoreceptors in the muscle that sense the degree of activity of the contracting muscles. The integrated response of the cardiovascular centers leads to decreased vagal traffic to the heart that causes increased heart rate. The increased sympathetic outflow leads to increased cardiac contractility, increased tone of the splanchnic, renal, and other resistance vessels, constriction of the splanchnic capacitance vessels, and release of catecholamines, mainly epinephrine, from the adrenal medulla. β-Adrenergic stimulation contributes to the heart rate response. As systemic blood pressure begins to rise, mechanoreceptors of the carotid sinus and aortic arch (and presumably atrial and ventricular deformation receptors also) are activated and may modify the increase in arterial pressure, heart rate, and cardiac output. The activation of the sympathetic nervous system results in elevated plasma norepinephrine, most of which is thought to constitute overflow from vascular receptors mediating vasoconstriction, especially in resting skeletal muscles. Catecholamine kinetics are complex, and plasma levels do not necessarily provide an accurate estimate of sympathetic nerve traffic. Metabolic vasodilatory activity in exercising muscles may override the α-mediated vasoconstriction. However, studies in normal subjects have demonstrated significant residual vasoconstrictor activity during maximal exercise that involves large muscle groups and requires rates of oxygen uptake and transport that equal or exceed maximal systemic capacity. Carbon dioxide and potassium released by the exercising muscle are among the most important local vasodilators. In addition, potassium released during exercise activates muscle afferents and modulates the reflex-induced increases in heart rate, cardiac output, contractile state, and arterial pressure.[81,82] Autonomic dysfunction is an important feature in congestive heart failure and plays a significant role in the effort intolerance and other symptoms as well as in the prognosis, as will be discussed in more detail later.

ASSESSMENT OF AUTONOMIC FUNCTION

The anatomic location of the ANS renders it relatively inaccessible to direct clinical testing, with the exception of intraneural recording of sympathetic activity in certain peripheral nerves.[9] A battery of tests assessing autonomic function has been established, based on measuring end-organ responses to standardized physiologic and pharmacologic perturbations or challenges, determining levels of neurotransmitters and neuromodulators in blood, cerebrospinal fluid, and urine, and quantifying autonomic receptor density and affinity.[11] In addition to autonomic reflex testing, evaluation of autonomic function by spectral analysis of heart rate as a means of assessing the relative magnitude and balance of sympathetic and parasympathetic activity has been increasingly used.[54,59,60,83,84] We will concentrate on the study of cardiovascular reflexes, in addition to which pupillometry, sweat testing, and urodynamic testing may be required in the evaluation of autonomic disorders. There are several detailed descriptions of ANS testing[4,67,85–91] that contain details of technique and normal values in relation to

age, which modifies autonomic responses, as described in the Physiology section. Some tests are more readily quantifiable, such as assessment of respiratory R-R variation by standard deviation of R-R index,[92] standard deviation of mean R-R interval,[93] vectorial analysis of R-R variability,[94] and spectral analysis of heart rate.[54,59,60] Some tests, mediated via baroreflex arcs (Valsalva, postural tests) or independent of them (sinus arrhythmia with deep breathing, handgrip, cold pressor, cortical arousal by mental arithmetic or delayed auditory stimulation), are particularly applicable in the clinical setting because of their relative simplicity.[67,86] Instantaneous heart rate monitoring and blood pressure measurement are always required (indirect "indices" based solely on heart rate provide insufficient information). Blood pressure can be measured noninvasively by sphygmomanometer (automated or not), or continuous recording of finger blood pressure by means of a FINAPRES instrument, employing the volume clamp method of Penaz.[95] Noninvasive cardiac output by Doppler technique with computation, finger blood flow by finger plethysmography with infrared flow probe, capillary blood flow by laser-Doppler flowmeter, and respiratory rate by nasal thermistor are highly desirable measures in more sophisticated ANS evaluation.[86] Reproducibility of these tests has been established.[93,96–98] Simplicity of execution, reproducibility, and standardization of the challenge to the ANS are not synonymous with simplicity of interpretation in autonomic reflex testing.[99,100]

Certain tests that have provided highly precise information, especially on human baroreceptor function, such as lower body negative pressure to induce volume shifts similar to orthostatic stress,[45,101] application of pressure (positive or negative) to the neck to evaluate carotid baroreceptor response,[102] evaluation of pressor responses to infusion of phenylephrine or angiotensin II,[103] and multiunit recording of peripheral sympathetic nerve traffic,[9] are best performed in a research laboratory setting, with special precautions to avoid emotional interference in test results. Further analysis of some specific tests of frequent use may be helpful.

Postural Test

After 30 minutes of quiet recumbency, the subject (not exposed to caffeine, nicotine, or cardioactive drugs) undergoes gravitational stress either by standing or by passive tilt (motorized table, to which the subject is loosely attached by a broad waistband to avoid falling, tilted to 70 or 80 degrees). We have chosen 80 degrees because the hydrostatic effect of tilt governing the translocation of blood from the central volume is proportional to the sine of the angle between the table and the horizontal. Thus, 80 degrees is similar (98 percent) to standing or to the effect of 40 to 50 mmHg lower body negative pressure.[104] The early changes in heart rate (first 20 seconds) due to abrupt inhibition of cardiac vagal tone triggered by voluntary muscle contraction upon standing are absent or very blunted during passive tilt with a footrest. The "unloading" of low pressure baroreceptors, and later the arterial receptors, causes a very rapid decrease of vagal tone (very short latency) and later an increase in sympathetic tone (more prolonged latency)[29] that are responsible for the heart rate increase and the vasomotor change that maintain arterial blood pressure. A persistent fall in systolic pressure larger than 20 mmHg, in diastolic pressure larger than 5 mmHg, or both is considered abnormal even in elderly subjects.[88] A non-neurogenic disturbance caused by de-

creased blood volume is likely to cause a fall in systolic blood pressure only, whereas autonomic failure involves both the systolic and diastolic pressures. The steady-state heart rate response (after 1 to 2 minutes of standing) depends predominantly on increased activity of the sympathetic system[105] and an excessive heart rate response indicates excessive adrenergic drive to the sinus node.[104] An abnormal heart rate response cannot be fully evaluated without monitoring the concomitant blood pressure responses. This fundamental concept applies to the interpretation of all abnormal heart rate responses that are known to be baroreflex-mediated.[99] Abnormalities of the response to tilt due to autonomic dysfunction are fundamental in the evaluation of orthostatic hypotension and syncope. In that case, the usual 3-minute head-up tilt is prolonged to 45 to 60 minutes or is combined with isoproterenol infusion. Analysis of heart rate and blood pressure after return to the horizontal position is also valuable.[67]

Valsalva Maneuver

After a deep inspiration, the supine subject performs a sustained forced expiration through a mouthpiece connected to an aneroid manometer (30 mmHg, which most subjects can maintain) for 12 to 15 seconds. Blood pressure falls initially, but should cease to fall after the first few seconds if peripheral sympathetic vasoconstriction is normal. On release from blowing there is normally a pressure overshoot. The heart rate changes opposite to the blood pressure changes during the Valsalva maneuver depend primarily on vagal innervation.[98] Some precautions in interpretation have been emphasized by Bennett.[106]

Heart Rate Studies

The change of heart rate with breathing (sinus arrhythmia) is dependent on the vagus,[107] and lessening or absence of this variation is indicative of vagal denervation.[108] With the subject in the supine position, sinus arrhythmia is assessed by R-R or heart rate change with a single deep breath, the mean measurement of 5 or more breaths at 6 bpm synchronized by metronome or oscilloscope signal,[92,109] the standard deviation of R-R, or the vectorial analysis of R-R variation.[94] Sinus arrhythmia varies with age, so it is fundamental to compare carefully obtained age-related normal values.[110,111] Spectral analysis of continuously recorded heart rate by Fourier or autoregressive analysis of R-R variability is yielding valuable information on autonomic regulation in ambulatory subjects.[54,59,60,84] Simpler measures, from 24-hour electrocardiogram (ECG) recording such as the mean hourly R-R interval, have been advocated for clinical use.[87] The heart rate and blood pressure response (increase) to a 15-second maximal *handgrip* assesses parasympathetic tone because it is due to its withdrawal in response to a reflex triggered by muscle ergoreceptors. The response to 90- or 180-second sustained handgrip at 30 percent maximal force assesses sympathetic activity. Thus this test is useful for testing for vagal and sympathetic dysfunction independently of the integrity of the baroreceptor reflex mechanisms.[35] The short latency of the parasympathetic nervous system (PNS) and the longer latency of the sympathetic nervous system (SNS) allow this dual evaluation.[29] Since 1981 we have used the *"echo"* stress test (direct cortical arousal induced by out-of-phase reproduction of a prerecorded reading via earphones to the subject while reading aloud the same paragraph), suggested to us by Dr. John T. Shepherd,

for the assessment of central and efferent sympathetic response independent of baroreceptor mechanisms.[67] Heart rate and blood pressure increase monitored during the immediate reaction are measures of acute sympathetic stimulation, caused by the delayed auditory feedback (0.15-second delay), which is a more reliable stimulus than mental arithmetic and does not lose its effect by habit.[112] Application of negative or positive *pressure to the neck* to change the transmural pressure in the common carotid arteries, which modifies their diameter and alters the degree of activation of the carotid sinus baroreceptors, has been accomplished either by enclosing the neck in a chamber or cuff or by applying a cup over the carotid sinus region. This technique has allowed the study of the relationships among changes in carotid transmural pressure, arterial blood pressure, heart rate, and resistance in systemic vascular beds.[7] The alterations of arterial blood pressure induced by changes in carotid sinus baroreceptors will affect aortic baroreceptors (and possibly receptors in the left ventricle) in an opposite manner. In order to obviate this effect, this approach has been refined by Eckberg and his associates[7] to evaluate the vagally mediated effects on heart rate. A computer-controlled system delivers an ECG-triggered ramp of neck collar pressures. Each pressure level is imposed only during a single cardiac cycle, and the effect is measured by the R-R change of the following cardiac cycle, as the reflex response time is very short. The pressure ramp is easily repeated, and stimulus-response curves can be based on multiple measurements.[7] A combination of direct sympathetic nerve recording and this neck pressure technique has confirmed, by ingenious research, that both carotid and aortic baroreceptor reflexes participate in the control of arterial pressure in human subjects and has suggested that the aortic reflex is more powerful than the carotid in humans. The greater sensitivity applies to the control of both heart rate and adrenergic vasoconstrictor activity.[113,114]

Plasma Catecholamine

Plasma catecholamine concentrations, frequently used in the clinical assessment of autonomic function, are assayed by readily available and precise techniques.[115] They reflect the function of the adrenergic system in a complex manner dependent on release and uptake kinetics,[116,117] the regional nature of sympathetic activation, the richness of adrenergic innervation in a given circulatory territory (and its extension), and on the subject's age.[118,119] They require evaluation during precise physiologic stresses.[120,121] Plasma levels of epinephrine reflect adrenal activity quite accurately. Norepinephrine concentration in a mixed venous sample represents a minute fraction of the neurotransmitter released as the result of sympathetic nerve activation and is not necessarily an accurate indicator of sympathetic neural activity. As sympathetic discharge is differentiated, neural activity to a given target organ may be poorly reflected in the pooled venous sample.[122]

CARDIOVASCULAR MANIFESTATIONS OF AUTONOMIC DYSFUNCTION

Faulty autonomic regulation can easily lead to inappropriate tachycardia or bradycardia, orthostatic hypotension, dyspnea,[123] reduced effort tolerance, fatigability, chest pain,[123] and rhythm disturbances.[124–128] Autonomic dysfunction or dysautonomia may be caused by (A) changes affecting the basic functional characteristics of the autonomic nervous system (structural disturbance of autonomic reflexes and pathways) or (B) abnormal patterns of activation or modulation of "normal reflexes" (functional dysautonomia). We will analyze the cardiovascular abnormalities resulting from multiple conditions associated with autonomic dysfunction.

Orthostatic Hypotension

Hypotension is a common and frequently disabling condition of both neurogenic and nonneurogenic origin.[35] Blomqvist, in a comprehensive recent review,[129] has suggested that the conventional terminology of sympaticotonic or hyperadrenergic orthostatic hypotension (OH), and asympaticotonic or hypoadrenergic OH, be changed because it only focuses on the responses mediated by the sympathetics NS and ignores other reflex abnormalities and changes of volemia. He proposes the terms *normovolemic hyporeactive OH* and *hypovolemic hyperreactive OH*. The former typically results from autonomic failure (type A dysfunction; see above) and the latter from a nonstructural dysfunction (type B; see above).

A change in body position from supine to standing or sitting initiates a well-defined sequence of events and the corresponding reflex adjustments: a blood volume shift from the central volume to the lower body (700 to 800 ml), a fall of cardiac filling pressures, and decrease of stroke volume by 20 to 30 percent. An equally large fall in arterial pressure is prevented by rapid baroreflex-induced increases in heart rate and vascular resistance (of arterioles and systemic and splanchnic veins). Cerebral perfusion pressure is kept within the autoregulatory range. Cerebral blood flow usually starts to decrease significantly when driving pressure (mean arterial pressure at the eye level) falls below 50 mmHg. Consciousness may be lost when cerebral blood flow falls below 25 percent of normal, which usually occurs at a mean pressure of about 40 mmHg[130] in the absence of obstructive cerebral arterial lesions. As in the upright position, cerebral arterial pressure is ±30 mmHg lower than that in the aortic arch; this corresponds to a mean brachial pressure of 70 mmHg (or blood pressure 80/65). A significant shift of the autoregulatory range to the left frequently "protects" patients with OH due to chronic autonomic dysfunction.[131] Short-term regulation of blood pressure is accomplished mainly by neural mechanisms. The fall in intravascular and intracardiac pressures causes a decrease in activation of carotid, aortic, and cardiopulmonary mechanoreceptors that results in decreased afferent traffic to the nucleus tractus solitarius. Such lessened traffic decreases both central inhibitory activity and parasympathetic efferent drive and increases sympathetic drive. The end result is an increase in heart rate and contractility; arteriolar vasoconstriction that reduces blood flow to skin, inactive skeletal muscle, and renal and splanchnic regions; and release of renin from juxtaglomerular cells and vasopressin from the neurohypophysis. There is controversy about the relative role of active reflex-mediated venomotor changes. Active venoconstriction may occur in the skin and splanchnic region. Veins supplying skeletal muscle are poorly innervated. The deep veins have thin walls, and venous compliance is largely determined by the characteristics of skeletal muscle. Young persons with OH and syncope have lower intramuscular pressure in the leg at rest and subnormal increase of that pressure during tilt.[132] A combination of magnetic resonance imaging and occlusion plethysmography has shown that at hydrostatic pressures equivalent to that of the upright position more than one-half of the increase in leg volume is accommodated by the deep veins.[133] Vasoconstriction with decreased limb blood flow occurs in humans in response to local venous distention, mediated by a local (axonal) sympathetic reflex.[134] Streeten et al.[135] have measured gravitational pooling of blood in the legs and reduction of blood in the head by external gamma counting of autologous erythrocytes labeled with sodium pertechnetate Tc^{99m} through ports in fixed positions over the leg and the temple assessed as a percent change from recumbency values.

Normovolemic Hyporeactive Orthostatic Hypotension

Normovolemic hyporeactive OH is caused fundamentally by disorders of the central nervous system and the peripheral nerves, encompassed in the causes of primary and secondary autonomic failure in Sir Roger Bannister's comprehensive classification.[136] Irwin Schatz[137] has classified it as "orthostatic hypotension due to organic derangements." The monographs of Bannister, Schatz, and Low[136-138] contain excellent in-depth coverage of autonomic failure and OH. OH, the cardinal feature of autonomic failure (AF), has been defined by various criteria of blood pressure change. A drop on standing (within a maximum of 10 minutes) of systolic blood pressure of 25 mmHg or more and diastolic pressure 10 mmHg or more is considered diagnostic by Schatz.[137] It is important to characterize OH clinically by the fall in upright blood pressure that results in symptoms due to inadequate cerebral perfusion (light-headedness, blurring of vision, pain in the back of the neck, and finally transient loss of consciousness that recovers on assuming the supine position). Chronic OH is accompanied by a change in cerebrovascular autoregulation that enables many patients to stand without symptoms of cerebral hypoperfusion with a systolic blood pressure of 60, whereas most normal subjects require no less than 80 mmHg. Time to appearance of symptoms is an important marker of severity of OH, which also helps in assessing the effect of therapy. It may be necessary to measure BP on arising in the morning or after meals to document the diagnosis. Evaluation of the heart rate response is very important, since patients with neurogenic or structural OH display minimal or no increase in heart rate. David Streeten,[139] in his monograph on orthostatic disorders of the circulation, defined the following normal ranges of orthostatic change from the study of 92 healthy subjects of both sexes, aged 17 to 61 years:

Systolic blood pressure	-19 to $+11$ mmHg
Diastolic blood pressure	-9 to $+22$ mmHg
Pulse pressure	-27 to $+6$ mmHg
Heart rate	-6 to $+27$ bpm

Tests of autonomic function, described above, may impart a better understanding of the pathologic process, its natural course and prognosis. Although precise anatomic localization may not be possible, the portion of the reflex arc that is impaired may often be identified by judicious use of autonomic function testing combined with knowledge of relevant clinical data. In the absence of a specialized laboratory for autonomic function testing, the clinician can verify autonomic failure by some simple bedside tests. The presence of sinus arrhythmia (described in the section on Testing) is an indication of adequate parasympathetic innervation to the heart and is usu-

ally absent in patients with true AF. Heart rate is monitored with an electrocardiogram while the patient takes six deep breaths per minute. The fastest heart rate during each inspiratory phase is divided by the slowest heart rate during each expiratory phase. A mean ratio of 1.2 or more is normal. Heart rate response to the Valsalva maneuver can be measured with an ECG. Heart rate normally increases as the patient strains (reflex tachycardia due to reduction in blood pressure) and decreases immediately following the maneuver (reflex bradycardia due to blood pressure overshoot). A ratio between the highest heart rate during strain and the lowest rate after release of 1.4 or more is considered normal. An increase of blood pressure of 15 mmHg or more after 3 minutes of sustained handgrip is normal. This response is absent in AF with sympathetic efferent deficiency. A careful medical evaluation should allow the exclusion of aggravating factors (diuretics, vasodilators, tricyclic antidepressants) and causes of secondary AF, especially diabetic or alcoholic neuropathy and paraneoplastic neuropathy (especially bronchogenic carcinoma). As therapies become increasingly diversified, the precise knowledge of the autonomic dysfunction may play an ever increasing role in the choice of treatment.

There is a wide spectrum of neurogenic causes of OH. Bannister distinguishes (1) primary autonomic failure due to disease processes with well-defined involvement of a limited number of structural elements [pure autonomic failure (PAF), AF with multiple system atrophy (MSA), and AF with Parkinson's disease]; (2) secondary AF, in which involvement of the nervous system is part of a more general process (general medical disorders, autoimmune diseases, metabolic diseases, hereditary disorders, CNS infections, CNS lesions, neurotransmitter defects and aging); and (3) drug-induced AF (tranquilizers, antidepressants, vasodilators, adrenergic blocking agents, angiotensin-converting enzyme inhibitors.[90,129,136] Schatz classified the neurogenic causes of OH according to the anatomic site of the principal defect into (1) afferent lesions (diabetic neuropathy, alcoholic neuropathy, tabes dorsalis, Holmes-Adie syndrome); (2) central disorders (idiopathic parkinsonism, familial dysautonomia—Riley-Day syndrome—parasellar and posterior fossa tumors, posterior fossa surgery, multiple cerebral infarcts, and Wernicke's encephalopathy); and (3) efferent defects [pure AF, the Bradbury-Eggleston syndrome (formerly called idiopathic OH), AF with multiple system atrophy (Shy-Drager syndrome)]. Diabetes and chronic alcoholism cause both afferent and efferent lesions.[137]

Most forms of autonomic failure due to chronic neurologic disorders are insidious in onset, with mild symptoms that may be concealed for some time (even years) because of autonomic compensatory mechanisms. Initial symptoms may be vague weakness, postural dizziness, or faintness and may be easily overlooked or misdiagnosed as psychosomatic. The importance of measurement of standing blood pressure cannot be overemphasized. Overt OH and syncope do not go unrecognized. Some patients first complain of bladder dysfunction, impotence, or bowel dysfunction. Symptoms of OH are strikingly worse in the early morning, after meals, in hot weather, or after exercise or ingestion of alcohol, all of which cause redistribution of blood volume (vasodilatation). Supine hypertension is frequent (loss of baroreflex control). Partial or complete loss of thermoregulatory sweating is very frequent. Involuntary inspiratory gasps or "cluster breathing," probably of central origin, may become associated with sleep apnea and respiratory arrest.[140,141]

PAF is characterized by features of denervation-hypersensitivity to direct-acting catecholamines, decreased response to tyramine, low peripheral catecholamine stores, and increased α-adrenergic receptor density. The pathologic lesion consists of marked cell loss in the intermediolateral columns, the site of sympathetic preganglionic cell bodies. AF with MSA is a more diffuse pathologic process with degeneration in locus ceruleus, nucleus tractus solitarius, and preganglionic vagal neurones. Olivopontocerebellar atrophy and degeneration of corticobulbar, extrapyramidal, and cerebellar tracts may also exist.[142] Polinsky[143] has recently reviewed his extensive experience in neurotransmitter and neuropeptide function in AF. Patients with MSA generally have normal or slightly elevated recumbent norepinephrine levels. In patients with PAF, levels are lower than normal, with the exception of the patients reported by Esler et al.[117] with decreased clearance of norepinephrine. No significant increase in plasma norepinephrine concentration is observed after standing for 5 to 10 minutes in patients with PAF or MSA, whereas in patients with hypovolemic hyperreactive OH, the increase is normal or exaggerated. There is virtual absence of norepinephrine in plasma, urine, and cerebrospinal fluid in the congenital deficiency of dopamine-β-hydroxylase, which leads to absence of norepinephrine in noradrenergic nerve terminals. This causes isolated sympathetic noradrenergic failure with OH, with normal sympathetic cholinergic function (preserved sweating) and normal parasympathetic function.[10]

In addition to the alteration of autonomic control of the circulation, studies have shown that patients with AF have inadequate conservation of sodium during low sodium intake. This has serious consequences, as inadequate venous return in the upright posture plays such a key role in the pathophysiology of AF. Supine hypertension probably contributes to nocturnal diuresis (pressure diuresis). Nocturnal loss of intravascular and interstitial fluid leads to relative hypovolemia that worsens OH in the morning.[144,147] The abnormalities of sodium and water homeostasis in AF are complex.[149] They are probably partly due to decreased adrenergic activity in the kidney (decreased renal vasoconstriction and decreased activation of the renin-angiotensin system), as sympathetic nerve stimulation promotes reabsorption of sodium. Besides, significantly increased levels of atrial natriuretic factor have been documented in patients with AF, especially when supine.[150]

Therapy for Chronic OH of the "Normovolemic" Hyporeactive Type. Comprehensive approaches to treatment have been formulated in several recent reviews.[137,144–148]

General Recommendations. Trivial stresses can produce symptomatic hypotension, including straining during micturition or defecation, isometric exercises in general, exposure to a warm environment, and having an ordinary meal (carbohydrates are more likely to induce hypotension than fats or protein, perhaps via release of insulin and vasodilator gastrointestinal hormones). Caffeine can minimize postprandial hypotension,[151] so coffee has been recommended with meals, particularly with breakfast.[147] Vasoactive drugs should be avoided (even cold preparations and diet pills) because of the exaggerated response to dilators and constrictors (risk of hypertension due to denervation hypersensitivity). Salt intake should be liberal. Exercise should be encouraged as tolerated, especially swimming with appropriate precautions and walking submerged to above-the-waist level, which can minimize blood pooling (exiting the water must be done very carefully). Nocturnal diuresis and volume loss, described above, must be reduced by elevating the head of the bed with 6- to 9-inch blocks to approximately 5 to 20°. This head-up tilt improves the early morning accentuation of orthostatic symptoms and may even increase circulating volume enough to lead to significant improvement of blood pressure during the day. In addition, it plays an important role in avoiding nocturnal (supine) hypertension. External support in the form of a custom-fitted elastic support garment (which must be waist-high to avoid pooling in the lower abdomen as well as the legs) is quite effective in many patients, but not comfortable to wear. We have had success with less cumbersome thigh-high elastic stockings plus a well-fitted elastic abdominal girdle. Elastic supports should not be worn in the supine position.

Pharmacologic Approaches. The review articles cited[144–148] contain detailed tables of the numerous agents that have been used. Unfortunately, by the very nature of these diseases, many agents have only been used in small groups of patients. Fluorohydrocortisone (fludrocortisone acetate) is the most widely used pharmacologic agent. Its multiple actions include plasma volume expansion (substituting for the diminished aldosterone) and sensitization of vascular receptors to pressor amines, perhaps by increasing the number of adrenergic receptors. The vascular effects help in understanding the benefit in patients who have only small increases in blood volume.[152–154] This drug, as all others for patients with AF, should be started in very small doses (e.g., 0.1 mg/day). Divided doses, morning and evening, may provide smoother blood pressure control. The dose can be slowly increased to 0.4 mg/day (very rarely 0.8 mg) with careful monitoring for supine hypertension and hypokalemia. Potassium supplements may sometimes be required. Dihydroergotamine is a direct acting α-adrenergic agonist that may preferentially cause venoconstriction, which has been used in patients who do not have coronary or peripheral vascular disease. It has poor bioavailability when given by mouth but may be effective by inhalation (0.36 mg). Ergotamine tartrate (2 to 6 mg/day) has been used successfully in very small series of patients. Small doses of short-acting sympathomimetics such as phenylpropanolamine (12.5 mg), immediately prior to activity, have also been advocated.[147] The new α-receptor agonist midodrine was reported to be of considerable benefit in five patients with PAF or MSA.[155] Studies are now in progress to evaluate this agent in a large cohort of patients. Special precautions are required to avoid supine hypertension. It appears that with proper dosing it may provide significant help, even in very incapacitated patients.[156] The value of inhibitors of prostaglandin synthesis in AF is still unclear, despite some enthusiastic reports. Indomethacin, 50 mg t.i.d., has occasionally been helpful, but sustained benefit seems rare. Finally, a word of caution: even minute doses of nitrates or furosemide may precipitate severe hypotensive episodes. β-Agonists, such as those used in the treatment of asthma, may induce hypotension, as patients with neurogenic OH are more sensitive to β-receptor stimulation (vasodilatation).[13]

Hyperreactive Hypovolemic Orthostatic Hypotension

Hyperreactive hypovolemic OH is due to autonomic dysregulation produced by abnormal patterns of activation or modulation of circulatory reflexes, without structural or organic derangements of the ANS. Schatz[137] has classified it as "orthostatic hypotension due to functional derangements." We will confine the discussion to "chronic hyperreactive hypovolemic OH," excluding OH due to acute reduction of circulating volume (hemorrhage, dehydration, burns, etc.), impairment of reflex adjustments due to expected effects of pharmacologic agents, adrenal insufficiency, and electrolyte derangements. All these conditions must be ruled out by careful evaluation of the patient before OH can be attributed to functional autonomic dysregulation. In chronic hyperreactive "hypovolemic" OH, the hypovolemia may represent actual decrease of intravascular volume or a reduction of "effective circulating volume," due to excessive pooling of blood within the capacitance vessels in the upright posture that induces appropriately excessive physiologic responses. Streeten[139] has termed these the "venous pooling syndromes" that may result from abnormal regulation of venous function or from the effect of a circulating vasodilator (bradykinin, histamine, prostaglandins). Patients with hyperreactive OH characteristically have an exaggerated increase in heart rate that accompanies the drop of upright blood pressure, as opposed to the deficient heart rate response seen in patients with neurogenic or hyporeactive OH. This is often a clue to the clinician. The venous pooling syndromes are characterized by orthostatic diastolic hypertension, orthostatic systolic hypotension, orthostatic narrowing of pulse pressure, and orthostatic tachycardia. At the Uihlein Autonomic Research Laboratory of the University of Alabama (UAB), we have identified an interesting subset of patients in the group of 25 percent of the patients with mitral valve prolapse syndrome (the combination of mitral valve prolapse diagnosed by strict criteria and symptomatic autonomic dysfunction); these patients have orthostatic intolerance and do not have the expected orthostatic tachycardia. They have minimal increases in heart rate during head-up tilt and marked oscillation of their heart rate throughout the test. The inadequate response is not likely to be due to faulty sensing by cardiopulmonary receptors, because on returning to the horizontal position they respond to the central translocation of blood volume with an inappropriately exaggerated bradycardia. Tests of sympathetic function independent of the baroreceptor mechanism, such as the "echo-stress test" (see section on Heart Rate Studies, p. 301), show normal sympathetic responsiveness.[67] Our data suggest that these patients have abnormal parasympathetic regulation. During the Valsalva maneuver, the vagally mediated bradycardia response to the blood pressure overshoot following release is normal or exaggerated, but it persists long after the blood pressure has returned to baseline.

Several conditions may produce abnormal response to gravitational forces (orthostatic intolerance) and, potentially, hyperreactive OH. We will review the most clinically relevant. There is an excellent recent review by Gunnar Blomqvist.[129] Aging and "excessive physical conditioning," although not classic for hyperreactive OH, deserve special mention as examples of orthostatic intolerance due to autonomic dysregulation without structural diseases that can certainly cause OH.

Aging. Cardiovascular control mechanisms are less efficient even in generally healthy older persons. Changes in arterial blood pressure produce a smaller heart rate response, suggesting a blunting of the arterial baroreflex response.[157] This may be due to decreased distensibility of the arterial wall of the baroreceptor site.[158] Heart rate variability and respiratory sinus arrhythmia decrease with age. Changes in catecholamines, nerve traffic, and adrenoreceptors have been

discussed on p. 295). Orthostatic hypotension is more prevalent in the elderly population. An orthostatic fall of systolic blood pressure of more than 20 mmHg was found in 17 percent and more than 40 mmHg in 5 percent of 100 patients in a geriatric hospital.[159] Caird and associates[160] studied 496 ambulatory men and women aged 65 and older and found a decrease in upright systolic blood pressure of 20 mmHg or more in 24 percent and 30 mmHg or more in 9 percent. Subjects whose blood pressure dropped usually had a combination of causes such as hypovolemia, effect of drugs that impair autonomic control (levodopa, phenothiazines, tricyclic antidepressants, vasodilators), varicose veins, or structural neurologic lesions. Orthostatic hypotension becomes symptomatic in the elderly subjects with failure of cerebral autoregulation.[161] Less than 10 percent of the population in Caird's study had organic brain syndrome. Prompt correction of hypovolemia and infection, elastic support stockings to avoid pooling in varicose veins, moderate dynamic exercise (walking), efforts to maintain or build muscle tone and mass, avoidance of prolonged recumbency, and 10- to 20-degree elevation of the head of the bed (to avoid deactivation of postural reflexes and decline of blood volume) when recumbency is necessary all help avoid OH. Postprandial hypotension has been documented in the elderly without evidence of autonomic neuropathy.[4] Avoidance of large meals, especially those rich in carbohydrates, is advisable. We have occasionally required small doses of fludrocortisone with careful monitoring of blood pressure and serum potassium.

Excessive Physical Conditioning. Most, but not all investigators, have reported fitness-related differences in orthostatic tolerance.[162] Fit persons have been shown to have attenuated heart rate and vasoconstrictor responses to orthostatic stress.[163] Blomqvist[129] has emphasized the importance of mechanisms related to ventricular diastolic mechanics (pressure-volume curve), and has suggested that this may explain why the very fit and the unfit tend to have orthostatic intolerance, which is absent in the midrange of fitness. This has great importance in aviation and space medicine, particularly with the high G-forces imposed by modern high-performance military aircraft. Healthy fighter pilots who develop excessive parasympathetic responsiveness from exaggerated running programs develop decreased acceleration tolerance (J. E. Whinnery, personal communication), similar to that of pilots with mitral valve prolapse in an otherwise totally healthy condition.[164] Exaggerated vagal tone has caused marked bradycardia as well as first- and second-degree heart block (Mobitz I) in excessively conditioned subjects. All these effects are reversed by decreasing the level of exercise training.

Conditions Associated with more Classic Hyperreactive Orthostatic Hypotension

Prolonged Bed Rest and Related Conditions. Prolonged bed rest is a common cause of orthostatic intolerance due to a hypovolemic (generally 300- to 500-ml decline) hyperreactive cardiovascular regulation. It has generally been attributed to prolonged physical inactivity, but considerable evidence now suggests that abnormalities occur rather rapidly as a result of redistribution of body fluids, which resembles that occurring in the microgravity environment of space flight.[104] The degree of cardiovascular dysfunction is similar after a 3-week bed rest period and after 20 hours of −5-degree head-down tilt.[165] In addition to a change in reflex regulation, there is a significant inhibition of vasopressin, renin, and aldosterone. A negative fluid balance

is established within hours of initiation of head-down tilt. Blood volume loss during bed rest can be prevented by administration of fludrocortisone, but this does not totally restore normal hemodynamics.[104] Blomqvist and Stone[104] have pointed out that once the hemodynamics of subjects adapted to bed rest (or head-down tilt) becomes similar to the upright pattern, the subject loses the capacity to deal with the fluid shift that occurs during the change from supine to upright position. The development of orthostatic intolerance from supine bed rest is prevented by periods of sitting or standing, but not by exercise in the supine position. Research on the preventive effects of periods of moderate lower body negative pressure is being carried out in space flights.

Mitral Valve Prolapse with Symptomatic Autonomic Dysfunction. A subset of patients with carefully proven mitral valve prolapse have faulty control of their circulation,[166–168] similar in many ways to the abnormalities documented in earlier studies of "neurocirculatory asthenia," which Starr attributed, with keen wit, to "clumsiness of the circulation."[169] Clumsiness, in the sense of lack of precise and physiologically appropriate control, is a prominent feature of subjects with or without mitral valve prolapse and symptomatic autonomic dysfunction or dysautonomia (Fig. 10-3). The combined experience of several investigators has been reviewed in detail.[170] Some patients with mitral valve prolapse have either markedly attenuated[167] or exaggerated vagally mediated cardiovascular responses to common stimuli.[166] It has been suggested that many patients have a primary hyperadrenergic state.[171] Most of Gaffney et al.'s[167] patients had normal supine catecholamines and response to isoproterenol infusion. In a subset of 200 patients from a cohort of 2,000 totally similar patients, we only found purely

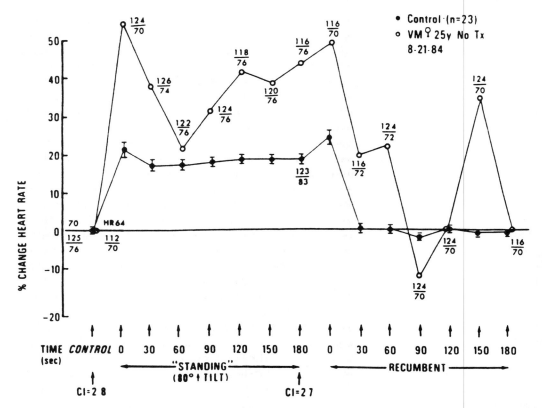

Fig. 10-3. Comparison between the blood pressure and heart rate response during head-up tilt in 23 healthy controls (closed circles) and in a patient with autonomic dysfunction (open circles). The extremely variable circulatory regulation in autonomic dysfunction is evident and represents what Starr[172] termed "clumsy circulation." (From Coghlan,[67] with permission.)

hyperadrenergic cardiovascular responses (to a battery of autonomic reflex tests) in 10 percent.[67] Reduced total blood volume[170] and abnormal reduction of left ventricular filling in the upright posture both at rest and during exercise[67] has been documented and plays a key role in orthostatic intolerance, poor exercise performance, and effort tolerance.[172–174] The exact contribution of abnormal venous return and reduced blood volume is undefined. Our experience suggests that abnormal upright venous pooling plays an important role in the exaggerated standing tachycardia and effort intolerance and fatigue of many patients

who are symptomatic due to dysautonomia. Some of these patients clearly resemble those with the "venous pooling syndrome" described by Streeten et al.[135] with excessive orthostatic tachycardia, intolerance of diuretic therapy, and bluish discoloration of the legs when standing (without visible varicose veins or signs of venous insufficiency). They may have a supine blood pressure of 90/64 mmHg and heart rate of 65 bpm and standing blood pressure of 157/118 with a heart rate of 159.

Orthostatic hypotension was present in 25 percent of our 200 symptomatic mitral valve prolapse patients,[67] in 17 percent of

Weissman et al.'s[175] series, and was frequent in the patients described by Santos et al.[176] Gaffney and associates[174] have identified patients who have hypovolemia and a true α-adrenergic hyperreactivity in the upright posture, such that their daily activity with sitting, standing, and walking produces a chronic hyperadrenergic state, reminiscent of patients with pheochromocytoma, in whom excessive catecholamines cause a volume-contracted state. They postulate a vicious cycle in which hypovolemia and reduction in left ventricular end-diastolic volume cause further reduction in forward stroke volume during upright rest and exercise, and mediate a further increase in catecholamine release, which enhances the chronic vasoconstriction and leads to further decrease in blood volume.[170] Pasternac et al.[177] have measured blood volume, atrial natriuretic factor (ANF), and plasma norepinephrine and epinephrine in 16 patients. The seven patients with elevated ANF values had significantly lower blood volume and higher standing plasma norepinephrine concentrations than the patients with normal ANF values. Hypovolemia has also been found in patients with severe chronic stress directly related to serious somatic disease. Such patients have been described as having "the missing blood syndrome."[178] Fouad et al.[179] described 11 patients with orthostatic intolerance and an average reduction in blood volume of -27 percent, with no evidence of pheochromocytoma or hypoaldosteronism, a condition they termed idiopathic hypovolemia.

Therapy. Reassurance is fundamental. Orthostatic hypotension causes great anxiety, which magnifies the adrenergic responses (central "modulation of reflexes" resembling the fight-flight pattern) and enhances tachycardia, which causes further fear of serious disease. These patients often have very low exercise capacity and may derive little benefit from attempted physical training until therapy improves the abnormal cardiovascular regulation. We have used small doses of clonidine, as well as small doses of diltiazem, which have vasodilator effects (but not as exaggerated as nifedipine) quite successfully for years in the treatment of patients with excessive vasoconstriction and adrenergic responses. Gaffney et al.[180] used this centrally acting α-agonist with secondary peripheral adrenergic activity at our suggestion; they performed a thorough study demonstrating that clonidine, titrated very slowly, starting at 50 μg at bedtime and gradually increasing to doses as high (in some patients) as 0.4 mg/day or to side effects, improved symptoms and orthostatic tolerance and caused a 12 percent expansion of plasma volume.[170,180] We have also frequently combined small doses of fludrocortisone (100 μg q A.M. or 50 μg b.i.d.) to help restore blood volume and enhance vascular response to norepinephrine,[153,154] which may reduce the requirement for sympathetic efferent activation for a given degree of required "compensatory vasoconstriction." We avoid sodium restriction but we feel that increased salt and fluid intake per se are not particularly beneficial. We encourage very gradual exercise conditioning, beginning with supine exercises to enhance muscle tone in very symptomatic patients, followed by swimming (with a life vest to allay fear of weakness or syncope and enhance safety), because it allows physical conditioning without the added orthostatic stress. As soon as feasible, a balanced program designed to improve aerobic fitness and skeletal muscle strength (and mass) is implemented. Patients with severe "venous pooling syndrome" very often benefit from long elastic support hose plus a well-fitted elastic abdominal girdle.

Syncope of Uncertain or Unexplained Etiology

Consciousness is maintained by a complex interplay between multiple biologic mechanisms including autonomic neural controls, central global neurologic function, cardiac factors, and peripheral hemodynamic adjustments. Syncope, defined as a sudden and transient loss of consciousness with loss of postural tone, which subsides spontaneously and without localizing neurologic deficit, is a prevalent, potentially dangerous condition of vast psychosocial impact. Failure of one or more of the controlling mechanisms mentioned above may lead to transient global cerebral hypoperfusion, frequently the final common pathophysiologic pathway of syncope. The evaluation of recurrent syncope, no doubt one of the most dramatic cardiovascular symptoms, is frequently enormously expensive and unfortunately may fail to produce a clear etiologic diagnosis in over 40 percent of patients.[181–183] Up to 60 percent of patients continue to have symptoms at 1 year,[184] and over 50 percent of patients may have injured themselves by the time they seek medical advice.[185] Syncope accounts for 1 to 6 percent of medical admissions and 3 percent of emergency room visits.[186,187] In the prolonged follow-up of the Framingham population (aged 30 to 62 years at entry), 3 percent of men and 3.5 percent of women experienced syncope.[188] One-year mortality in unexplained syncope is 6 percent, lower than the 30 percent for proven cardiovascular causes.[182]

We will confine the discussion to recurrent syncope of unexplained origin, excluding syncope that results from easily demonstrable orthostatic hypotension (see preceding section) and the multiple important causes of cardiac syncope and other etiologies that are readily identified

by a thorough medical, cardiologic, and neurologic evaluation. A large number of studies during this last decade have revealed that abnormal cardiovascular performance due to autonomic dysfunction or dysregulation is a frequent and identifiable cause of syncope of undetermined etiology, and one that can be treated with considerable success, following appropriate study of the pathophysiology with relatively simple "provocative tests." The diagnostic work-up of syncope unfortunately is a difficult task, due to the complexity of the underlying mechanisms and etiologies, its intermittent nature, and the frequent absence of diagnostic abnormalities during the remission period. This led to the search for provocative tests designed to disclose predisposing abnormalities and reproduce the clinical picture of the reported spontaneous syncope, a prerequisite to the acceptance of a demonstrable abnormal physiology as a plausible cause for the patient's clinical condition. Our discussion will include presyncope—a sensation of loss of strength with the feeling of impending loss of consciousness and generally with blurring of vision—as a lesser degree of the same problem, because the pathophysiology is entirely similar (Fig. 10-4).

The study of the integrity and efficiency of blood pressure-controlling mechanisms in patients with syncope of unknown origin had largely been ignored. In the recent decade, head-up tilt has become established as a useful diagnostic test in adults[185,189–200] as well as children and adolescents.[201] Manual or electrically driven tilt tables with footrests have been used, and different authors have utilized 60-, 70-, or 80-degree upright tilt alone (baseline head-up tilt or HUT-B) or preceded by isoproterenol infusion (HUT-ISO) and lasting 10 to 60 minutes, as a challenge to the reflexes responsible for adaptation to orthostatic

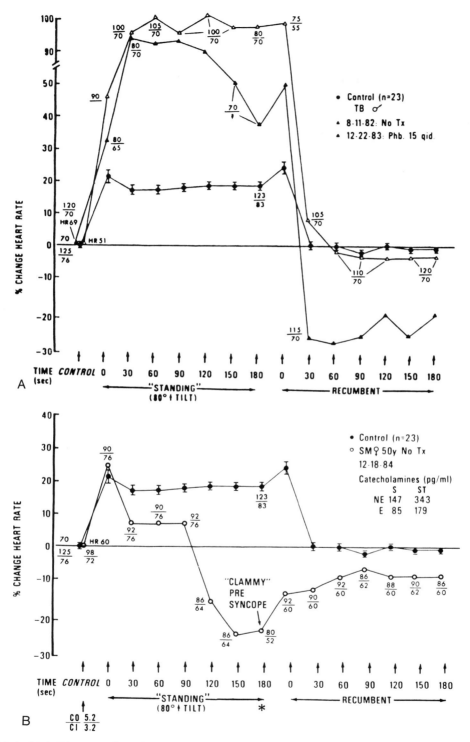

Fig. 10-4. (**A & B**) Examples of the results of head-up tilt as a provocative test for the diagnosis of syncope of undetermined etiology. Both patients had experienced multiple syncopes with a "negative evaluation." The abnormal autonomic responses caused presyncope during a short 80-degree head-up tilt, at which point the patients were returned to the horizontal position. The normal response of heart rate and blood pressure is represented by the closed circles. Most patients require more prolonged tilt tests to reproduce their clinical picture (see text). (Fig. A from Coghlan,[67] with permission.)

stress. In one study of pediatric patients, quiet motionless standing replaced passive tilt.[202] The day-to-day reproducibility of the test for eliciting susceptibility to "neurally mediated syncope" is 71 to 80 percent.[195,196,198,199,203] Janosik et al.[204] reported that a 20-minute tilt at 80 degrees even with isoproterenol titrated to increase heart rate 25 percent above resting heart rate failed to reproduce syncope in a 30-year-old patient with recurrent syncope, whereas 52 minutes of passive tilt without isoproterenol reproduced his clinical syncope. She warned that studies using a short duration of tilt could seriously underestimate the number of positive tests. A duration of 60-degree tilt of at least 45 minutes has been suggested to reduce the possibility of false-negative results.[198] Almquist et al.[191] provoked syncope in only 27 percent of patients with 10 minutes of 80-degree HUT. Infusion of 1 to 5 μg/min of isoproterenol during 80-degree HUT increased the percentage of positive tests to 87 percent, suggesting an important synergistic effect of gravity-induced hypovolemia and drug-enhanced contractility in initiating neurally mediated syncope.[191] Several studies have shown a low prevalence of positive tests (0 to 11 percent) in small groups of normal controls. Kapoor and Brant,[200] after studying 40 controls matched by age and sex with their patient group, have warned that the test with isoproterenol may not be quite specific, as they found 31 percent positive responses in controls.

Abi-Samra et al.[190] completed a study with 60 percent HUT of 20-minute duration in 151 patients (mean age, 56 years) with syncope of unknown origin. Assessment of blood volume and gravitational volume shift (change of cardiopulmonary volume measured by nuclear medicine techniques) and additional autonomic testing were performed. Sixty-three patients (42 percent) developed syncope, 53 patients (35 percent) had normal responses to HUT, and 35 patients (23 percent) had an abnormal blood pressure, heart rate, or volume distribution response (20 percent decrease in cardiopulmonary volume during HUT, the normal being 8 to 10 percent), but did not develop syncope. None of the 15 healthy controls developed syncope. One of the 63 patients who developed syncope had a separate cause (pacemaker syndrome). Eight patients (12.5 percent) manifested a pattern of autonomic dysfunction characterized by prompt, persistent, and progressive decrease first in diastolic and then in systolic blood pressure after HUT, with minimal or no change in heart rate. Forty patients (64 percent) had vasovagal syncope, defined as syncope associated with sudden marked decrease in blood pressure and heart rate, 14 patients (22 percent) had vasodepressor syncope, characterized as syncope associated with sudden marked decrease in blood pressure without a change in heart rate. Other authors have described vasovagal syncope as one entity (sudden hypotension-bradycardia after an initial period of normal circulatory adjustment to HUT) with three profiles: vasodepression, cardioinhibition, and mixed, depending on the degree of bradycardia.[205,206] These same authors have added a third type to the dysautonomic and vasovagal responses to HUT—the psychosomatic response characterized as syncope with no alteration of vital signs and accompanied by a rising level of plasma norepinephrine during the course of symptoms.[205]

Of the 35 patients in the very important study of Abi-Samra et al.[190] who had abnormal response to HUT but no syncope, 8 (23 percent) had absent chronotropic response (an increase of 3 bpm or less over baseline), and 25 (71 percent) had an exaggerated chronotropic response (an increase of 30 percent or $\geq$ 20 bpm over baseline heart rate). These percentages bear a striking resemblance to the distribution of autonomic subsets in our study of dysautonomic patients[67]: 33 percent cardioinhibitory or hypervagal and 64 percent hyperadrenergic or mixed responsiveness. It is noteworthy that 15 of 19 patients with exaggerated chronotropic response to HUT had hypovolemia or marked venous pooling. In the 40 patients with vasovagal syncope, hypotension preceded bradycardia in 85 percent of patients and occurred simultaneously in 13 percent. Only one patient had bradycardia before hypotension. Nine of the 40 patients with vasovagal syncope demonstrated severe bradycardia, with sinus arrest in 7 (5 to 73 seconds) and transient high-grade AV block in 2. This subset represents what has been termed by Maloney et al.[207] the malignant vasovagal syndrome. The clinical presentation is one of sudden complete loss of consciousness that occurs without warning. Patients with this syndrome tend to have more frequent episodes than patients who do not respond with asystole of more than 4 seconds to HUT. They frequently sustain bodily injury, which is distinctly rare in patients who do not develop asystole. During HUT their periods of asystole also occur with little or no prodromata.[208]

It is interesting that vagal inhibition of the heart as the primary cause of syncope was postulated by Foster in 1888.[209] Sir Thomas Lewis[210] introduced the term "vasovagal" after his astute observations documenting that the main cause of the fall in blood pressure was vasodilatation rather than bradycardia. Elegant studies by Epstein et al.[211] using 80-degree HUT-B revealed two phases in the typical vasovagal syncope: phase I, a gradual decline in arterial pressure without significant change in forearm vascular resistance and of highly variable duration; and phase II, characterized by an abrupt fall in arterial pressure (a fall of mean ar-

terial pressure from 74 to 34 mmHg) and heart rate (from an average of 84 to 47 bpm), and an average fall in forearm vascular resistance of 62 percent. The authors emphasized that these circulatory changes were "obtained only during syncopal reactions precipitated by the orthostatic position, by lower body negative pressure, venesection or applications of tourniquets to the thighs, all of which lead to decrease in effective circulatory volume." They also postulated that syncope induced by fear, emotional stimuli, pain, and other forms of psychic trauma might have somewhat different circulatory changes.

Goldstein et al. studied vasodepressor syncope precipitated by threatening situations in which neither "fight [n]or flight is possible; they showed that the severe hypotension was unresponsive to cardiac pacing or atropine but improved immediately with assumption of the supine posture, suggesting that pooling of blood in the lower body caused a reduction of effective circulating volume. They presented evidence in support of significant decrease of total peripheral resistance. Furthermore, they showed that the same painful stimulus did not cause syncope if applied while the patient was being distracted. This led them to the hypothesis that the vasodepressor syncope resulted from a "coordinated pattern of central nervous origin, in response to the threatening situation, resembling the 'playing dead' reaction." Interestingly, such vasovagal syncopes may occur in the supine position,[213] which further supports a possible central origin.[4]

Recent studies of vasovagal syncope induced by HUT using continuous noninvasive assessment of cardiac output and stroke volume by impedance cardiography[205] have confirmed the observations of Epstein et al.[211] Phase I, slowly falling blood pressure, coincides with a fall in stroke volume and cardiac outp along with rising heart rate and maintenance of mean arterial blood pressure. In phase II, diastolic and mean arterial blood pressure fall rapidly along with a marked drop in total peripheral resistance and an even greater fall in forearm vascular resistance. Plasma norepinephrine increases 100 percent preceding syncope but falls 30 percent at the onset of syncope, along with an increase of epinephrine of 827 ± 154 percent from baseline. The normal reflex adjustments to orthostatic stress were discussed on page 302. During vasovagal or vasodepressor syncope the cutaneous circulation is usually vasoconstricted, but the marked dilatation in skeletal muscle causes the marked reduction in systemic resistance. Paradoxic vasodilatation and bradycardia also occur in severe hemorrhagic shock in subjects with normal circulatory reflexes. Data obtained by direct recording of peroneal sympathetic outflow to skeletal muscle (using tungsten microelectrodes) during syncope induced by standing or by nitroprusside infusion showed an increase in traffic prior to syncope and an abrupt interruption of sympathetic outflow 20 seconds after the onset of blood pressure decrease. The recovery of nerve traffic after syncope was slow.[9,214]

Blomqvist[129] has reviewed the most likely mechanism of the circulatory changes of vasovagal syncope. He feels that conflicting inputs from arterial and cardiopulmonary baroreceptors play a key role. Cardiac receptors with nonmyelinated (C-fiber) vagal afferents are inhibitory and form the afferent limb of the Bezold-Jarisch reflex. Some receptors respond to chemical stimuli and some to mechanical (deformation) stimuli. Stimulation of this reflex increases parasympathetic activity and inhibits sympathetic activity, producing bradycardia, vasodilatation, and hypotension.[76] These left ventricular receptors, preferentially distrib-

uted in the inferoposterior wall of the left ventricle, are normally activated by increased intracavitary pressure, volume, or both (increased wall stress). A progressive reduction in ventricular volume occurs during the presyncopal stage. Echocardiographic studies have demonstrated gradually decreasing left ventricular volumes with increasing degrees of peripheral venous pooling.[215,216] The left ventricular endocardial receptors eventually become activated by direct compression of the small ventricle with vigorous contraction due to sympathetic stimulation resulting from unloading of arterial and atrial baroreceptors with declining venous return. The salient stimulus is deformation, but the sensing system "cannot differentiate" between compression associated with low volume in addition to pressure from enhanced contraction and distension caused by high ventricular pressure or volume.[129] Activation of ventricular deformation receptors by high ventricular transmural pressure or direct contact is likely to cause syncope in aortic stenosis and hypertrophic cardiomyopathy and cavity obliteration with or without outflow obstruction.[76]

Calkins et al.[217] suggested that a hypercontractile ventricle with a small end-systolic volume might stimulate receptor discharge by inducing intraventricular pressure gradients. The importance of the combined effect of reduced volume and adrenergically mediated hypercontractility in orthostatic intolerance, such as is documented by HUT studies, is supported by research showing a clear improvement in orthostatic tolerance in subjects deconditioned by bed rest with β-blocker therapy.[218] We suspect that enhanced sympathetic discharge coupled with gravitational stress may cause syncope in occasional patients with dysautonomic response to HUT who do not manifest syncope on tilt-testing, but who have spontaneous episodes proved not to be arrhythmic. The likely mechanism of this pathophysiology, which mimics that of vasovagal syncope, could be a sudden adrenergic discharge due to what Penfield[219] described as diencephalic autonomic epilepsy in a patient who proved to have a localized tumor. Subsequent reports on such patients have documented paroxysmal catecholamine release described as mimicking pheochromocytoma, which was carefully ruled out.[220,221] Our patients presented with syncope of threateningly sudden onset, without prodromata, always in an upright or sitting position for a certain period of time. They had no orthostatic symptoms at other times and no orthostatic hypotension on HUT. Syncope was suppressed and has remained so for years either by carbamazepine (interestingly, only after reaching a therapeutic level), by clonidine (which similarly has been shown to control this autonomic epilepsy[221]), or by clonazepam alone or combined with clonidine in small doses (50 μg b.i.d. or t.i.d.). We have only managed to document seizure activity by repeated studies with nasopharyngeal leads in one of our patients.

The unstable circulatory control immediately preceding syncope induced by HUT manifests by increased oscillation of subcutaneous microvascular blood flow, monitored by laser-Doppler flowmetry.[68] Continuous monitoring of blood flow velocity in the middle cerebral artery by transcranial Doppler during vasovagal syncope produced by HUT showed a 75 percent decrease in diastolic velocity and 73 $\pm$ 34 percent increase in resistance index, concomitant with the development of hypotension and bradycardia. Patients who did not develop syncope as well as control subjects had no significant alteration in cerebral flow pattern.[222] Subsequent tilt-table tests in the 20 initially positive patients, after pharmacologic therapy successfully prevented syncope, showed normal cranial flow pattern.

The marked reduction in cerebral blood flow during syncope may occasionally cause myoclonic jerks, tonic spasm, and even sphincter incontinence, making the differential diagnosis with epilepsy difficult.[4] The circumstances of the "attacks," a history of visual blackout, and the observation of a pale, ashen or white face at the time of loss of consciousness may suggest a diagnosis of syncope.[223] Electroencephalograms (EEGs) recorded during syncope induced by ocular compression, with asystole lasting more than 8 seconds, have shown bilateral synchronous slow wave activity, during which there may be jerks, followed by electrical silence accompanied by tonic spasm.[224] Clinical differentiation may be difficult, especially as temporal lobe seizures may be accompanied by pallor. Continuous ambulatory simultaneous EEG and ECG recording has been very helpful.[225] Goldstein et al.[212] also reported no epileptiform activity on EEG recorded during vasovagal syncope with asystole, in a patient who had tonic or clonic movements in some of her episodes. Gastaut and Fischer-Williams[224] emphasized that no patients had a rhythmic clonic phase as observed in generalized epileptic seizures.

The third type of response on HUT, the psychosomatic response, characterized by loss of consciousness with no alteration of hemodynamics, also described as psychogenic syncope, has been extensively studied by Linzer and colleagues.[205,206] Two such patients had rising plasma levels of norepinephrine during the symptoms induced by HUT, and three subjects showed no abnormality of simultaneously recorded EEG or of cerebral blood flow assessed by transcranial Doppler during HUT-induced syncope.[205,206] Neurally mediated syncope, conversion reaction, or other as yet undetermined mechanisms have been invoked in these patients, who generally have major depression or anxiety disorder; they can be treated successfully with psychotropic medications after careful diagnostic evaluation to rule out other causes of syncope, (in particular undetected arrhythmias) and a thorough psychiatric evaluation.[206] Like Linzer and associates, we have found continuous ambulatory EEG and ECG monitoring (and patient-activated memory-loop ECG recorders in patients with prodromata) combined with HUT very useful in the study of these patients. Kapoor et al.[226] also emphasized psychiatric illness as a possible cause in a proportion of patients with syncope of undetermined origin.

Treatment of Recurrent Neurally Mediated Syncope

Knowledge of the pathophysiologic mechanisms, although not definitive and all-inclusive, has allowed therapeutic strategies designed to curb the excessive vagal response, moderate the adrenergic response, correct hypovolemia, or decrease venous pooling. These therapies have been reported in several not very extensive series of patients. They had the important feature, however, that therapeutic results were evaluated by ascertaining noninducibility of syncope: the baseline or head-up tilt if necessary was repeated, using the same dose of isoproterenol that caused the diagnostic test to become positive.

Vagolytic Therapy. Scopolamine (transcutaneous patch changed every other day) was administered to 10 patients with vasovagal/vasodepressor syncope, without underlying volume abnormality.[190] Nine of 10 patients remained free of syncope, and 1 had decreased frequency and milder episodes with some warning, for an average of 10 months (4 to 16 months) follow-up. Only two discontinued ther-

apy due to side effects, with recurrence of syncope. Response to HUT was normalized or markedly improved in all. A central modulating effect has also been postulated.[190,207] Propantheline bromide (7.5 to 15 mg t.i.d./q.i.d.), a vagolytic recommended on the basis of electrophysiologic demonstration of excessive vagal tone, was administered to 12 patients. Six experienced no further presyncope or syncope with a follow-up of 3 to 67 months. Three patients continued to have syncope. One required a permanent pacemaker.[227] Benditt et al.[228] reported a beneficial effect of theophylline in patients with recurrent bradycardias. In 3 of 15 patients with syncope on HUT, the test was negative 7 days later after transdermal scopolamine.[197] Milstein et al.[229] have proposed disopyramide (150 mg t.i.d.), with repeat HUT testing (using isoproterenol in some patients) to document its effect. Disopyramide has a potent antichlorinergic and a negative inotropic effect. It may also directly increase peripheral vascular resistance. Nine of Milstein et al.'s 10 patients remained asymptomatic during a follow-up of 20 ± 5 months.

β-Blockers. Almquist et al.[191] suggested the use of β_1-adrenergic blocking drugs to prevent the sympathetically mediated inotropic/chronotropic response that plays an important role in precipitating neurally mediated syncope. Nine of 15 patients with positive HUT became tilt-table negative on metoprolol 50 mg b.i.d. and remained asymptomatic for up to 16 months of follow-up in the series of Grubb et al.[197] Thilenius reported on 12 pediatric patients treated with atenolol (25 to 50 mg/day) as well as 3 patients who were treated with long-acting propranolol (80 mg/day). All except one had no further syncope.[201] Tamboli et al.[230] reported that β-blockers (30 patients) and disopyramide (9 patients) controlled neurocardiogenic syncope in 94 percent of their population followed for 16 ± 5 months.

Volume/Vascular Response Modifying Therapies. Hydrofluorocortisone has been used in the treatment of patients with idiopathic or essential hypovolemia[179] and in patients with neurally mediated syncope. In two patients whose HUT became negative on hydrofluorocortisone (0.1 mg/day), there was no recurrence of syncope in 16 months.[197] Similar good results were reported in two pediatric patients who objected to β-blockers because they wished to remain very active.[201] We have had similar good results in over 20 patients with fluorohydrocortisone, sometimes combined with Donnatal or Robinul for vagolytic effect. Waist-high elastic support or long stockings plus an adjustable abdominal elastic support have also been very beneficial in our experience, alone or as adjuncts to pharmacotherapy. Midodrine is presently being evaluated. Raviele reported on six patients who had no recurrence of syncope for 9 to 16 months on oral etilephrine 15 to 30 mg/day. This α-agonist prevented syncope induced by HUT and had a sustained effect, presumably on blood pooling. One patient had to discontinue the drug and had recurrence of syncope.[196] Malignant vasovagal syndrome[207] with prolonged asystole provoked by HUT poses special problems. Grubb et al.[208] found that 10 of 50 consecutive patients evaluated for recurrent unexplained syncope had ventricular asystole of 4 seconds or more (7 on HUT alone and 3 on HUT-ISO). Four patients became tilt-table negative on metoprolol 50 mg b.i.d., two patients became negative on sustained-release disopiramide 100 mg b.i.d., and four patients required permanent DDD pacemaker implantation. Over a follow-up of 21 ± 6 months, no further syncopal episodes occurred. Maloney et al.[207] felt that patients could be treated with transdermal scopolamine,

but warned that permanent pacing should be considered the prime therapy in severe cases, in which sudden severe hypotension and asystole might have serious effects on ventricular function and vulnerability (lowering the threshold for ventricular fibrillation). Milstein et al.[231] and Engle[232] postulated that severe vasovagal syncope could be a potential mechanism for sudden death in some patients. In fact, 3 of 10 patients of Grubb et al.[208] had received bystander cardiopulmonary resuscitation, and 2 had spontaneous episodes, with asystole of 12 and 22 seconds, while being monitored in the hospital. In two of four patients, AV sequential pacing did not prevent syncope on HUT, but converted the episodes from a sudden dramatic loss of consciousness without warning to a gradual decrease in blood pressure over a 10-minute period, which allowed the patients to take 2 mg sublingual ergotamine tartrate to abort the hypotensive episodes.[208]

Special Forms of Syncope (Abnormal Afferent Signals)

Carotid Sinus Syncope
Middle-aged or elderly patients, usually men, may have an abnormal sensitivity to manual pressure or massage of the carotid sinus area. Carotid sinus syncope, however, is a rare condition (5 to 20 percent only of patients who respond to massage with cardiac asystole ≥3 seconds or a drop of blood pressure to ≥50 mmHg). Sinus node dysfunction and arrhythmias must be ruled out, due to the age and frequent coexistence of coronary or other vascular pathology, as well as local pathology capable of causing compression. Carotid massage is carried out after careful exclusion of carotid disease by examination and ultrasound if indicated. Technique is not standardized, but it has been recommended that duration be limited to 5 seconds, with continuous ECG moni-

toring and resuscitation equipment present, one side at a time. There may be syncope or minor symptoms, such as near fainting, dizziness, light headedness, weakness, and confusion. The cardiovascular response to carotid sinus stimulation may be "cardioinhibitor" (bradycardia or asystole without hypotension), "vasodepressor" (hypotension without cardiac slowing), or "mixed." The pure vasodepressor type is rare (10 to 15 percent). Vagolytic agents are rarely effective or well tolerated due to patient age. Well-documented carotid sinus syncope is best treated with AV sequential permanent pacing. Three recent reviews are recommended.[233-235] Transient increase in nerve traffic from the carotid sinus leading to hypotension and bradycardia may occur following carotid endarterectomy.[236,237] Electroneurograms of human carotid sinus nerve (bipolar silver-silver chloride electrode) showed increased activity. In five of six patients who had decreases of diastolic blood pressure of 30 mmHg or more, blood pressure rose within 5 minutes of application of local anesthetic (lidocaine) to the sinus node area.[237] The hypotension is usually transient and can be controlled with volume and pressors.

Glossopharyngeal Neuralgia

Episodic severe bradycardia and even asystole, as well as hypotension, preceded by paroxysmal unilateral pain and dysesthesia in the territory of the glossopharyngeal nerve (pharynx, tonsillar area, base of the tongue, and ear) may be associated with syncope due to enhanced vagal tone and paroxysmal withdrawal of sympathetic efferent traffic, with profound vasodilatation that requires energetic therapy.[238] It may be precipitated by chewing, swallowing, or coughing. Abnormal stimuli from the sensory territory of the glossopharyngeal nerve may be due to neck tumors or lym-

phoma.[238-241] Occasionally, as in trigeminal neuralgia, no apparent structural lesion is found. Afferent fibers from the trigger zone run in the glossopharyngeal nerve, which also carries the afferent fibers from the carotid sinus. It is thought that a pathologic synapse (ephapse) may develop between these fibers, allowing stimuli to be misdirected to the baroreceptor fibers, which then carry the strong stimulus to the nucleus tractus solitarius and cause the inhibitory response. Atropine reverses the bradycardia, but hypotension persists unless volume and often pressors are administered. We have seen patients with a decrease of systolic blood pressure to 40 mmHg, supine. Wallin et al.[238] documented the abrupt cessation of sympathetic nerve outflow in the peroneal nerve during an episode that occurred while nerve traffic was being recorded. Implantation of a demand pacemaker has not prevented syncope, which is caused by the sympathetic withdrawal. Glossopharyngeal nerve sectioning has been required, in several patients, to control syncope. Carbamazepine has controlled pain and occasionally syncope.[242]

NEUROLOGIC DISORDERS AFFECTING THE HEART AND CIRCULATORY CONTROL

Acute Inflammatory Demyelinating Polyradiculoneuropathy (Guillain-Barré Syndrome)

Autonomic dysfunction is well recognized and accompanies most cases of Guillain-Barré syndrome, causing special problems in patient care during the acute phase, particularly while ventilatory support is being used. The mechanism of autonomic dysfunction is not clearly established, but pathologic studies have demonstrated demyelinating lesions in the glossopharyngeal and vagus nerve, the brain stem, the intermediolateral columns of the spinal cord, the sympathetic ganglia, and the white rami. The severity of the involvement of the ANS does not appear to be related to the degree of motor or sensory disturbance. In many patients, the consequences of involvement of the ANS are not serious, but they may become severe and even life-threatening. Relative tachycardia is universal. OH and hypertension are frequent, difficult to treat, and can complicate the management of patients with respiratory compromise. Death can occur suddenly following unexplained fluctuations in blood pressure, acute profound bradycardia or asystole (presenting spontaneously or induced by bronchial aspiration or mobilization), or cardiac arrhythmias. Autonomic dysfunction may produce pupillary disturbances, neuroendocrine disturbances, peripheral pooling of blood and poor venous return, low cardiac output, and cardiac arrhythmias.

The varying combinations of increased sympathetic activity, decreased sympathetic activity, deranged vagal activity, and denervation hypersensitivity result from the mosaic of pathologic involvement of neural structures of the afferent and efferent limbs of the baroreceptor mechanism, central dysfunction of vasomotor control, and unbalanced and heterogeneous sympathetic and vagal efferent traffic to the heart. Altered activity of sympathetic and parasympathetic cardiac traffic may also produce ECG abnormalities that include flat or inverted T waves (even widespread and deep T-wave inversions), QT prolongation, and bursts of tachycardia or bradycardia. Sinus arrhythmia with quiet and deep breathing should be followed closely, as the loss of

this R-R variation, which signifies loss of vagal control, identifies the patients at risk of sympathetically mediated ventricular tachycardia or fibrillation (similar to diabetic autonomic neuropathy and, likewise, a marker of arrhythmic risk).[243–248] Sympathetic overactivity has been confirmed by direct microelectrode recording of muscle sympathetic nerve activity[249] during the acute phase, in patients with hypertension and tachycardia. Increased central nervous system catecholaminergic and serotoninergic neurotransmitter synthesis has been demonstrated by Durocher et al.[248]

The manifestations of sympathetic overactivity (hypertension, tachycardia, and diaphoresis) may become severe and require therapy. They may be treated with agents that are readily titratable because of their very short half-life, such as esmolol. These patients respond like subjects with denervation hypersensitivity. Thus pharmacologic measures, when they absolutely must be used, need to be administered in fractions of the usual dose, titrated with very close supervision and without the usual loading dose. We prefer to start with 10 μg/kg/min of esmolol and titrate up cautiously. Whenever possible, blood pressure changes should be treated by adjusting the head of the patient's bed. Esmolol is also particularly helpful in controlling ventricular arrhythmias due to sympathetic overactivity. Adequate maintenance of high normal serum magnesium and potassium levels is very important to avoid electrical instability of the heart. If hypotension does not respond to position and fluids, cautious administration of phenylephrine or dopamine may be required. Pneumatic compression (antiembolism) stockings are very useful to reduce the risk of venous thrombosis and to promote better venous return. One must remain alert to detect signs of autonomic dysfunction even in patients whose course is improved by plasmapheresis. Nursing care is of paramount importance. Extreme care is essential in performing suction and body position should be changed very gently, to avoid precipitating vasodepressor responses from vagal afferent reflexes of upper and lower airway[70] or from painful or emotional stimuli.

Diabetic Autonomic Neuropathy

It has been almost two decades since Wheeler and Watkins[250] proposed the systematic evaluation of autonomic function in diabetics and three decades since Sharpey-Schafer and Taylor[251] first reported "absent circulatory reflexes in diabetic neuritis." The development of standardized tests of autonomic nervous system function (p. 299) has revealed that autonomic dysfunction with important effects on the cardiovascular system is common in type I diabetes mellitus, and is frequently present early,[252,253] before the commonly recognized manifestations [OH, neurogenic impotence, and diabetic diarrhea (nocturnal) and bladder dysfunction] become present.

The risk for development of cardiovascular autonomic neuropathy is particularly high among persons with the HLA antigens DR3 and DR4.[254] In addition to OH, which can be severely incapacitating, cardiovascular autonomic neuropathy causes resting tachycardia, silent myocardial infarction (33 to 42 percent), silent myocardial ischemia, an increased risk of sudden cardiac death, and exercise intolerance, as reviewed in two recent publications.[254,255] In a study of 100 nonketotic diabetics, two-thirds of whom were insulin dependent, 25 percent had OH.[256] It may occur despite normal or raised plasma norepinephrine response to standing. Most of the autonomic tests assess autonomic cardiac innervation, but

there is no proof that the degree of cardiac neuropathy reflects autonomic neuropathy as a whole. The usual tests define ANS function by heart rate variability, especially during breathing (the absence of which documents vagal neuropathy), and response to orthostatic stress (p. 301). In addition to the important increase in sudden cardiac death,[257] autonomic neuropathy may produce cardiorespiratory arrest due to defective respiratory reflexes, chemoreceptor denervation, or vagal denervation of the lungs.[258] Special caution should be observed in the use of respiratory depressant drugs and general anesthesia. Persistent sinus tachycardia may be disturbing to patients. It is greatest with pure vagal neuropathy. As sympathetic neuropathy develops, it may decrease somewhat. Diabetes and chronic alcoholism cause both afferent and efferent lesions. Treatment of orthostatic hypotension is similar to that of OH with autonomic failure (p. 306). There is no effective therapy for deficient vagal function, but symptomatic excessive sinus tachycardia may be treated with low-dose β-blockers or clonidine, with close observation in order to withdraw this therapy if significant sympathetic deficiency develops. It is likely that such therapy may offer some protection against sympathetically mediated cardiac arrhythmias, but I am not aware of a formal published study.

Alcoholic Neuropathy

Acutely, alcohol stimulates the sympathetic nervous system, causing tachycardia and other arrhythmias (including atrial flutter and fibrillation) and hypertension.[259] Klatsky et al.[260] emphasized the link between alcohol and cardiovascular deaths. Chronic alcoholics, who have evidence of peripheral neuropathy affecting motor or sensory nerves, tend to have an elevated resting heart rate due to vagal damage that also causes impaired heart rate response to Valsalva maneuver, deep breathing, change in posture, neck suction, and atropine.[261] Such patients have pathologic evidence of parasympathetic damage in the vagus, in parasympathetic pathways to the eye, and in sacral outflow. The parasympathetic abnormality is rarely associated with the major sympathetic failure that causes OH. Distal sympathetically mediated sweating loss is more frequent. Some patients have shown improvement following months of complete abstinence. It is possible that autonomic neuropathy may predispose affected alcoholics to sudden death.[35] An increased mortality, predominantly from cardiovascular causes, has been reported in alcohol abusers with vagal neuropathy.[262] A possible contribution of autonomic dysfunction to the development of alcoholic cardiomyopathy has been suggested.[4]

Chronic Renal Failure

Peripheral neuropathy associated with chronic renal failure may involve autonomic nerves and cause disorders of sweating and faulty cardiovascular reflex control. Disturbances in cardiovascular reflexes may be caused by lesions in afferent pathways.[263] Autonomic neuropathy may be a contributory factor to hypotension occurring during and following hemodialysis.[264] Nies et al.[265] have demonstrated normal efferent sympathetic function in these patients, suggesting that the most likely sites of primary damage are the baroreceptors, or their afferent fibers or central nervous system connections. They have emphasized that autonomic neuropathy does not appear to be the sole explanation of the sustained hypotension that occurs in some hemodialysis patients. Hypotension and cramps are related to rates of ultrafiltra-

tion and usually respond to injections of small amounts of hypertonic fluids, such as 0.3 M NaCl or 20 percent mannitol. Along with autonomic insufficiency, diminished cardiac function and hypotensive drugs play a causative role. Slowing ultrafiltration may prevent hypotension.

Autonomic Neuropathy in Chronic Liver Disease

Hendrickse et al.[266] found autonomic dysfunction, by autonomic testing, in 27 of 60 patients with "well compensated chronic liver disease." Vagal neuropathy was equally common in patients with alcohol-related and non-alcohol-related liver disease. The cumulative 4-year mortality rate was 30 percent in patients with vagal neuropathy and 6 percent in those with normal autonomic function. The autonomic neuropathy of chronic liver disease,[267] by altering the afferent input from central volume receptors and baroreceptors,[268] has been postulated to result in defective responses to stressful events, causing an increased mortality from bleeding and sepsis. Two patients with autoimmune chronic hepatitis and one abstinent alcohol abuser showed improvement of autonomic responses, suggesting a potential for reversal of vagal neuropathy with improvement in hepatic function, similar to that observed in vagal neuropathy associated with chronic alcohol abuse and prolonged abstinence.[269]

Major Heredofamilial Neuromyopathic Disorders

Friedreich's Ataxia

Friedreich's ataxia is associated with cardiac abnormalities in 90 to 100 percent of cases.[270] Patients characteristically present with progressive congestive heart failure, angina, and arrhythmias (both supraventricular—particularly atrial fibrillation—and ventricular), as well as conduction disturbances. The ECG frequently shows widespread T-wave inversion and pathologic Q waves. A recent study[271] revealed obstructive disease of the large coronary branches, mostly due to fibromuscular dysplasia, and widely distributed focal lesions of small coronary arteries, consisting of medial degeneration, intimal proliferation, fibromuscular dysplasia, and subintimal deposition of an amorphous Schiff-positive material. There was extensive focal degeneration of myelinated and unmyelinated cardiac nerves and cardiac ganglia (parasympathetic). There was focal degeneration and fibrosis of the sinus node, with lesser disease of the atrioventricular node and sparing of the His system. Hypertrophy, focal degeneration, and fibrosis of the myocardium were present. Extracardiac neural abnormalities have also been described that may contribute to disturbances of cardiac rhythm and conduction and may cause dysautonomia and labile hypertension.[272] Neural control of the heart profoundly influences every component of its function but is especially effective upon the processes governing repolarization and thus the appearance of the ST segment and T wave.[273] Cardioneuropathy could also affect myocardial contractility and coronary vasomotor control and cause abnormal excitatory or inhibitory reflexes originating in the heart (see section on physiology). James et al.[271] proposed that the cardiac abnormalities of Friedreich's ataxia could result from the interplay of molecular faults, cardiomyopathy, cardioneuropathy, and coronary disease. Cardiac disease is often the cause of death.[270]

Kearns-Sayre Syndrome
Kearns-Sayre Syndrome is defined as progressive external ophthalmoplegia with pigmentary retinopathy and heart block. Clinically overt cardiac disease is the exception. Cardiac involvement primarily affects the specialized conduction pathways and causes a propensity to complete heart block, requiring pacemaker implantation. Two derangements of cardiac conduction coexist: (1) gradually progressive impairment of infranodal conduction (left anterior hemiblock, right bundle branch block, complete heart block) and (2) concomitant enhancement of AV nodal conduction (identified by His bundle electrocardiography).[274,275]

Duchenne's Muscular Dystrophy
A sex-linked recessive disorder, Duchenne's muscular dystrophy occurs in 1 of 5,000 male births. Rapidly progressive preterminal heart failure may follow years during which the only suspicion of cardiac involvement is an abnormal ECG. Prolonged ambulatory ECG recording has shown that the most common rhythm disturbance is inappropriate sinus tachycardia, which may be labile and gradual or abrupt in onset. It has been attributed to autonomic dysfunction.[276] Disease of the sinoatrial node may be the cause of abnormal sinus node automaticity, sinus node reentry, and labile sinus tachycardia of abrupt onset.[277] Atrial arrhythmias (including atrial flutter, a common preterminal arrhythmia) are more common than ventricular arrhythmias. Significant ventricular electrical instability seldom occurs, despite regional left ventricular dystrophy (which characteristically involves the posterobasal and lateral wall of the left ventricle). Infranodal conduction abnormalities may present with a left posterior fascicular block pattern.

Myotonic Muscular Dystrophy
Far less frequent than Duchenne's disease, myotonic muscular dystrophy (Steinert's Disease) is noted for selective involvement of the sinus node, AV node, His bundle, and bundle branches; such

involvement causes sinus bradycardia, premature atrial beats, atrial flutter, atrial fibrillation, ventricular premature beats, and ventricular tachycardia. The most common electrocardiographic abnormalities (prolongation of PR interval, left anterior fascicular block, and increased QRS duration) reflect the His-Purkinje disease, which can infrequently progress rapidly to complete, life-threatening AV block. Sudden death also occurs from ventricular tachycardia.[278]

Acute Cerebral Disorders Accompanied by Cardiovascular Abnormalities

Raised Intracranial Pressure

Raised intracranial pressure may be accompanied by an increase of arterial pressure, bradycardia, and slow irregular respirations, a triad recognized by Harvey Cushing in 1902[279] as a danger signal requiring immediate action. The response may occur with relatively small increases in intracranial pressure, if there is an acute distortion of the lower brain stem affecting the vasomotor area.[280] Hypertension is particularly likely to occur with space-occupying lesions of the posterior fossa; it demands immediate treatment. Paroxysmal hypertension has been reported in the following posterior fossa lesions: astrocytomas, cerebellar tumors, and basilar artery aneurysms. The paroxysmal hypertension is associated with increased catecholamine release. Posterior fossa lesions should be considered in any patient with paroxysmal hypertension in whom a pheochromocytoma cannot be demonstrated.

Acute Brain Injury Caused by Cerebrovascular Accidents

Acute brain injury caused by subarachnoid hemorrhage, intracerebral hematoma, cerebral infarction, and cranio-cerebral trauma may be accompanied by hypertension. Eighty-four percent of 334 patients admitted with acute stroke manifested hypertension during the first 24 hours.[281] Only one-half of those patients had a prior history of hypertension. Catecholamine concentrations become raised in plasma, cerebrospinal fluid, and urine. In subarachnoid hemorrhage, this sympathetic overactivity has been attributed to an irritative effect of blood on autonomic centers within the hypothalamus or to hypothalamic damage.[282] The autonomic dysfunction produced by acute brain injury also causes ECG abnormalities and electrical instability of the heart, myocardial injury, neurogenic pulmonary edema, and cardiopulmonary arrest. Approximately 90 percent of patients with acute cerebral accidents—most notably spontaneous cerebral or subarachnoid hemorrhage or acute cerebral trauma—exhibit electrocardiographic abnormalities that consist mainly of disturbances of cardiac rhythm and repolarization. Disturbances of rhythm include sinus bradycardia (sometimes profound), sinus tachycardia, atrial arrhythmias (ectopic beats, fibrillation, flutter, supraventricular tachycardia), junctional rhythms, and ventricular arrhythmias (ectopic beats, ventricular tachycardia, or fibrillation). Conduction disturbances include first-, second-, and third-degree heart block. Repolarization abnormalities closely resemble those of ischemic heart disease and consist mainly of abnormal ST and T waves, prominent U wave, and QT prolongation. ST segments may be dramatically elevated and T waves dramatically inverted (25 mm in some cases, in precordial leads), producing a "pseudoinfarction pattern."[283–290]

There is substantial evidence that the autonomic dysfunction, with its marked increase in catecholamine release from sympathetic nerve endings in the heart, may produce myocardial damage reflected in elevation of serum cardiac enzymes (CK-MB), left ventricular wall motion abnormalities detected by echocardiography, and microscopic evidence of myofibrillar degeneration and subendocardial injury.[287,291] Glucocorticoids may add to the effect of catecholamines in producing the "stress myocardial injury." A justified concern has been raised around the fact that donors for heart or heart-lung transplantation are motor vehicle accident or gunshot wound victims who have suffered massive cerebral injury; they probably have varying degrees of catecholamine- and stress-induced myocardial injury.

Neurogenic pulmonary edema similar to that observed in experimental animals sometimes accompanies acute cerebral injury.[292] Cerebrogenic cardiac arrhythmias[293,294] and neurogenic pulmonary edema have been reported in patients with tonic-clonic epileptic seizures, and without acute cerebral injury. The postulated altered efferent discharge of cardiac sympathetic and parasympathetic nerves has been well documented in the cat during pentylenetetrazol-induced epileptogenic activity.[295] It offers an explanation for the high incidence of sudden unexpected death in epileptic subjects. Like the clinical picture in patients with acute brain injury, there are manifestations of excessive vagal activity (bradycardia, heart block) as well as excessive sympathetic tone. Thus, we have used intravenous atropine or short-acting β-blockers like esmolol IV in the management of hypertension and arrhythmias. Esmolol is ideal because it can be easily titrated to avoid the excessive drop in blood pressure that would jeopardize cerebral perfusion pressure (particularly since autoregulation is deranged in the setting of acute brain injury). The beneficial effect of adrenergic blockade has been analyzed by Walter et al.[296]

Cardiac Denervation

Cardiac denervation represents the extreme degree of cardiac dysautonomia. The most common cause is cardiac transplantation. It has been suggested that the donor heart be considered decentralized, rather than denervated, because there is postganglionic separation from central sympathetic centers but preganglionic separation from central parasympathetic centers. Partial sympathetic reinnervation has been documented.[297] The transplanted heart has been considered a special model for studying autonomic control of the heart[298] and for elegant electrophysiologic and pharmacologic studies without the confounding effect of pharmacologic autonomic blockade.[299] Despite the absence of autonomic reflex control, exercise performance may be quite adequate.[300] Heart rate response is gradual, as prompt vagal withdrawal and sympathetic neural enhancement are absent, and is mediated by circulating catecholamines from extracardiac sympathetic nerve endings and adrenal medulla. Maximal heart rate is less, so cardiac output response depends more on increase of stroke volume. There is supersensitivity to norepinephrine (and administered isoproterenol) due to upregulation of β-receptors and loss of norepinephrine uptake by postganglionic sympathetic neurons of the donor heart.[301] These studies nicely confirm the predictions from the experimental animal model.[302] Chagas' disease, with its highly selective damage to cardiac autonomic nerves and epicardial parasympathetic ganglia,[303] is a disease-induced model of cardiac denervation.[304] Defective parasympathetic control, manifested by abnormal responses to autonomic tests, has been reported in patients who have not yet reached the stage of myocardial involvement with fibrosis and apical aneurysm formation. It has been attributed to the severe degenerative lesions of parasympathetic cardiac ganglia[305] and may play a key role in the arrhythmias, conduction disturbances, and tendency to sudden death of affected patients. Progressive increase in plasma catecholamines occurs with progression of the cardiac autonomic neuropathy, enhancing the arrhythmic risk. Electrical instability and sudden death have been well documented in other forms of cardiac neuropathy.[19,21]

CARDIOVASCULAR DISORDERS IN WHICH AUTONOMIC DYSFUNCTION PLAYS AN IMPORTANT ROLE

Heart Failure

Autonomic dysfunction is an important feature of congestive heart failure (CHF). Changes that affect the basic functional characteristics of the ANS, as well as abnormal patterns of activation of autonomic reflexes, are present and affect the responses mediated by both sympathetic and parasympathetic systems. Heart failure is characterized by an excessive neurohumoral activation, as indicated by increased circulatory levels of catecholamines, plasma renin, angiotensin II, and vasopressin.[306,307] Direct evidence of increased central sympathetic outflow has been obtained from intraneural recordings in the human peroneal nerve.[308] This neurohumoral activation, which in normal subjects constitutes an appropriate response to a decrease in cardiac output, such as that caused by gravitational stress in upright activity, may exacerbate and accelerate the manifestation of CHF.[309] An excessive sympathoadrenal drive has been described in patients with

CHF during muscular exercise.[310] Plasma norepinephrine levels in CHF are markedly elevated at intensities of exercise that produce little change in normal subjects. The rate of release of norepinephrine is determined by relative (percent of individual maximum) rather than absolute work load. Oxygen uptakes during exercise at 2 to 4 times resting levels correspond to loads well below 50 percent of maximal capacity in normal subjects, but are maximal in patients with severe CHF.[78] However, in some patients with advanced CHF, resting plasma levels of epinephrine and norepinephrine and heart rate are higher than in normal subjects, whereas they are significantly lower during exercise.[311]

Reduced ability of arterial and cardiopulmonary mechanoreceptors to inhibit the vasomotor center and sympathetic outflow has been demonstrated in CHF. How this occurs is not yet known. In patients who have undergone cardiac transplantation, the diminished circulatory control by the carotid and aortic baroreceptors is reversed as early as 2 weeks after surgery, suggesting that depressed baroreflex sensitivity is not due to structural damage to the mechanoreceptors in the vessel wall but might be due to central changes. Normally the mechanoreceptors in the cardiac chambers with unmyelinated vagal afferents tonically inhibit the vasomotor centers, and those in the atria with myelinated vagal afferents also regulate the release of vasopressin from the posterior pituitary gland. Normal subjects develop reflex arterial vasoconstriction in the forearm with peripheral venous pooling (lower body negative pressure), whereas patients with left ventricular dysfunction have a paradoxical reflex vasodilatation.[312] The impaired chronotropic response to physiologic stimuli,[313] and the attenuated response to endogenous or exogenous catecholamines in the failing heart do not occur in the vascular system. While adrenergically mediated vasoconstriction normally occurs in vessels supplying the kidneys and splanchnic viscera during exercise, neurogenic vasoconstriction is even more marked in patients with CHF and limited augmentation of cardiac output with exercise.[314,315]

The control of multiple vascular beds has been extensively studied in the conscious dog model.[316] In patients with CHF, β-adrenoceptors on lymphocytes and α-adrenoceptor on platelets are "downregulated" (presumably due to prolonged elevation of norepinephrine). Myocardium obtained from patients with CHF shows a marked reduction in β-adrenoceptor density, in isoproterenol-mediated adenylate cyclase stimulation, and in contractility.[317] The beneficial effect of the administration of low doses of the relatively specific β₁-receptor antagonist metoprolol, in patients with CHF due to dilated cardiomyopathy, has been attributed to reversal of the downregulation of the receptors.[318] Norepinephrine content of ventricular myocardium obtained by endomyocardial biopsy in patients with CHF is markedly reduced in those with severe ventricular dysfunction.[319] In the norepinephrine-depleted failing heart, fluorescence is absent in the terminal varicosities of adrenergic fibers in close association with cardiac myocytes. This has been documented noninvasively by the decreased uptake of ^{123}I-metaiodobenzylguanidine myocardial scintigraphy in patients with dilated cardiomyopathy.[320]

Defective parasympathetic control of the heart in CHF was demonstrated as early as 1971.[321] The parasympathetic restraint on sinoatrial node automaticity is markedly reduced in patients with CHF, who also exhibit less heart rate slowing for any given elevation of systemic arterial pressure. This represents reduced baroreceptor reflex sensitivity, which has also been demonstrated in the conscious dog model.[322] Power spectral analysis of heart rate variability in response to respiration (sinus arrhythmia) and to baroreceptor modulation by blood pressure changes, studied in ambulatory patients with severe heart failure, showed evidence of diminished vagal but relatively preserved sympathetic modulation of heart rate.[323] The Multicenter Postinfarction Research Group noted that the standard deviation of the R-R interval over 24 hours, an index of vagal tone, was a very strong determinant of subsequent survival after acute myocardial infarction.[348] The study of the standard deviation of R-R interval in the 25 patients with severe heart failure showed that, like the frequency-specific measures of heart rate variability, it was markedly decreased in the patients with CHF whose median survival was only 5 months. Cohn et al.[324] reported a markedly reduced survival in patients with chronic CHF whose resting plasma norepinephrine levels were 400 pg/ml or more. This enhanced adrenergic activity not only increases afterload, with an obviously deleterious effect on the course of chronic CHF, but also increases the risk of arrhythmogenesis, an important cause of poor survival. It was formerly thought that ventricles were insensitive to both parasympathetic stimulation and acetylcholine. It is now apparent that cholinergic nerves supply the ventricles and conducting tissues of the His-Purkinje system.[325] The inhibitory effects of cholinergic stimulation on the ventricles and His-Purkinje system are much more prominent following β-adrenergic stimulation, so that parasympathetic stimulation blunts the response to sympathetic stimulation,[49] exerting a protective effect against arrhythmogenesis that is deficient or lost in the patients with severe CHF, thus explaining the above observations.

Verrier and Lown[127] demonstrated the important effect of the sympathetic-parasympathetic interaction on ventricular electrical stability. The harmful effect of ventricular arrhythmias on survival in patients with CHF was emphasized by Dargie et al.[326] Increased levels of plasma catecholamines may also cause hypokalemia and hypomagnesemia, both of which increase electrical instability.[327,328] These electrolyte abnormalities are enhanced by diuretic therapy.[329]

It is not possible to enhance parasympathetic (protective) activity by a straightforward pharmacologic approach. The therapy of CHF should have as one of its fundamental goals that of reducing the enhanced adrenergic activity. Vasodilator therapy, especially with angiotensin-converting enzyme (ACE) inhibitors which increase cardiac output, tends to reverse the pathophysiologic mechanisms that lead to the hyperadrenergic state. In addition, the reduction of angiotensin II removes the central and peripheral sympathetic-enhancing effect of angiotensin II. ACE inhibitors exert a beneficial effect directly in the myocardium, where angiotensin II promotes myocardial hypertrophy and activation of interstitial fibroblasts. As anxiety magnifies the adrenergic response, reassurance and a caring, supporting attitude are fundamental. Assessment of autonomic function by the study of heart rate variability and other autonomic tests is likely to become an integral part of the diagnostic and prognostic evaluation of CHF.

Myocardial Ischemia and Myocardial Infarction

The overwhelming majority of patients with acute myocardial infarction show evidence of autonomic disturbances during the first 30 to 60 minutes of the attack.[330,331] Approximately 55 percent of patients have bradyarrhythmias, hypotension, or both (parasympathetic overactivity), and 36 percent have sinus tachycardia, hypertension, or both (sympathetic overactivity) in the early phase of myocardial infarction. Webb et al.[330] demonstrated that the type of autonomic disturbance is related to the site of infarction. Bradycardia or hypotension occurs much more commonly in patients with inferoposterior infarction, whereas tachycardia or hypertension occur more commonly in patients with anterior infarction.

Similar observations were made by Perez-Gomez et al.[75] during transmural myocardial ischemia in patients with Prinzmetal's angina (caused by coronary spasm) in angiographically defined territories. Heart rate decreased significantly during pain in the patients with inferior ischemia, whereas it increased significantly during pain in patients with anterior ischemia. In addition, the incidence of ectopic arrhythmias was significantly greater in patients with anterior ischemia. There was a high incidence of atrioventricular block in patients with posterior ischemia.

Robertson et al.[77] reported on 2,240 episodes of transmural myocardial ischemia in 12 patients with well-documented single vessel coronary spasm. The pattern of hemodynamic response was remarkably uniform for a given patient and location of ischemia. Of seven patients with inferoposterior ischemia, six had associated bradycardia or hypotension, a response that only occurred in one of the five patients with anterior ischemia. Of the other four patients with anterior ischemia, two had a hypertensive, tachycardia response. Experimental studies and the clinical observations referred to above have provided considerable insight into the mechanisms of the autonomic disturbances that accompany myocardial ischemia and infarction. An excellent review has been published by Mark.[76] Stimulation of cardiac receptors with nonmyelinated (C-fiber) vagal afferents (distributed preferentially in the inferoposterior wall of the left ventricle) by systolic deformation or "bulging" of the ischemic or recently infarcted myocardium feeds afferent signals into the nucleus tractus solitarius of the medulla; these signals cause parasympathetic activation and sympathetic withdrawal (the Bezold-Jarisch reflex). Bradycardia, reduction of arteriolar resistance, enhancement of venous capacitance (which cause hypotension and reduction of venous return with a decline in preload) and possibly nausea or vomiting from activation of vagal fibers to the stomach characterize the response to the Bezold-Jarisch reflex, most commonly seen in inferoposterior ischemia.

Anterior myocardial ischemia or infarction activates cardiac receptors with sympathetic afferent fibers, leading to tachycardia and hypertension. A cardiogenic hypertensive chemoreflex[332] may contribute to bradycardia and hypertension (there is simultaneous vagal and sympathetic efferent discharge) during myocardial ischemia. Chemoreceptors with a blood supply from the initial portion of the left coronary artery (proximal left anterior descending and circumflex) are activated by serotonin from platelet thrombi. The afferent fibers travel in the vagus, whereas the efferent limb extends through both vagal and sympathetic fibers. The chemoreceptors have been demonstrated in both canine and human hearts.[333] The Bezold-Jarisch reflex is triggered also by injection of angiographic contrast into the posterior coronary circulation.[334] It is caused by the osmotic contrast, not by changes in vascular pressure.[335] Other causes of this reflex are myocardial reperfusion following thrombolytic therapy in patients with acute myocardial infarction, particularly of the posteroinferior wall,[336] changes in wall stress in the syncope of patients with aortic stenosis,[76] and vasovagal syncope.[129] Digitalis[337] and nitroglycerine[338] sensitize the cardiac receptors from which the Bezold-Jarisch reflex is elicited. In order to counteract this reflex in treating patients, it is generally necessary to block the parasympathetic with intravenous atropine and "substitute" for the withdrawn sympathetic traffic to arterioles by pressor agents, and to the capacitance system by careful volume expansion. Atropine alone will promptly correct the bradycardia or the conduction disturbance but not the hypotension.

A caveat: atropine should be used cautiously and only if required by hemodynamic deterioration, because tachycardia in the presence of ischemia, which increases ventricular electrical instability, may precipitate ventricular tachycardia or fibrillation.[339,340] Doses of less than 0.8 mg do not appear to be associated with increased ventricular irritability.[341] A parasympathomimetic effect, which can cause slowing of heart rate and atrioventricular conduction disturbance, can occur initially[85] and transiently before the parasympatholytic effect becomes established. Epstein et al.[299] presented strong evidence that low-dose atropine causes bradycardia by a central effect.

The circadian variation of autonomic tone is important in determining diurnal changes in arterial vasomotor tone as well as changes in blood pressure and coronary vasomotor responses. There is a probable relationship to the well-established circadian frequency distribution of acute cardiovascular disorders such as transient myocardial ischemia, myocardial infarction, sudden cardiac death, and stroke. These issues were discussed on page 295 and are well described in the references cited.[52–58]

Some Aspects of Cardiac Arrhythmias in Myocardial Ischemia and Myocardial Infarction Influenced by Autonomic Dysfunction

The influence of sympathetic-parasympathetic interaction on ventricular electrical stability has been analyzed in detail by Verrier and Lown.[127] In the experimental animal, there is a surge in sympathetic neural[349] and humoral[343] activity during the first few minutes after coronary artery occlusion. In a study of patients on entry to a coronary care unit, patients with infarction who subsequently developed ventricular fibrillation had higher concentrations of noradrenaline and particularly adrenaline than patients who did not develop fibrillation.[344] Experimentally, the protection afforded by vagal activation was considerably less than that provided by β-adrenergic blockade. Further research, however, showed that augmented sympathetic activity increases the ventricular vulnerability to fibrillation, and this effect can be neutralized by an increase in vagal activity.[345,346] The vagal effect depends on the existing sympathetic tone, as it is mediated principally by antagonizing the influence of the prevailing sympathetic activity.[49] In patients with acute myocardial infarction followed in our Myocardial Infarction Research Unit, we observed with Mantle (unpublished observation) that the onset of ventricular tachycardia or fibrillation was preceded by a marked decrease in respiratory heart rate variability, monitored by constant computer-measured R-R. Therefore, decrease in this index of vagal tone clearly appeared to precede the increase of ventricular vulnerability in the clinical setting.

Lombardi et al.[347] studied heart rate variability by power spectral analysis in 40 patients with myocardial infarction and 18 control subjects at 2 weeks and 6 and 12 months after acute myocardial infarction. Their analysis revealed that the enhanced sympathetic activation of the early period declined over the time of observation, along with a progressive recovery of the vagal tone. The Multicenter Post-Infarction Research Group demonstrated that the standard deviation of the R-R interval over 24 hours, a reliable index of vagal tone, was the strongest determinant of subsequent survival after acute myocardial infarction in a group of unselected patients.[348]

Beyond these general autonomic considerations, arrhythmias in ischemic heart disease are complex. The anatomic substrate of infarcted-ischemic-scarred myocardium is highly heterogenous and is favorable to the appearance of varied regional reentry circuits. The distribution of vagal afferent and efferent fibers in the myocardium (dog) is mostly subendocardial, whereas the corresponding sympathetic fibers are primarily epicardic and course along coronary arterial pathways and then penetrate the myocardium. Myocardial infarction can damage autonomic fibers and cause denervation distal to the infarct zone, setting up areas of denervation hypersensitivity that also influence the propensity to arrhythmias. A complete review has been published recently by Zipes.[349]

This abnormality of adrenergic function, which extends beyond the area of abnormal myocardial perfusion defined by T1-201 myocardial scintigraphy, was documented by ^{123}I-labeled metaiodobenzylguanidine scintigraphy in 27 patients, 10 ± 4 days after acute myocardial infarction.[16] Anterior myocardial infarction was associated with greater disruption of adrenergic function. The severity of adrenergic abnormality correlated with the degree of left ventricular dysfunction. Significant ventricular ectopy was detected in 11 patients, all of whom had significantly higher scintigraphy "defect scores" than the patients without evidence of ventricular arrhythmia. In addition to these special features of adrenergic function, we must consider that the vagal effects predominate in heart control, whereas sympathetic effects predominate in the control of atrioventricular conduction;[18] and that autonomic input to the heart has a certain sidedness, such that the right sympathetic and vagus nerves affect the sinus node more than the atrioventricular node, whereas the left sympathetic and vagus nerves affect the atrioventricular node more than the sinus node.[349] Imbalance of autonomic input to the heart is arrhythmogenio.[350] Myocardial infarction produces damage to cardiac plexus and epicardial cardiac neural ganglia (parasympathetic) as well as the mediastinal cardiac plexus, leading to arrhythmias in a manner entirely similar to that of cardioneuropathies of viral or other etiology that have caused sudden death, serious arrhythmias, and long QT syndrome (acquired).[19–21,351]

This broad pathophysiologic spectrum explains why our therapeutic armamentarium must include avoidance of fear and anxiety, β-blockers specific antiarrhythmic agents (often determined by electrophysiologic evaluation) ablation of arrhythmogenic foci by regional alcohol injection or by application of radiofrequency (for the destruction of arrhythmia-generating abnormal myocardium) cryosurgery and other surgical procedures, automatic implantable cardioverter-defibrillators.

ACKNOWLEDGEMENTS

I am deeply indebted to my wonderful wife and children for their love and forebearance; to Mr. and Mrs. Joseph Uihlein for their generous support of our Autonomic Research Laboratory, to Dr. Gerald Pohost and my colleagues in the Division of Cardiology for their support and encouragement, to Leona Walker and Loren Levson for their invaluable collaboration in the Autonomic Laboratory, to Dr. Joseph Donnelly, PhD and the personnel in the Lister Hill Library for bibliographic assistance, and especially to Mrs. Jean Gray and Barbara Jolley for their expert and devoted secretarial help.

REFERENCES

1. Leonardo da Vinci: Quaderni di Anatomia II (VIII, F.3 Royal Library of Windsor). p. 576. In Favaloro G (ed): Ricerche Embriologiche ed Anatomiche Intorno al Cuore dei Vertebrati. Drucker, Padua, 1914

1a. De Cyon E, Ludwig C: Die Reflexe eines der Sensibelch Blutgetässe. Ber Sacchs Ges Wiss 18:307, 1866

2. Appenzeller O: Clinical Autonomic Failure. Elsevier, Amsterdam, 1986

3. Plum F: Autonomic disorders and their management. p. 2105. In: Cecil Textbook of Medicine, 18th Ed. WB Saunders, Philadelphia, 1988

4. Johnson RH, Lambie DG, Spalding JMK: Neurocardiology. WB Saunders, London, 1984

5. Natelson BH: Neurocardiology. An interdisciplinary area for the 80s. Arch Neurol 42:178, 1985

6. Kulbertus HE, Franck G: Neurocardiology. Futura Publishing, Mount Kisco, NY, 1988

7. Kasting GA, Eckberg DL, Fritsch JM, Birkett CL: Continuous resetting of the human carotid baroreceptor-cardiac reflex. Am J Physiol 252: R732, 1978

8. Hagbarth KE, Valbo AB: Pulse and respiratory grouping of sympathetic impulses in human muscle nerves. Acta Physiol Scand 74:96, 1968

9. Wallin BG: Intraneural recordings of

normal and abnormal sympathetic activity in man. p. 177. In Bannister R (ed): Autonomic Failure: A Textbook of Clinical Disorders of the Autonomic Nervous System, 2nd Ed. Oxford University Press, Oxford, 1988

10. Robertson D, Goldberg MR, Onrot J et al: Isolated failure of autonomic noradrenergic neurotransmission: evidence for impaired β-hydroxylation of dopamine. N Engl J Med 314:1494, 1986

11. Lefkowitz RJ: Direct binding studies of adrenergic receptors: biochemical, physiologic and clinical implications. Ann Intern Med 91:450, 1979

12. Davies IB, Sever PS: Adrenoceptor function. p. 348. In Bannister R (ed): Autonomic Failure: A Textbook of Clinical Disorders of the Autonomic Nervous System, 2nd Ed. Oxford University Press, Oxford, 1988

13. Robertson D, Hollister AS, Carey EL et al: Increased vascular beta $_2$-adrenoceptor responsiveness in autonomic dysfunction. J Am Coll Cardiol 3:850, 1984

14. Schatz IJ, Ramanathan S, Villagomez R, McLean C: Orthostatic hypotension, catecholamines and α-adrenergic receptors in mitral valve prolapse. West J Med 152:37, 1990

15. Kline RC, Swanson DP, Weiland DM et al: Myocardial imaging in man with I-123 meta-iodobenzylguanidine. J Nucl Med 22:129, 1981

16. McGhie AI, Corbett JR, Akers MS et al: Regional cardiac adrenergic function using I-123 meta-iodobenzylguanidine tomographic imaging after acute myocardial infarction. Am J Cardiol 67:236, 1991

17. Inoue H, Zipes DP: Changes in atrial and ventricular refractoriness and in atrioventricular nodal conduction produced by combinations of vagal and sympathetic stimulation that result in a constant spontaneous cycle length. Circ Res 60:942, 1987

18. Urthaler F, James TN: Cholinergic and adrenergic control of the sinus node and AV junction. p. 249. In Randall WC (ed): Neural Regulation of the Heart. Oxford University Press, New York, 1977

19. James TN: Primary and secondary cardioneuropathies and their functional significance. J Am Coll Cardiol 2:983, 1983

20. James TN: Sir Thomas Lewis redivivus: from pebbles in a quiet pond to autonomic storms. Br Heart J 52:1, 1984

21. Rossi L: Cardioneuropathy and extracardiac neural disease. J Am Coll Cardiol 5:66B, 1985

22. Spyer KM: Central nervous system control of the cardiovascular system. p. 56. In Bannister R (ed): Autonomic Failure: A Textbook of Clinical Disorders of the Autonomic Nervous System, 2nd Ed. Oxford University Press, Oxford, 1988

23. Shepherd JT: The heart as a sensory organ. J Am Coll Cardiol 6:83B, 1985

24. Korner PI: Central nervous control of autonomic cardiovascular function. In Berne RM, Sperelakis N (eds): Handbook of Physiology: The Cardiovascular System. Vol. I. American Physiological Society, Bethesda, MD, 1979

25. Abboud FM, Thames MD: Interaction of cardiovascular reflexes in circulatory control. p. 675. In Shepherd JT, Abboud FM, Geiger SR (eds): Handbook of Physiology: The Cardiovascular System. Vol. III. American Physiological Society, Bethesda, MD, 1983

26. Mancia G, Mark AL: Arterial baroreflexes in humans. p. 755. In Shepherd JT, Abboud FM, Geiger SR (eds): Handbook of Physiology: The Cardiovascular System. Vol. III. American Physiological Society, Bethesda, MD, 1983

27. Mark AL, Mancia G: Cardiopulmonary baroreflexes in humans. p. 795. In Shepherd JT, Abboud FM, Geiger SR (eds): Handbook of Physiology: The Cardiovascular System. Vol. III. American Physiological Society, Bethesda, MD, 1983

28. Bishop VS, Malliani A, Thorén P: Cardiac mechanoreceptors. p. 497. In Shepherd JT, Abboud FM, Geiger SR (eds): Handbook of Physiology: The Cardiovascular System. Vol. III. American Physiological Society, Bethesda, MD, 1983

29. Shepherd JT, Mancia G: Reflex control of the human cardiovascular system. Rev Physiol Biochem Pharmacol 105:1, 1986

30. Shepherd JT: Reflex control of the venous system in man. p. 247. In Kovach AGB, Sandor P, Kollai M (eds): Advances in Physiological Sciences: Cardiovascular Physiology, Neural Control Mechanisms. Pergamon Press, New York, 1981

31. Shepherd JT, Vanhoutte PM: Neurohumoral regulation. p. 107. In Shepherd JT, Vanhoutte PM (eds): The Human Cardiovascular System, Facts and Concepts. Raven Press, New York, 1979

32. Folkow B, Neil E: Nervous control of the circulation. p. 307. In Folkow B, Neil E (eds): Circulation. Oxford University Press, New York, 1971

33. Shepherd RFJ, Shepherd JT: Control of blood pressure and the circulation in man. p. 80. In Bannister R (ed): Autonomic Failure: A Textbook of Clinical Disorders of the Autonomic Nervous System, 2nd Ed. Oxford University Press, Oxford, 1988

34. Joyner MJ, Shepherd JT: Autonomic control of circulation. p. 55. In Low PA (ed): Clinical Autonomic Disorders. Little, Brown, Boston, 1993

35. Johnson RH, Lambie DG, Spalding JMK: The autonomic nervous system. p. 1. In Baker AB, Joynt RJ (eds): Clinical Neurology. Vol. 4. Harper and Row, Philadelphia, 1986.

36. Manning JW: Intracranial mechanisms of regulation. p. 189. In Randall WC (ed): Neural Regulation of the Heart. Oxford University Press, New York, 1977

37. Smith OA: Reflex and central mechanisms involved in the control of the heart and circulation. Annu Rev Physiol 36:93, 1974

38. Reid JL: Central and peripheral autonomic control mechanisms. p. 44. In Bannister R (ed): Autonomic Failure: A Textbook of Clinical Disorders of the Autonomic Nervous System, 2nd Ed. Oxford University Press, Oxford, 1988

39. Mancia G, Zanchetti A: Hypothalamic control of autonomic functions. p. 147.

In Panskeep PJ, Morgane J (eds): Handbook of Hypothalmus. Marcel Dekker, New York, 1981

40. Reis DJ, Granata AR, Joh TH et al: Brain stem catecholamine mechanisms in tonic and reflex control of blood pressure. Hypertension, 6(suppl II):II-7, 1984

41. Abboud FM: Effects of sodium, angiotensin and steroids on vascular reactivity in man. Fed Proc 33:143, 1974

42. Lee WB, Ismay MJ, Lumber ER: Mechanism by which angiotensin II affects heart rate of conscious sheep. Circ Res 47:286, 1980

43. Hedwall PR, Abdel-Sayed WA, Schmid PG, Abboud FM: Inhibition of vasoconstrictor responses by prostaglandin E1. Proc Soc Exp Biol Med 135:757, 1970

44. Brody MJ, Kadowitz PJ: Prostaglandins as modulators of the autonomic nervous system. Fed Proc 33:48, 1974

45. Rowell LB: Human Circulation: Regulation During Physical Stress. Oxford University Press, New York, 1986

46. Hall JE: Symposium: Arterial pressure and body fluid homestasis. Fed Proc 45:2862, 1986

47. Levy MN: Sympathetic-parasympathetic interactions in the heart. Circ Res 29:437, 1971

48. Vanhoutte PM, Levy MN: Prejunctional cholinergic modulation of adrenergic neurotransmission in the cardiovascular system. Am J Physiol 238:H275, 1980

49. Levy MN: Sympathetic-parasympathetic interactions in the heart. p. 85. In Kulbertus HE, Frank G (eds): Neurocardiology. Futura Publishing, Mt. Kisco, NY, 1988

50. Krnjevic K: Central cholinergic pathways. Fed Proc 28:113, 1969

51. Folkow B, Langston J, Oberg B, Prerovsky E: Reactions of the different series-coupled vascular sections upon stimulation of the hypothalamic sympatho-inhibitory area. Acta Physiol Scand 61:476, 1964

52. Panza JA, Epstein SE, Quyyumi AA: Circadian variation in vascular tone and its relation to *a*-sympathetic vasocon-

strictor activity. N Engl J Med, 325:986, 1991

53. Millar-Craig MW, Bishop CN, Raftery EB: Circadian variation of blood pressure. Lancet 1:795, 1978
54. Furlan R, Guzzetti S, Crivellaro W et al: Continuous 24-hour assessment of the neural regulation of systemic arterial pressure and RR variabilities in ambulant subjects. Circulation 81:537, 1990
55. Verdecchia P, Schillaci G, Guerrieri M et al: Circadian blood pressure changes and left ventricular hypertrophy in essential hypertension. Circulation 81:528, 1990
56. Rocco MB, Barry J, Campbell S et al: Circadian variation of transient myocardial ischemia in patients with coronary artery disease. Circulation 75:395, 1987
57. Mulcahy D, Keegan J, Cunningham D et al: Circadian variation of total ischemic burden and its alteration with anti-anginal agents. Lancet 2:755, 1988
58. Muller JE, Tofler GH, Stone PH: Circadian variation and triggers of onset of acute cardiovascular disease. Circulation 79:733, 1989
59. Hayano J, Sakakibara Y, Yamada M et al: Diurnal variations in vagal and sympathetic cardiac control. Am J Physiol 258:H642, 1990
60. Pagani M, Lombardi F, Guzzetti S et al: Power spectral analysis of heart rate and arterial pressure variabilities as a marker of sympatho-vagal interaction in man and conscious dog. Circ Res 59:178, 1986
61. Kelly J, O'Malley K: Adrenoceptor function and ageing. Clin Sci 66:509, 1984
62. Kalbfleisch JH, Stowe DF, Smith JJ: Evaluation of the heart rate response to the valsalva maneuver. Am Heart J 95:707, 1978
63. Lee TD, Linderman RD, Yiengst MJ, Shock NW: Influence of age on the cardiovascular and renal responses to tilting. J Appl Physiol 21:55, 1966
64. Kino M, Lance VQ, Shahamatpour A, Spodick DH: Effects of age on responses to isometric exercise. Am Heart J 90:575, 1975
65. Collins KJ, Exton-Smith AN, James MH, Oliver DJ: Functional changes in autonomic nervous responses with ageing. Age Ageing 9:17, 1980
66. Low PA: The effect of aging on the autonomic nervous system. p. 685. In Low PA (ed): Clinical Autonomic Disorders. Little, Brown, Boston, 1993
67. Coghlan HC: Autonomic dysfunction in the mitral valve prolapse syndrome: the brain-heart connection and interaction. p. 389. In Boudoulas H, Wooley CF (eds): Mitral Valve Prolapse and the Mitral Valve Prolapse Syndrome. Futura Publishing, Mt. Kisco, NY, 1988
68. Chen MY, Yu GY, Buetikofer J et al: Increased microvascular blood flow oscillation frequency: a predictor of syncope during head-up tilt testing, abstracted. Circulation, 82(suppl III):III-707, 1990
69. Jordan D, Spyer KM: Brainstem integration of cardiovascular and pulmonary afferent activity. p. 295. In Cervero F, Morrison JBF (eds): Progress in Brain Research. Vol. 67. Elsevier Science Publishing, Amsterdam, 1986
70. Cunningham ET Jr, Ravich WJ, Jones B, Donner MW: Vagal reflexes referred from the upper aerodigestive tract: an infrequently recognized cause of common cardiorespiratory responses. Ann Intern Med 116:575, 1992
71. Honig CR: Functions and organization of neural controls. p. 267. In Honig CR (ed): Modern Cardiovascular Physiology. Little, Brown, Boston, 1981
72. Hageman GR, Coghlan HC, James TN, Neely BH: Influence of atrial mechanoreceptors upon the sympathetic efferent activity elicited during a cardiogenic chemoreflex in the dog. J Autonom Nerv Syst 9:637, 1983
73. Thoren P: Activation of left ventricular receptors with non-medullated vagal afferents during occlusion of a coronary artery in the cat. Am J Cardiol 37:1046, 1976
74. Thames MD, Klopfenstein HS, Abboud FM et al: Preferential distribution of inhibitory cardiac receptors with vagal afferents to the inferoposterior wall of the left ventricle activated during coronary

occlusion in the dog. Circ Res 43:512, 1978

75. Perez-Gomez F, Martin de Dios R, Rey J, Garcia Aguado A: Prinzmetal's angina: reflex cardiovascular response during episode of pain. Br Heart J 42:81, 1979

76. Mark AL: The Bezold-Jarisch reflex revisited: clinical implications of inhibitory reflexes originating in the heart. J Am Coll Cardiol 1:90, 1983

77. Robertson D, Hollister AS, Forman MB, Robertson RM: Reflexes unique to myocardial ischemia and infarction. J Am Coll Cardiol 5:99B, 1985

78. Blomqvist CG: Physiology and pathophysiology of exercise. p. 1. In Parmley WW, Chatterjee K (eds): Cardiology. Vol. 1. JB Lippincott, Philadelphia, 1988

79. Shepherd JT, Blomqvist CG, Lind AR et al: Static (isometric) exercise. Retrospection and introspection. Circ Res (suppl 1) 48:I179, 1981

80. Mitchell JH: Cardiovascular control during exercise: central and reflex neural mechanisms. Am J Cardiol 55:34D, 1985

81. Wildenthal K, Mierzwiak DS, Skinner NS Jr, Mitchell JH: Potassium-induced cardiovascular and ventilatory reflexes from the dog hindlimb. Am J Physiol 215:542, 1968

82. Tibes U: Reflex inputs to the cardiovascular and respiratory centers from dynamically working canine muscles: Some evidence for involvement of group III or IV nerve fibers. Circ Res 41:332, 1977

83. Akselrod S, Gordon D, Ubel FA et al: Power spectrum analysis of heart rate fluctuation: a quantitative probe of beat-to-beat cardiovascular control. Science 213:220, 1981

84. Pomeranz B, Macauley RJB, Caudill MA et al: Assessment of autonomic function in humans by heart rate spectral analysis. Am J Physiol 248:H151, 1985

85. Robertson D: Clinical pharmacology: assessment of autonomic function. p. 86. In Baughman KL, Greene BM (eds): Clinical Diagnostic Manual. Williams & Wilkins, Baltimore, 1981

86. Bannister R, Mathias C: Testing autonomic reflexes. p. 289. In Bannister R (ed): Autonomic Failure: A Textbook of Clinical Disorders of the Autonomic Nervous System, 2nd Ed. Oxford University Press, Oxford, 1988

87. Ewing DJ: Recent advances in the non-invasive investigation of diabetic autonomic neuropathy. p. 667. In Bannister R (ed): Autonomic Failure: A Textbook of Clinical Disorders of the Autonomic Nervous System, 2nd Ed. Oxford University Press, Oxford, 1988

88. Wieling W: Standing, orthostatic stress, and autonomic function. p. 308. In Bannister R (ed): Autonomic Failure: A Textbook of Clinical Disorders of the Autonomic Nervous System, 2nd Ed. Oxford University Press, Oxford, 1988

89. Shepherd JT, Vanhoutte PM, Joyner MJ: The sensory systems involved in cardiovascular regulation. p. 166. In Giuliani ER, Fuster V, Gersh BJ et al: Cardiology. Fundamentals and Practice. Mosby-Year Book, St. Louis, 1991

90. Freeman R: Autonomic nervous system. p. 1984. In Stein JH (ed): Internal Medicine. Little, Brown, Boston, 1990

91. Low PA, Pfeifer MA: Standardization of clinical tests for practice and clinical trials. p. 287. In Low PA (ed): Clinical Autonomic Disorders. Little, Brown, Boston, 1993

92. Ewing DJ, Borsey DQ, Bellavere F, Clarke BF: Cardiac autonomic neuropathy in diabetes: comparison of measures of R-R interval variation. Diabetologia 32:18, 1981

93. Pfeifer MA, Cook D, Brodsky J et al: Quantitative evaluation of cardiac parasympathetic activity in normal and diabetic man. Diabetes 31:339, 1982

94. Weinberg CR, Pfeifer MA: An improved method for measuring heart-rate variability: assessment of cardiac autonomic function. Biometrics 40:855, 1984

95. Molhoek GP, Wesseling KH, Settels JJ et al: Evaluation of the Penáz servo-plethysmo manometer for the continous, non-invasive measurement of finger blood pressure. Basic Res Cardiol 79:598, 1984

96. Baldwa VS, Ewing DJ: Heart rate response to Valsalva manoeuver. Reproducibility in normals, and relation to

variation in resting heart rate in diabetics. Br Heart J 39:641, 1977

97. Ewing DJ: Practical bedside investigation of diabetic autonomic failure. p. 371. In Bannister R (ed): Autonomic Failure: A Textbook of Clinical Disorders of the Autonomic Nervous System. Oxford University Press, Oxford, 1983

98. Johnson RH, Spalding JMK: The nervous control of the circulation and its investigation. p. 35. In Johnson RH, Spalding JMK (eds): Disorders of the Autonomic Nervous System. FA Davis, Philadelphia, 1974

99. Eckberg DL: Parasympathetic cardiovascular control in human disease: a critical review of methods and results. Am J Physiol H581, 1980

100. Low PA: Pitfalls in autonomic testing. p. 355. In Low PA (ed): Clinical Autonomic Disorders. Little, Brown, Boston, 1993

101. Bennett T, Hosking DJ, Hampton JR: Cardiovascular responses to graded reductions of central blood volume in normal subjects and in patients with diabetes mellitus. Clin Sci 58:193, 1980

102. Eckberg DL: Temporal response patterns of the human sinus node to brief carotid baroreceptor stimuli. J Physiol 258:769, 1976

103. Smyth HS, Sleight P, Pickering GW: Reflex regulation of arterial pressure during sleep in man: a quantitative method of assessing baroreflex sensitivity. Circ Res 24:109, 1969

104. Blomqvist CG, Stone HL: Cardiovascular adjustments to gravitational stress. p. 1025. In Shepherd JT, Abboud FM, Geiger SR (eds): Handbook of Physiology: The Cardiovascular System. Vol. 3. American Physiological Society, Bethesda, MD, 1983

105. Marin Neto JA, Gallo L Jr, Manco JC et al: Mechanisms of tachycardia on standing: studies in normal individuals and in chronic Chagas' heart patients. Cardiovasc Res 14:541, 1980

106. Bennett T: Physiological investigation of diabetic autonomic failure. p. 406. In Bannister R (ed): Autonomic Failure: A Textbook of Clinical Disorders of the

Autonomic Nervous System. Oxford University Press, Oxford, 1983

107. Fouad FM, Tarazi RC, Ferrario CM et al: Assessment of parasympathetic control of heart rate by a non-invasive method. Am J Physiol 246:H838, 1984

108. Wheeler T, Watkins PJ: Cardiac denervation of diabetics. Br Med J 4:584, 1973

109. Hilsted J, Jensen SB: A simple test for autonomic neuropathy in juvenile diabetics. Acta Med Scand 205:385, 1979

110. Smith SA: Reduced sinus arrhythmia in diabetic autonomic neuropathy: diagnostic value of an age-related normal range. Br Med J 285:1599, 1982

111. Wieling W, van Brederode JFM, de Rijk LG et al: Reflex control of heart rate in normal subjects in relation to age: a data base for cardiac vagal neuropathy. Diabetologia 22:163, 1982

112. Badian M, Appel E, Palm D et al: Standardized mental stress in healthy volunteers induced by delayed auditory feedback (DAF). Eur J Clin Pharmacol 16:171, 1979

113. Ferguson DW, Abboud FM, Mark AL: Relative contribution of aortic and carotid baroreflexes to heart rate control in man during steady state and dynamic increases in arterial pressure. J Clin Invest 76:2265, 1985

114. Sanders JS, Ferguson DW, Mark AL: Arterial baroreflex control of sympathetic nerve activity during elevation of blood pressure in normal man: dominance of aortic baroreflexes. Circulation 77:279, 1988

115. Hjemdahl P, Daleskog M, Kahan T: Determination of plasma catecholamines by high performance liquid chromatography with electrochemical detection: comparison with a radioenzymatic method. Life Sci 25:131, 1979

116. Esler M: Assessment of sympathetic nervous function in humans from noradrenaline plasma kinetics. Clin Sci 62:247, 1982

117. Esler M, Jackman G, Kelleher D et al: Norepinephrine kinetics in patients with idiopathic autonomic insufficiency. Circ Res 46(suppl. I):I47, 1980

118. Folkow B, Di Bona GF, Hjemdahl P et al: Measurements of plasma norep-

inephrine concentrations in human primary hypertension: a word of caution on their applicability for assessing neurogenic contributions. Hypertension 5:399, 1983

119. Goldstein DS, Lake CR, Chernow B et al: Age-dependence of hypertensive-normotensive differences in plasma norepinephrine. Hypertension 5:100, 1983

120. Robertson D, Johnson GA, Robertson RM et al: Comparative assessment of stimuli that release neuronal and adrenomedullary catecholamines in man. Circulation 59:637, 1979

121. Eckberg DL, Harkins SW, Fritsch JM et al: Baroreflex control of plasma norepinephrine and heart period in healthy subjects and diabetic patients. J Clin Invest 78:366, 1986

122. Brown MJ, Jenner DA, Allison DJ, Dollery CT: Variations in individual organ release of noradrenaline measured by an improved radioenzymatic technique: limitations of peripheral venous measurements in the assessment of sympathetic nervous activity. Clin Sci 61:585, 1981

123. Hayase S: Neurocirculatory asthenia—an approach to its pathogenesis. Jpn Heart J 9:431, 1968

124. Hageman GR, Goldberg JM, Armour JA, Randall WC: Cardiac dysrhythmias induced by autonomic nerve stimulation. Am J Cardiol 32:823, 1973

125. Hageman GR, Randall WC, Armour JA: Direct and reflex cardiac bradydysrhythmias from small vagal nerve stimulations. Am Heart J 89:338, 1975

126. Abildskov JA: The nervous system and cardiac arrhythmias. Circulation 51(suppl. III):III-116, 1975

127. Verrier RL, Lown B: Sympathetic-parasympathetic interactions and ventricular electrical stability. p. 75. In Schwartz PJ, Brown AM, Malliani A, Zanchetti A (eds): Neural Mechanisms in Cardiac Arrhythmias. Raven Press, New York, 1978

128. James TN, McLean WAH: Paroxysmal ventricular arrhythmias and familial sudden death associated with neural lesions in the heart. Chest 78:24, 1980

129. Blomqvist CG: Orthostatic hypotension. p. 1. In Parmley WW, Chatterjee K (eds): Cardiology. Vol. 1. JB Lippincott, Philadelphia, 1988

130. Hainsworth R: Fainting. p. 142. In Bannister R (ed): Autonomic Failure: A Textbook of Clinical Disorders of the Autonomic Nervous System, 2nd Ed. Oxford University Press, Oxford, 1988

131. Bannister R, Mathias C: Management of postural hypotension. p. 569. In Bannister R (ed): Autonomic Failure: A Textbook of Clinical Disorders of the Autonomic Nervous System, 2nd Ed. Oxford University Press, Oxford, 1988

132. Mayerson HS, Burch CE: Relationship of tissue (subcutaneous and intramuscular) and venous pressure to syncope induced in man by gravity. Am J Physiol 128:258, 1940

133. Buckey JC, Peshock RM, Blomqvist CG: Deep venous contribution to hydrostatic blood volume changes in the leg. Am J Cardiol 62:449, 1988

134. Henriksen O, Sejrsen P: Local reflex in neurocirculation in human skeletal muscle. Acta Physiol Scand 99:19, 1977

135. Streeten DHP, Auchincloss JH Jr, Anderson GH Jr et al: Orthostatic hypertension. Pathogenetic studies. Hypertension 7:196, 1985

136. Bannister R: Introduction and classification. p. 1. In Bannister R (ed): Autonomic Failure: A Textbook of Clinical Disorders of the Autonomic Nervous System, 2nd Ed. Oxford University Press, Oxford, 1988

137. Schatz IJ: Orthostatic Hypotension. FA Davis, Philadelphia, 1986

138. Low PA: Clinical Autonomic Disorders. Little, Brown, Boston, 1993

139. Streeten DHP: Orthostatic Disorders of the Circulation. Mechanisms, Manifestations and Treatment. Plenum, New York, 1987

140. Bannister R: Clinical features of autonomic failure. A. Symptoms, signs and special investigations. p. 267. In Bannister R (ed): Autonomic Failure: A Textbook of Clinical Disorders of the Autonomic Nervous System, 2nd Ed. Oxford University Press, Oxford, 1988

141. Chokroverty S: Sleep apnoea and respi-

ratory disturbances in multiple system atrophy with autonomic failure. p. 432. In Bannister R (ed): Autonomic Failure: A Textbook of Clinical Disorders of the Autonomic Nervous System, 2nd Ed. Oxford University Press, Oxford, 1988

142. Oppenheimer D: Neuropathology and neurochemistry of autonomic failure. p. 451. In Bannister R (ed): Autonomic Failure: A Textbook of Clinical Disorders of the Autonomic Nervous System, 2nd Ed. Oxford University Press, Oxford, 1988

143. Polinsky RJ: Neurotransmitter and neuropeptide function in autonomic failure. p. 321. In Bannister R (ed): Autonomic Failure: A Textbook of Clinical Disorders of the Autonomic Nervous System, 2nd Ed. Oxford University Press, Oxford, 1988

144. Bannister R, Mathias C: Management of postural hypotension. p. 569. In Bannister R (ed): Autonomic Failure: A Textbook of Clinical Disorders of the Autonomic Nervous System, 2nd Ed. Oxford University Press, Oxford, 1988

145. Polinsky RJ: Neurogenic orthostatic hypotension: concepts in diagnosis and management. IM 4:120, 1983

146. Onrot J, Goldberg MR, Hollister AS et al: Management of orthostatic hypotension. Am J Med 80:454, 1988

147. Paul S, Zygmunt D, Haile V et al: Chronic orthostatic hypotension. Compr Ther 14:58, 1988

148. Fealey RD, Robertson D: Management of orthostatic hypotension. p. 731. In Low PA (ed): Clinical Autonomic Disorders. Little, Brown, Boston, 1993

149. Wilcox CS, Aminoff MJ, Slater JDH: Sodium homeostasis in patients with autonomic failure. Clin Sci Mol Med 53:321, 1977

150. Hollister AS, Biaggioni I, Robertson D et al: Posture modulates plasma atrial natriuretic factor in orthostatic hypotensive patients, abstracted. Circulation 76 (suppl IV):IV-319, 1987

151. Onrot J, Goldberg MR, Biaggioni I et al: Hemodynamic and humoral effects of caffeine in human autonomic failure: therapeutic implications for postpran-

dial hypotension. N Engl J Med 313:549, 1985

152. Schatz IJ, Miller MJ, Frame B: Corticosteroids in the management of orthostatic hypotension. Cardiology 61 (suppl 1):280, 1976

153. Davies B, Bannister R, Sever P, Wilcox C: The pressor actions of nonadrenalin, angiotensin II and saralasin in chronic autonomic failure treated with fludrocortisone. Br J Clin Pharmacol 8:253, 1979

154. Davies B: Adrenergic receptors in autonomic failure. p. 174. In Bannister R (ed): Autonomic Failure: A Textbook of Clinical Disorders of the Autonomic Nervous System. Oxford University Press, Oxford, 1983

155. Schirger A, Sheps SG, Thomas JE, Fealey RD: Midodrine—a new agent in the management of idiopathic orthostatic hypotension and Shy Drager syndrome. Mayo Clin Proc 56:429, 1981

156. Jankovic J, Gilden JL, Hiner BC et al: Neurogenic orthostatic hypotension: a double blind, placebo-controlled study with midodrine. Am J Med 95:38, 1993

157. Bristow JD, Gribbin B, Hanour AJ et al: Diminished baroreflex sensitivity in high blood pressure and aging man. J Physiol 202:45P, 1969

158. Winson M, Heath D, Smith P: Extensibility of the human carotid sinus. Cardiovasc Res 8:58, 1974

159. Johnson RH, Smith AC, Spalding JMK, Wollner L: Effect of posture on blood pressure in elderly patients. Lancet 1:731, 1965

160. Caird FI, Andrews GR, Kennedy RD: Effect of posture on blood pressure in the elderly. Br Heart J 35:527, 1973

161. Wollner L, McCarthy ST, Soper NDW, Macy DJ: Failure of cerebral autoregulation as a cause of brain dysfunction in the elderly. Br Med J 1:1117, 1979

162. Convertino VA: Aerobic fitness, endurance training and orthostatic tolerance. Exerc Sport Sci Rev 15:223, 1987

163. Raven PB, Rohm-Young D, Blomqvist CG: Physical fitness and cardiovascular response to lower body negative pressure. J Appl Physiol 56:138, 1984

164. Whinnery JE: Acceleration tolerance of asymptomatic aircrew with mitral valve

prolapse. Aviat Space Environ Med 57:986, 1986

165. Gaffney FA, Nixon JV, Karlsson ES et al: Cardiovascular deconditioning produced by 20-hour bed rest with head-down tilt (−5°) in middle-aged men. Am J Cardiol 56:634, 1985

166. Coghlan HC, Irwin PK, Cowley MJ et al: Abnormal heart rate response in mitral valve prolapse syndrome: results with valsalva and tilt testing, abstracted. Clin Res 25:45A, 1977

167. Gaffney AF, Karlsson ES, Campbell W et al: Autonomic dysfunction in women with mitral valve prolapse syndrome. Circulation 59:894, 1979

168. Coghlan HC, Phares PK, Cowley MJ et al: Dysautonomia in mitral valve prolapse. Am J Med 67:236, 1979

169. Starr I: Ballistocardiographic studies of draftees rejected for neurocirculatory asthenia. War Med (Chicago) 5:155, 1944

170. Gaffney FA, Blomqvist CG: Mitral valve prolapse and autonomic nervous system dysfunction: a pathophysiological link. p. 447. In Boudoulas H, Wooley CF (eds): Mitral Valve Prolapse and the Mitral Valve Prolapse Syndrome. Futura Publishing, Mt. Kisco, NY, 1988

171. Boudoulas H, Reynolds JC, Mazzaferri E, Wooley CF: Metabolic studies in mitral valve prolapse syndrome. A neuroendocrine cardiovascular process. Circulation 61:1200, 1980

172. Bashore TM: Mitral valve prolapse syndrome: dynamic changes with exercise and posture. p. 465. In Boudoulas H, Wooley CF (eds): Mitral Valve Prolapse and the Mitral Valve Prolapse Syndrome. Futura Publishing, Mt. Kisco, NY, 1988

173. Bashore TM, Grines CL, Utlak D et al: Postural exercise abnormalities in symptomatic patients with mitral valve prolapse. J Am Coll Cardiol 11:499, 1988

174. Gaffney FA, Bastian BC, Lane B et al: Abnormal cardiovascular regulation in the mitral valve prolapse syndrome. Am J Cardiol 52:316, 1983

175. Weissman NJ, Shear MK, Kramer-Fox R, Devereaux RB: Contrasting patterns of autonomic dysfunction in patients with mitral valve prolapse and panic attacks. Am J Med 82:880, 1987

176. Santos AD, Mathew PK, Hilal A, Wallace A: Orthostatic hypotension: a commonly unrecognized cause of symptoms in mitral valve prolapse. Am J Med 71:746, 1981

177. Pasternac A, Latour JG, Leger-Gauthier C et al: Stability of hyperadrenergic state, atrial natriuretic factor and platelet abnormalities in mitral valve prolapse syndrome. p. 445. In Boudoulas H, Wooley CF (eds): Mitral Valve Prolapse and the Mitral Valve Prolapse Syndrome. Futura Publishing, Mt. Kisco, NY, 1988

178. Valeri DR, Altschule MD: Hypovolemic Anemia of Trauma: The Missing Blood Syndrome. CRC Press, Boca Raton, FL, 1981

179. Fouad FM, Tadena-Thome L, Bravo EL, Tarazi RC: Idiopathic hypovolemia. Ann Intern Med 104:298, 1986

180. Gaffney FA, Lane LB, Pettinger W, Blomqvist CG: Effects of clonidine administration on the hemodynamic and neuroendocrine postural responses in patients with dysautonomia. Chest 83S:436, 1983

181. Silverstein MD, Singer DE, Mulley AG et al: Patients with syncope admitted to medical intensive care units. JAMA 248:1185, 1982

182. Hess DS, Morady F, Scheinman MM: Electrophysiologic testing in the evaluation of patients with syncope of undetermined origin. Am J Cardiol 50:1309, 1982

183. Kapoor WN, Karpf M, Masher Y et al: Syncope of unknown origin. The need for a more cost-effective approach to its diagnostic evaluation. JAMA 247:2687, 1982

184. Kapoor WN, Karpf M, Wieand S et al: A prospective evaluation and follow-up of patients with syncope. N Engl J Med 309:197, 1983

185. Kenney RA, Ingram A, Bayliss J, Sutton R: Head-up tilt. A useful test for investigating unexplained syncope. Lancet 1:1352, 1986

186. Day SC, Cook EF, Funkenstein H,

Goldman L: Evaluation and outcome of emergency room patients with transient loss of consciousness. Am J Med 73:15, 1982

187. Gendelman HE, Linzer M, Gabelman M et al: Syncope in a general hospital patient population. NY State J Med 83:1161, 1983

188. Savage DD, Corwin L, McGee DL et al: Epidemiologic features of isolated syncope: the Framingham Study. Stroke 16:626, 1985

189. Grossi D, Nozzoli C, Roca M et al: Head-up tilt for triggering and diagnosing syncope. Funct Neurol 11:457, 1987

190. Abi-Samra F, Maloney JD, Fouad-Tarazi FM, Castle L: The usefulness of head-up tilt testing and hemodynamic investigations in the workup of syncope of unknown origin. PACE 11:1202, 1988

191. Almquist A, Goldenberg IF, Milstein S et al: Provocation of bradycardia and hypotension by isoproterenol and upright posture in patients with unexplained syncope. N Engl J Med 320:346, 1989

192. Strasberg B, Rechavia, E, Sagie A et al: The head-up tilt table test in patients with syncope of unknown origin. Am Heart J 118:923, 1989

193. Waxman MB, Yao L, Cameron DA: Isoproterenol induction of vasodepressor-type reaction in vasodepressor-prone persons. Am J Cardiol 63:58, 1989

194. Chen MY, Goldenberg IF, Milstein S et al: Cardiac electrophysiologic and hemodynamic correlates of neurally mediated syncope. Am J Cardiol 63:66, 1989

195. Fitzpatrick A, Sutton R: Tilting towards a diagnosis in recurrent unexplained syncope. Lancet 1:658, 1989

196. Raviele A, Gasparini G, DiPede F et al: Usefulness of head-up tilt test in evaluating patients with syncope of unknown origin and negative electrophysiologic study. Am J Cardiol 65:1322, 1990

197. Grubb BP, Temesy-Armos P, Hahn H, Elliott L: Utility of upright tilt-table testing in the evaluation and management of syncope of unknown origin. Am J Med 90:6, 1991

198. Fitzpatrick AP, Theodorakis G, Vardas P, Sutton R: Methodology of head-up tilt testing in patients with unexplained syncope. J Am Coll Cardiol 17:125, 1991

199. Brignole M, Menozzi C, Gianfranchi L et al: Carotid sinus massage, eyeball compression, and head-up tilt test in patients with syncope of uncertain origin and in healthy control subjects. Am Heart J 122:1644, 1991

200. Kapoor WN, Brant N: Evaluation of syncope by upright tilt testing with isoproterenol. A nonspecific test. Ann Intern Med 116:358, 1992

201. Thilenius OG, Quinones JA, Husayni TS, Novak J: Tilt test for diagnosis of unexplained syncope in pediatric patients. Pediatrics 87:334, 1991

202. Ross BA, Hughes S, Anderson E, Gillette P: Abnormal responses to orthostatic testing in children and adolescents with recurrent unexplained syncope. Am Heart J 122:748, 1991

203. Chen XC, ChenMY, Remole S et al: Reproducibility of head-up tilt-table testing for eliciting susceptibility to neurally mediated syncope in patients without structural heart disease. Am J Cardiol 69:755, 1992

204. Janosik D, Genovely H, Fredman C: Discrepancy between head-up tilt test results utilizing different protocols in the same patient. Am Heart J 123:538, 1992

205. Hackel A, Linzer M, Anderson N, Williams R: Cardiovascular and catecholamine responses to head-up tilt in the diagnosis of recurrent unexplained syncope in elderly patients. J Am Geriat Soc 39:663, 1991

206. Linzer M, Varia I, Pontinen M et al: Medically unexplained syncope: Relationships to psychiatric illness. Am J Med 92:1A18S, 1992

207. Maloney J, Jaeger F, Fouad-Tarazi F, Morris H: Malignant vasovagal syndrome: prolonged asystole provoked by head-up tilt. Cleve Clin J Med 55:542, 1988

208. Grubb BP, Temesy-Armos P, Moore J et al: Head-upright tilt-table testing in evaluation and management of the malignant vasovagal syndrome. Am J Cardiol 69:904, 1991

209. Foster M: Text Book of Physiology. Macmillan, London, 1888.

210. Lewis T: Vasovagal syncope and the carotid sinus mechanism with comments on Gower's and Nothnagel's syndrome. Br Med J 1:873, 1932

211. Epstein SE, Stampfer M, Beiser D: Role of capacitance and resistance vessels in vasovagal syncope. Circulation 37:524, 1968

212. Goldstein DS, Spanarkel M, Pitterman A et al: Circulatory control mechanisms in vasodepressor syncope. Am Heart J 104:1071, 1982

213. Verrill PJ, Aellig WH: Vasovagal faint in the supine position. Br Med J 4:348, 1970

214. Wallin BG, Sundlöf G: Sympathetic outflow to muscles during vasovagal syncope. J Autonom Nerv Syst 6:287, 1982

215. Ahmad M, Blomqvist CG, Mullins CB, Willerson JT: Left ventricular function during lower body negative pressure. Aviat Space Environ Med 48:512, 1977

216. Shalev Y, Gal R, Tchow PJ et al: Echocardiographic demonstration of decreased left ventricular dimensions and vigorous myocardial contraction during syncope induced by head-up tilt. J Am Coll Cardiol 18:746, 1991

217. Calkins H, Kadish A, Sousa J et al: Comparison of responses to isoproterenol and epinephrine during head-up tilt in suspected vasodepressor syncope. Am J Cardiol 67:207, 1991

218. Sandler H, Goldwater DJ, Popp RL et al: Beta blockade in the compensation for bed-rest cardiovascular deconditioning: physiologic and pharmacologic observations. Am J Cardiol 55:114D, 1985

219. Penfield W: Diencephalic autonomic epilepsy. Arch Neurol Psychiatry 22:358, 1929

220. Geoghegan T, Mueller EJ: Diencephalic autonomic attacks. Report of case with predominantly sympathetic manifestations. N Engl J Med 247:841, 1952

221. Metz SA, Halter JB, Porte D, Robertson RP: Autonomic epilepsy: clonidine blockage of paroxysmal catecholamine release and flushing. Ann Intern Med 88:189, 1978

222. Grubb BP, Gerard G, Roush K et al: Cerebral vasoconstriction during head-upright tilt-induced vasovagal syncope. A paradoxic and unexpected response. Circulation 84:1157, 1991

223. Aita JF: Facial color and syncope. JAMA 248:2238, 1982

224. Gastaut H, Fischer-Williams M: Electroencephalographic study of syncope: its differentiation from epilepsy. Lancet 2:1018, 1957

225. Lai CW, Ziegler DK: Syncope problem solved by continuous ambulatory simultaneous EEG/ECG recording. Neurology 31:1152, 1981

226. Kapoor W, Fortunato M, Sefcik T, Schulberg H. Psychiatric illnesses in patients with syncope, abstracted. Clin Res 37:316A, 1989

227. McLaran CJ, Gersh BJ, Osborn MJ et al: Increased vagal tone as an isolated finding in patients undergoing electrophysiological testing for recurrent syncope: response to long term anticholinergic agents. Br Heart J 55:53, 1986

228. Benditt DG, Benson DW Jr, Kreitt J et al: Electrophysiologic effects of theophylline in young patients with recurrent symptomatic bradyarrhythmias. Am J Cardiol 52:1223, 1983

229. Milstein S, Buetikofer J, Dunnigan A et al: Usefulness of disopyramide for prevention of upright tilt-induced hypotension-bradycardia. Am J Cardiol 65:1339, 1990

230. Tamboli HP, Sra JS, Jazayeri MR et al: Long term follow-up in patients with neurocardiogenic syncope treated with beta adrenergic blocker or disopyramide, abstracted. Circulation 82 (suppl III):III-708, 1990

231. Milstein S, Buetikofer J, Lesser J et al: Cardiac asystole. A manifestation of neurally mediated hypotension-bradycardia. J Am Coll Cardiol 14:1626, 1989

232. Engle GL: Psychologic stress, vasodepressor (vasovagal) syncope and sudden death. Ann Intern Med 89:403, 1987

233. Strasberg B, Sagie A, Erdman S et al: Carotid sinus hypersensitivity and the

carotid sinus syndrome. Prog Cardiovasc Dis 5:379, 1989

234. Sugrue DD, Gersh BJ, Holmes DR Jr et al: Symptomatic "isolated" carotid sinus hypersensitivity: natural history and results with anticholinergic drugs or pacemaker. J Am Coll Cardiol 7:158, 1986

235. McIntosh SJ, Lawson J, Kenny RA. Clinical characteristics of vasodepressor, cardioinhibitory, and mixed carotid sinus syndrome in the elderly. Am J Med 95:203, 1993

236. Tarlow E, Schmidek H, Scott RM et al: Reflex hypotension following carotid endarterectomy: mechanism and management. J Neurosurg 39:323, 1973

237. Angell-James JE, Lumley JSP: The effects of carotid endarterectomy on the mechanical properties of the carotid sinus and carotid sinus nerve activity in atherosclerotic patients. Br J Surg 61:805, 1974

238. Wallin BG, Westerberg CE, Sundlöf G: Syncope induced by glossopharyngeal neuralgia: sympathetic outflow to muscle. Neurology 24:522, 1984

239. Dykman TR, Montgomery EB Jr, Gerstenberger PD et al: Glossopharyngeal neuralgia with syncope secondary to tumor. Am J Med 71:165, 1981

240. Cicogna R, Bonomi FG, Ferretti C et al: Reflex cardiovascular syndromes involving the glossopharyngeal nerve. J Autonom Nerv Syst 30: S43, 1990

241. Fraioli B, Esposito V, Ferrante L et al: Microsurgical treatment of glossopharyngeal neuralgia: case reports. Neurosurgery 25:630, 1989

242. Jacobsen RR, Russell RWR: Glossopharyngeal neuralgia with cardiac arrhythmias: a rare but treatable cause of syncope. Br Med J 1:379, 1979

243. Appenzeller O, Marshall J: Vasomotor disturbances in the Guillain-Barré syndrome. Arch Neurol 9:368, 1968

244. Lichtenfeld P: Autonomic dysfunction in the Guillain-Barré syndrome. Am J Med 50:772, 1971

245. Mitchell PL, Meilman E: Mechanism of hypertension in the Guillain-Barré syndrome. Am J Med 42:986, 1965

246. Oakley CM: The heart in the Guillain-Barré syndrome. Br Med J 288:94, 1984

247. Palferman TG, Wright I, Doyle DV, Amiel S: Electrocardiographic abnormalities and autonomic dysfunction in Guillain-Barré syndrome. Br Med J 284:1231, 1982

248. Durocher A, Servais B, Caridroix M: Autonomic dysfunction in the Guillain-Barré syndrome. Hemodynamic and neurobiochemical studies. Intens Care Med 6:3, 1980

249. Fagius J, Wallin BG: Microneurographic evidence of excessive sympathetic outflow in the Guillain-Barré syndrome. Brain 106:589, 1983

250. Wheeler T, Watkins PJ: Cardiac denervation in diabetes. Br Med J 4:584, 1973

251. Sharpey-Schafer EP, Taylor PJ: Absent circulatory reflex in diabetic neuritis. Lancet 1:559, 1960

252. Sundkvist G: Autonomic nervous function in asymptomatic diabetic patients with signs of peripheral neuropathy. Diabetes Care 4:529, 1981

253. Pfeifer MA, Weinberg CR, Cook DL et al: Autonomic neural dysfunction in recently diagnosed diabetic subjects. Diabetes Care 7:447, 1984

254. Barzilay J, Warram JM, Rand LI et al: Risk of cardiovascular autonomic neuropathy is associated with the HLA-DR 3/4 phenotype in Type I diabetes mellitus. Ann Intern Med 116:544, 1992

255. Acharya DV, Shekhar YC, Aggarwal A, Anand IS: Lack of pain during myocardial infarction in diabetes—is autonomic dysfunction responsible. Am J Cardiol 68:793, 1991

256. Cryer PE, Silverberg AB, Santiago JV, Shah SD: Plasma catecholamines in diabetes. Am J Med 64:407, 1978

257. Ewing DJ, Clarke BF: Diabetic autonomic neuropathy: present insights and future prospects. Diabetes Care 9:648, 1986

258. Page MM, Watkins PJ: Cardiorespiratory arrest and diabetic autonomic neuropathy. Lancet 1:14, 1978

259. Grassi GM, Somers VK, Renk WS et al: Effects of alcohol intake on blood pres-

sure and sympathetic nerve activity in normotensive humans: a preliminary report. J Hypertens 7 (suppl 6):S20, 1989

260. Klatsky AL, Armstrong MA, Friedman GD: Alcohol and cardiovascular deaths, abstracted. Circulation 80 (suppl II): II-614, 1989

261. Duncan G, Johnson RH, Lambie DG, Whiteside EA: Evidence of vagal neuropathy in chronic alcoholics. Lancet 2:1053, 1980

262. Johnson RH, Robinson BJ: Mortality in alcoholics with autonomic neuropathy. J Neurol Neurosurg Psychiatry 5:476, 1988

263. Lilley JJ, Golden J, Stone RA: Adrenergic regulation of blood pressure in chronic renal failure. J Clin Invest 57:1190, 1976

264. Kersh ES, Kronfield SJ, Unger A et al: Autonomic insufficiency in uremia as a cause of hemodialysis-induced hypotension. N Engl J Med 290:650, 1974

265. Nies AS, Robertson D, Stone WJ: Hemodialysis hypotension is not the result of uremic peripheral autonomic neuropathy. J Lab Clin Med 94:395, 1979

266. Hendrickse MT, Thuluvath PJ, Tiger DR: Natural history of autonomic neuropathy in chronic liver disease. Lancet 339:1462, 1992

267. Thulervath PJ, Tiger DR: Autonomic neuropathy in chronic liver disease. Q J Med 72:737, 1989

268. Satchell PM: Pathophysiology of the vagus. p. 159. In Bannister R (ed): Autonomic Failure: A Textbook of Clinical Disorders of the Autonomic Nervous System, 2nd Ed. Oxford University Press, New York, 1988

269. Tan ETH, Johnson RH, Lambie DG, Whiteside EA: Alcoholic vagal neuropathy: recovery following prolonged abstinence. J Neurol Neurosurg Psychiatry 47:1335, 1984

270. Child JS, Perloff JK, Bach PM et al: Cardiac involvement in Friedreich's ataxia: a clinical study of 75 patients. J Am Coll Cardiol 7:1370, 1986

271. James TN, Cobbs BW, Coghlan HC et al: Coronary disease, cardioneuropathy,

and conduction system abnormalities in the cardiomyopathy of Friedreich's ataxia. Br Heart J 57:446, 1987

272. Margalith D, Dunn HG, Carter JE, Wright JM: Friedreich's ataxia with dysautonomia and labile hypertension. Can J Neurol Sci 11:73, 1984

273. Abildskov JA: Adrenergic effects of the QT interval of the electrocardiogram. Am Heart J 92:210, 1976

274. Roberts NK, Perloff JK, Kark P: Cardiac conduction in Kearns-Sayre syndrome. Am J Cardiol 44:1396, 1979

275. Clark DS, Myerburg RJ, Morales RR et al: Heart block and Kearns-Sayre: electrophysiologic-pathologic correlation. Chest 68:727, 1975

276. Miller G, D'Orsogna L, O'Shea JP: Autonomic function and the sinus tachycardia of Duchenne muscular dystrophy. Brain Dev 11:247, 1989

277. Perloff JK: Cardiac rhythm and conduction in Duchenne muscular dystrophy. J Am Coll Cardiol 3:1263, 1984

278. Grigg LE, Chan W, Mond HG et al: Ventricular tachycardia and sudden death in myotonic distrophy: clinical electrophysiologic and pathologic features. Am J Cardiol 6:254, 1985

279. Cushing H: Some experimental and clinical observations concerning states of increased intracranial tension. Am J Med Sci 124:375, 1902

280. Thompson RK, Malina S: Dynamic axial brain-stem distortion as a mechanism explaining the cardio-respiratory change in increased intracranial pressure. J Neurosurg 16:664, 1959

281. Wallace JD, Levy LL: Blood pressure after stroke. JAMA 246:2177, 1981

282. Doshi R, Neil-Dwyer G: A clinicopathological study of patients following a subarachnoid hemorrhage. J Neurosurg 52:295, 1980

283. Yamour BJ, Sridharam MR, Rice JF, Flowers NC: Electrocardiographic changes in cerebrovascular hemorrhage. Am Heart J 99:294, 1980

284. McLeod AA, Neil-Dwyer G, Meyer CHA et al: Cardiac sequelae of acute head injury. Br Heart J 47:221, 1982

285. Myers MG, Norris JW, Hachinski VC et

al: Cardiac sequelae of acute stroke. Stroke 13:838, 1982

286. Samuels MA: Electrocardiographic manifestations of neurologic disease. Semin Neurol 4:453, 1984

287. Tobias SL, Bookatz BJ, Diamond TH: Myocardial damage and electrocardiographic changes in acute cerebrovascular hemorrhage. A report of three cases and review. Heart Lung 16:521, 1987

288. Goldberger AL. Recognition of ECG pseudoinfarct patterns. Mod Concepts. Cardiovasc Dis 49:13, 1980

289. Taylor AL, Fozzard HA: Ventricular arrhythmias associated with CNS disease. Arch Intern Med 142:232, 1982

290. Carruth JE, Silverman ME: Torsades de pointes atypical ventricular tachycardia complicating subarachnoid hemorrhage. Chest 78:886, 1980

291. Pollick C, Cujec B, Parker S, Tator C: Left ventricular wall motion abnormalities in subarachnoid hemorrhage: an echocardiographic study. J Am Coll Cardiol 12:600, 1988

292. Schell AR, Shenoy MM, Friedman SA, Patel AR: Pulmonary edema associated with subarachnoid hemorrhage. Arch Intern Med 147:591, 1987

293. Fredberg U, Bötker HE, Römer FK: Acute neurogenic pulmonary edema following generalized tonic clonic seizure. A case report and a review of the literature. Eur Heart J 9:933, 1988

294. Oppenheimer SM, Cechetto DF, Hachinski VC: Cerebrogenic cardiac arrhythmias. Arch Neurol 47:513, 1990

295. Lathers CM, Schraeder PL: Autonomic dysfunction in epilepsy: characterization of autonomic cardiac neural discharge associated with pentylenetetrazol-induced epileptogenic activity. Epilepsia 23:633, 1982

296. Walter P, Neil-Dwyer G, Cruickshank JM: Beneficial effects of adrenergic blockade in patients with subarachnoid hemorrhage. Br Med J 284:1661, 1982

297. Wilson RF, Christensen BV, Olivari MT: Evidence for structural sympathetic reinnervation after orthotopic cardiac transplantation in humans. Circulation 83:1210, 1991

298. Kent KM, Cooper T: The denervated heart: a model for studying autonomic control of the heart. N Engl J Med 291:1017, 1974

299. Epstein AE, Hirschowitz BI, Kirklin JW et al: Evidence for a central site of action to explain the negative chronotropic effect of atropine: studies on the human transplanted heart. J Am Coll Cardiol 15:1610, 1990

300. Kavanagh T, Jacoub MH, Martens DJ et al: Cardiorespiratory responses to exercise training after orthotopic cardiac transplantation. Circulation 77:162, 1988

301. Borow KM, Neumann AA, Arensman FW, Jacobs MH: Cardiac and peripheral vascular responses to adrenoceptor stimulation and blockage after cardiac transplantation. J Am Coll Cardiol 14:1229, 1989

302. Shepherd JT, Vanhoutte PM: Nervous control. Cardiac denervation. p. 264. In Shepherd JT, Vanhoutte PM (eds): The Human Cardiovascular System. Facts and Concepts. Raven Press, New York, 1979

303. Mott KE, Hagstrom JWC: The pathologic lesions of the cardiac autonomic nervous system in chronic Chagas' myocarditis. Circulation 31:273, 1965

304. Oliveira JSM: A natural human model of intrinsic heart nervous system denervation. Chagas' cardiomyopathy. Am Heart J 110:1092, 1985

305. Amorim DS, Olsen EGJ: Assessment of heart neurons in dilated (congestive) cardiomyopathy. Br Heart J 47:11, 1982

306. Dzau VJ, Colucci WS, Hollenberg NK, Williams GH: Relationship of the renin-angiotensin-aldosterone system to clinical state in congestive heart failure. Circulation 63:645, 1981

307. Goldsmith SR, Francis GS, Cowley AW Jr et al: Increased plasma arginine vasopressin levels in patients with congestive heart failure. J Am Coll Cardiol 1:1385, 1983

308. Leimbach WN, Wallin BG, Victor RG et al: Direct evidence from intraneural recordings for increased central sympa-

thetic outflow in patients with heart failure. Circulation 73:913, 1986

309. Packer M: Neurohumoral interactions and adaptations in congestive heart failure. Circulation 77:721, 1988

310. Chidsey CA, Harrison DC, Braunwald E: Augmentation of the plasma norepinephrine response to exercise in patients with congestive heart failure. N Engl J Med 267:650, 1962

311. Lewis SF, Taylor WF, Graham RM et al: Cardiovascular responses to exercise as functions of absolute and relative work loads. J Appl Physiol 54:1314, 1983

312. Ferguson DW, Abboud FM, Mark AL: Selective impairment of baroreflex-mediated vasoconstrictor responses in patients with ventricular dysfunction. Circulation 69:451, 1984

313. Colucci WS, Rebeiro JP, Rocco MB et al: Impaired chronotropic response to exercise in patients with congestive heart failure. Role of postsynaptic beta-adrenergic desensitization. Circulation 80:314, 1989

314. Kubo SH, Rector TS, Heaifetz SM, Cohn JN: a_2-Receptor-mediated vasoconstriction in patients with congestive heart failure. Circulation 80:1660, 1989

315. Leier CV, Binkley PF, Cody RJ: a-Adrenergic component of the sympathetic nervous system in congestive heart failure. Circulation 82(suppl I):I-68, 1990

316. Higgins CB, Vatner SF, Millard RW et al: Alterations in regional hemodynamics in experimental heart failure in conscious dogs. Trans Assoc Am Physicans 85:267, 1972

317. Bristow MR: The adrenergic nervous system in heart failure. N Engl J Med 311:850, 1984

318. Heilbrunn SM, Shah P, Bristow MR et al: Increased beta-receptor density and improved hemodynamic response to catecholamine stimulation during long-term metoprolol therapy in heart failure from dilated cardiomyopathy. Circulation 79:483, 1989

319. Schofer J, Tews A, Langes K et al: Relationship between myocardial norepinephrine content and left ventricular function—an endomyocardial biopsy study. Eur Heart J 8:748, 1987

320. Schofer J, Spielman R, Schuchert A et al: Iodine-123 metaiodobenzylguanidine scintigraphy: a noninvasive method to demonstrate myocardial adrenergic nervous system disintegrity in patients with idiopathic dilated cardiomyopathy. J Am Coll Cardiol 12:1252, 1988

321. Eckberg DL, Drabinsky M, Braunwald E: Defective cardiac parasympathetic control in patients with heart disease. N Engl J Med 285:877, 1971

322. Higgins CB, Vatner SF, Eckberg DL, Braunwald E: Alterations in the baroreceptor reflex in conscious dogs with heart failure. J Clin Invest 51:715, 1972

323. Saul JP, Arai Y, Berger RD et al: Assessment of autonomic regulation in chronic congestive heart failure by heart rate spectral analysis. Am J Cardiol 61:1292, 1988

324. Cohn JN, Levine TB, Olivari MT et al: Plasma norepinephrine as a guide to prognosis in patients with chronic congestive heart failure. N Engl J Med 311:819, 1984

325. Loffenholz K, Pappano AJ: The parasympathetic neuroeffector junction of the heart. Pharmacol Rev 37:1, 1985

326. Dargie HJ, Cleland JG, Leckie BJ et al: Relation of arrhythmias and electrolyte abnormalities to survival in patients with severe chronic heart failure. Circulation 75:98, 1987

327. Seelig M: Cardiovascular consequences of magnesium deficiency and loss: pathogenesis, prevalence and manifestations—magnesium and chloride loss in refractory potassium repletion. Am J Cardiol 63:4G, 1989

328. Brown MJ, Brown DC, Murphy MB: Hypokalemia from beta$_2$-receptor stimulation by circulating epinephrine. N Engl J Med 309:1414, 1983

329. Dyckner T, Wester PO: Potassium/magnesium depletion in patients with cardiovascular disease. Am J Med 82:(suppl 3A):11 1987

330. Webb SA, Adgey AAJ, Pantridge JF: Autonomic disturbances at onset of acute myocardial infarction. Br Med J 3:89, 1972

331. Pantridge JF: Autonomic disturbances at the onset of acute myocardial infarc-

tion. p. 7. In Schwartz PJ, Brown AM, Malliani A, Zanchetti A (eds): Neural Mechanisms in Cardiac Arrhythmias. Raven Press, New York, 1978

332. James TN, Isobe JH, Urthaler F: Analysis of components in a cardiogenic hypertension chemoreflex. Circulation 52:179, 1975

333. James TN, Urthaler F, Hageman GR, Isobe JH: Further analysis of components in a cardiogenic hypertensive chemoreflex. p. 251. In Schwartz PJ, Brown AM, Malliani A, Zanchetti A (eds): Neural Mechanisms in Cardiac Arrhythmias. Raven Press, New York, 1978

334. Perez-Gomez F, Garcia-Aguado A: Origin of ventricular reflexes caused by coronary arteriography. Br Heart J 39:967, 1977

335. Eckberg DL, White CW, Kioschos JM, Abboud FM: Mechanisms mediating bradycardia during coronary arteriography. J Clin Invest 54:1445, 1974

336. Wei JY, Markis JE, Malagold M, Braunwald E: Cardiovascular reflexes stimulated by reperfusion of ischemic myocardium in acute myocardial infarction. Circulation 67:796, 1983

337. Thames MD, Waickman LA, Abboud FM: Sensitization of cardiac receptors (vagal afferents) by intracoronary acetylstrophanthidin. Am J Physiol 239: H628, 1980

338. Come PC, Pitt B: Nitroglycerin-induced severe hypotension and bradycardia in patients with acute myocardial infarction. Circulation 54:624, 1976

339. Cooper MJ, Abinader MG: Atropine-induced ventricular fibrillation: a case report and review of the literature. Am Heart J 97:225, 1979

340. Massumi RA, Mason DT, Amsterdam EA et al: Ventricular fibrillation and tachycardia after intravenous atropine for treatment of bradycardias. N Engl J Med 287:336, 1972

341. Schweitzer P, Mack H: The effect of atropine on cardiac arrhythmias and conduction. Am Heart J 100:255, 1980

342. Malliani A, Schwartz PJ, Zanchetti A: A sympathetic reflex elicited by experimental coronary occlusion. Am J Physiol 217:703, 1969

343. Straszewska-Barczak J: The reflex stimulation of catecholamine secretion during the acute stage of myocardial infarction in the dog. Clin Sci 41:419, 1971

344. Bertel O, Bühler FR, Baitsch G et al: Plasma adrenaline and noradrenaline in patients with acute myocardial infarction. Chest 82:64, 1982

345. Kolman BS, Verrier RL, Lown B: The effect of vagus nerve stimulation upon vulnerability of the canine ventricle; role of sympathetic-parasympathetic interactions. Circulation 52:578, 1975

346. Lown B, Verrier RL: Neural activity and ventricular fibrillation. N Engl J Med 294:1165, 1976

347. Lombardi F, Sandrone G, Pernpruner M et al: Sympatho-vagal interaction in the first year after myocardial infarction, abstracted. Circulation 72(suppl III): III-242, 1985

348. Kleiger RE, Miller JP, Bigger JT et al: Decreased heart rate variability and its association with increased mortality after acute myocardial infarction. Am J Cardiol 59:256, 1987

349. Zipes D: Cardiac innervation and its importance in the genesis of some cardiac arrhythmias. p. 1. In Rackley CE (ed): Challenges in Cardiology I. Futura Publishing, Mount Kisco, NY, 1992

350. Randall WC, Thomas JX, Euler DE, Rozanski GJ: Cardiac dysrhythmias associated with autonomic nervous system imbalance in the conscious dog. p. 123. In Schwartz PJ, Brown AM, Malliani A, Zanchetti A (eds): Neural Mechanisms in Cardiac Arrhythmias. Raven Press, New York, 1978

351. Rossi L: Neuroanatomopathology of the cardiovascular system. In Kulbertus HE, Franck G (eds): Neurocardiology. p. 25. Futura Publishing, Mount Kisco, NY, 1988

11

Cardiovascular Consequences of AIDS

Judith Hsia

Reports of an acquired syndrome of immune deficiency in young homosexual men appeared in the summer of 1981,[1,2] harbingers of a disease that has since generated widespread fear in the international community and has had a serious adverse impact on health care costs in the United States and around the world. Soon thereafter, the etiologic agent of the acquired immunodeficiency syndrome (AIDS), the human immunodeficiency virus type 1 (HIV), was identified[3] and isolated.[4] Despite the rapid identification and characterization of HIV, international efforts to prevent or slow dissemination of the virus have met with modest success. As the AIDS pandemic enters its second decade, the rate of increase in AIDS cases reported to the Centers for Disease Control is slowing; however, about one-half million United States residents have been diagnosed with AIDS; three-quarters of them have died.[5]

Worldwide, the disease now predominantly affects heterosexuals, particularly in developing countries; the World Health Organization estimates that 9 to 11 million adults have been infected by HIV; 3 to 5 million are women. In some sub-Saharan nations, the prevalence of HIV infection in adults is thought to be 15 to 20 percent; by conservative estimates 15 to 20 million people will be infected with HIV by the turn of the century.[6]

Clearly any disease entity as widespread as HIV infection that has so dramatically captured public attention will be the focus of research efforts in the medical community. During the first decade of the AIDS pandemic, substantial resources were directed toward the study and management of manifestations of HIV infection. HIV affects virtually every organ, and the cardiovascular system is no exception; endocrine, renal, pulmonary, and other manifestations of HIV infection may secondarily affect the heart as well.

The peak incidence of new AIDS cases is expected in the mid-1990s, and AIDS will inevitably remain a major disease problem in the United States for years to come in view of the steady rise in heterosexual transmission. Presumably, these increases in numbers of AIDS cases will lead to parallel increases in HIV-associated heart disease.

PATHOLOGY

In evaluating reports of clinical manifestations of HIV infection, it is helpful to bear in mind two aspects of the disease that have evolved substantially during the past 12 years: (1) the epidemiologic shift from a disease predominantly affecting homosexuals to one including increasing numbers of intravenous drug users and heterosexuals and (2) the switch from diagnosis by purely clinical criteria[7] to use of sensitive molecular biologic methods such as the polymerase chain reaction. Diagnostic criteria have inevitably affected the descriptions of sequelae of HIV infection. Pathologic findings in hearts of patients dying with HIV infection are summarized in Table 11-1.

Kaposi's Sarcoma and Lymphoma

The initial description of cardiac findings at necropsy in 10 subjects was included in a report from the National Institutes of Health published prior to identification of the etiologic agent of AIDS.[8] Since serologic testing was not yet available, diagnosis at that time was based on clinical criteria defined by the Centers for Disease Control; thus opportunistic infections and Kaposi's sarcoma figured prominently in the case descriptions. Cardiac involvement was confined to epicardial Kaposi's sarcoma, and no infectious organisms were identified. The hearts of all 10 subjects (8 homosexuals, 1 intravenous drug user, and 1 Haitian) were normal in size, and none of the patients had symptoms referable to the heart during life. In a later report the same investigators found Kaposi's sarcoma involving the heart in 5 of 18 patients with AIDS, none with apparent cardiac dysfunction.[9]

The next several necropsy series were

Table 11-1. Cardiac Pathology in HIV Infection

Malignancies
  Kaposi's sarcoma
  Lymphoma
Endocarditis
  Marantic (nonbacterial thrombotic)
  Infectious due to bacteria or *Aspergillus*
Cardiomyopathy
  Right ventricular dilation/hypertrophy
  Biventricular dilation with or without
    myocarditis
Myocarditis
  Lymphocytic infiltration with myocardial necrosis without identification of potential pathogen
  Lymphocytic infiltration with concurrent identification of *Mycobacterium tuberculosis* or *avium intracellulare*, *Pneumocystis carinii*, *Candida albicans*, *Coccidioides immitis*, *Toxoplasma gondii*, *Cryptococcus neoformans*, *Aspergillus fumigatus*, *Histoplasma capsulatum*, HIV, cytomegalovirus, herpes simplex, coxsackievirus
Pericardial disease.
  Fibrinous pericarditis without identified pathogen
  Infectious pericarditis with *Staphylococcus aureus*, *Mycobacterium tuberculosis* or *avium intracellular*, herpes simplex, *Histoplasma capsulatum*, *Cryptococcus neoformans*, *Nocardia*
  Malignant pericarditis
  Pericardial effusion without identified pathogen
Myocardial fibrosis without lymphocytic infiltration

from California. As of June, 1983, about 80 deaths attributable to AIDS had been reported in the San Francisco Bay area, 36 (45 percent) of which were included in an autopsy series.[10] The group included 2 children and 34 men, 32 of whom were known to be homosexual. No cardiovascular abnormalities were identified in the children. Among the adults, (average age, 39 years), two hearts had acute myocardial necrosis and six others showed focal interstitial fibrosis. Kaposi's sarcoma involved the heart in three and the aorta in two others, consistent with the previous reports. Significant numbers of AIDS cases were occurring in the Los Angeles area as well during the early 1980s. Cardiac involvement was found in 10 of 41 autopsies on patients dying of AIDS,[11] 9 of whom were homosexual and one Haitian. Kaposi's sarcoma was identified in four hearts, nonbacterial thrombotic endocarditis in three, cryptococcal myocarditis in one, and isolated fibrinous pericarditis in two. Despite disseminated *Mycobacterium avium intracellulare* infection in 13 of the 41 subjects, no acid-fast organisms were detected in the myocardium.

The definition of AIDS at that time required either opportunistic infection or unusual malignancy; thus, the frequency with which Kaposi's sarcoma was detected at autopsy is not surprising. In reports published after the identification of HIV as the causative agent of AIDS and the development of serologic tests to diagnose HIV infection, the proportion of AIDS patients dying with Kaposi's sarcoma involving the heart has been 5 to 10 percent.[12–14]

Although Kaposi's sarcoma was the predominant malignancy involving the heart in these early reports, lymphoma, the other malignancy defining AIDS, has been identified as well.[15–20] In two cases reported by Balasubramanyam et al.,[15] the heart was the primary site of tumor involvement, and both patients had symptomatic cardiac dysfunction. The first patient had a pericardial effusion, and gated blood pool scan antemortem showed inferior wall akinesis. The second patient had both supraventricular and ventricular arrhythmias and subsequently developed complete heart block. In both cases, large intramyocardial and subendocardial tumor masses were found. More commonly, the heart is one of several sites involved with lymphoma. Symptoms have ranged from none to sudden death,[21] and have included a range of arrhythmias, pericarditis, cardiac tamponade, and congestive heart failure.

Myocarditis and Pericarditis

The spectrum of cardiac pathology in early reports of AIDS appeared fairly narrow among homosexuals; as autopsy findings of patients with other risk factors for AIDS were reported, a wider range of cardiac pathology became apparent. An autopsy series on 54 residents of the Miami area dying of AIDS before December, 1983, included intravenous drug users, Haitians, and a hemophiliac, as well as homosexual men. This group differed from previous autopsy series in detecting frequent myocarditis.[12] Lymphocytic infiltration with or without myocardial necrosis was observed in 11, and tachyzoites of *Toxoplasma gondii* in 6 with adjacent myocardial necrosis.

The relationship between AIDS and myocarditis has been complicated by evolving criteria for pathologic diagnosis of myocarditis,[22] but it received widespread recognition following two reports of 26 and 71 consecutive autopsies from Milan and Washington, DC in which myocarditis was found in 35 percent and 52 percent, respectively.[13,23] The inflammatory stimulus in HIV-associated myocarditis remains controversial. A variety of pathogens were identified in myocardial sections, including acid-fast bacilli, gram-positive cocci, *Toxoplasma gondii*, *Histoplasma capsulatum*, and characteristic cytomegaloviral inclusion bodies. In most cases, however, the inflammatory stimulus was unclear. Other pathogens reported in heart tissue of HIV-infected individuals include *Cryp-*

tococcus neoformans,[24,25] coxsackievirus,[26] *Candida,*[14,27] *Mycobacterium tuberculosis*[28] and *avium intracellulare,*[29,30] *Sarcosporidium,*[23] *Coccidioides immitis, Pneumocystis carinii,* herpes simplex,[31] and the HIV itself.[33–35]

The possibility that observed myocarditis was attributable to intravenous drug use rather than HIV infection was raised in light of suggestive differences in myocarditis prevalence in differing risk groups. This hypothesis can be assessed by comparing the frequency of lymphocytic infiltrates in intravenous drug users with and without AIDS. Microscopic examination of the heart from 15 HIV-seronegative intravenous drug users revealed active myocarditis in a third and borderline myocarditis in another third.[36] The frequency of myocarditis in association with HIV infection has varied from a few percent[14] to Anderson et al.'s[13] report of 52 percent. The proportion of intravenous drug users in these series is variable, and depends to a great extent on the accuracy of risk factor reporting. Myocarditis has certainly been identified in HIV-infected patients who were not intravenous drug users,[37] but its appearance in hearts of HIV-infected subjects may be linked significantly to intravenous drug use. In children, myocarditis with and without identifiable pathogens has been identified as well.[38,39] Epicarditis and vasculitis have also been reported, particularly involving the conduction system,[39] findings that appear to differ from those in adults.

Isolated fibrinous pericarditis was reported in 1985 in two AIDS patients without apparent cardiac infection or malignancy.[11] In autopsy series, pericarditis has been observed in both the presence and absence of infectious agents; culprit organisms have included *Mycobacterium tuberculosis,*[40] *Staphylococcus,*[41] and herpes simplex.[42] When reports of autop-sies were pooled, pericardial effusions were detected in 64 percent.[14]

Endocarditis

Both marantic and infectious endocarditis have been observed in autopsy studies of patients with AIDS.[11,14] Marantic endocarditis commonly involved multiple valves, and in some cases, it was associated with systemic embolization.

Although infectious endocarditis might be anticipated in an immunosuppressed population that includes significant numbers of intravenous drug users, it has turned out to be uncommon. Occasional reports of bacterial and fungal endocarditis have appeared.[14,43] In contrast, nearly one-half of 168 opiate addicts without AIDS had active or healed infectious endocarditis.[44] The pathophysiologic basis for this paradox is unknown.

Cardiomyopathy

Dilated cardiomyopathy, which has turned out to be an important clinical entity, was not mentioned in pathologic reports during the early years of the AIDS era. Right ventricular hypertrophy, which might be anticipated in view of the frequent pulmonary complications in HIV infection, was initially reported in 1984[45]; biventricular dilatation with clinical cardiomyopathy was reported in 1986 in adults[46] and subsequently in children.[47,48] Subsequent large series found dilated cardiomyopathy in 2 of 115 autopsies,[14] none of 96,[49] and 3 of 58.[50] Thus, from past reports, cardiomyopathy does not appear to be a leading cause of death among individuals dying from complications of HIV infection. As prevention and treatment of infectious complications improves, cardiomyopathy may figure more prominently. Certainly echocardiographic studies suggest that the frequency of cardiac dysfunction is higher than it has appeared from autopsy series.

To summarize, the pathologic findings in the hearts of HIV-infected individuals include Kaposi's sarcoma, lymphoma, pericarditis, myocarditis (particularly among intravenous drug users), a variety of pathogens that may or may not cause tissue damage, right ventricular hypertrophy, dilated cardiomyopathy, and marantic as well as (rarely) infective endocarditis.

CLINICAL MANIFESTATIONS

Despite the pathologic evidence of cardiac involvement in AIDS, a minority of the patients included in autopsy studies died from cardiac complications. Reports of clinical heart disease in HIV infection lagged behind the autopsy studies by several years; the initial report of congestive cardiomyopathy in a patient with AIDS appeared in 1986.[46]

Subsequent reports have broadened the range of clinical manifestations of heart disease in AIDS to include congestive cardiomyopathy, ventricular and supraventricular arrhythmias, endocarditis, intracardiac masses and abscesses, and pericardial tamponade (Table 11-2). Women remain significantly understudied[51] despite the rise in both absolute numbers and proportion of women among seropositive adults.[52] Women comprised 16 percent of new reported cases of AIDS in 1992,[53] yet most clinical information about heart disease associated with HIV infection is based on studies in men. Cardiac sequelae of HIV infection appear to differ in adults and children, conduction system abnor-

Table 11-2.   Cardiac Manifestations of HIV Infection

In adults
   Congestive cardiomyopathy with or without associated arrhythmia
   Pericardial effusion and cardiac tamponade due to infection, malignancy or unknown cause
   Intracardiac masses with or without obstruction
   Endocarditis, infectious and noninfectious
   Arrhythmias without cardiomyopathy (heart block, supraventricular and ventricular tachycardia, and sudden death)

In children
   Congestive cardiomyopathy
   Pericardial effusion
   Arrhythmia (heart block, ventricular and supraventricular tachycardia)

malities being more prominent in the latter.

Cardiomyopathy

Ventricular dysfunction associated with HIV infection includes (1) impaired left ventricular systolic function, (2) abnormal diastolic function, and (3) right ventricular abnormalities.

Left Ventricular Dysfunction
Following the initial report of cardiomyopathy by Cohen et al.,[54] a number of case reports reinforced the view that this was a definite manifestation of HIV infection, not an unrelated event.[55,56] The prevalence of cardiomyopathy was initially assessed through retrospective analysis of hospitalized patients. An early report on patients diagnosed by clinical criteria prior to 1984 included predominantly homosexuals, three intravenous drug users, and a Haitian woman. Three

patients had echocardiographic, but apparently not clinical, evidence of left ventricular dysfunction.[57] At that time the National Institutes of Health was following a large number of HIV-infected individuals and reported clinical cardiac manifestations in a group of predominantly homosexual men studied from 1981 to 1986.[50] Congestive heart failure was reported in 4 of 58 patients from that study group undergoing autopsy, all of whom met the Dallas criteria for myocarditis.[22] One of these patients died from cardiac decompensation and the others from infectious complications. An additional noteworthy observation was that 22 other patients had myocarditis without clinical heart failure.

A group of patients that included 40 percent intravenous drug users and eight women, underwent echocardiography between 1983 and 1986. The group was reported on jointly from Paris and from a Miami Veterans Administration Hospital.[58] Echocardiographic wall motion abnormalities were detected in 13 of 86 (15 percent), although it was not apparent that any had clinical heart failure.

Prospective echocardiography of consecutive hospitalized patients identified low shortening fraction in 9 of 60 HIV-seropositive subjects (15 percent) in Washington, DC.[59] Systolic dysfunction was more common among patients with AIDS than those without prior AIDS-defining illnesses (that is, opportunistic infection or characteristic malignancy). In a comparable group of consecutive hospitalized patients referred for echocardiography in San Francisco, 8 of 25 (32 percent) had dilated cardiomyopathy; clinical congestive heart failure was diagnosed and treated in 4.[60] In contrast, none of 45 outpatients from the same community referred for echocardiography had ventricular dysfunction. These findings underscored the limitations of studies including only hospitalized patients re-

ferred for diagnostic procedures because of suggestive symptoms, but also supported the value of echocardiography in hospitalized HIV-infected patients with cardiorespiratory symptoms. Especially during the early years of the HIV epidemic, opportunistic pneumonia was the primary consideration in HIV-infected patients with dyspnea, which may have resulted in treatment delay and unnecessary bronchoscopy in those with congestive heart failure.

The importance of congestive cardiomyopathy in HIV infection is best assessed through prospective follow-up of patients without heart disease. In one such study, during 22-month follow-up of 256 HIV-infected subjects in Washington, DC who started out with normal echocardiograms, left ventricular dilatation developed in 22 (9 percent) and clinical cardiomyopathy in 8 (3 percent).[61] Figure 11-1 shows serial evaluation of left ventricular contractility over a 2-year interval in an asymptomatic HIV-infected man.

Congestive cardiomyopathy is a problem in HIV-infected children as well as adults.[62] Among 31 pediatric patients reported from Boston, symptomatic dilated cardiomyopathy was observed in 4,[63] a finding similar to that reported by others.[38] During serial follow-up of HIV-infected children, progressive left ventricular dilatation was observed with compensatory hypertrophy. Hypertrophy appeared inadequate to maintain wall stress, resulting in impaired ventricular performance. Many children with echocardiographic abnormalities, however, did not have symptomatic congestive heart failure.[64]

Diastolic Dysfunction

Diastolic dysfunction developed in a proportion of HIV-infected subjects undergoing serial echocardiography as participants in natural history studies of heart

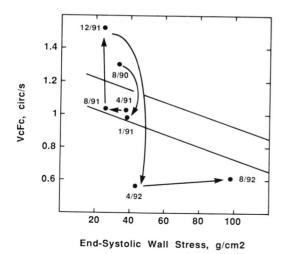

Fig. 11-1. Serial evaluation over 2 years of left ventricular contractility in an asymptomatic HIV-seropositive homosexual man. Heart rate-corrected velocity of fiber shortening is plotted against end-systolic wall stress to produce a measure of contractility that is preload independent and incorporates afterload. Parallel lines indicate 95 percent confidence limits for left ventricular contractility. The patient's contractility started out and remained in the normal range until a precipitous fall in contractility in April, 1992. Increased wall stress in August, 1992 failed to return contractility into the normal range.

disease in HIV infection. It has been suggested that diastolic dysfunction may be associated with cocaine use in this population, although this has not been borne out in studies of cocaine users with unknown HIV status.[65]

Right Ventricular Dysfunction

Right heart failure had been anticipated in view of the susceptibility of HIV-infected patients to pulmonary infection, but it has proved to be fairly uncommon. Over a 7-year period, six men with AIDS were identified in the San Francisco area with pulmonary hypertension and cor pulmonale, an estimated incidence of 0.5

percent.[65] A limited number of cases of pulmonary hypertension in HIV-infected individuals have subsequently been reported, with plexogenic arteriopathy as the most common pathologic finding.[67,68]

In addition to case reports and pathology studies, evaluation of pulmonary artery pressure by Doppler echocardiography has been carried out. Prospective evaluation of 74 HIV-infected subjects (53 homosexuals and 21 intravenous drug users) with cardiopulmonary complaints identified 6 with pulmonary hypertension.[69] A recent retrospective analysis of 60 hospitalized black patients, which include 42 percent women, found echocardiographic evidence of pulmonary hypertension in 8 (13 percent), suggesting that this may be a fairly common finding among HIV-infected African-Americans.[70] Evaluation of subjects with cardiopulmonary symptoms and hospitalized patients may, however, provide a misleading view of the prevalence of pulmonary hypertension in HIV infection.

In the District of Columbia study population of 256 seropositive subjects, symptomatic right heart failure was observed in a single individual with an obstructing right atrial mass.[71] Thus, despite the frequency of infectious and infiltrating lymphocytic pneumonitis in individuals infected with HIV, right heart abnormalities of clinical relevance appear to be comparatively infrequent. Pulmonary hypertension and cor pulmonale have been reported in pediatric HIV infection, but appear to be similarly uncommon.[72]

Arrhythmias

Rhythm disturbances in HIV infection are attributable to many causes including ventricular inflammation and scarring, drug effects, electrolyte and hormonal abnormalities, and malignancy. Cardiac arrhythmia was first mentioned in Cohen et al.'s[46] report of three patients with cardiomyopathy, one of whom had unspecified rhythm abnormalities shortly before death. Subsequent reports have described refractory ventricular tachycardia and sudden death either with or without accompanying myocarditis or congestive heart failure.[37,57,59] The frequency of clinically significant arrhythmias was assessed in the District of Columbia study population in whom serial signal averaged electrocardiograms were performed prospectively.[73] Although late potentials were observed in 59 of 225 HIV-infected subjects, symptomatic ventricular tachycardia developed in only 3, 2 of whom had developed clinical cardiomyopathies during follow-up. Late potentials were transient in about 40 percent, a striking difference from patients with ischemic heart disease, in whom transient late potentials are common only during the first few days after myocardial infarction. One hypothesis suggested to account for the unexpectedly frequent presence of late potentials was that conduction was affected by focal myocarditis, which might be subclinical and transient. Bradyarrhythmias including heart block appear rare, having only been reported in patients with infiltration of the conducting system by tumor.[15]

In addition to rhythm disturbances attributable to tumor, cardiomyopathy, or myocarditis, drugs have been implicated as contributing agents. Perhaps the most widely observed drug-induced ventricular tachycardia in HIV infection is attributable to treatment of *Pneumocystis carinii* pneumonia with pentamidine isoethionate, which is associated with a syndrome of QT prolongation along with hypomagnesemia and torsades des pointes.[74–79] A characteristic electrocardiogram with marked QT prolongation is shown in Figure 11-2. During repletion of magnesium, the patient developed torsades des pointes with hypotension (Fig. 11-3), from which he was resuscitated. A

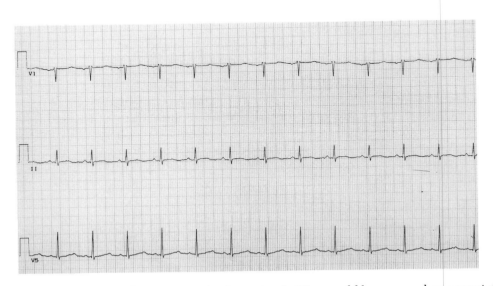

Fig. 11-2. Marked QT prolongation on rhythm strip of a 29-year-old homosexual man receiving home treatment for *Pneumocystis carinii* pneumonia and systemic *Mycobacterium avium intracellulare* infection with amikacin, acyclovir, clofazamine, clarithromycin, and pentamidine. He was admitted with persistent fever; serum magnesium was 0.5 mEq/L.

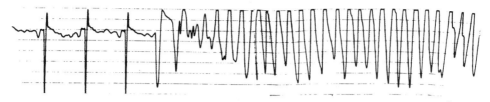

Fig. 11-3. The same patient shown in Figure 11-2 developed torsades des pointes shortly thereafter during magnesium replacement.

number of renal[80] and endocrine abnormalities[81] seen in patients with HIV infection, as well as infectious diarrhea and AIDS enteropathy,[82] lead to electrolyte abnormalities in this population; such abnormalities can also provide an arrhythmogenic substrate in individuals with or without cardiac pathology.

Arrhythmias are a more common finding in children than in adults. Ventricular tachycardia was detected in 3 of 30 HIV-infected children in Boston, supraventricular tachycardia in 1, first-degree heart block in 3, and second-degree heart block in 1.[62,63] These clinical observations are consistent with the pathologic infiltration of the conducting system observed in HIV-infected children, which seems a more conspicuous feature of the disease than in adults.

of organs including the brain, lung, and heart.[11,84] Disseminated intravascular coagulation has also been reported in association with nonbacterial thrombotic endocarditis in AIDS.[81]

Infectious endocarditis has not been a frequent finding in HIV infection despite the increased risk associated with indwelling venous catheters and the immune deficiency. Healed bacterial endocarditis has been observed, but may reflect prior clinical events in a group that includes substantial numbers of intravenous drug users. One case of *Aspergillus fumigatus* mitral endocarditis with a paravalvular abscess was reported.[43] This patient had no heart murmur, but did suffer a hemiparetic stroke, a well-known complication of infectious endocarditis.

Endocarditis

Both infectious and marantic endocarditis have been reported in patients with AIDS. Nonbacterial thrombotic endocarditis, so-called marantic endocarditis, is commonly associated with chronic inflammatory illnesses and malignancies and may involve left- or right-sided valves.[11,12,83] The vegetations may be large enough to cause hemodynamically significant valvular insufficiency and may also embolize systemically or through the pulmonary circulation. Embolic infarction in conjunction with HIV-associated marantic endocarditis may affect a variety

Intracardiac Masses

Neoplastic invasion of the heart by Kaposi's sarcoma or lymphoma was reported initially in autopsy studies with antecedent clinical symptoms, including tachyarrhythmias, heart block,[15,17] right ventricular hypokinesis,[19] pericardial effusion,[11] and congestive heart failure.[15] Although palliative treatment has been provided, appearance of an intracardiac mass appears to be associated with a uniformly poor prognosis.

A right atrial mass that developed in a young homosexual man with a previously normal echocardiogram is shown in Fig-

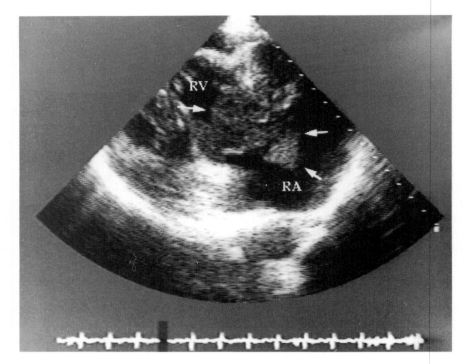

Fig. 11-4. Right atrial mass in a 36-year-old, HIV-infected homosexual man with a normal echocardiogram 4 months earlier. This large right atrial mass (*arrows*) prolapsed through the tricuspid valve, causing tricuspid outflow obstruction. RV, right ventricle; RA, right atrium.

ure 11-4. The mass grew rapidly and obstructed the tricuspid valve, leading to his death within a few months.

Pericardial Effusion and Tamponade

As a practical matter, pericardial effusions can be characterized as either asymptomatic or symptomatic. Effusions are common among patients referred for echocardiography because of cardiomegaly on chest roentgenography or cardiorespiratory symptoms; as is the case for cardiomyopathy, series of hospitalized patients referred for echocardiography may provide a misleading view of the prevalence of pericardial effusion. For example, effusions were identified in 7 of

25 hospitalized HIV-infected patients in San Francisco,[60] and in none of 45 ambulatory patients evaluated. A study of outpatients in San Diego provided contrasting data; 15 of 70 outpatients had effusions, although none were symptomatic.[85]

The predominantly homosexual population in studies from California can be compared with HIV-infected populations with intravenous drug use as the primary risk factor. In one such study, 62 subjects, 93 percent of whom were intravenous drug users, underwent echocardiography for clinical indications, mostly fever. Pericardial effusions were detected in 46 percent although none had tamponade.[86]

During prospective follow-up of 256 HIV-seropositive subjects with initially normal echocardiograms in the District of

Columbia, pericardial effusions developed at the rate of about 5 percent annually.[86a]

Infectious pericarditis might be anticipated in an immunosuppressed population, and this expectation is, to an extent, borne out by observations in AIDS. Among the agents identified are herpes simplex,[42] *Mycobacterium tuberculosis*[28,87] and *avium intracellulare*,[88,89] *Staphylococcus aureus*,[87] *Cryptococcus neoformans*,[90,91] and *Nocardia asteroides*.[92]

In children, pericardial effusions without tamponade were seen in 8 of 31 HIV-seropositive patients undergoing prospective echocardiographic follow-up.[62] No pathologic organisms were detected in pericardial fluid samples.

Pericardial tamponade is a life-threatening complication of HIV infection; pericardiocentesis may be nondiagnostic but has yielded both infectious[87,88] and malignant diagnoses.[87,93,94] Figures 11-5 to 11-7 demonstrate typical echocardiographic findings in a young homosexual man with AIDS; pericardiocentesis was nondiagnostic.

PATHOPHYSIOLOGY

Several pathophysiologic bases for HIV-associated cardiomyopathy have been proposed, including myocardial infection with HIV or other pathogens, autoimmune damage, electrolyte abnormalities, and drug toxicity (Table 11-3).

Although a variety of pathogens, as described above, had been detected in heart tissue, no consistent relationship was apparent between these agents and adjacent myocardial necrosis, and either

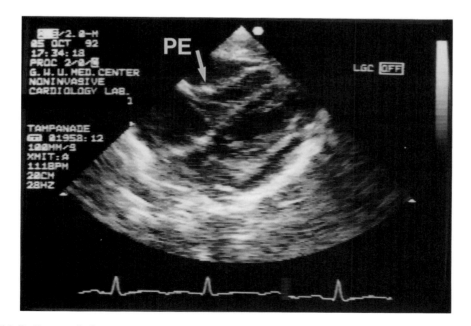

Fig. 11-5. Pericardial tamponade in a young homosexual man with HIV infection. He presented with dyspnea; cardiomegaly was noted on chest roentgenogram, and he was referred for echocardiography. A large circumferential pericardial effusion (PE) with right atrial and ventricular collapse (*arrow*) is shown in the subxiphoid view.

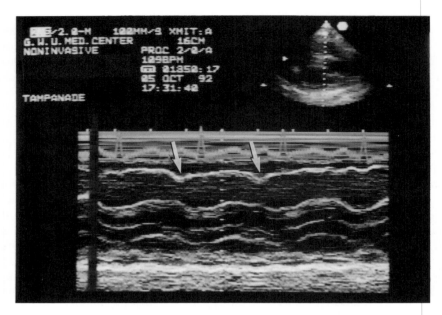

Fig. 11-6. Cyclic diastolic right ventricular collapse (*arrows*) is demonstrated on M-mode in the same patient shown in Figure 11-5.

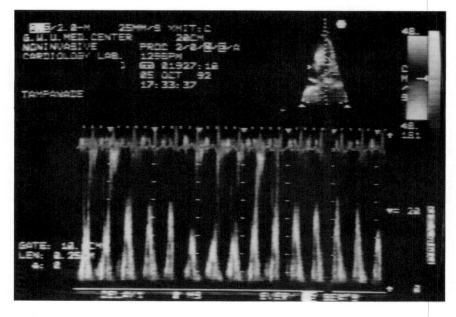

Fig. 11-7. Respiratory variation in mitral outflow velocity is demonstrated in the same patient shown in Figure 11-5. Pericardiocentesis was nondiagnostic.

Table 11-3. Pathophysiology of HIV-Associated Cardiomyopathy

Infection-induced myocardial damage
    HIV
    Cytomegalovirus
    Coxsackievirus
    Other pathogens

Autoimmune tissue damage
    Induced by infection
    Induced by abnormal expression or
      recognition of myocardial proteins

Nutritional deficiency

Drug toxicity
    α-Interferon
    Zidovudine (AZT)
    Didanosine (ddI)
    Zalcitabine (ddC)

---

clinical or pathologic evidence of ventricular dysfunction. Particularly in view of the prevalence of myocarditis in some autopsy series, viruses, which might not be evident by light microscopy, came under scrutiny.

In the first report of HIV detection in myocardium, endomyocardial biopsy tissue from a homosexual man with congestive cardiomyopathy was cocultured with HIV-negative phytohemagglutinin-stimulated peripheral blood mononuclear cells; reverse transcriptase activity, the hallmark of retroviruses, was detected in the culture supernatant.[32] A limitation of this approach is that the reverse transcriptase activity might be attributable to contaminating lymphocytes carried into culture with the biopsy sample rather than to infection of cardiac cells per se. Available molecular biologic techniques have grown increasingly sophisticated during the past decade, leading to subsequent identification of HIV nucleotide sequences[33,95] and proteins[96] in heart tissue from adults and a child,[34] although the specific cell types infected could not be determined by these methods.

In a study by Rodriguez et al.,[35] individual myocytes and dendritic cells were microdissected from endomyocardial biopsy samples taken from HIV-infected patients with and without cardiomyopathy. Dendritic cells are CD4-receptor-bearing interstitial cells that were present in increased numbers in heart tissue from patients with cardiomyopathy. DNA was extracted from nuclei and amplified using a highly specific, nested polymerase chain reaction. HIV sequences were identified using a labeled probe against a sequence internal to the primers; sequences against the gag or pol gene were detected in every patient studied, including those without apparent heart disease. These findings, in conjunction with those of other investigators, support the view that HIV itself may be a stimulus for tissue damage in the heart.

Other viruses proposed as etiologic candidates were cytomegalovirus, which is widespread in patients with AIDS, and coxsackievirus. Characteristic cytomegaloviral inclusion bodies[13,45,81] have been reported in heart tissue, but efforts to identify cytomegalovirus DNA by in situ hybridization have been unrewarding. Similarly, in situ hybridization studies seeking RNA from picornaviruses such as coxsackievirus have been negative (unpublished observations). In one patient with cardiomyopathy and normal endomyocardial biopsy, serum titers against coxsackievirus B2 rose from 1:128 to 1:512,[26] but this relationship has not been reported since. The paucity of evidence for pathogens other than HIV in the heart supports the view that HIV may be the culprit. Unanswered questions remain: (1) what is the mechanism whereby HIV causes tissue damage? and (2) if all these patients' hearts are infected with HIV, why don't they all develop cardiomyopathy?

Immune activation has been proposed to cause the observed myocardial necrosis through either direct tissue injury or a bystander effect.[97] The autoimmune response could be directed against myocytes, interstitial cells, lymphocytes, or macrophages infected with viruses or other pathogens, or against abnormally expressed heart antigens.[94] Hershkowitz and colleagues[98,99] have carried out a number of studies evaluating autoimmune-mediated tissue damage in hearts of HIV-infected patients. CD8[+] lymphocytes were identified in the lymphocytic infiltrates in endomyocardial biopsies of HIV-infected patients. Furthermore, a variety of induced class I and II antigens were identified on the arteriolar endothelium, suggesting local secretion of cytokines such as α- and β-interferon. These observations were consistent with cell-mediated autoimmune injury to the heart in HIV infection; whether the stimulus to this immune response was the HIV or something else remains to be determined.

The wasting syndrome in AIDS leads to metabolic disturbances[100] including selenium deficiency, which has been associated with cardiomyopathy in children.[101] Whether selenium or other nutritional deficiency plays a role in HIV-associated cardiomyopathy is not known.

Antiretroviral agents may also be cardiotoxic. Three patients receiving prolonged, high-dose treatment with α-interferon developed congestive heart failure that resolved upon discontinuation of the drug.[102] Zidovudine (AZT) is well known to cause skeletal myopathy and myositis[103] and was temporally associated in one patient with development of cardiomyopathy after 17 months of treatment; the cardiomyopathy improved upon discontinuation of the drug.[104] Heart failure has also been reported in association with didanosine (ddI)[103] and zalcitabine (ddC).[103,105] With a variety of plausible mechanisms proposed for the tissue damage observed at autopsy and

by endomyocardial biopsy in HIV-infected patients with cardiomyopathy, chances are that this entity is multifactorial in origin.

MANAGEMENT

Management of HIV infection is a highly specialized, rapidly changing field best undertaken by physicians with both interest and experience in the field. Even asymptomatic HIV-seropositive individuals require counseling, staging, and monitoring, until their CD4-bearing lymphocyte counts fall to a level triggering anti-retroviral therapy and prophylaxis against opportunistic infections. With the development of new antiretrovirals, treatment at the time of diagnosis may be instituted soon, a change in management strategy that will affect current serologic screening practices.

Management of cardiac manifestations of HIV infection such as cardiomyopathy and pericardial effusion differs little from management in non-HIV-infected patients, since no studies of specific therapies directed at heart disease in HIV infection have been carried out. In general, the most valuable step a clinician can take is early consideration of heart disease in a patient known or suspected to be infected with HIV. Thus, patients with dyspnea and abnormal chest x-ray should undergo echocardiography to exclude congestive cardiomyopathy prior to bronchoscopy or institution of pentamidine treatment for presumptive *Pneumocystis carinii* pneumonia.

Congestive Cardiomyopathy

The mainstays of medical treatment for congestive heart failure remain afterload reduction, diuretics, and inotropes. No trials of these therapies have been conducted in HIV-infected populations, but anecdotal reports suggest they are as efficacious in HIV-associated cardiomyopathy as in the population at large.[46,50,55,56,106]

Occasionally a patient with new onset heart failure will be found to have active myocarditis on endomyocardial biopsy. In the absence of prior opportunistic infections, immunosuppressive therapy may be considered. Evidence supporting a role for immunosuppression in HIV-associated myocarditis is even more meager than for non-HIV-associated myocarditis; however, when little else can be offered, such treatment has occasionally been successful.[37]

Pericardial Effusion

Some controversy has surrounded the question of the frequency with which infectious organisms and malignancies can be identified in HIV-infected patients with cardiac tamponade, and hence the clinical utility of pericardiocentesis. In an analysis of all patients with AIDS or AIDS-related complex and pericardial effusions discharged from San Francisco General Hospital between 1984 and 1990, 10 of 25 had incidental pericardial effusions, 10 had clinical pericarditis, and 8 had tamponade.[107] Pericardiocentesis was performed in 10, with subsequent pericardial window in 2 and autopsy in 3; all the pericardial fluid samples were exudates, and none were diagnostic. Not all experiences with pericardial fluid in this population have been as unrewarding, however.[86] Some diagnoses obtainable by pericardiocentesis are treatable, so an effort to identify individuals with those diagnoses is worthwhile.

Tamponade is a clear indication for intervention, whether in the form of pericardiocentesis or pericardial window. Purulent pericarditis may be a cause of antibiotic-resistant sepsis; thus early pericardiocentesis may be indicated in such individuals. AIDS patients commonly suffer multiple, concurrent infections; identification of one organism in the presence of a pericardial effusion documented by echocardiography does not permit assumption that the effusion is attributable to the same organism. Furthermore, the heart can be the sole site of either infection or malignancy, so diagnoses may be missed altogether without pericardial fluid sampling.

From a somewhat different perspective, tamponade is unusual in young adults, especially without known malignancy, so serologic testing for HIV is indicated in such individuals once consent for HIV testing has been obtained.

LABORATORY TESTING

Electrocardiography

Electrocardiographic abnormalities in HIV infection have included nonsinus rhythm, premature atrial and ventricular beats, bundle branch block, repolarization abnormalities, pericarditis, QRS alternans, QT prolongation, and pathologic Q waves.[50,59] The latter, along with intraventricular conduction delays, and nonspecific ST-T wave abnormalities, are common in patients with cardiomyopathy. QT prolongation is seen predominantly as a drug effect, particularly with pentamidine. Typical changes of pericarditis and occasionally QRS alternans can be observed in patients with large pericardial effusions.

The value of screening electrocardiography would be enhanced if development of electrocardiographic abnormalities preceded echocardiographic findings. During prospective 22-month follow-up of HIV-infected subjects with normal echocardiograms and abnormal electrocardiograms, 14 percent developed new echocardiographic abnormalities.[61]

Holter Monitoring

Twenty-four-hour ambulatory electrocardiographic monitoring was carried out in HIV-infected patients to determine the frequency of occult arrhythmias. Although unsuspected, ventricular tachycardia was detected in several patients, all of these individuals had evident cardiac involvement, with abnormal echocardiograms and 12-lead electrocardiograms.[59]

Echocardiography

A number of studies have demonstrated a high yield from echocardiograms performed in HIV-infected individuals with cardiopulmonary symptoms.[59,60] The value of echocardiography in asymptomatic patients is not established. In a group of 27 homosexual men with AIDS in New York, in whom heart disease was not suspected, abnormally low shortening fraction was detected in 8 (30 percent) and pericardial effusions in 7 (26 percent).[108] In the control group of 9 HIV-seronegative and 12 seropositive homosexual men without AIDS-defining illness, one subject with low shortening fraction and one with a pericardial effusion were identified ($P < 0.05$). This study suggested that "screening" echocardiograms might be useful in AIDS. A contrasting viewpoint is suggested, however, by results of a natural history study of heart disease in 300 HIV-infected men and women in the District of Columbia.[61] Among those with normal echocardiograms at baseline and no cardiac symptoms, only 7 percent developed cardiomyopathy or pericardial effusion during mean follow-up of 17 months.

Overall, if the treatment plan will not be affected by detection of a small pericardial effusion or asymptomatic wall motion abnormality, across-the-board echocardiography may not be cost effective.

A separate but related issue is the value of HIV serologic testing and early echocardiography in young adults with cardiopulmonary symptoms who are not known to be seropositive. With the increasing prevalence of HIV infection among heterosexuals, screening should not be limited to members of traditional HIV risk groups. Cardiomyopathy and pericardial effusion are not that common in adults in their late 30s, the mean age in most studies of HIV-infected patients. Detection of these abnormalities by echocardiography should trigger serologic testing.

Radionuclide Ventriculography

In general, echocardiography has superceded radionuclide ventriculography for evaluation of ventricular function. Depressed right ventricular ejection fraction was detected in 3 of 12 and left ventricular ejection fraction in 2 of 12 HIV-infected subjects; most of them had AIDS and past intravenous drug use.[109] The drawbacks of this approach are failure to provide information about pericardial and valvular disease in a population with comparatively high prevalence of these abnormalities.

Pericardiocentesis

Reports of the yield of pericardiocentesis for diagnosis of etiology of pericardial effusions have varied from 0[62,108] to 100 percent.[87] Therapeutic pericardial drainage is clearly indicated for tamponade, and probably for febrile HIV-infected patients with large pericardial effusions. Beyond that, there is little evidence on which to base a decision. These patients are likely to have concurrent lymphoma, drug reactions, and multiple infections, so one cannot presume an etiology of pericardial effusion on the basis of concurrent disease.

Endomyocardial Biopsy

There are no widely accepted standards for performance of endomyocardial biopsy in HIV-infected patients with new cardiomyopathies.[110] Since treatment generally does not depend upon biopsy findings, and the procedure is not risk-free, biopsy seems unwarranted in most situations. There may be an occasional patient with an acutely disastrous downhill course, such as one requiring constant defibrillation for refractory ventricular tachycardia,[37] in whom the diagnosis of myocarditis might provoke immunosuppressive treatment. In carefully thought through situations that have been discussed in advance with the patient, the family, or with both, biopsy may lead to helpful and life-prolonging treatment.

Other Invasive Evaluation

The life expectancy of individuals with HIV infection has grown considerably since the onset of the pandemic and currently exceeds 10 years. Under these circumstances, individuals who meet generally accepted standards for invasive evaluation should receive that evaluation. Indeed since the current practice is to assume that every patient on whom one is performing an invasive procedure is HIV infected, there is no basis to deny known HIV-infected patients appropriate care.

FUTURE ISSUES

Cardiac manifestations in HIV infection fortunately do not approach infectious complications in frequency, inevitability, or mortality. However, as HIV-seropositive patients live longer and their infectious complications are treated better, the frequency of cardiac disease should rise[111] and in fact appears to be increasing. At a minimum, it is being recognized more frequently. Further, new pharmacologic agents to treat the retrovirus and secondary infections are under development and may demonstrate cardiotoxicity as their use becomes more widespread. A high index of suspicion in young adults with or without known HIV infection who present with dypsnea or chest pain will prevent delay in diagnosis and appropriate treatment.

Consideration of HIV-related heart disease in young adults, even those not belonging to traditional risk groups, is warranted if they present with cardiopulmonary symptoms. Serologic testing for HIV and echocardiography are safe and probably cost-effective approaches in this group. As heterosexual transmission of HIV represents a proportionately greater number of new cases, HIV-associated cardiomyopathy will no doubt manifest in an increasingly diverse population.

REFERENCES

1. Masur H, Michelis MA, Greene JB et al: An outbreak of community-acquired *Pneumocystis carinii* pneumonia. Manifestations of cellular immune dysfunction. N Engl J Med 305:1431, 1981
2. Gottlieb MS, Schroff R, Schanker HM et al: *Pneumocystic carinii* pneumonia and mucosal candidiasis in previously healthy homosexual men. Evidence of a

new acquired cellular immunodeficiency. N Engl J Med 305:1425, 1981

3. Barré-Sinoussi F, Chermann JC, Rey F et al: Isolation of a T-lymphocyte retrovirus from a patient at risk for acquired immune deficiency syndrome (AIDS). Science 220:868, 1983

4. Gallo RC, Sarin PS, Kramarsky B et al: First isolation of HTLV-III. Nature 321:119, 1986

5. CDC: Projections of the number of persons diagnosed with AIDS and the number of immunosuppressed HIV-infected persons—United States, 1992–4. MMWR 41:RR-18, 1992

6. Chin J, Remenyi MA, Morrison F, Bulatao R: The global epidemiology of the HIV/AIDS pandemic and its projected demographic impact in Africa. World Health Stat Q 45:220, 1992

7. Revision of the case definition of acquired immunodeficiency syndrome for national reporting—United States. MMWR 34:373, 1985

8. Reichert CM, O'Leary TJ, Levens DL et al: Autopsy pathology in the acquired immune deficiency syndrome. Am J Pathol 112:357, 1983

9. Silver MA, Macher AM, Reichert CM et al. Cardiac involvement by Kaposi's sarcoma in acquired immune deficiency syndrome (AIDS). Am J Cardiol 53:983, 1984

10. Welch K, Finkbeiner W, Alpers CE et al: Autopsy findings in the acquired immune deficiency syndrome. JAMA 252:1152, 1984

11. Cammarosano C, Lewis W: Cardiac lesions in acquired immune deficiency syndrome (AIDS). JACC 5:703, 1985

12. Roldan EO, Moskowitz L, Hensley GT: Pathology of the heart in acquired immunodeficiency syndrome. Arch Pathol Lab Med 111:943, 1987

13. Anderson DW, Virmani R, Reilly JM et al: Prevalent myocarditis at necropsy in the acquired immunodeficiency syndrome. J Am Coll Cardiol 11:792, 1988

14. Lewis W: AIDS: cardiac findings from 115 autopsies. Prog Cardiovasc Dis 32:207, 1989

15. Balasubramanyam A, Waxman M, Kazal HL, Lee MH: Malignant lymphoma of the heart in acquired immune deficiency syndrome. Chest 90:243, 1986

16. Guarner J, Brynes RK, Chan WC et al: Primary non-Hodgkin's lymphoma of the heart in two patients with the acquired immunodeficiency syndrome. Arch Pathol Lab Med 111:254, 1987

17. Kelsey RC, Saker A, Morgan M: Cardiac lymphoma in a patient with AIDS. Ann Intern Med 115:370, 1991

18. Goldfarb A, King CL, Rosenzweig BP et al: Cardiac lymphoma in the acquired immunodeficiency syndrome. Am Heart J 118:1340, 1989

19. Andress JD, Polish LB, Clark DM, Hossack KF: Transvenous biopsy diagnosis of cardiac lymphoma in an AIDS patient. Am Heart J 118:421, 1989

20. Ioachim HL, Cooper MC, Hellman GC: Lymphomas in men at high risk for acquired immune deficiency syndrome (AIDS): a study of 21 cases. Cancer 56:2831, 1985

21. Roh T, Paparo G: Primary malignant lymphoma of the heart in sudden unexpected death. J Forensic Sci 27:718, 1982

22. Aretz T, Edwards W, Factor S et al: Myocarditis: a histopathologic definition and classification. Am J Cardiovasc Pathol 1:3, 1986

23. Baroldi G, Corallo S, Moroni M et al: Focal lymphocytic myocarditis in acquired immunodeficiency syndrome (AIDS): a correlative morphologic and clinical study in 26 consecutive fatal cases. J Am Coll Cardiol 12:463, 1988

24. Lewis W, Lipsick J, Cammarosano C: Cryptococcal myocarditis in acquired immune deficiency syndrome. Am J Cardiol 55:1240, 1985

25. Lafont A, Wolff M, Marche C et al: Overwhelming myocarditis due to *Cryptococcus neoformans* in an AIDS patient. Lancet 2:1145, 1987

26. Dittrich H, Chow L, Denaro F, Spector S: Human immunodeficiency virus, coxsackievirus, and cardiomyopathy. Ann Intern Med 108:308, 1988

27. Lafont A, Marche C, Wolff M et al: Myocarditis in acquired immunodefi-

ciency syndrome (AIDS): etiology and prognosis, abstracted. J Am Coll Cardiol 11:196A, 1988

28. D'Cruz IA, Sengupta EE, Abrahams C et al: Cardiac involvement, including tuberculous pericardial effusion, complicating acquired immune deficiency syndrome. Am Heart J 112:1100, 1986

29. Cantwell AR, Jr: Necroscopic findings of variably acid-fast bacteria in a fatal case of acquired immunodeficiency and Kaposi's sarcoma. Growth 47:129, 1983

30. Hui AN, Koss MN, Meyer PR: Necropsy findings in acquired immunodeficiency syndrome: a comparison of premortem diagnoses with post-mortem findings. Hum Pathol 15:670, 1984

31. Acierno LJ: Cardiac complications in acquired immunodeficiency syndrome. J Am Coll Cardiol 13:1144, 1989

32. Calabrese LH, Profitt MR, Yen-Lieberman B et al: Congestive cardiomyopathy and illness related to the acquired immunodeficiency syndrome (AIDS) associated with isolation of retrovirus from myocardium. Ann Intern Med 107:691, 1987

33. Grody WW, Cheng L, Lewis W: Infection of the heart by the human immunodeficiency virus. Am J Cardiol 66:203, 1990

34. Lipshultz SE, Fox CH, Perez-Atayde AR et al: Identification of human immunodeficiency virus-1 RNA and DNA in the heart of child with cardiovascular abnormalities and congenital acquired immune deficiency syndrome. Am J Cardiol 66:246, 1990

35. Rodriguez ER, Nasim S, Hsia J et al: Cardiac myocytes and dendritic cells harbor human immunodeficiency virus in infected patients with and without cardiac dysfunction: detection by multiplex, nested, polymerase chain reaction in individually microdissected cells from right ventricular endomyocardial biopsy tissue. Am J Cardiol 68:1511, 1991

36. Turnicky RP, Goodin J, Smialek JE et al: Incidental myocarditis with intravenous drug abuse: The pathology, immunopathology, and potential implications for human immunodeficiency virus-associated myocarditis. Hum Pathol 23:138, 1992

37. Levy WS, Varghese PJ, Anderson DW et al: Myocarditis diagnosed by endomyocardial biopsy in human immunodeficiency virus infection with cardiac dysfunction. Am J Cardiol 62:658, 1988

38. Stewart JM, Kaul A, Gromisch DS et al: Symptomatic cardiac dysfunction in children with human immunodeficiency virus infection. Am Heart J 117:140, 1989

39. Bharati S, Joshi VV, Connor EM et al: Conduction system in children with acquired immunodeficiency syndrome. Chest 96:406, 1989

40. Moskowitz LB, Kory P, Chan JC et al: Unusual causes of death in Haitians residing in Miami. JAMA 250:1187, 1983

41. Stechel PR, Cooper DJ, Greenspan J et al: Staphylococcal pericarditis in a homosexual patient with AIDS-related complex. NY State J Med 86:592, 1986

42. Freedberg RS, Gindea AJ, Dietrich DT et al: Herpes simplex pericarditis in AIDS. NY State J Med 1987:304

43. Henochowicz S, Mustafa M, Laivrinson WE et al: Cardiac aspergillosis in acquired immune deficiency syndrome. Am J Cardiol 55:1239, 1985

44. Dressler FA, Roberts WC: Modes of death and types of cardiac diseases in opiate addicts: analysis of 168 necropsy cases. Am J Cardiol 64:909, 1989

45. Guarda LA, Luna MA, Smith JL et al: Acquired immune deficiency syndrome: postmortem findings. Am J Clin Pathol 81:549, 1984

46. Cohen IS, Anderson DW, Virmani R et al: Congestive cardiomyopathy in association with the acquired immune deficiency syndrome. N Engl J Med 315:628, 1986

47. Joshi VV, Gadol C, Connor E et al: Dilated cardiomyopathy in children with acquired immunodeficiency syndrome: a pathologic study of five cases. Hum Pathol 19:69, 1988

48. Issenberg HJ, Cho S, Rubinstein A: Cardiac pathology in children with acquired

immune deficiency. Pediatr Res 20:295A, 1986

49. Magno J, Margaretten W, Cheitlin M: Myocardial involvement in acquired immunodeficiency syndrome: incidence in a large autopsy study, abstracted. Circulation 78:II–459, 1988

50. Reilly JM, Cunnion RE, Anderson DW et al: Frequency of myocarditis, left ventricular dysfunction and ventricular tachycardia in the acquired immune deficiency syndrome. Am J Cardiol 62:789, 1988

51. Mitchell JL, Tucker, J, Loftman PO, Williams SB: HIV and women: current controversies and clinical relevance. J Women's Health 1:35, 1992

52. Morlat P, Parneix P, Douard D et al: Women and HIV infection: a cohort study of 483 HIV-infected women in Bordeaux, France, 1985–1991. AIDS 6:1187, 1992

53. Centers for Disease Control and Prevention. HIV/AIDS Surveillance Report. February:1, 1993

54. Cohen IS, Anderson DW, Virmani R et al: Congeative cardiomyopathy in association with the acquired immunodeficiency syndrome. N Engl J Med 315:628, 1986

55. Kaminski HJ, Katzman M, Wiest PM et al: Cardiomyopathy associated with the acquired immune deficiency syndrome. J Acquir Immune Defic Syndr 1:105, 1988

56. Miller RF, Gilson R, Hage C et al: HIV-associated dilated cardiomyopathy. Genitourin Med 67:453, 1991

57. Fink L, Reichek N, St. John Sutton MG: Cardiac abnormalities in acquired immune deficiency syndrome. Am J Cardiol 54:116, 1984

58. Monsuez J-J, Kinney EL, Vittecoq D et al: Comparison among acquired immune deficiency syndrome patients with and without clinical evidence of cardiac disease. Am J Cardiol 62:1311, 1988

59. Levy WS, Simon GL, Rios JC, Ross AM: Prevalence of cardiac abnormalities in human immunodeficiency virus infection. Am J Cardiol 63:86, 1989

60. Himelman RB, Chung WS, Chernoff DN et al: Cardiac manifestations of human immunodeficiency virus infection: a two-dimensional echocardiographic study. J Am Coll Cardiol 13:1030, 1989

61. Hsia JA, McQuinn LB: AIDS Cardiomyopathy. 39:21, 1993

62. Steinherz LJ, Brochstein JA, Robins J: Cardiac involvement in congenital acquired immunodeficiency syndrome. Am J Dis Child 140:1241, 1986

63. Lipshultz SE, Chanock S, Sanders SP et al: Cardiovascular manifestations of human immunodeficiency virus infection in infants and children. Am J Cardiol 63:1489, 1989

64. Lipshultz SE, Orav EJ, Sanders SP et al: Cardiac structure and function in children with human immunodeficiency virus infection treated with zidovudine. N Engl J Med 327:1260, 1992

65. Chakko S, Fernandez A, Mellman TA et al: Cardiac manifestations of cocaine abuse: a cross-sectional study of asymptomatic men with a history of long-term abuse of "crack" cocaine. J Am Coll Cardiol 20;1168, 1992

66. Himelman RB, Dohrmann M, Goodman P et al: Severe pulmonary hypertension and cor pulmonale in the acquired immunodeficiency syndrome. Am J Cardiol 64:1396, 1989

67. Mette SA, Palevsky HI, Pietra GG et al: Primary pulmonary hypertension in association with human immunodeficiency virus infection. A possible viral etiology for some forms of hypertensive pulmonary arteriopathy. Am Rev Respir Dis 145:1196, 1992

68. Polos PG, Wolfe D, Harley RA et al: Pulmonary hypertension and human immunodeficiency virus infection. Two reports and a review of the literature. Chest 101:474, 1992

69. Speich R, Jenni R, Opravil M et al: Primary pulmonary hypertension in HIV infection. Chest 100:1268, 1991

70. Webber JD, Lewis JF, Mody V: Cardiovascular abnormalities by echocardiography in patients with human immunodeficiency virus infection: influence of race and gender, abstracted. J Am Coll Cardiol 21:395A, 1993

71. Mohanty N, Adams S, Hsia J: Cardiac

problems in persons with AIDS. Choices Cardiol 6:1, 1993

72. Rhodes J, Schiller MS, Montoya CH, Fikrig S: Severe pulmonary hypertension without significant pulmonary parenchymal disease in a pediatric patient with acquired immunodeficiency syndrome. Clin Pediatr October:629, 1992

73. Hsia J, Colan SD, Adams S, Ross AM: Late potentials and their relation to ventricular function in human immunodeficiency virus infection. Am J Cardiol 68:1216, 1991

74. Wharton JM, Demopulos PA, Goldschlager N: Torsades de pointes during administration of pentamidine isethionate. Am J Med 83:571, 1987

75. Mitchell P, Dodek P, Lawson L et al: Torsades de pointes during intravenous pentamidine isethionate therapy. Can Med Assoc J 140:173, 1989

76. Pujol M, Carratala J, Mauri J, Viladrich P: Ventricular tachycardia due to pentamidine isethionate. Am J Med 84:980, 1988

77. Bibler MR, Chou T-C, Toltzis RJ, Wade PA: Recurrent ventricular tachycardia due to pentamidine-induced cardiotoxicity. Chest 94:1303, 1988

78. Stein KM, Haronian H, Mensah GA et al: Ventricular tachycardia and torsades de pointes complicating pentamidine therapy of Pneumocystis carinii pneumonia in the acquired immunodeficiency syndrome. Am J Cardiol 66:888, 1990

79. Stein KM, Fenton C, Lehany AM et al: Incidence of QT interval prolongation during pentamidine therapy of Pneumocystis carinii pneumonia. Am J Cardiol 68:1091, 1991

80. Bourgoignie JJ: Renal complications of human immunodeficiency virus type 1. Kidney Int 37:1571, 1990

81. Grinspoon SK, Bilezikian JP: HIV Disease and the endocrine system. N Engl J Med 327:1360, 1992

82. Smith PD: Gastrointestinal infections in AIDS. Ann Intern Med 116:63, 1992

83. Niedt GW, Schinella RA: Acquired immunodeficiency syndrome. Clinicopath-

ologic study of 56 autopsies. Arch Pathol Lab Med 109:727, 1985

84. Snider WD, Simpson DM, Nielsen S et al: Neurological complications of acquired immune deficiency syndrome: analysis of 50 patients. Ann Neurol 14:403, 1983

85. Blanchard DG, Hegenhoff C, Chow LC et al: Reversibility of cardiac abnormalities in human immunodeficiency virus (HIV)-infected individuals: a serial echocardiographic study. J Am Coll Cardiol 17:1270, 1991

86. Kinney EL, Brafman D, Wright RJ, II: Echocardiographic findings in patients with acquired immunodeficiency syndrome (AIDS) and AIDS-related complex (ARC). Cathet Cardiovasc Diagn 16:182, 1989

86a. Hsia J, Ross AM: Pericardial effusion and pericardiocentesis in human immunodeficiency virus infection. Am J Cardiol, in press

87. Dalli E, Quesada A, Juan G et al: Tuberculous pericarditis as the first manifestation of acquired immunodeficiency syndrome. Am Heart J 114:905, 1987

88. Woods G, Goldsmith J: Fatal pericarditis due to Mycobacterium avium-intracellulare in acquired immunodeficiency syndrome. Chest 95:1355, 1989

89. Turco M, Seneff M, McGrath BJ, Hsia J: Cardiac tamponade in the acquired immunodeficiency syndrome. Am Heart J 120:1467, 1990

90. Schuster M, Valentine F, Holzman R: Cryptococcal pericarditis in an intravenous drug user. J Infect Dis 153:842, 1985

91. Brivet F, Livartowski J, Herve P et al: Pericardial cryptococcal disease in acquired immune deficiency syndrome. Am J Med 82:1273, 1987

92. Holtz MA, Lavery DP, Kapila R: Actinomycetes infection in the acquired immunodeficiency syndrome. Ann Intern Med 102:203, 1985

93. Stotka JL, Good CB, Downer WR, Kapoor WN: Pericardial effusion and tamponade due to Kaposi's sarcoma in acquired immunodeficiency syndrome. Chest 95:1359, 1989

94. Steigman CK, Anderson DW, Macher

AM et al: Fatal cardiac tamponade in acquired immunodeficiency syndrome with epicardial Kaposi's sarcoma. Am Heart J 116:1105, 1988

95. Flomembaum M, Soeiro R, Udem SA et al: Proliferative membranopathy and human immunodeficiency virus in AIDS hearts. J Acquir Immune Defic Syndr 2:129, 1989

96. Cotton P: AIDS giving rise to cardiac problems. JAMA 263:2149, 1990

97. Ho DD, Pomerantz RJ, Kaplan JC: Pathogenesis of infection with human immunodeficiency virus. N Engl J Med 317:278, 1987

98. Beschorner WE, Baughman K, Turnicky RP et al: HIV-associated myocarditis. Pathology and immunopathology. Am J Pathol 137:1365, 1990

99. Herskowitz A, Willoughby SB, Ansari AA et al: High risk profile for the development of congestive heart failure in HIV-related cardiomyopathy, abstracted. Circulation 84:II-3, 1991

100. Grunfeld C, Feingold KR: Metabolic disturbances and wasting in the acquired immunodeficiency syndrome. N Engl J Med 327:329, 1992

101. Kavanaugh-McHugh A, Rowe S, Benjamin Y et al: Selenium deficiency and cardiomyopathy in malnourished pediatric AIDS patients, abstracted. Fifth International Conference on AIDS. Montreal, section B:329, 1989

102. Deyton LR, Walker RE, Kovacs JA et al: Reversible cardiac dysfunction associated with interferon alfa therapy in AIDS patients with Kaposi's sarcoma. N Engl J Med 321:1246, 1989

103. Dalakas MC, Illa I, Pezeshkpour GH et al: Mitochondrial myopathy caused by long-term zidovudine therapy. N Engl J Med 322:1098, 1990

104. Herskowitz A, Willoughby SB, Baughman KL et al: Cardiomyopathy associated with antiretroviral therapy in patients with HIV infection: a report of six cases. Ann Intern Med 116, 311, 1992

105. Salgo M, Lieberman J: Cardiomyopathy or congestive heart failure (CHF) in patients on nucleoside: anti-retrovirals including ddC. Information Amendment to Principal Investigators of Clinical Trials Units. Hoffman-LaRoche, September 17, 1991

106. Corboy JR, Fink L, Miller WT: Congestive cardiomyopathy in association with AIDS. Radiology 165:138, 1987

107. Galli FC, Cheitlin MD: Pericardial disease in AIDS: frequency of tamponade and therapeutic and diagnostic use of pericardiocentesis, abstracted. J Am Coll Cardiol 19:266A, 1992

108. Hecht SR, Berger M, Van Tosh A, Croxson S: Unsuspected cardiac abnormalities in the acquired immune deficiency syndrome. An echocardiographic study. Chest 96:805, 1989

109. Raffanti SP, Chiaramida AJ, Sen P et al: Assessment of cardiac function in patients with the acquired immunodeficiency syndrome. Chest 93:592, 1988

110. Case records of the Massachusetts General Hospital: case 44-1992. N Engl J Med 327:1370, 1992

111. Jacob AJ, Boon NA: HIV cardiomyopathy: a dark cloud with a silver lining? Br Heart J 66:1, 1991

Index

Page numbers followed by f indicate figures; those followed by t indicate tables.

A

Acebutolol, for hypertension, 179
  in diabetic patients, 147
Acetaminophen, thrombocytopenia induced by, 233
Acetazolamide
  anemia associated with, 232
  thrombocytopenia induced by, 233
Acetohexamide, for diabetic patients, 126
Acetylcholine, for primary pulmonary hypertension, 41
N-Acetylprocainamide, excretion and dose modification in end-stage renal disease, 191t
Acquired immunodeficiency syndrome
  arrhythmias in, 355–358
  cardiac involvement in
    antiviral agents and, 362
    clinical manifestations of, 353–362
    echocardiography of, 364
    electrocardiography in, 363–364
    endomyocardial biopsy of, 365
    future issues in, 365
    Holter monitoring of, 364
    laboratory testing of, 363–365
    management of, 362–363
    pathophysiology of, 359, 361–362
    pericardiocentesis of, 364–365
    radionuclide ventriculography of, 364
  cardiomyopathy in, 352–353
  cardiovascular effects of, 349–370
  diastolic dysfunction in, 354–355
  endocarditis in, 352, 357
  intracardiac masses in, 357–358, 358f
  Kaposi's sarcoma in, cardiac involvement in, 350–351
  left ventricular dysfunction in, 353–354
  lymphoma in, cardiac involvement in, 350–351
  metabolic disturbances in, 362
  mortality from, 349
  myocarditis in, 351–352
  pericarditis in, 351–352
  right ventricular dysfunction in, 355
  worldwide incidence of, 349
Acromegaly, 92–95

cardiovascular effects of, 93–94
cause of, 92
clinical features of, 93
diagnosis of, 94
mortality from, 93
mutations in, 92–93
symptoms of, 93
Action potentials, late, in Duchenne's muscular dystrophy, 57
Acute inflammatory demyelinating polyradiculoneuropathy, autonomic dysfunction in, 320–322
Acute myocardial infarction. *See also* Myocardial infarction
  atypical presentations of, 122–123
  in diabetic patients, 122–123
    management of, 129
  during pregnancy, 6
  in sickle cell anemia, 200
Acute respiratory distress syndrome, in acute pulmonary heart disease, 32
Advanced glycation end products, in diabetic patients, 118–119
Afterload
  increased, and ventricular function, 12f, 13f
  stroke volume and, 185
AGEs. *See* Advanced glycation end products
Airway(s)
  diseases affecting, 23t
  obstruction of, in pulmonary heart disease, 13
Albuminuria, as risk factor for atherosclerotic cardiovascular disease, 121
Alcohol
  cardiovascular effects of, 83–86
    negative, 83–84
    protective, 83
  cirrhosis caused by, 84–86
  holiday heart syndrome and, 86
  hypertensive effects of, 83–84
  myocardial damage from, 84, 84f
  restriction of, in diabetic patients, 125
Alcoholic hepatitis, portal hypertension in, 77
α-Adrenergic blocking agents
  antihypertensive effects of, 180